Marginalization in Globalizing Delhi:
Issues of Land, Livelihoods and Health

Sanghmitra S. Acharya · Sucharita Sen
Milap Punia · Sunita Reddy
Editors

Marginalization in Globalizing Delhi: Issues of Land, Livelihoods and Health

Springer

Editors
Sanghmitra S. Acharya
Centre of Social Medicine
and Community Health,
School of Social Sciences
Jawaharlal Nehru University
New Delhi
India

Sucharita Sen
Centre for the Study of Regional
Development, School of Social Sciences
Jawaharlal Nehru University
New Delhi
India

Milap Punia
Centre for the Study of Regional
Development, School of Social Sciences
Jawaharlal Nehru University
New Delhi
India

Sunita Reddy
Centre of Social Medicine
and Community Health
Jawaharlal Nehru University
New Delhi
India

ISBN 978-81-322-3857-7 ISBN 978-81-322-3583-5 (eBook)
DOI 10.1007/978-81-322-3583-5

Printed on acid-free paper

This Springer imprint is published by Springer Nature
The registered company is Springer (India) Pvt. Ltd.

Foreword

The relationship between urban space and people, an issue with a long preoccupation of urban experts, has been constantly theorized. Cities have historically played an important role not only in the economic and social transformation of the nation states, but also served at the same time as an instrument of hegemony, power and wealth for some classes, and of marginalization, peripheralization, and exploitation of others. Internal morphology of cities transform and their relationship with peripheries result in enormous changes in the land use, creation of real estates and uneven development of infrastructure influencing livelihoods, living conditions and health of the people in these spaces.

This study provides detailed empirical evidences from both urban and peri-urban Delhi, keeping people who are at the margins at the center of the analysis. The book brings together multidisciplinary, multi-dimensional work, and offers insights and research inputs for students and researchers interested in urban issues from disciplines like Geography, Sociology, Economics, Demography, Anthropology, and Public Health.

R. B. Bhagat
Professor and Head
Department of Migration and Urban Studies
International Institute for Population Sciences
Mumbai

Preface

It gives us immense pleasure to share our journey in compiling this volume *Marginalization in Globalizing Delhi: Issues of Land, Livelihoods and Health.* This journey was initiated with our participation in a workshop organized by the Institute for Housing and Urban Development Studies (IHS), in Rotterdam, the Netherlands in 2012, on "Urban Development(s) and Emerging Issues of Inclusion, Governance and Sustainability in India".

The conference not only enriched us academically but was also an experience, which invigorated and stimulated our minds. The vibrant discussions and exchange of ideas at the workshop culminated in this comprehensive and interdisciplinary volume. During the tea breaks between the sessions of the conference, over the cups of hot beverages of our choices, and while breathing in the freshness of the morning air into our lungs during the walks, we discovered ourselves drawn together to work on this manuscript with a new camaraderie. A realization of common academic interests despite different specializations propelled this idea further. The commonalities and similar interests, which brought us together for this innovative, productive, and memorable journey, have since then multiplied manifold!

Jawaharlal Nehru University is known for interdisciplinary studies. What could be a better illustration than four colleagues with different areas of expertise from two different centers coming together to initiate, develop, and compile a volume, involving young scholars who have worked with them? This is also a reflection of a productive culmination of an academic relationship, which evolved during the shaping of dissertations and theses, in a more innovative and creative way.

This book is a collation of ideas to trigger the discourse on the processes of globalization which a city undergoes to change the dynamics of land, livelihoods and health, with a focus on people at the margins of society.

New Delhi, India

Sanghmitra S. Acharya
Sucharita Sen
Milap Punia
Sunita Reddy

Acknowledgements

This book would not have been possible without the vision of Prof. Amitabh Kundu who was instrumental in the collaboration between Institute for Housing and Developmental Studies (IHS), Rotterdam, the Netherlands and Jawaharlal Nehru University, New Delhi. He encouraged our participation in the workshop on "Urban Development(s) and Emerging Issues of Inclusion, Governance and Sustainability in India" organized under this collaboration which triggered our academic thinking into shaping this book. We wish to put on record our gratitude to him. We are also grateful to the participants in the Rotterdam workshop, interaction with whom gave the direction to our idea of this book.

We also wish to thank all the scholars who readily agreed to contribute. We would like to specially thank all the research scholars who took out time from their research, to write the papers based on their M.Phil. and Ph.D. works. We highly appreciate their efforts to revise the papers after getting suggestions and comments. The delays on our part were put up by the contributors in good spirit and revisions done with patience. We highly appreciate their endeavor to improve and produce the best.

To facilitate the process of putting the volume together, we held a review workshop on 20–21 December 2014, which was sponsored by the Indian Council of Social Science Research (ICSSR) and Jawaharlal Nehru University, New Delhi. A panel of experts discussed the papers and gave their valuable comments and suggestions. This helped in enriching the quality of the papers. We express our heartfelt gratitude to Profs. P.M. Kulkarni, Saraswati Raju, Sachidanand Sinha, R.B. Bhagat, Shrawan K. Acharya, Ritu Priya, Talat Munshi, Dr. Attiqur Rehman and Dr. Abdul Shaban for their efforts.

Special thanks are due to our dedicated and enthusiastic students. Without their support, it would have been difficult to bring this endeavor to fruition. Dr. Ranvir Singh, Kanhaiya Kumar, Golak B. Patra, and Ajit K. Lenka, for their support in organizing the workshop and shaping the manuscript. We also thank Dr. Lakhan Singh for managing the accounts, Mr. Kaushal for logistics, and Mr. Sukant for making arrangements for the food during the workshop. We also thank CSRD, SSS for providing the seminar hall for conducting the workshop.

Our acknowledgment will remain incomplete without mentioning the patience with which the editorial team of Springer acceded to our request of pushing the deadlines more than twice. We are extremely grateful for this considerate gesture.

Sanghmitra S. Acharya
Sucharita Sen
Milap Punia
Sunita Reddy

Contents

Abbreviations

AAP	Aam Admi Party
AIIMS	All India Institute of Medical Sciences
ANM	Auxiliary Nurse Midwife
AOI	Area of Interest
APL	Above Poverty Line
AUNAU	Area Under Non-Agricultural Use
AWW	Anganwadi Worker
AYUSH	Ayurveda, Yoga, Unani, Siddha and Homeopathy
BOCW	Building and Other Construction of Workers (BOCW) Act
BPL	Below Poverty Line
BPO	Business Process Outsourcing
BUA	Built-Up Area
CBI	Central Bureau of Investigation
CD Blocks	Community Development (CD) Blocks
CEDAW	The Convention on the Elimination of all Forms of Discrimination Against Women
CGHS	Central Government Health Scheme
CHC	Community Health Center
CII	Confederation of Indian Industry
CONTAG	Contagion index
CONTIG_AM	Area weighted mean contiguity index
CPCB	Central Pollution Control Board
CR	Census Reports
CS	Coefficient of Sensitivity
CSR	Corporate Social Responsibility
CT	Census Towns
D	Doctors
DAC	Department of Agriculture and Cooperation
DAM	Districts Around Metropolitan Cities
DCA	Double Cropped Area
DCB	Delhi Cantonment Board

DDA	Delhi Development Authority
DDF	Devki Devi Foundation
DEDA	Delhi Energy Development Agency
DGHS	Directorate General of Health Services
DJB	Delhi Jal Board
DLHS	District Level Household and Facility Survey
DNES	Department of Non-Conventional Energy Sources
DTC	Delhi Transport Corporation
DTCP	Department of Town and Country Planning
EBTC	European Business and Technology Centre
EPR	Extended Producer Responsibility
ESA	European Space Agency
ESI	Employee State Insurance
ESV	Ecosystem Service Value
FDI	Foreign Direct Investment
FGD	Focus Group Discussion
FICCI	Federation of Indian Chambers of Commerce and Industry
FRAC_AM	Area weighted mean Fractal Dimension Index
GDP	Gross Domestic Product
GIS	Geographic Information System; Geographical Information System
GMC	Gurgaon Municipal Corporation
GOI	Government of India
GTB	Gautam Budhha Nagar
GYRATE_AM	Area Weighted Mean radius of gyration
H1	Kalawati Saran Children's Hospital
H2	Lok Nayak Hospital
Ha	Hectare
HTC	Hanuman Temple Children
ICDS	Integrated Child Development Scheme
ICRMW	International Convention on the Rights of Migrant Workers and their Families
IGAS	Institute of Global and Area Studies
IHD	Institute for Human Development
IPD	Inpatient Department
IRS P6 LISS3	Indian Remote Sensing Satellites P6 *Linear Imaging* Self Scanning Sensor
ISM	Indian System of Medicine
ITES	Information Technology Enabled Services
IVF	In Vitro Fertilization
JCI	Joint Commission of International Accreditation
JJ	Jhughi Jhopri
JnNURM	Jawaharlal Nehru National Urban Mission
JNU	Jawaharlal Nehru University
JSY	Janani Suraksha Yojna

Km	Kilometer
KMP	Kundli–Manaser–Palwal
KTJC	Karpuri Thakur Janjeevan Camp
Landsat TM	Landsat Thematic Mapper
LHV	Lady Health Visitor
LISS IV	Linear Imaging Self Scanning IV
LNJP	Lokanayak Jai Prakash Narayan hospital
LPG	Liquid Petroleum Gas
LPI	Largest Patch Index
LULC	Land Use Land Cover
MC	Municipal Corporation
MCD	Municipal Corporation Delhi
MCH	Maternal and Child Health
MDA	Meerut Development Authority
MDG	Millennium Development Goal
MDM	Mid-Day Meal
MGD	Million Gallon Daily
MLC	Medico-Legal Case
MNC	Multi National Corporation
MoEF	Ministry of Environment and Forest
MP	Master Plan
MPCE	Monthly Per-Capita Consumption Expenditure
MT	Medical Tourism
NABH	National Accreditation Board for Hospitals and Health Care Providers
NABL	National Accreditation Board for Testing and Calibration Laboratories
NCEUS	National Commission for Enterprise in the Unorganized Sector
NCR	National Capital Region
NCRPB	National Capital Region Planning Board
NCT	National Capital Territory
NCTD	National Capital Territory of Delhi
NDC	New Delhi Railway Station Children
NDMA	New Delhi Municipal Corporation
NDMC	New Delhi Municipal Council
NELM	New Economics of Labour Migration
NFHS	National Family Health Survey
NGO	Non Government Organization
NH	National Highway
NHFS	National Health and Family Surveys
NRSC	National Remote Sensing Centre
NRWQMSP	National Rural Drinking Water Quality Monitoring and Surveillance Programme
NSA	Net Sown Area
NSSO	National Sample Survey Organisation

OBC	Other Backward Castes
ODF	Open Defecation Free
OPD	Out Patient Department
ORNL	Oak Ridge National Laboratory
PAHO	Pan American Health Organization
PDS	Public Distribution System
PHC	Primary Health Center
PIL	Public Interest Litigation
PPP	Public Private Partnership
PR	Patch Richness
PRC	Provisional Regularisation Certificates
PTI	Press Trust of India
PWC	Price Water Cooper
RCH	Reproductive and Child Health
RDF	Refuse Derived Fuel
RMP	Registered medical practioner
RSBY	Rashtriya Swastya Bima Yojana
SBA	Swachh Bharat Yojona
SBT	Salam Balak Trust
SC	Scheduled caste
SCA	Single Cropped Area
SECC	Socio Economic Caste Census
SEZ	Special Economic Zone
SFS	Self Financing Scheme
SHDI	Shannon's Diversity index
SPCB	State Pollution Control Board
ST	Scheduled tribe
STI	Sexually Transmitted Infection
SUB- C	Sub Center
SWM	Solid waste management
TB	Tuberculosis
TBA	Traditional Birth Attendant
TCL	Total Cultivable Land
TFP	Total Factor Productivity
TM	Thematic Mapper
UDPFI	Urban Development Plan Formulation and Implementation
UK	United Kingdom
ULB	Urban Local Bodies
UN	United Nations
UNICEF	United Nations Children's Emergency Fund
UPAVP	Uttar Pradesh Awas Vikas Parishad
UPS	Usual Principal Status
UPSIDC	Uttar Pradesh State Industrial Development Corporation
UPSS	Usual Principal and Subsidiary Status

US	United States
USSR	United States of Soviet Russia
VC	Value Coefficient
VHW	Village Health Worker
WHO	World Health Organization
WPR	Work Participation Rate
Yr	Year

Editors and Contributors

About the Editors

Sanghmitra S. Acharya is Professor at the Centre of Social Medicine and Community Health, School of Social Sciences JNU and is currently deputed as Director to Indian Institute of Dalit Studies, New Delhi. She has been a Visiting Fellow at CASS, China, Ball State University, USA and UPPI, Manila, East West Center, Honolulu, Hawaii and University of Botswana. She was awarded the Asian Scholarship Foundation fellowship in 2005. She has delivered lectures, chaired sessions and contributed in national and international conferences in various Institutions within the country and abroad. Her research includes health and discrimination; vulnerability among youth; gender in urban spaces; and caste gender intersectionality. She has published in national and international journal and has three books to her credit.

Sucharita Sen is Professor in the Centre for the Study of Regional Development, School of Social Sciences, Jawaharlal Nehru University. She was a Nehru-Fulbright Fellow in 2009–2010 and was associated with Ohio State University, Columbus, Ohio, USA during this period. She is an economic geographer and has published in areas of land resources, its acquisition and effect of dispossession on rural livelihoods, rural employment, the impact of watershed development programs as a means for sustaining rural livelihoods. She is currently working on one major project other than the 'Gender Atlas' funded by the Department of Science and Technology (DST), which is the Inter University Consortium on Cryosphere and Climate Change (IUCCCC) project of 'Himalayan Cryosphere: Science and Society', also funded by the DST. She also regularly contributes to the geography curriculum in school (Central Board of Higher Secondary Education) through her association with the National Council of Educational Research and Training, New Delhi.

Milap Punia is Professor of Geography in the Centre for the Study of Regional Development, School of Social Sciences, Jawaharlal Nehru University, New Delhi, India. He did his postdoctoral research work on urban studies from School of Forestry and Environment Studies, Yale University, USA. He has served as scientist in Photogrammetry and Remote Sensing Division, Indian Institute of Remote Sensing-ISRO, Dehradun from 2002 to 2006, and Adjunct Faculty of Centre for Space Science and Technology Education in Asia and the Pacific (Affiliated to the UN). His areas of research include urban studies, spatial data analysis for urban planning and regional development; sustainability, land use change, disaster management, spatial aspects of governance, and to bridge research gap between social sciences and remote sensing discipline. He is involved in various research projects of international (Subaltern Urbanization-ANR, remapping of global South-DAAD and of national repute (Snow Spectral Properties and Regional Climate -Hyperspectral Mapping, Geovisualisation of Landscape-DST-GOI) and Spatial aspects of Governance for Decentralised Local Bodies-Indian Council of Social Science and Research (ICSSR).

Sunita Reddy is Associate Professor at the Centre of Social Medicine and Community Health, School of Social Sciences, Jawaharlal Nehru University, New Delhi, India. She is an anthropologist, specializing in medical anthropology. She has researched on various issues of women and child health; breastfeeding practices, tribal women's health, childbirth and child rearing practices among the tribes. She has researched on disaster issues from social science perspectives and published a book *Clash of Waves: Post Tsunami Relief and Rehabilitation in Andaman and Nicobar Islands* (2013) Indos publishers, New Delhi. This book is a based longitudinal study using anthropological research techniques. Her current area of research is 'Medical Tourism and Reproductive Tourism', 'Surrogacy' issues. She has published articles in peer-reviewed journals, contributed papers for edited volumes and disseminated her research work in various universities abroad. She is a founder member of 'Anthropos India Foundation' a trust which promotes visual and action anthropology and has a dynamic website: www.anthroposindiafoundation.com. She is also an honorary president of an organization called 'SATAT', which works for empowering women and children.

Contributors

Sweta Bhusan is presently working as Consultant with CARE India at their Head Office in Delhi. Her doctoral thesis is on Family Structure and Well-Being of the Elderly: A Study on Urban West Bengal and was awarded from the Centre for the Study of Regional Development, School of Social Sciences, Jawaharlal Nehru University, New Delhi. She also completed her M.Phil. from the same Centre. She graduated as a Bachelor of Science in Geography from Lady Brabourne College under the University of Calcutta and did her postgraduation from the Department of Geography, Banaras Hindu University. She has worked in three projects funded by DST, UGC, and ICSSR under capacities of Senior Research Fellow, Research Associate, and Project Fellow. She has to her credit several research publications in reputed journals and has also presented her research findings in various national and international seminars. Her academic interest is focused on population aging, urbanization, migration, economic development, human and physical geography.

Pritha Chatterjee has completed her doctoral research on cities and social space, from the Centre for the Study of Regional Development, School of Social Sciences, Jawaharlal Nehru University. She is a social geographer by training and a development professional, currently engaged as Research Consultant with Citizens Rights' Collective (Urban Poverty Knowledge Activist Hub of ActionAid India). Her interest areas are urban space, social inclusion, and sustainable development.

Ankita Choudhary is a Research Scholar in the Centre for the Study of Regional Development, School of Social Sciences, Jawaharlal Nehru University, New Delhi. Her research interest includes urban issues and regional development.

Bhaswati Das is currently Associate Professor at the Centre for the Study of Regional Development, School of Social Sciences in Jawaharlal Nehru University New Delhi. She did her graduation from Presidency College, Kolkata and continued her higher education at Jawaharlal Nehru University, New Delhi where she had completed her MA in Geography and M.Phil. in Population Studies. She was awarded Ph.D. on 'Study of Fertility Behaviour in a Transitional Socio-Economic Condition'. She has started her career in leading NGO in Delhi and worked on several projects on women and child health issues for Government of India and for United Nations. She has more than 30 publications in peer-reviewed journals of repute in her credit on the issues of population and development. Her book Gender Issues in Development from Rawat Publications is well acclaimed. Recently she has completed her project on "Gender dimensions in Ageing in India" under the aegis of University Grants Commission India. Currently she is editing an academic magazine in Bengali language.

Nanda Dulal Das, after completing M.Phil. and Ph.D. from Jawaharlal Nehru University, New Delhi, is presently working in the government sector. His areas of research in the doctoral and pre-doctoral level varied from issues relating to convergence between MGNREGS and Watershed Development Programmes to expansion of urban centers and loss of farmlands in the periphery of large urban centers. He also has extensively used the techniques of Remote Sensing and GIS in his research to explain the spatial change process in finer details.

Dipendra Nath Das did his B.Sc. from Presidency College, Kolkata and MA and Ph.D. from Jawaharlal Nehru University (JNU), New Delhi. Currently he is a faculty in the Centre for the Study of Regional Development (CSRD), JNU. His areas of research interests are pattern and processes of urbanization and migration, problems in access to basic amenities and socioeconomic and health issues of elderly. He teaches courses on population studies, remote sensing, and geographic information system (GIS). In his more than 15 years of teaching he has authored two books and published a large number of articles/chapters in reputed journals and books.

Chandrani Dutta is an Assistant Professor at the Indian Institute of Dalit Studies, New Delhi. She obtained her Ph.D. from the Centre for the Study of Regional Development, School of Social Sciences, Jawaharlal Nehru University, New Delhi. Her areas of research include marginal communities living in slums, contemporary urban policies and development of dalits.

G. Dilip Diwakar is currently working as Assistant Professor at the Department of Social Work, Central University of Kerala. He has more than 10 years of experience in the research, program management, and teaching. Before he joined CUK, he had worked with Indian Institute of Dalit Studies (IIDS), New Delhi as Associate Fellow for 5 years. His other work experience includes engagement with both National and International development organizations like ActionAid, Aide-et-Action, Centre for Equity Studies at various capacities for about 6 years. He has co-authoured a book "Caste, Discrimination and Exclusion in Modern India", Sage 2015. He has published more than 15 research articles in both national and international peer-reviewed journals and chapters in books. He had completed ten research projects for government and various other funding organizations.

Yogi Joseph is affiliated to the Centre for Urban Equity at CEPT University, Ahmedabad. He is also Visiting Assistant Professor at the University's Faculty of Planning. He is trained as an architect and urban planner and is keen on studying issues of equity and accessibility, especially from the perspective of vulnerable groups such as women, children, and the differently-abled. Contact details: Yogi Joseph, Research Associate, Centre for Urban Equity, CEPT University, Navrangpura, Ahmedabad, 380009, Gujarat, India.

Vishavpreet Kaur is Public Health Research Scholar, pursuing Ph.D. from Centre of Social Medicine and Community Health, school of Social Sciences JNU, New Delhi. She is currently associated with Safai Karmachari Andolan as Programme Officer. Her interest areas include urbanization, migration, and politics of world-class cities, social exclusion, and public health.

Kanhaiya Kumar is Research Scholar at Jawaharlal Nehru University, New Delhi. He did M.Phil and is pursuing his Ph.D. in Public Health from JNU. He was awarded *ICSSR Institutional Doctoral Fellowship (2013–2015)* from Institute of Economic Growth under the aegis of Indian Council of Social Science Research (ICSSR), New Delhi, India. He had worked more than 2 years in research institutes. He has also published papers and contributed chapters in various books. The main areas of his research work are patterns of social exclusion with special reference to gender and health issues and evaluation of developmental programs for of dalits and migrants.

Sunita Kumari is a Research Scholar in Centre for the Study of Regional Development, School of Social Sciences, Jawaharlal Nehru University, New Delhi. Her research interest includes social vulnerability mapping.

Ajit Kumar Lenka is currently working as Research Scholar, Centre of Social Medicine and Community Health, School of Social Sciences, Jawaharlal Nehru University, New Delhi-110067. He completed his MA in Sociology, PG Diploma in Rural Development from Pondicherry Central University. He has cleared UGC National Eligibility Test (NET) in sociology. He had completed his M.Phil. from Centre of Social Medicine and Community Health, Jawaharlal Nehru University. His interests include urbanization, issues in slum, water and sanitation, social exclusion and public health.

Chinmoyee Mallik is a geographer and graduated from Presidency College, Kolkata and completed her M.Phil. and Ph.D. degrees from the Centre for the Study of Regional Development, Jawahrlal Nehru University. She worked on livelihood issues in relation to land dispossession in the periurban areas of Delhi and Kolkata. Following her postdoctoral research at IIM Calcutta that was focused on understanding of the political economy of livelihood transition in India, she joined Birati College Kolkata as Assistant Professor of Geography in 2014. Her specific areas of interest span employment, peri-urbanization, agricultural and economic geography. In addition to research articles that are published in various journals like Indian Journal of Labour Economics, Indian Journal of Agricultural Economics, she is also the author of a book entitled *Employment in the Globalizing Rural Peripheries in Indian Mega-cities*. Her present thrust of research focuses on the political economy of land policy in India.

Tarun Prakash Meena is a Research Scholar at the Centre for the Study of Regional Development, School of Social Sciences, Jawaharlal Nehru University, New Delhi. His area of research interest includes vulnerability of people and places.

Chandra Prakash Morya is a Research Scholar at the Centre for the Study of Regional Development, School of Social Sciences, Jawaharlal Nehru University, New Delhi and currently working as Assistant Professor in the Department of Geography, University of Rajasthan, Jaipur. His area of research interest is ecosystems and cities, Livelihood and vulnerability in desert environments.

Talat Munshi is Associate Professor and also co-ordinates the Master in Urban and Regional Planning program at the Faculty of Planning, CEPT University, India. Prior to his current employment (since 2007), he worked as Lecturer in Transport at ITC, at TERI University in Delhi, India and as Lecturer at Faculty of Planning (then School of Planning), CEPT University. His interests are to teach and advocate spatial and non-spatial tools and methods that help in taking urban and regional planning decisions for the larger benefit of the society. He did his Ph.D. from University of Twente and has two master's degrees: in Planning, from CEPT University and in Urban Infrastructure Management from Faculty of ITC, University of Twente, the Netherlands. Undergraduate degree is in Construction Technology also from CEPT. Contact details: Faculty of Planning CEPT University, Navrangpura, Ahmedabad.

Navin Narayan is a development professional and works with Knowledge Activist Hub-Democratisation of ActionAid-an international anti-poverty agency based in New Delhi. He had been a researcher with the Indian Institute of Dalit Studies. The research he was engaged in is now published as a book, *Social Justice Philanthropy: Strategies and Approaches of Funding agencies in India* by Rawat Publication (2009). His interests of areas are issues related to poverty, exclusion, and marginalization, access of health services, democratization of public institutions, entitlement and full citizenship rights of marginalized and de-notified communities. He has presented articles in seminars and conferences written on these subjects. Some of them are published in magazines and edited books. He is actively engaged with social movements. Presently he is writing his Ph.D. thesis for Centre for Social Medicine and Community Health, JNU, New Delhi, India.

Golak B. Patra is pursuing his Ph.D. in the Centre of Social Medicine and Community Health, School of Social Sciences, Jawaharlal Nehru University, New Delhi 110067. His area of research is urban planning and urban health. His research interests include urban health, urban planning, urban process, migration and workers' health, and dalit human rights.

Jagdev C. Sharma is Assistant Professor in Government College, Sarahan, Sirmaur, Himachal Pradesh. He is pursuing his Ph.D. in Waste management and Health Concerns of the Workers in the Centre of Social Medicine and Community Health, JNU. His research interests are urban health and workers engaged in hazardous occupations.

Ranvir Singh received his Ph.D. in Public Health from JNU. He works mainly on spatial disparity in health care provisioning and its access as well as on social determinants and equity issues in health at urban centres. He has expertise in management information systems for efficient data modeling, monitoring and assessment. His experience in participatory rapid appraisals cuts across diverse states and he has conducted action research on social determinants and equity issues in health at urban centres such as Mumbai and Delhi. After an experience of more than 5 years in the development sector with diverse expertise, currently he is placed in a senior position in Fiinovation (a solution enabler for civil society and corporate social responsibility partnerships) where he is heading the research proposal division.

Zia-Ul-Haque is Urban Planner at the Regional Centre for Urban & Environmental Studies (MoUD GOI), Lucknow, visiting faculty in Masters of Architecture Programme at Faculty of Architecture, Dr. A.P.J. Abdul Kalam Technical University and Partner at Studio: Collaborative for Urban Research in Environments. His interests are spatial planning, urban design interventions, exploring historic precincts, cultural contexts, and research in traditional settlements, which help in taking multidisciplinary approach in his architecture and planning decisions for holistic decision-making. He is a graduate in Urban & Regional Planning from CEPT University and has received an undergraduate degree in Architecture from Government College of Architecture, Lucknow.

List of Figures

Marginalization and Socio-ecological Transformation in New Urban Peripheries: A Case Study of Gurgaon

Ecosystem Services in NCT Delhi

Examining Equity in Spatial Distribution of Recreational and Social Infrastructure in Delhi

Neo-Liberal Urbanization, Work Participation and Women: Comparing the Urban and Peri-urban Contexts of Delhi with Mumbai and Kolkata

Embedded or Liberated? An Exploration into the Social Milieu of Delhi

Gender Violence in Delhi: Perceptions and Experience

Migrant Women Workers in Construction and Domestic Work: Issues and Challenges

Revealing the Vulnerabilities of Population and Places at Risk in Delhi

Vulnerabilities of Relocated Women, A Case of Resettlement in Bawana JJ Colony, Delhi

Social Vulnerability Mapping for Delhi

Disrupted Megacities and Disparities in Health Care

Access to Maternal and Child Health Care: Understanding Discrimination in Selected Slum in Delhi

Life on Streets: Health and Living Conditions of Children in Delhi

Socio-Economic Disparities Among Youth in Delhi: Issues and Challenges

Condition of the Aged in National Capital Territory of Delhi

Water and Sanitation and Public Health Issues in Delhi

Living in Blight in the Globalized Metro: A Study on Housing and Housing Conditions in Slums of Delhi

List of Tables

Marginalization and Socio-ecological Transformation in New Urban Peripheries: A Case Study of Gurgaon

Ecosystem Services in NCT Delhi

Examining Equity in Spatial Distribution of Recreational and Social Infrastructure in Delhi

Land Acquisition Policy and Praxis: The Case of Peri-urban Delhi

Neo-Liberal Urbanization, Work Participation and Women: Comparing the Urban and Peri-urban Contexts of Delhi with Mumbai and Kolkata

Embedded or Liberated? An Exploration into the Social Milieu of Delhi

Gender Violence in Delhi: Perceptions and Experience

Migrant Women Workers in Construction and Domestic Work: Issues and Challenges

Revealing the Vulnerabilities of Population and Places at Risk in Delhi

Social Vulnerability Mapping for Delhi

Disrupted Megacities and Disparities in Health Care

Changing Health Care Dynamics: Corporatization and Medical Tourism in National Capital Region

Access to Maternal and Child Health Care: Understanding Discrimination in Selected Slum in Delhi

Life on Streets: Health and Living Conditions of Children in Delhi

Socio-Economic Disparities Among Youth in Delhi: Issues and Challenges

Condition of the Aged in National Capital Territory of Delhi

Water and Sanitation and Public Health Issues in Delhi

Solid Waste Management and Health of Workers

Living in Blight in the Globalized Metro: A Study on Housing and Housing Conditions in Slums of Delhi

List of Maps

Embedded or Liberated? An Exploration into the Social Milieu of Delhi

Land, Livelihoods and Health: Marginalization in Globalizing Delhi

Sanghmitra S. Acharya, Sucharita Sen, Milap Punia and Sunita Reddy

Introduction

Historically cities have evolved as an outcome of the process of urban growth; trade and economy; movement of people, industrialization and trade; and administration. Cities first emerged in Syria, Mesopotamia, Egypt and India 5000–6000 years ago long before the growth of modern factory. These cities were, on the one hand centres of religion, political administration and on the other, represented growth centres, stimulated by international trade in spices, gold, cloth and precious goods. The pre-industrialization city was smaller, less densely populated, built within protective walls, and often organized around a central storage and a place of worship. In contrast, the industrial city that began to emerge by the end of eighteenth century, was more dynamic, and had complex social system requiring new means of mass communication. Subsequently, such cities were ridden with a host of social problems such as poverty, pollution, crime (Ong 2011; Smith 2015).

S.S. Acharya (✉) · S. Reddy
Centre of Social Medicine and Community Health, School of Social Sciences,
Jawaharlal Nehru University, New Delhi, India
e-mail: sanghmitra.acharya@gmail.com

S. Reddy
e-mail: sunitareddyjnu@gmail.com

S. Sen · M. Punia
Centre for the Study of Regional Development, School of Social Sciences,
Jawaharlal Nehru University, New Delhi, India
e-mail: ssen.jnu@gmail.com

M. Punia
e-mail: milap.punia@gmail.com

S.S. Acharya
Indian Institute of Dalit Studies, Delhi, India

S.S. Acharya et al. (eds.), *Marginalization in Globalizing Delhi: Issues of Land, Livelihoods and Health*, DOI 10.1007/978-81-322-3583-5_1

Though many great cities grew up with modern industry drawing workers from the rural hinterland, Industrialization alone has not been responsible for urbanization. With the passage of time, cities have experienced transformations. Political unrest in the hinterland, over population, lack of economic opportunities in rural areas, resulted in city-ward push. Some of the fastest growing cities in the world are in the semi-industrialized developing countries (Hall and Raumplaner 1998).

As regards urbanization, a large number of countries in the Latin America have already reached the 75 % mark by 2014. China has crossed the 50 % mark, while India, though growing fast, has a moderate 34 % living in cities. The factor that is appreciably scarce for expansion of urbanization, in contrast, is land. In most cases, the acquisition of land depends on the state and policies of the nation state. Second, the capital investment had to take innovative and new forms and expand unfettered for its own multiplication. Much of this takes the shape of public–private partnerships, where commonly, the public component takes the risk and the private gets more of the profit (Harvey 2012). Thus, both the role of the private sector and the state in the urbanization process and the resultant outcomes of large metropolitan centres deserve attention.

Cities, particularly metropolitan, are known to exert pull on their surrounding regions leading to in-migration creating pressure on the existing resources and services. Cities are limited in their provisioning of resources and services to their citizens for various reasons: the nature of development processes, lack of political will, poor governance and meager resource base often leave the city incapable of meeting the demands of the people. In addition, social gradients such as class, gender, region, religion and ethnicity of the populations act as enhancers for some and barriers for the others in accessing services and resources. Cities in Indian subcontinent also encounters a unique determinant of discrimination, that is often based, not only on the economic but also the social identity, that emanates from complex intersectionalities of caste, ethnicity, gender, region and religion. Notably, such discriminations are the result of the way public fund is distributed, and the barriers to access basic services of life in the city (Jain 2011). In recent times, inequalities of access to basic services and means of livelihoods have become even starker due to centrality of growth in our development paradigm that has pushed back the distribution agenda.

This book attempts to study Delhi and its suburban localities as a social observatory in terms marginalization, peripheralization of social vulnerabilities and systemic approach to understand loss of ecosystem services over period of three decades, land use change and increase in built environment. The central theme of this edited volume is to understand urban growth, changing landscapes, changing livelihoods, growth in the health sector; and access to resources and services in Delhi. The central argument we make is that in the process of globalization and urban growth, disparities have increased, leading to marginalization, discrimination and exclusions along various gradients. Delhi, the capital city of India is taken as a case study to understand this process. The primary focus of the book is to understand, whether development as we understand it today, some causes of elation to the people at the margin, or has caused exclusion and alienation among them, while favouring others that enjoy the benefits of this growth-centric process. Adopting a political economy framework, the book attempts to analyze changing landscape and thereby livelihoods and the nature of physical, economic and social impacts on different groups of people. It also analyzes changing nature of health care services and access to health care in Delhi and the National Capital Region (NCR). This book is based on collated work of the four editors from interdisciplinary areas of Geography, Geographical Information System (GIS), Remote Sensing, Anthropology and Public Health, and that of their colleagues and research scholars associated with them.

Like in case of many other cities in India, the changes in Delhi's metropolitan character has become particularly noticeable since the neo-liberal policies of the 1990s (Veltz 2004). The way Delhi stands out, however, is its locational adjacency with two states, both of which lend it agriculturally rich hinterland. The urban expansions leading to significant land use changes due to investments in infrastructure and real estate impacts the rural surroundings in a way that is significantly different from the case of say, Mumbai, Bangalore and Hyderabad, that do not intrude into high value agricultural land. The expansions and changes within the core city of Delhi, not only reorganized the marginalized within the city, but led to a differential impact on the peri-urban space with redefined patterns of livelihoods, employment and health care to the populace in the peri-urban area that were earlier in profitable professions due to their engagements in highly productive agriculture. An emerging phenomenon that one observes in the recent mode of city building is that of peri-urbanization, that can be interpreted both as a process and as a marginalized space occupied by much of the poor. This section of the population plays an important role in providing the labour force needed to expand the cities. The expansion of the city, however, often alter patterns of rural natural resource use, that cause far-reaching social, cultural and economic changes for the people living in the peri-urban regions of large metropolitan cities (Narain 2009). Delhi and its peripheries have been experiencing new patterns of investments and infrastructure changes, emerging imbalances in rural and urban livelihood patterns, and bipolarity of health care services that on one hand aims to target the neo-rich groups from India and abroad as part of Medical Tourism with state of the art technology and denies basic health services to the marginalized (Aggarwal 2009).

Gobalization is building and rebuilding cities. Most of the nation states now provide primacy to growth, rather than 'development'. Often assuming that the former will lead to the latter. The role of the state, thus, has changed significantly, from being that of a *regulator* or watchdog of the way development progresses to a *facilitator* that ensures efficiency in the market. The cities and their governance get significantly impacted as a result of this distinct change in the role of the state. The forms that cities would take are being organized globally and developed locally (Castells 2002) which is really defined by movement of capital, as opposed to that of labour (Jain 2011). Globalization is facilitated by information and communication technology (ICT). This technology has been brought about to facilitate the deepening of globalization and it is a fallacy to assume that the ICT has driven and shaped globalization.

With the reducing regulation by the government, as is inevitable and consistent with the neo-liberal policies, the private and corporate sector has taken up not only in the consumer goods sector, but also basic goods and services such as agriculture, health and education. Globalization has diverted focus on the metropolis, megalopolis and extended megacities that remain the centre of attention of the growth led development and the target of multiple schemes, infrastructure support and governance reforms, ignoring the rural 'other'. This has increased social vulnerabilities of deprived groups and have often pushed them to the peripheries of the city, often without a foothold there in terms of their livelihoods. As per National Sample Survey Organisation (NSSO 2009) 64th round, about 49 thousand slums were estimated to be in existence in urban India in 2008–09, 24 % of them were located along *nallahs* and drains and 12 % along railway lines. The changes in urban landscape is not just pushing and showing the poor to the margins, but also privatization of essential resources, which adds to the vulnerabilities of population. Like in the case of other metropolitan cities, the state has not only passively made way for the private players in the social sectors of water and electricity, but have actively brought in various regulatory urban reforms that have pushed the poor out of the city, that led scholars from diverse disciplines to argue for the right to the city of the poor and vulnerable.

Evolution of Urban Delhi

The scale of urbanization for Delhi initiated from the pre-mercantile through mercantile, industrial and post-industrial period. In the pre-mercantile period, there were few small and scattered urban centres, which were environmentally determined. As their number and size increased, they became less dependent on environment, but were still sustainable during the mercantile period. As industrialization set in, high growth was evident through physical spread of the city and growth of population size. Diverse impacts on the environment were also evident. Post industrialization brought in high urbanization, stabilization and decentralization. Environmental concerns were also addressed. Institutions responsible also transformed during this period. The palace and military of the pre-mercantile period, allowed entry of the religious institutions, guilds, and forts during mercantile period. This further consolidated during industrial period through industrial associations and guilds, trade unions and state parliamentary democracy. In the post-industrial period, the role of the State has been decreasing. There emerged a plurality of institutions that ranged from civil society-based organization, financial and information related ones along with the market and multinationals emerged in Delhi.

The morphology of Delhi also changed through these periods. Public spaces like markets and the 'Citadel' was the core of the city. The grid plan of the core city merged with the unplanned suburban city. Land use was based on social rank. Multiple use of land was evident during the pre-mercantile period. Multiple use of land also marked social segregation of rich and poor on the basis different ethnic groups, occupations and kinships. The rich were located in the centre, and the richness reduces towards periphery, which was inhabited by the poorest (Hasan 2015; Miller 2008).

Delhi has grown in ever expanding roughly concentric circles. Urban sprawl defines the land use. Environmentally determined revitalization and conservation of inner city and planned development of suburbs has become important. The social processes responsible for animating this growth can be attributed to 'differentiation' and 'ecological succession' (Hawley 1950). Differentiation is a process by which urban populations and their activities become more complex and heterogeneous over time. Ethnic, racial, socio-economic classes may enter into competition with each other for dominance in particular areas. For example, businesses may push residents out of certain areas to establish commercial zones (Jain 2015; Miller 2008).

Contemporary Delhi is undergoing a multiplicity of processes, which superimpose one on the other. Transforming from primitive mercantile to post-colonial modern identity, the 'new city' has been continuously redefining itself. Laws established by capitalism and colonialism construct the histories, cultures and aspirations that the city has grown to strive for. Delhi has wielded power of different kinds from historical times. From the tenth century Lal Kot of the Tomar rulers through Quila Rai Pithora of Prithviraj Chauhan, Tughlaqabad of the Tughlaqs and the Shahjahanabad of the Mughals to the nineteenth century Delhi of the British, histories and flows of cultures have shaped the aspirations of the city. Today, it sprawls as a conurbation, extending itself into the districts of all the neighbouring states. It has grown much beyond the functional classification (Mitra 1974) of the 1970s, which listed it as an administrative city. Functions influence city life, its growth and morphology. Delhi's functions are mostly related to non-primary activities like manufacturing, trade-commerce, transport, communication and administration. Which are often grouped under secondary and tertiary categories. Other services like professional (education, medical), personal (hotel) recreation, financial (banking, insurance), public administration (capital, defence), public utility services (electricity, drinking water, sanitation), and sociocultural (religious, literary philosophical). These functions can be grouped under three broad categories: (1) basic (2) non-basic and (3) centripetal and centrifugal. Of these basic, centripetal and centrifugal functions play major role in the evolution and development of urban centres.

Delhi exemplifies the attributes listed for the cities of the developing world. Delhi with 168 million population in 2011 is most urbanized state in India with 97.5 % of urban population (Census of India 2011). While it is vying for global attention along with Singapore and Shanghai, it has sprawled all around its original core like no other metropolitan city in the country. Many of the conditions which plagued the industrial city-poverty, inadequate housing, and structural employment are still evident in the city today. However, since 1970s a new urban phenomenon has emerged alongside the legacy of old urban forms- the post-modern city which are increasingly privatized, aspiring to be the part of a global city, and

Table 1 Shrinking rural and expanding urban spaces of Delhi

	1961	1971	1981	1991	2001	2011
Rural population	–	–	–	9.49	–	4.19
No. of villages	300	–	–	209	165	112
Growth in Urban areas	–	–	–	–	–	**20.44**
Census towns	–	3	–	29	–	110
Rural area	–	–	–	–	558.32 sqkm	369.35 sqkm

Source Census of India, various years

is essentially fragmented characterized with a high degree of social segmentation. This has led to the reduction of public spaces and being converted to use of those who can afford to pay for the use of these spaces. Delhi, in many ways is a post-modern city, therefore, is more fragmented than the corporate city. It lacks a single way of life such as urbanism or sub-urbanism. Variety of lifestyles and subcultures proliferate in the post-modern city that is Delhi. They are based on race, ethnicity, immigrant status, class, sexual orientation, caste region and religion. Post-modern city is more **globalized** than the corporate city. They are world centres of economic and financial decision-making which is fairly evident in the economic and commercial activities of the National Capital Territory (NCT) of Delhi. These are also sites of innovation, where new products and fashions originate. They are the command posts of globalized economy and its culture. Delhi presents a reflection of all this through its economic growth rate of 8.5 % per year in 1994–2001. The Gross State Domestic Product (GSDP) of Delhi at current prices during 2014–15 was Rs. 45,1154 crores, which recorded a growth of 15.35 % over the previous year.

As regards the physical spread, the total area of the NCT of Delhi, which came into force in January 1992 is 1483 km^2. With the rapid pace of urbanization and growth of urban population, the rural population and rural area is continuously decreasing as confirmed by successive Census Reports. Delhi's rural population has decreased from 9.49 lakh in 1991, to 4.19 lakh in 2011. On the other hand, the number of villages in Delhi has reduced from 300 in 1961 to 165 in 2001 and 112 in 2011. Correspondingly, rural area of Delhi reduced from 558.32 m^2 in 2001 to 369.35 m^2 in 2011. On the other hand, the number of census towns has increased from 3 in 1971 to 29 in 1991 and 110 in 2011. The growth in urban area during 2001–2011 was 20.44 % (Table 1).

Changing Composition of Rural–Urban Space

During 1950s–1960s many homes in low income and minority group areas were torn down. While agriculture land gave way to urban land use, these houses in urban areas were replaced by high-rise apartment buildings and office towers in the city core. During 1970s–1980s some middle class people moved into run-down areas and restored them through the process of *gentrification*. Most of the pockets of the core remained in the state of decay. Number of people living in high poverty doubled as recessions and economic restructuring closed factories in inner city. The physical structures of the inner city improved during the economic boom of 1990s, which was an expression of capital accumulation within the city core. The city expanded outwards with visible signs of *sub-urbanism,* leading to development of urbanized area outside the political boundaries of cities. Such peri-urban space around Delhi, thus has on the one hand *gated communities* characterized by expensive, upper middle class residential developments, and shanties inhabited by the working class responsible for the reconstruction of the cities. It also has *exurbs*—rural residential areas within commuting distance of the city; and the *Edge Cities*—the exurban clusters of malls, offices and entertainment complexes that often arise at the convergence point of major highways. Delhi also exemplifies *urban sprawl*—the spread of city into larger expanses of the surrounding countryside. The middle class moving into what was earlier the run-down areas of the inner city, restored later can be observed in Delhi and is evident in urban villages like Pilanji, Mohommedpur and Ber Sarai.

Many of the conditions, which plagued the industrial city—poverty, inadequate housing, and structural employment, are still evident in cities today. However, since 1970s, a new urban phenomenon has emerged alongside the legacy of old urban forms. The changes that have been taking place in the recent decades are expressions of growth and investment in the post-reform Delhi that is increasingly becoming privatized. The outcome of such privatization, is often seen as access to formerly public spaces becoming increasingly limited to those who can afford to pay. Delhi has also been seen by scholars as lacking in a single way of life. Variety of lifestyles and subcultures based on race, ethnicity, immigrant status, class, sexual orientation, caste, have proliferated over time and differentially across city spaces. Delhi has increasingly become a world centre of economic and financial decision-making; and also a site of innovation, where new products and fashions originate, on the one hand, and creating marginalized spaces that are being moved towards the peripheries, to make the former possible (Roy and Ong 2011). One of the offshoots of such spatial segmentation in the neo-liberal city has found expression in the crime and violence reported in the city, specifically against girls and women.

Transforming Peripheries

The reorganization of spaces described above is essentially through changing character of land, both in the nature of access and the use that it is put to, as well as the change in the environmental services of the natural resources connected with land, like water. Thus land is a complex issue, particularly in the Indian context, since it is very densely knitted with a society that is extremely plural; in economic, social and cultural terms. Land is transacted for residential, commercial and industrial use through land acquisition laws and notifications of master plans for urban development. Pluralism of legality and institution involved in both these processes largely benefited the elite builders and the rich. At this junction, it is pertinent to understand and to investigate for what purpose land is being acquired and do farmers and landless laborers get fair compensations? Are dispossessed farmers able to cope up with loss of social networks, farm and non-farm employment and up to what level it distort their sociocultural milieu? Dispossessed marginal farmers and agricultural labourers dependent on the land that change hands, are often reduced to petty workers in this whole process and have to make their living through multiple jobs. Thus transforming peripheries degenerated enclaves of marginality in terms of increasing heterogeneity, loss of ecosystem services and every day contestation over land, water and food continues. However, farmers with larger land holdings, constructed buildings and thrive on rental income.

In south Asia, Roy (2003) explains the rapid peri-urbanisation that is unfolding at the edges of the world's largest cities (including Delhi) in a deliberated and considered informalized process, often in violation of Master Plans and state norms, but informally sanctioned by the state. The State policy intervenes in land in two ways—regulate land use, like control areas and direct physical growth through the master planning process to invest in infrastructure. These actions affect the patterns of land development as well as the characteristics of real estate market. Since the mid 1990s, the strategies of State for stimulating growth in and around cities included the creation of spatial enclaves and implementation of mega infrastructure projects especially transport corridors. The rural fringes adjoining cities are one of the sites for such interventions. Debroy and Bhandari (2009), Keivani and Mattingly (2007) articulated that land developers and highly connected people collude informally to assist and allow land conversion through state's intervention in the name of urbanization and growth. Typically this informality is maintained to facilitate the transfers of land from petty owners and tenants through the private sector. The important point to be maintained is that such transfers of land could not have taken place without the mediation of the State.

Livelihoods in the City in the Post-reform Period

The way the large cities in India has been reconfigured due to inflows of private capital, often mediated by the state has had a crucial bearing on the livelihood paths of the citizens of the cities. The land transfers from the common government spaces and petty owners to large corporates have shaped cities that are alienated from the needs of the local population. Bangalore, Gurgaon and Kolkata are developing for the sake of hi-tech firms and globetrotting population to produce cities that are deeply divided (Roy 2009). To quote Bhaduri (2007: 552)

> …the India that shines with its fancy apartments and houses in rich neighbourhoods, corporate houses of breathtaking size, glittering shopping malls, and hi-tech flyovers over which flows a procession of new model cars. These are the images from a globalized India on the verge of entering the first world. And then there is the other India…and children too small to walk properly, yet begging on the streets of shining cities.

Thus, in spite of the India experiencing an urban-centric growth, fuelled by existing large cities that overtly aspires to become global cities and smart cities, it is evident that there is a substantial underbelly of this shining urban India. The logic of the market overtly does not discriminate across caste, class, ethnicity and gender, but evidences reveal that the making of the modern post-globalization cities actually achieved their objectives by building cities that have essentially excluded not only people at the margin. For example, the labour arrangements like informalization and sub-contracting are on the one hand aiding the constructing the reconfigured cities, and on the other relegating the workers to margins of the city in terms of their lived and working spaces, both directly through demolition and relocation of slums and indirectly, through casualization and low wages.

Even when the vulnerable sections are not shifted out of the city core, the rich isolate themselves to buy 'protection' and 'safety' that can be observed in the increasing incidence of gated communities, while the poor become '*ghettoized by default*' (Harvey 2003). Such segregations are seen in slums and temporary migrant settlements in the city core, where cheap and flexible unskilled and semi-skilled labour is required in the vicinity of construction and other activities, or in the peripheral areas that Castells (2002) includes in the 'metropolitan areas' (as opposed to metropolitan regions) in resettlement colonies and 'unauthorized' settlements.

One of the major impacts on livelihood that cities in the post-globalization period have had is increased informalization of labour. The flow of capital, coupled by a liberalized financial sector has enabled effective chasing of a cheap labour pool. Unlike the Fordist model of employing labour directly within the domains of the primary labour market with high wage rates and secure jobs in a state regulated private sector, the post-globalization post-fordist era of flexible specialization is centrally about flexible deployment of labour. An example of the phenomenon pointed out by Roy (2009) can be seen in the dilution of labour laws like the Industrial Disputes Act of 1947 by the central and a few state governments in India in recent years. This indicates purposeful moves to promote informality, aided by which labour is not only re-entrenched into the greater marginalities, both economically and socially, but also gets restricted to the margins of the city, with the newly built high rises and hi-tech infrastructure of the city mostly staying out of their reaches.

Health: Infrastructure and Services

Health constitutes a core pillar of human development. It is therefore, considered as a key indicator for assessing achievements in capability enhancements and well-being. Health outcomes are considered as useful measures of how development policies and interventions have reduced deprivations and bridged social disparities. Thus, the starting point to understand health has been the demographic scenario in Delhi in our book, including the size, composition and characteristics of the population. The relationship between demography, health and health care is rooted in the parallel development of these three concepts (Pol and Thomas 2001). These three concepts are interdependent of each other in term of their changing nature over a period of time. Because of a good *health system,*[1] population's health status (which we usually measure through health indicator like life expectancy) increases and because of this change made through the former, demographic characteristics like mortality rate decreases (Aggarwal 2009). However, over the decades the mortality rates have decreased, morbidity and newer forms of diseases are on increase. Krass analyzed that megacities are often perceived as being burdened by numerous disadvantages—as the origins and motors of multiple problems as well as agents and victims of risks. In such disrupted environment, it is a challenging task to deliver health care services to the cities as entities, in entirety.

The milestone was laid by Primary Health Care conference in Alma Ata (1978) globally stirred a holistic vision to achieve a common goal, "Health for All". India's National Health Policy (1983) targeted "Health for All by 2000", with a vision to provide "health at people's doorsteps". But within a decade, the Alma Ata Declaration was abandoned by the State through National Health Policy 2002, which further legitimized privatization in health sector. The National Health Policy 2015 (Draft), follow the same path with loud assertions of strategic purchase of health care services from private sector. Within this whole context, the evolution of the public health care system can be imagined which lead to its existing fragmented state. Delhi being the national capital provided great opportunities to the private sector, subsidized by the state and the public health service systems getting less resources. Thus the access, availability and affordability to quality health care service for the poor remains a far cry.

Urbanization as an important development indicator, and its fast pace of growth has created a number of health care challenges. In the recent years, health needs of rural populations have been attempted under National Rural Health Mission (NRHM), while the National Urban Health Mission (NUHM) has been envisaged to address the same in socio-economic diverse urban population. This was a much needed effort when the number of towns increased by more than 50 % between 2001 and 2011 and the decadal change in population in urban areas (31.2 %) is far more than its rural counterpart (12.3 %). Since the conception of NUHM in 2010, its aim is to address the health concerns by facilitating equitable access to available health facilities by rationalizing and strengthening the capacity of the existing health care delivery system.

[1]Health System is the complex of interrelated elements that contribute health in homes, educational institutions, workplaces, public places, and communities, as well as in the physical and psychological environment and the health and the related sectors. It's a system that includes all the activities, whose purpose is to promote, restore and maintain health.

Sections and Chapters

The book is divided into three sections. The first section examines land and changing landscapes, followed by livelihoods and vulnerability and third section is about health and public facilities and civic amenities. Section one has six chapters.

Das's chapter compares the land use changes across large metropolitan cities and observes that in many cases the rate of post-reform growth of area under non-agricultural use has been faster than the pre-reform period. Using satellite data, Das shows that the built-up areas have consumed significant amounts of cropped area, even when there was availability of wasteland or underutilized land in the vicinity, sometimes greater than the amount of cropland converted. Large-scale land grab of the premium land around large metropolitan centres has resulted in not only the dispossession of land from the farming households, but a loss of livelihood for the tenant farmers and agricultural labourers. Till recently, the 1894 Act applied for land acquisition by the state whereby the eminent domain of state was recognized for such transfer for 'public purpose'. Increasingly, the understanding of public purpose was diluted and land was acquired in large scale for private enterprises.

Choudhary and Punia, in this volume analyzed urban forms and regional development in national capital region (NCR). They quantify spatial urban patterns from optical remote sensing datasets to describe forms, structures and changes in urban land use. Taking urban area as a spatial landscape unit, various landscape indices have been used to describe the urban form in the area. In order to test the effect of level of development on the urban form, a correlation was run between different class metrics, socio-economic development and infrastructural development for different towns of NCR showing more or less similar pattern for the urban form yet some differences which are mainly because of different level of economic development and location.

Punia using remote sensing datasets in his paper 'Marginalisation and Socio-Ecological Transformation in New Urban Peripheries: A Case Study of Gurgaon' examines marginalization from multiple dimensions such as assets, education, workforce participation, employment and land. Agriculture land loss was compensated for urban development, which led to changes in production of space in the post-globalization era. The paper analyzes sociopolitical meaning of this expansion and ways of life within the suburb.

Morya and Punia's paper 'Ecosystem services in NCT Delhi', quantify changes in land use/ land cover and ecosystem services due to urban sprawl in NCT Delhi. Using data provided by European Space agency over the period 1991, 2003, 2010, using 8 land use cover categories under built up, agriculture land and forests, the paper shows the continued decrease in ecosystem services. This led to lesser access of services at higher cost, especially to the poor.

Marginalization is measured by mismatch between infrastructure demand and supply. **Munshi, Haque and Joseph's** paper demonstrate that different areas within the same city enjoy variable amount of accessibility to social infrastructure like schools and parks. Sub-optimal levels of accessibility to social infrastructure have negative implications on human development leading to increased marginalization of communities. Also explores the changing landscape of Yamuna's river bed for the recreational purposes.

Mallik and Sen's paper 'Land Acquisition Policy and Praxis: the case of Peri-Urban Delhi' discusses the critical elements of the Land acquisition Act of 1894 in comparison to the new Act and through a case study of land acquisition in a village located in the urban fringe of Delhi, attempts to look into the nuances of the interlinkages between land dispossession and livelihood transformation. It also attempts to comments upon the implications of the livelihood outcomes of the farmer losing land to the state perpetrated land acquisition.

Section 2 of the book has 8 chapters, deals with the **livelihood, gender and vulnerability issues.** Given the numerous implications of the neo-liberal urban expansion on employment and livelihoods. The papers in this section deals with land dispossession and its impact on their livelihoods, adding to their vulnerabilities. Gender aspects of livelihoods and vulnerabilities are focused in set of four papers.

Mallik and Sen's paper attempts to understand the implications of the changes that were brought about first by the 2013 'Right to Fair Compensation and Transparency in Land Acquisition, Rehabilitation and Resettlement Act', and subsequently, of the 2014 proposed amendments to the 2013 Act. They argue that the amendments, if implemented would undo most of the progressive features of the 2013 Act, in particular through dilution of the consent clause and the mandatory social impact assessment to understand the impact of the acquisition on the people dependent on the land to be acquired. By the dilution of these clauses, the legal framework would nearly revert back to the 1894 Act, with the exception of a more reasonable compensation to the farmers. Finally, the paper, based on an exploratory fieldwork around Delhi, studies the impact on shifts in employment of population dependent on agricultural activities after land acquisition. It reveals that though the larger farmers have improved their employment status, the farmers at the lower end, and in particular the agricultural labourers have been rendered jobless in post-acquisition period.

Sen's paper 'Neo-Liberal Urbanization, Work Participation and Women: Comparing the Urban and Peri-Urban Contexts of Delhi with Mumbai and Kolkata' compare the three metropolitan cities of Delhi, Mumbai and Kolkata. It compares the employment patterns of men and women in city cores, peri-urban areas and the residual part of the respective states in which or adjacent to which these cities are located in. The paper concludes that though the urban locales of the peri-urban areas have been doing better in many respects vis-a-vis the urban cores, these benefits are not distributed equally. Women are worse off in terms of work opportunities and unemployment rates in the peri-urban areas, and such conditions can be explained by the social and demographic changes that have taken place in the peri-urban areas around the large metropolitan cities. With a smaller household size and a higher working age groups sex ratio compared to the interior districts (though lower than the urban core), the possible care burden on the adult women of the households could be a factor explaining their low work participation in these areas.

Pritha's paper on 'Embedded or liberated? An exploration into the social milieu of Delhi' looks into the economic opportunities that are sometimes provided through urban growth often are in contradiction with social embeddedness of the cities. This paper shows that in spite of the efforts of getting globally linked, Indian cities are socio-spatially embedded in their regional culture. It further explores whether metropolitan cities of India, particularly Delhi, emerge as socially liberated spaces rather than embedded entities within their rural surrounding. The analysis in this paper brings forth the point that patriarchal produced social relations between men and women, very typical of the northern social space, even in recent times shape the perceptions of the women respondents about their work status in Delhi.

The paper by **Reddy and Acharya** on 'Gender violence in Delhi: Perception and Experiences' shows the perception of fear across the young girls and women in accessing urban spaces in Delhi. The study reflect through the experiential evidences that patriarchal mind set, existing social values which internalize women as weak and dependent on men, perpetuate violence and crime against them, making the urban spaces difficult to navigate for them. In addition to the violence against women, there is also inadequate legal recourse, redresssal and surveillance mechanisms in the city. Multiculturalism in Delhi, and unfamiliarity with the nuances of the alieniating urban spaces, often leads to experiences of violence.

Acharya and Reddy's paper 'Migrant Women Workers in Construction and Domestic work: Issues and Challenges' analyzes the life of 1010 migrant women working in two sectors. It is the question of survival, which pushes them to the city like Delhi, however, assures them two square meals. The nature of work in both these sectors is exploitative, with no guarantee of minimum wages and also with no facilities such as toilets, crèche, clean drinking water at work place. They are also excluded and marginalized in accessing their rights and benefits, which are meant for them due to lack of awareness of the information and also inaccessibility. Both these sector have important role to play for any urban development, however, women especially from these unorganized sector are far behind reaping any fruits of development.

Meena and Punia in their paper 'Revealing the vulnerabilities of population and places at risk in Delhi' map the vulnerabilities of the population living near the flood prone areas of Yamuna River. Using GIS and land scan data from Oak Ridge National Laboratory (ORNL) the paper shows that increasing population pressure on land and lack of regulations related to construction activities on river bed, increases the risk of population and suggest an urgency in land policy and emphasis on disaster risk reduction through mitigation and preparedness.

Resettlement of the poor from the urban core has been an integral part of the reconstruction of Delhi in an effort to demonstrate it as a global city. **Kaur** in her study of resettlement colony Bawana, highlighted the implications of such changes on access to health care of the displaced women who were evicted from Yamuna Pushta to be resettled in Bawana. She addresses issue of repeated displacement due to settling and resettling of the slum dwellers, especially the life of voiceless excluded women. Most of the people, who are evicted, were left to fend for themselves with no or extremely few alternatives and choices. Her paper attempts to capture and document the painful experiences, and unheard voices of the poor women excluded throughout their lives.

Peripheralization of social vulnerability in national capital territory is evident from the paper by **Punia and Kumari**. They have analyzed mission convergence data of 1.1 million households across 274 municipal wards of Delhi. In the past unauthorized colonies have been regularized in Delhi. The total number of *Jhughi Jhopri* (JJ) clusters in 2011 were 687 and number of *Jhuggies* were 0.48 million (Delhi Shelter Board 2011). Delhi development report (DDR) 2013, reported reduction in poverty to single-digit Figs. (9.9 %) in 2011–2012, from approximately 13 % in 2004–05. Notwithstanding the wide concern over the present official poverty line, which is indeed an under-estimate of the state of vulnerability. To claim that there has certainly been a decline in absolute poverty levels in Delhi, can be critically looked at from the rest of the papers in this volume, which shows growing marginalization and disparities.

Section 3 has a set of 10 papers discussing on the issues of changing landscape in health care service sector, public amenities and public health services such as sanitation, water and housing. **Singh's** paper focuses on spatial expansion of the National Capital Territory of Delhi in recent times and evolution of health care services in the region. This paper further analyzes spatial coverage of health care institutions and the access to these institutions by the different socio-economic groups. There are spatial disparities in allocation of health care facilities, on one hand, some places are hotspots for hospitals and hospital beds' congestion, and contrarily other places are lacking healthcare facilities to the extreme of being non-existent in their surroundings. The clustered pattern of health facilities made urban poor more vulnerable especially when they are already situated at the lower end of social ladder. From central government to municipal bodies the multiplicity of key agencies involved in public healthcare makes an integrated health system difficult. This finding is in agreement with those of Chaplet et al. (2002) and Lefebvre (2004) who derived similar nuances for the private sector as well.

Reddy's paper 'Changing Health Care Dynamics: Corporatization and medical tourism in Delhi' analyzes the changing landscape of health care in Delhi and NCR. Post independence the landscape changed from public service oriented health care provisioning to privatized and corporatized health care, thanks to liberalization and health sector reforms. The paper discusses the growth of the corporate sector from critical public health perspective. Dovetailing with the Singh's paper on the distribution of health care services in Delhi, Reddy's paper focus on the growth of tertiary, super specialty corporate health care, giving rise to dichotomous health care provisioning. Ill-equipped, overburdened public hospital services for the poor and state-of-the-art, accredited, posh corporate health care sector for the rich, insured and foreign patients, under the catchy term 'Medical Tourism'.

The shift of public to private healthcare in not merely a structural change, as discussed in the two papers by Singh and Reddy, **Narayan** in his paper 'Health care providers in Metropolitan Cities' tried to examine health care providers in Delhi, their issues and concerns within a sociological perspective. He analyzed the objective attributes of doctors and their subjective perception of their status, in context of the larger society and within the occupational community of health personnel. The performance of any professional group partly depends on how far it has been able to change its pre-professional attitudes acquired during the period of primary socialization before entering in the professional training. Study is concerned with the medical professionals, who come from the upper strata of society and their process of socialization and high-tech education is different from that of the common man, to whom they provide the services.

Acharya and **Patra** in their paper 'Access to Maternal and Child Health Care: understanding discrimination in selected slum in Delhi' peeled one more layer of exclusion and discussed the issue of discrimination in accessing maternal and child healthcare by women and children. This paper aims to understand the nature and patterns of caste-based discrimination in access to health care practiced in different forms; and the consequences of such practices.

This volume also addresses the issue of vulnerability of different age groups in the city. **Diwakar's** paper focuses on the most marginalized lot, the 'street children' living in the streets of Delhi. This paper fills the gap in available literature on understanding the life at street and street children's experience in seeking care from public health institutions. Various factors interplay in determining the life of the street children. The poor living conditions and harassments on the streets, predispose them to high level of morbidity in the form of accidents, injuries and infectious diseases. The adverse experience with public health institutions leads to delayed health seeking, which in turn aggravates their health problems. Most of the time they seek treatment in emergency care unit.

Dutta and Kumar paper 'Socio-Economic Disparities among Youth in Delhi: Issues and Challenges', raised their concern about marginalization of youth in Delhi, where one-fifth of its main workforce is constituted by youth. They highlighted the disparity in their health status, gender based discrimination in sex ratios, and also unemployment of different social groups from different classes, in Delhi.

Another vulnerable, marginalized social group is the elderly; **Das** in her paper 'Conditions of aged in NCT of Delhi' discusses the conditions of the elderly population in the city. She observed that the capital has a relatively young age structure with lesser proportion of aged population than the country average. Elderly sex ratio also, which otherwise favours females is favouring males in the capital. Commensurate with previous studies, she observes that even in the capital city, women headship is low when they are in the union, which they get with increase in age and mostly when they are not in the union. High work participation may be linked with the low morbidity of the Delhi elderly where both the incidence and rate of hospitalization are substantially low.

Coming to public facilities, urbanization and rapid growth of population also raises water, sanitation and solid waste management issues among other amenities. Urban poor have poor access to such resources. **Lenka** discussed the challenges of water supply and sanitation with special reference to urban poor in Delhi. His paper attempts to examine the challenges of water supply to the vulnerable populations in the slums of Delhi and the monetary transactions involved between different stakeholders; quality of water supplied and events of illnesses with water quality.

Apart from water and sanitation, equal importance is to manage solid waste generated by the urban population. Delhi is the largest municipal solid waste producer in the country, which generates around 8,500 tonnes of solid waste daily. **Sharma's** paper 'Solid waste management and Health workers—Exploring situation in Delhi' is about the health concerns of solid waste management workers in Delhi. Though a less explored field especially to understand the impact on the health of workers engaged in solid waste management. It also addresses the poor management of solid waste in Delhi. Contractual system of their services makes their vulnerability two folds; they are under-paid and no protection gears leading to occupational health hazard.

Paper 'Living in blight in the globalized metro: A study on housing and housing conditions of Delhi' by **Das and Bhusan**, studied 13 slums, referred to as 'urban blight' in Delhi to show that they suffer from insufficiency of infrastructures and civic amenities. Filth and dingy ambience pose health hazards of the residents directly reflected in the type of dwelling unit, however, have regional variations in the conditions of slum dwellers, though seen as homogenous urban space.

Summing Up

It has been widely agreed that cities have historically been systems that encapsulate growth, innovation and human progress (Hall and Raumplaner 1998). Correspondingly, cities have also been sites of concentration of capital. The nature of investment of the capital and the ways in which the local population were accommodated therein had, in turn, shaped the cities. Cities have also been focus of creation and exchange of information and knowledge. The exchange of information and knowledge is manifested in the exchange of people, goods and services with a city's hinterland and other cities. Distance from the cities have traditionally been an important factor in determining the degree of this interaction, so much so, that Ullman (1980) proposed the mechanism of this interaction encapsulated in what was termed as the 'gravity' model (shaped loosely around Newton's laws of motion), where distance was given the primacy to explain interaction. Based on the similar principles, Francois Perroux (1950) and others conceptualized cities as growth-poles, an abstract economic space that has a field of influence on its surroundings resulting in a 'trickle-down' effect on its surrounding. This conceptualization was not without an intuitive appeal, and policy makers have historically interpreted cities as foci that transmit growth, and what was hoped would translate into 'development', in and around them.

People migrate to cities primarily for employment. To support their happy and comfortable living, they also need good quality housing, cost efficient physical and social infrastructure such as water, sanitation, electricity, clean air, education, health care, security, and entertainment. Industries are also located in the cities, because there are agglomeration economies that provide easy access to labour and other factors of production. However, the success of 'smart' Delhi rests on people's participation; and city's social and economic ecological frame. Energy saving and implementation of new technologies are some of the ways to make residential, commercial and public spaces sustainable. Absorption of the urban sprawl through the activities which connect the local with the global needs the same thrust. Delhi has come to a point in history where it needs to become smart, safe and sustainable global urban conurbation drawing people, investments and establishments from across local and global spaces albeit the construct of the millennium city embraces the concern for sustainable development through meaningful use and access to land, livelihood and health.

Delhi was always a city of hope for many. Population growth in the past century expanded the city from its core to the periphery. This expansion made it challenging to the local governing bodies to manage the public services' distribution. Economic disparity, inequality in the urbanization process and urban environment influence the health of the urban poor enormously. Continuous process of migration for livelihoods, scarcity of basic amenities, power equation, gender differences, specific age groups and unequal resource allocation are some major concerns of national capital addressed in this book.

References

Aggarwal, SK. (2009). Delhi: Towards a healthy city to live.in. Voquet, A (ed.) *Globalisation and Health. Manohar Publications*. New delhi pp 101–130.

Alma Ata (1978). Declaration of Alma-Ata. *International Conference on Primary Health Care*, Alma- Ata, USSR, 6–12 September 1978. Available at docs/almaata.html>.

Bhaduri, A. (2007). Development or developmental terrorism? *Economic and Political Weekly, 42*(7), 552.

Castells, M. (2002). Local and global: cities in the network society. *Tijdschriftvooreconomische en socialegeografie, 93*(5), 548–558.

Castells, M., & Portes, A. (1989). World underneath: The origins, dynamics, and effects of the informal economy. In L. Benton, et al. (Eds.), *the Informal Economy* (pp. 11–40). Baltimore, MD: Johns Hopkins University Press.

Census of India. (2011). *Provisional population totals (districts/Su-districts) NCT of Delhi.* Retrieved December 24, 2013, from http://www.censusindia.gov.in/2011-prov-results/paper2-vol2/data_files/Delhi/Provisional_Rural_Urban.pdf

Debroy, V., & Bhandari, L. (2009). Gurgaon and Faridabad—An Exercise in Contrasts, Center on Democracy, Development, and The Rule of Law Freeman Spogli Institute for International Studies.

Delhi Shelter Board. (2011). *JJ Cluster list, Govt of Delhi*. Retrieved December 13, 2013, from http://delhishelterboard.in

Hall, P., & Raumplaner, S. (1998). *Cities in civilization* (p. 291). New York: Pantheon Books.

Harvey, D. (2003). The right to the city. *International Journal of Urban and Regional Research, 27*(4), 939–941.

Harvey, D. (2012). *Rebel cities: From the right to the city to the Urban revolution*. Verso Books.

Hasan, A. (2015). Land contestation in Karachi and the impact on housing and urban development, *Environment and Urbanization*, *27*(1), 217–230.
Hawley, A. H. (1950). Human ecology: a theory of community structure. Ronald Press, New York.
Jain, A. K. (2011). *Sustainable Urban Mobilityin Southern Asia*. Regional Study. Sustainable Urban Mobility Gobal Report on Human Settlements 2010 UN Habitat. Nairobi.
Jain, A. K. (2015). Urban Housing ans Slums. jain Book Depot. New Delhi.
Keivani, R., & Mattingly, M. (2007). The interface of globalization and peripheral land in the cities of the south: Implications for Urban governance and local economic development. *International Journal of Urban and Regional Research, 31*(2), 459–474.
Lefebvre, B. (2004, June 19–20). The impact of metropolitanisation on public health care in Delhi. In *EGIRGHI Conference*. Maynooth, Iceland: NUI.
Miller, C. (2008). Sociable Cities: The Legacy of Ebenezer Howard Version of Record online: 28 JUN 2008*New Zealand Geographer*, *55*(2),76–77, October 1999.
Mitra, A. (1974). *A functional classification of India's Towns*. New Delhi: Institute of Economic Growth.
Narain, V. (2009). Growing city, shrinking hinterland: land acquisition, transition and conflict in peri-urban Gurgaon, India. *Environment and Urbanization*, *21*, 501–512.
NSSO. (2009). *64th round Report: Some Characteristics of Urban Slums, 2008–09*. Ministry of Statistics and Programme Implementation, Government of India.
Ong, A. (2011). Worlding cities, or the art of being global. Introduction. In A. Roy, & A. Ong (Eds.), *Worlding cities- Asian experiments and the art of being global* (p. 2). Chichester: Wiley Blackwell.
Perroux, F. (1950, February). Economic space: Theory and applications'. *The Quarterly Journal of Economics, 64*(1), pp. 89–104
Pol, L. G. & Thomas R. K. (2001). *The demography of health and health care* (second edition) byKluwer Academic/Plenum Publishers, New York.
Roy, A. (2003). *City Requiem, Calcutta: Gender and the Politics of Poverty*, University of Minnesota Press, Minnesota USA.
Roy, A. (2009). Why India cannot plan its cities: Informality, insurgence and the idiom of urbanization. *Planning Theory, 8*(1), 76–87.
Roy, A., & Ong, A. (Eds.). (2011). *Worlding Cities: Asian experiments and the art of being global New Delhi*. Oxford, UK: Wiley Blawell Publishing Ltd.
Smith, D. A. (2015). Mapping the Global Urban Transformation. *CityGegraphics- Urban Forms, Dynamics and Sustainability*. https://citygeographics.org/
Ullman, E. L. (1980). "*Geography as spatial interaction*". In R. B. Ronald (Ed.), Geography as Spatial Interaction University of Washington Press (13–27).
UN Habitat II. (1996, June 3–14) .*United Nations Conference on Human Settlements (Habitat II). GE.96-02500 (E)*. (Habitat II) in Istanbul, Turkey.
Veltz (2004). The Resurgent City- Keynote Address. *Leverhulme International Symposium*. London School of Economics.pp 19–21.

Part I
Land and Changing Landscape

Land-Use Dynamics of Peri-Urban Areas of Metropolitan Cities with Special Focus on Delhi

Nanda Dulal Das

Abstract Post-reform period has experienced increased flow of investment towards development of infrastructure around the large metropolitan cities in India. This has led to expansion of urban centres over the peripheral land-use classes which include productive croplands. This study seeks to find out the extent of growth of urban areas in the periphery of seven largest metropolitan cities in India and consumption of farmland by the process, with a special focus on Delhi. A trend of growing urban area is evident around almost all the metropolitan cities in the post-reform period. Though the cultivable area around the metropolitan cities has decreased in the post-reform period, the increase in net sown area in those areas signify more judicial utilization of land in the post-reform period in the peripheries of large urban centres. Though the growth of built-up area around Delhi metropolis has not followed any set pattern targeting consumption of any specific kinds of land for its expansion, large tracts of cultivable lands have disappeared in the process, despite the fact that wastelands or unutilized land remain which could have been converted for urban-centric land use. It has also been argued in this study that impact of conversion is more in areas closer to the urban centres and vice versa. A significantly high degree of negative correlation exists between the built-up area and distance from the city centre of Delhi. The analysis reveals that this process has been fairly prominent around the metropolitan city of Delhi.

Keywords Land-use dynamics · Peri-Urban · Metropolitan city · Centre-Periphery · Crop and wasteland

N.D. Das (✉)
Government Sector, Pune, India
e-mail: nandadulaldas@gmail.com

S.S. Acharya et al. (eds.), *Marginalization in Globalizing Delhi: Issues of Land, Livelihoods and Health*, DOI 10.1007/978-81-322-3583-5_2

Introduction

The process of economic reforms after 1991 has caused an intensification of private investment, especially Foreign Direct Investment (FDI) that is getting drawn towards the large urban centres. In the period between 1991 and 2004, Delhi and Mumbai together accounted for over 42 % of total incoming FDI. The concentration of high proportion of FDI saturates the urban core within a short period and is soon manifested in the outward dispersal of investment and urban infrastructure (Goldar 2007). Similar phenomena have been observed in the Class-I cities in China in recent years (Zhao et al. 2003). This "urban bias" also bends the public policies in favour of secondary and tertiary activities (Kydd 2002). Thus, urban areas grow at an unprecedented rate over an area previously occupied primarily by farming activities (Harvey and Clark 1965; Blobaum 1974; Hart 1976; Plaut 1980; Pachauri 1986; Alig and Healy 1987; Young 1999; Lopez et al. 2001). The emergence and continuous expansion of peri-urban regions is more of a recent phenomenon in India unlike the west, and thus, literature that seek to understand the dynamics of peri-urban land uses in India is not very extensive.[1] The increasing pressure on agricultural land particularly around the urban fringe could have some positive externalities for the area that remain under agriculture by enhancing investments and thereby increasing yield and altering the cropping pattern towards a high value combination due to presence of urban demand in its proximity (Gillies and Mittlebach 1958). However, loss of multi-cropped land with its associated impact on livelihood bases are a matter of concern, particularly if the urban processes fail to generate additional employment adequate to make up for such losses (Lal 2001). Thus understanding the dynamics of land-use changes is of crucial importance. The focus of the present study is to analyze the interactions between the agricultural and non-agricultural lands around Delhi metropolitan city in comparison to other large metropolitan cities in India between the pre-reform and post-reform period.

Focus, Data and Concepts

This study hypothesizes that increasing pressure of building infrastructure and built-up area around the large metropolitan centres in the post-reform period would be reflected in the loss of productive cropland in the peripheries of urban

[1]The dynamic interface at the periphery of urban boundary is characterized by gradually changing land-use from agricultural to other non-agricultural uses, changing populations, changing use of natural resources and changing processes of waste generation, etc. Changing population pressure and subsequent technological change and their impact on the dynamics of agricultural land-use has been extensively researched by some scholars (Boserup 1965). In the Indian context, peri-urban dynamics are recently being studied in detail (Shaw 2005; Sridharan 2006).

centres. The effect is expected to be more prominent in the areas closer to the urban centre. This study also assumes that with increasing pressure of urban expansion on the periphery and productive cropland, unproductive lands like wastelands would have been judiciously used in the post-reform period. Hence, this study seeks to find out the extent of conversion of different land-use classes into built-up area in a comparative perspective between the pre-reform and the post-reform period, in the peripheries of the large metropolitan centres with a special focus on the capital city of Delhi. To look into the urban-growth concentration around the large metropolitan cities in comparison to their respective larger regional perspectives, two specific sets are chosen. Districts around metropolitan (DAM) cities are chosen to represent the first set, i.e., urban periphery and the respective States have been chosen as the second set representing the larger regional backdrop.[2] To capture the impact of urban-growth phenomena, the extent of change in cultivable land area vis-à-vis area under non-agricultural use in the DAM and the respective states has been analysed in the pre-reform and post-reform period.[3] Seven large urban centres have been chosen for presenting a broad intra-regional and inter-regional pattern with a more detailed analysis of the peripheries of Delhi (Fig. 1).[4]

For the case study of the periphery of Delhi metropolitan region, a few community development (CD) Blocks have been extracted from the DAMs and within these Blocks; all the constituent villages have been studied (Fig. 2). Besides considering the loss of cultivable lands owing to increasing non-agricultural area, the extent of judicious utilization of wastelands in the periphery has also been looked in detail. The pattern of interaction among the different land-use classes has been analyzed to portray the "urban effect" in the peripheral region with the increasing distance from the urban centre. While the broader comparative analysis of the seven metropolitan centres is done based on the data published by the directorate of Economics and Statistics, the detailed analysis of Delhi is based on satellite images pertaining to two time periods, the data bases being of 1989-Landsat TM and 2006-IRS P-6, LISS-3. Numerous studies using the techniques of remote sensing and GIS have proven the phenomenon of cropland loss in the peri-urban areas effectively (Fazal 2000). Efforts have been made to classify the land utilization of the study region into standard land-use categories using satellite imagery

---

[2]Gurgaon, Sonepat, Jajjhar, Rohtak, Faridabad in Haryana and Ghaziabad in Uttar Pradesh; Thane and Raigad in Maharashtra; Haora, Hugli, N & S 24 Pargana in West Bengal; Chengalpattu-MGR and Thiruvallur in Tamilnadu; Rangareddy in Andhra Pradesh; Bangalore Rural in Karnataka; Kheda, Mahesana and Gandhinagar in Gujarat.

[3]For this dataset of Dept. of Agriculture & Cooperation (DAC) of the Ministry of Agriculture has been used. Triennium averages for 1978–'81, 1988–'91 and 1998–2001 have been used to reduce short-term fluctuations.

[4]Seven largest metropolitan cities according to the 2001 census have been selected for the study, namely, Mumbai, Kolkata, Delhi, Chennai, Hyderabad, Bangalore and Ahmadabad and respective states have also been chosen to represent the larger regional setting around the metropolitan cities.

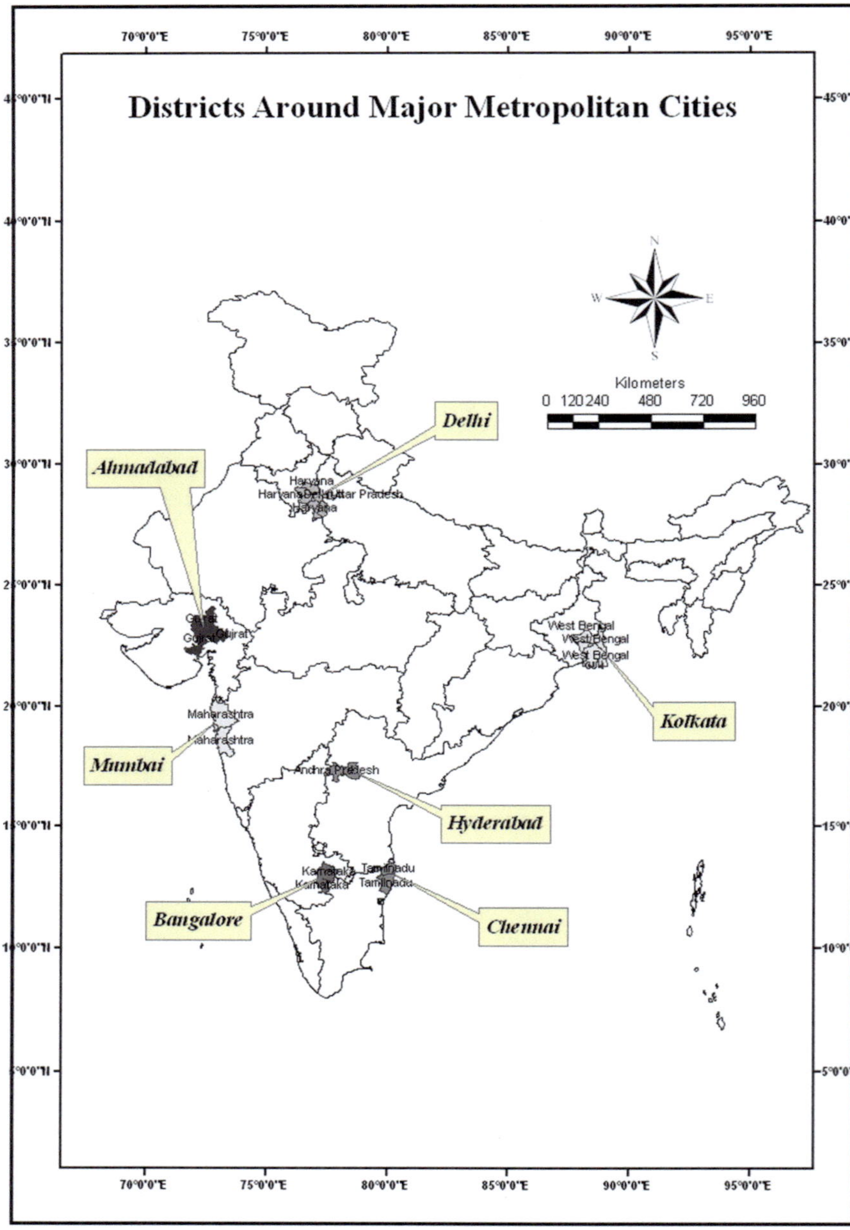

Fig. 1 Selected districts around the seven large metropolitan cities in India

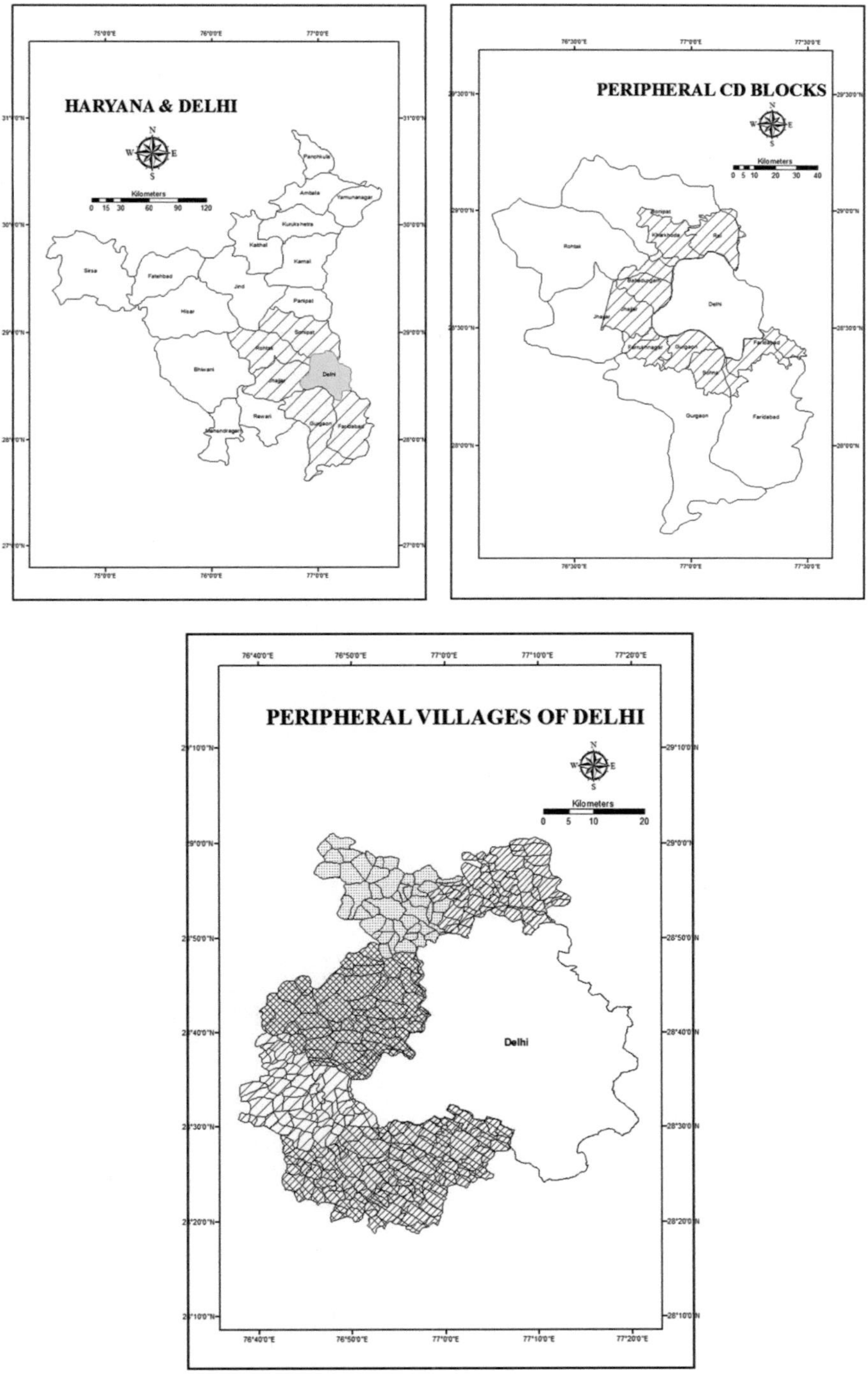

Fig. 2 Study area for microscopic analysis in the peripheral blocks and villages around Delhi (in the Haryana side)

(Anderson et al. 1976). Change detection between the two satellite imageries of two different years has been done using 'change vector study' (Coupin and Bauer 1996). The impact of land acquisition around Delhi on livelihood of farmers has been substantiated with field observations through an exploratory survey in a few villages around Delhi.

Dynamics of Land-Use in the Periphery of Large Metropolitan Cities

Several cities have witnessed a spill-over effect of urbanization around its peripheries in the post-reform period. This is more prominent around Hyderabad, Chennai, Delhi adjacent to Haryana and also Bangalore (Table 1).[5] Thus, the southern cities seem to have responded to the reform in a manner that was expected along with the areas adjacent to Delhi.

The peripheral areas have generally experienced higher increase in non-agricultural area that are faster than the respective states in the post-reform period. The only exceptions are Kolkata and Mumbai. The DAM of Chennai has experienced highest proportional increase of area under non-agricultural use (AUNAU) in the post-reform period than any other cities under consideration and this trend is consistent with the amount of investment it drew in the post-reform period.[6] This has happened despite the fact that it is having a base of AUNAU that is significantly higher than the other cities.

Several important patterns emerge out from the analysis of change in shares of net sown area (NSA) and total cultivable land (TCL) in the pre-and post-reform periods.[7] In most of the cases, proportion of both NSA and TCL is higher in the states than in the DAMs in both the pre-reform and post-reform period. Majority of the peripheries of metropolitan cities have improved in terms of extent of net sown area in the post-reform period in contrast to the pre-reform period. These are the same cities that had witnessed a decline in the extent of NSA in the pre-reform period. In contrast, periphery of Mumbai, Delhi (on the Haryana side) had registered a greater increase in NSA in the pre-reform period in comparison to the later period. Except for Hyderabad and Mumbai, peripheries of most of the other cities experienced continued decrease in proportion of total cultivable land (TCL), a process which had started from before the reforms. In spite of some increase in NSA in the post-reform period in many cases, none of them could revert back to their

[5]In 1989, 'Bangalore Rural' district was carved out from Bangalore and thus data for Bangalore Rural district was not available in 1981 separately.

[6]Source: Data from CAPEX, CMIE (Centre for Monitoring the Indian Economy), February 2005. (as presented in Shaw et al. 2006).

[7]Cultivable Land has been calculated by summing up the areas under Culturable Wasteland, Current Fallow Land and Fallow Other than Current Fallow Land and Net Sown Area; especially the lands having potentiality of producing agricultural crops.

Table 1 Decadal Percentages of AUNAU, NSA and TCL in the DAMs and respective states (1980–2000) (% to reporting area)

		Mum	MH	Kol	W.B.	Del	Har	Del	U.P.	Hyd	A.P.	Chen	T.N.	Bang	KNT	Ahm	Guj
AUNAU	('80)	6.4	3.4	21.5	14.3	10.8	8.5	12.1	7.5	9.2	7.8	23.7	13.2	NA	5.5	9.4	5.7
	('90)	7.8	3.6	24.3	18.4	11.1	6.9	14.1	8.2	10.1	8.4	25.4	14.0	7.5	6.2	9.9	5.9
	('00)	8.5	4.3	25.6	20.0	14.4	8.4	15.3	8.6	11.6	9.5	30.6	15.1	9.9	6.8	10.0	6.0
NSA	('80)	27.8	59.0	53.3	62.6	74.3	81.8	73.1	57.9	42.2	39.6	40.5	45.7	NA	53.4	75.4	50.9
	('90)	33.0	60.0	48.1	60.3	77.6	81.2	71.1	57.9	39.5	40.2	36.2	43.0	52.3	55.3	72.6	49.7
	('00)	32.0	57.5	49.9	61.5	75.4	81.0	71.7	59.0	39.7	39.7	36.9	42.1	51.0	54.5	74.9	50.7
TCL	('80)	38.1	67.8	54.7	68.7	83.7	86.3	82.0	68.2	65.9	56.5	59.5	63.9	NA	65.2	81.6	66.1
	('90)	45.1	69.7	52.6	66.5	82.9	86.0	80.7	68.1	66.4	57.4	58.9	63.2	61.5	66.0	80.6	65.6
	('00)	41.8	68.7	51.4	65.4	81.4	86.1	80.4	68.0	66.6	56.8	54.7	61.9	60.9	66.2	80.4	65.8

Source Calculated from the land-utilization statistics of Directorate of Economics and Statistics, Ministry of Agriculture, GOI. [Abbreviations: AUNAU-Area under Non-Agricultural Use, NSA-Net Sown Area, TCL-Total Cultivable Land] position of 1980. Thus, there was a net outflow of area under plough in those cases compared to the 1980s However, generally speaking, a decrease in total cultivable land on one hand and increase in NSA, on the other, in the post-reform period around many of the large metropolitan cities indicates better utilization of limited stock of agricultural land in the post-reform period. This general trend, however, needs to be studied in greater details, because the exact dynamics of urban expansion and the resultant land use changes cannot be understood by looking at the net inflows and outflows.

This section reveals to us that frequently, peripheries of all metropolitan cities have been more rooted to the larger regions in which they are located, rather than taking on a monolithic urban 'metropolitan' character. The difference in the patterns of land use changes in the large cities located in different regional contexts reveal that the geographical contexts and the socio-cultural and regional economic contexts are important in shaping these changes.

Dynamics of Land-Use in the Periphery of Delhi: A Detailed Analysis

Delhi has experienced a multipolar urbanization with Gurgaon and Faridabad merging with Delhi in terms of urban area expansion. From the analysis done in the earlier section, the peripheries of Delhi have the unique feature of experiencing a decline in both the net sown area and total cultivable land in the post-reform period. Also, Delhi is surrounded by multi-cropped productive area, both in Haryana and Western Uttar Pradesh. These characteristics make Delhi an ideal case to explore in greater depth.

The nature of transfer of land from one land-use class to another cannot be understood clearly from the analysis in the previous section. Use of satellite imageries of two periods for Delhi's peripheries has enabled change detection with higher certainty. The status of land utilization in the post-reform period (up to 2006), in the delineated study area, shows that none of the CD Blocks studied here is having more than 40 % of double-cropped area. Expectedly, in Gurgaon, total net sown area accounts for only 50 % (within which only 20 % are double cropped) and area under built-up use is reasonably higher than any other blocks under consideration. On the other hand, the block of Jhajjar possesses a great prospect for future growth of built-up area as proportion of built-up area is among the lowest and it is also having over 5 % of wasteland which presents a possibility of future expansion of built-up area at lesser costs than any other blocks.

The summary of land-use categories as derived from satellite data has been shown in Table 2. This provides us with the existing pattern of land utilization. An effort to address the question of how have different land-use classes been converted to built-up area in the post-reform period has been made by comparing the available imageries of Kharif seasons between 1989 and 2006. The following paragraphs give a detailed analysis of such conversion process.

Table 2 Percentage of areas under different land-use/land cover classes in CD Blocks (2006)

CD Block	Area (ha)	DCA	SCA	BUA	Vegetation	Wasteland	Water	Dry and sandy soil
Rai	27,373	39.8	9.9	32.0	15.5	1.6	2.4	0.1
Kharkhoda	30,355	36.4	18.6	27.7	12.5	3.1	1.5	0.2
Bahadurgarh	48,838	32.0	21.6	32.7	9.3	3.9	2.6	0.3
Jhajjar	30,534	31.6	38.7	19.4	2.5	5.1	1.0	1.8
Farrukhnagar	29,004	35.3	44.8	12.4	3.0	2.2	0.7	0.8
Gurgaon	27,795	20.2	30.6	33.2	7.4	2.7	4.8	1.1

Source Table generated from the land-use classification operation using two satellite imageries (IRS P-6 LISS-3 Path-96 Row-51) of 12/02/2006 (Rabi) and 10/10/2006 (Kharif) ,respectively and overlaying of maps of the six blocks of Haryana surrounding Delhi. The administrative boundaries of the districts and CD blocks have been taken from the Town and Village Directory of the Census of India (1991). N.B. DCA and SCA stand for double-and single-cropped area, respectively, while BUA stands for built-up area (Figures generated from supervised classification of satellite imagery)

The possibility of change detection between two periods of time is possible partially as imagery of two Kharif growing seasons are available (1989 & 2006). After performing supervised imagery-classification, overlaying and change detection techniques have been used for the analysis. To grasp the process of conversion more accurately, a comparison of different types of classes, which were converted into built-up area between 1989 and 2006, has been shown in terms of amount of area consumed from a village and also the percentage of one particular land-use/cover class converted to the built-up use in the respective villages (Figs. 3 and 4). Among all the peripheral blocks of Delhi, Gurgaon has experienced tremendous growth of area under built-up category and land-use types being consumed for the purpose of built-up area is quite diverse and extensive. The Case of Bahadurgarh block is almost similar to that of Gurgaon. Field study confirms high level of growth of built-up area in the post-reform period in both the blocks, especially around the cities of Gurgaon and Bahadurgarh.

Statistical analysis points to few prominent features of land conversion. First, land from almost all the land-use classes have been more or less converted into urban use. Second, land-use units occupying larger area (more than 100 ha) were converted mainly from uses like cropped area, seasonal fallow, vegetative cover other than agriculture and wasteland. Third, the overall conversion, irrespective of land-use classes, however, has happened mainly for the smaller units of use (Table 3). Thus, individual housing has probably outweighed large scale acquisition of land by Government and private owners.

Further, we could see that no one land-use class dominated in the process of conversion. Croplands, both cropped land and seasonal fallow combined, alone account for about 29 % of total conversion. Loss of area under croplands to the extent of 30–40 % has taken place in many villages, which is a matter of concern given its potential impact on those dependent on agriculture.

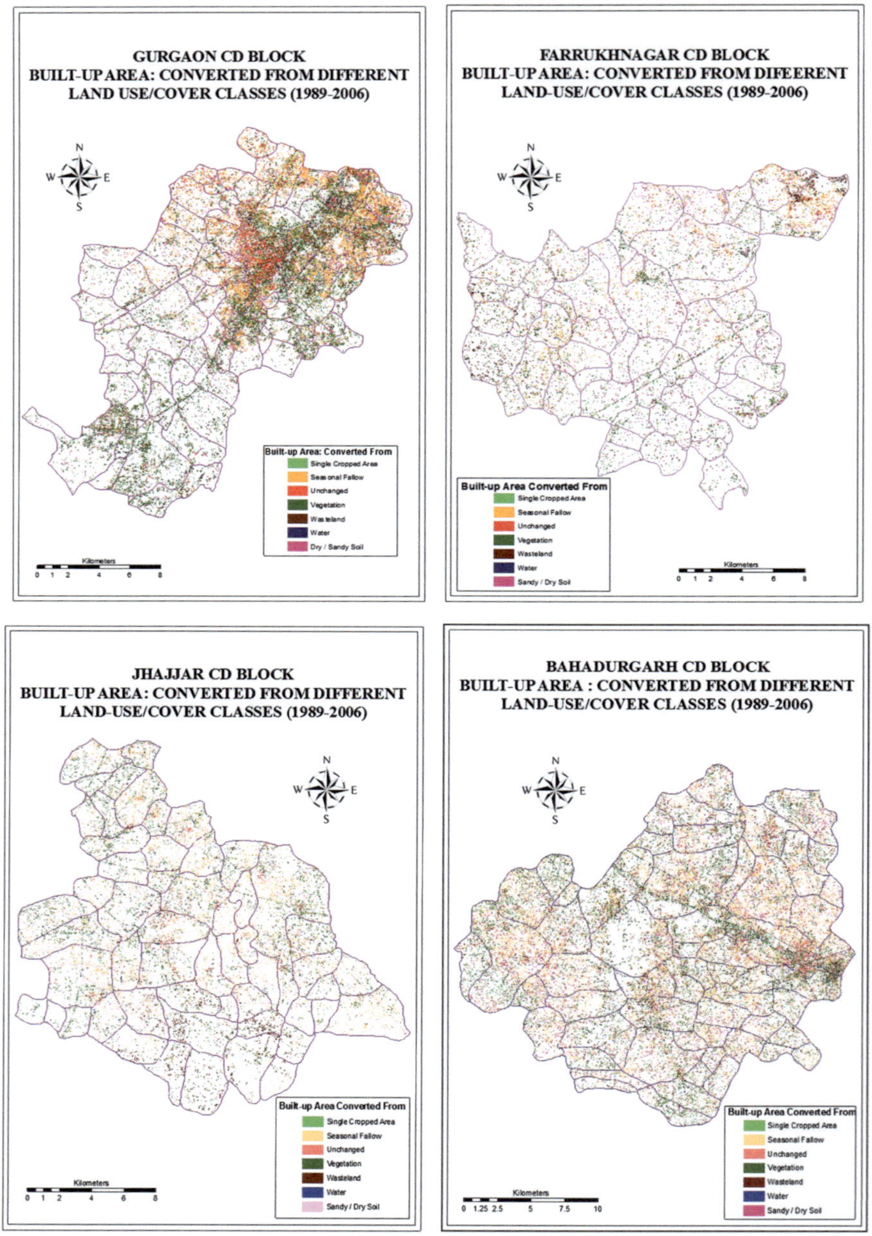

Fig. 3 Conversion of different land-use/cover classes to Built-up Area (1989–2006). (CD Blocks of Gurgaon, Farrukhnagar, Bahadurgarh and Jhajjar clockwise from the *top left*)

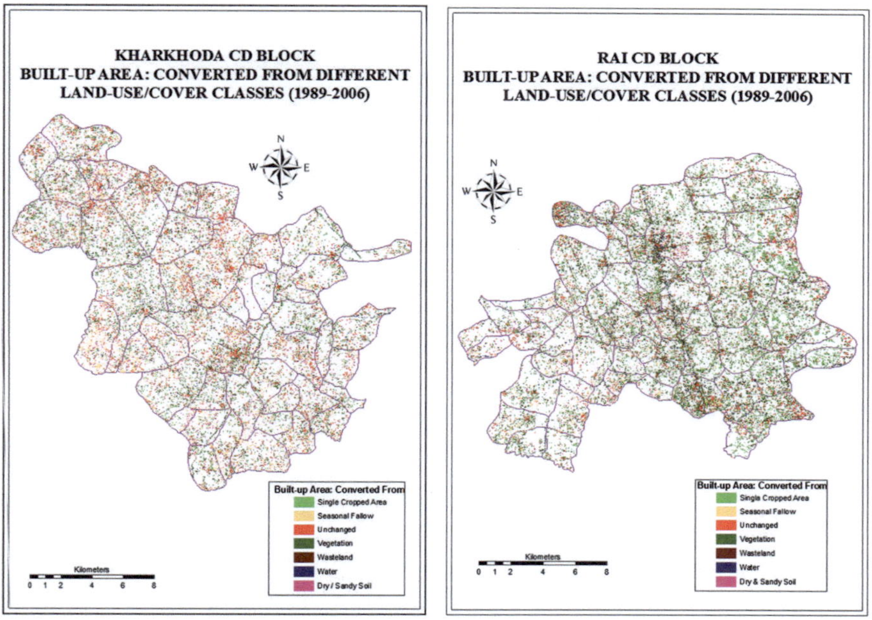

Fig. 4 Conversion of different land-use/cover classes to Built-up Area (1989–2006). (CD Blocks of Kharokhoda and Rai)

Table 3 Area-wise conversion of major land-use/cover types into built-up area in different peripheral CD blocks of Delhi (1989–2006)

			Area converted to built-up area (%)						Total (%)
			1.00	2.00	3.00	4.00	5.00	6.00	
Built-up area converted from	Cropped area	% of changed cases	63.8	17.8	10.9	6.6	0.9	0.0	100.0
		% of total conversion	**9.1**	2.5	1.6	0.9	0.1	0.0	**14.3**
	Seasonal fallow	% of changed cases	33.5	15.6	24.4	18.2	5.7	**2.6**	100.0
		% of total conversion	**4.8**	2.3	**3.5**	2.6	0.8	0.4	**14.4**
	Wasteland	% of total conversion	90.4	6.1	2.6	0.9	0.0	0.0	100.0
		% of total conversion	**12.8**	0.9	.4	0.1	0.0	0.0	**14.1**

Source Table generated from the land-use classification operation using two satellite imageries (IRS P-6 LISS-3 Path-96 Row-51) of 10/10/2006 (Kharif) and Landsat TM Path-147, Row-40 of 09/10/1989 (Kharif), respectively and overlaying of these classified imageries along with maps of the six blocks of Haryana surrounding Delhi to obtain change detection between different classes. The administrative boundaries of the districts and CD blocks have been taken from the Town and Village Directory of the Census of India (1991). N.B.: Column title marked as 1.00, 2.00, 3.00, 4.00, 5.00, and 6.00 represent the area of a single land-use converted from a single village and their absolute values are −10 ha and less, 10–20, 20–40, 40–100, 100–200 and 200 ha and more, respectively. All the figures are approximate

The study also finds that among the different blocks in the periphery of Delhi metropolitan area, there was a large area under wastelands still unaffected that could have been converted in the post-reform period and at the aggregate level, loss of cropland could have been restricted. There are also some blocks where even extensive croplands' conversion could not feed the rapid urban-growth experiences in the post-reform period. Table 4 and Fig. 5 gave the extent of croplands that could have been saved had wastelands been converted to urban use. While the limitation that the distribution of wasteland may not fit into the land demands for built-up area extension is understood, the argument that the intrusion on farmland is inevitable due to lack of availability of any other kinds of land gets discounted.

Dynamics of Land-Use with Increasing Distance from Urban Centre of Delhi

To identify the effect of metropolitan expansion on the land-use pattern of the villages in the peripheral blocks of Delhi, owing to the higher investment made in the post-reform period, different buffer areas at increasing distances from the urban centre have been delineated and the phenomena of conversion of productive cropland and other important land-use classes have been considered. The areas so delineated have been shown in Fig. 6a. Following paragraphs focuses on the process of land-use change that had actually happened to those villages in the state of changing demand for land with increasing distance from the urban centre.

Table 4 Extent of converted croplands and remaining wastelands in the periphery of Delhi in the post-reform period (1989–2006) (Area in hectares)

CD blocks	Converted croplands	Remaining wastelands	Croplands (that could have been saved)
Bahadurgarh	6362	2188	4174
Farrukhnagar	871	2376	−1504 (No cropland conversion was needed)
Gurgaon	2843	786	2057
Jhajjar	1981	2819	−838 (No cropland conversion was needed)
Kharkhoda	2818	1021	1797
Rai	2719	418	2301

Source Table generated from the land-use classification operation using two satellite imageries (IRS P-6 LISS-3 Path-96 Row-51) of 10/10/2006 (Kharif) and Landsat TM Path-147, Row-40 of 09/10/1989 (Kharif), respectively and overlaying of these classified imageries along with maps of the six blocks of Haryana surrounding Delhi to obtain change detection between different classes. The administrative boundaries of the districts and CD blocks have been taken from the Town and Village Directory of the Census of India (1991)

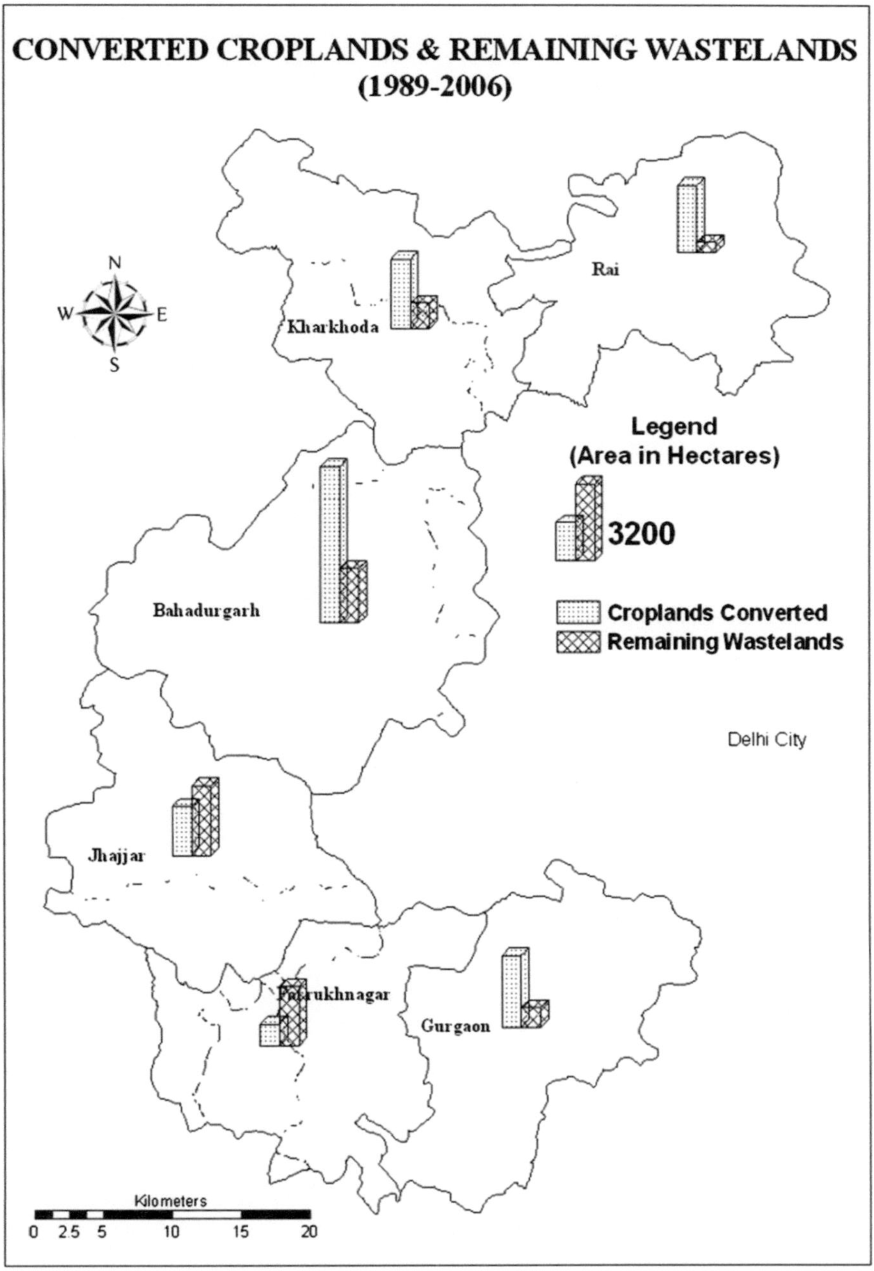

Fig. 5 Extent of remaining wastelands and converted croplands in the post-reform period in the periphery of Delhi

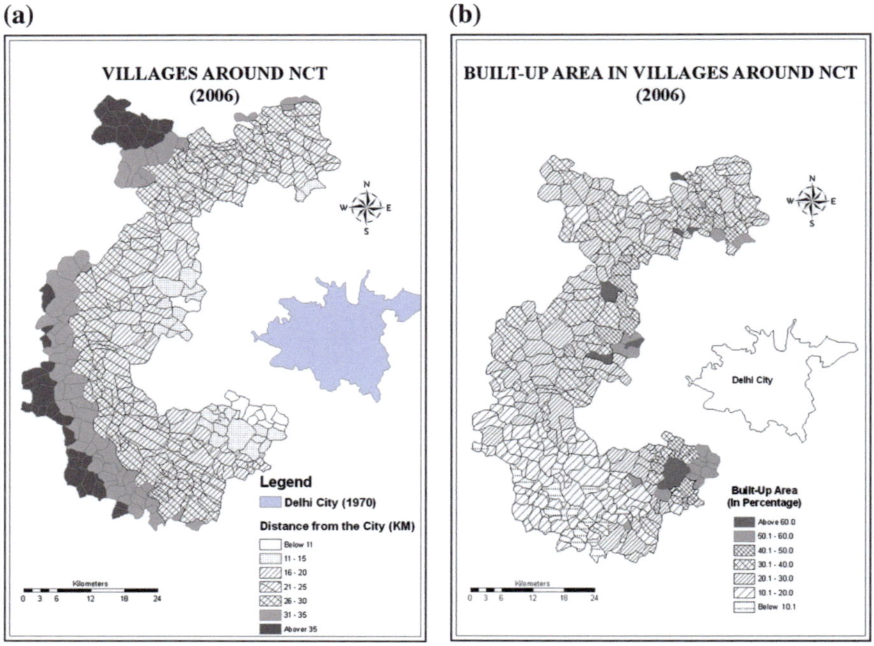

Fig. 6 **a** Villages at different distances (shown in *different colour*) from the urban centre of Delhi and **b** present status (2006) of built-up area in the villages

As the map of built-up area suggests that the concentration of area under this use increases as distance from urban centre declines (Fig. 6b). It can be observed that wherever the city centre approaches the villages' boundary, the occurrence of built-up area is significantly high; most of the villages having more than 60 % of built-up area within them are located within 20 km from the city centre and the villages with lower percentage of built-up area within them are reasonably far away from the city centre. There exists a significantly high degree of negative correlation between the built-up area and distance from the city centre. It implies that with increasing distance from the city centre of Delhi, the percentage of built-up area in the villages' decreases and vice versa. It supports the very basics of this study which assumes that increased level of investment in the post-reform period in and around large metropolitan centres will necessitate enhancement of infrastructure and other developmental activities what would be reflected in the expansion of built-up area in the periphery of large urban metropolitan centres. The foregoing analysis reveals that this process has been fairly prominent around the metropolitan city of Delhi.

Analyzing the present distribution of built-up area does not serve our purpose completely as long as we do not look into the process of transfer of land from different uses, especially from cropland, to built-up area during the period 1989–2006. Such transfer tells about the rationale of land-use change processes as a reflection of local land-use decisions and motives of different players involved.

As far as the conversion of single-cropped area is concerned, the percentage change of single-cropped area, between the two periods, into built-up area has been considered here in correlation with changing distance from the city centre (Table 5 and Fig. 7a).[8] A fair degree of significant negative correlation is found between these two land-use classes. High proportion of conversion of cropped area into built-up area occurring closer to the urban area has left meagre amount of available total stock of cultivable land in the nearby villages to the urban centre. Similar kind of phenomena has been found in a study around the urban centres of Mumbai, Kolkata and Delhi (Chadha et al. 2004).

To have a better understanding of the phenomena, percentage loss in single-cropped area to built-up area has been extracted and analyzed in relation with distance with the distance centre. Table 5 suggests that highest number of villages where higher percentage of single-cropped area has been converted into built-up area lie nearest to the urban centre and vice versa. It is found that higher number of villages where low to moderate level conversion to built-up area has happened lie between 25 and 35 km from the city centre. However, if we extend the analysis to the conversion of seasonal fallow land, a higher level of correlation is found between the percentage change in area under seasonal fallow and distance from the city centre. In this case also, villages experiencing higher percentage of conversion are found in the closest three belts of the city centre. Thus, one thing becomes very clear here, i.e. increasing built-up area has not worked in the rationale of saving precious croplands for the future. There exists significant negative correlation (−0.480) between these two variables (seasonal fallow/single cropped land and distance from the city centre). Figure 7a, b gives a clear understanding of the process.

The rationale of sustainable land-use practice can be viewed from one more perspective, i.e. how the wastelands were used in the process of conversion with increasing distance from the city centre. There exists again a significant negative correlation (−0.493) of higher degree between the level of conversion of wasteland and their distance from the city centre. With increasing distance from the city centre there is again a trend of lower proportion of conversion. Highest proportions of wastelands conversion in villages are concentrated within the distance of 20 km from the city centre (See Fig. 8). This partly shows that urban pressure has worked well in many peripheral villages to convert large plots of wastelands into built-up area and this satisfies our assumption.

When we look at the proportion of different classes that were converted to built-up area with increasing distance from the city centre in the post-reform period (1989–2006), we see that seasonal fallow lands contributed highly in the villages

[8]These farmland areas, as has been found in the kharif season imagery of 1989, could also possibly be considered as double-cropland area and also what has been seen as fallow lands in the 1989 imagery, can be considered as single cropped area here to ease the analysis. During our field survey to some of the villages in and around Delhi, it was found that, lands may remain fallow in the Kharif season if it is actually there; otherwise what has been cultivated in the Kharif season, in all the cases those were cultivated in the rabi season also. Thus, this assumption is backed by evidences from field study.

Table 5 Percentages of double and single-cropped area converted to BUA in villages with increasing distance from the city centre

			Percentage of double cropped area (DCA) and single-cropped area (SCA) consumed (%)					Total (%)
			1.00	2.00	3.00	4.00	5.00	
Distance from the city centre (in km)	10	Percentage of DCA	0.0	18.2	18.2	18.2	***45.5***	100.0
		Percentage of SCA	0.0	0.0	9.1	**27.3**	**63.6**	100.0
	15	Percentage of DCA	6.9	34.5	24.1	20.7	13.8	100.0
		Percentage of SCA	0.0	27.6	31.0	10.3	***31.0***	100.0
	20	Percentage of DCA	10.3	31.0	51.7	3.4	3.4	100.0
		Percentage of SCA	8.8	26.3	***40.4***	14.0	10.5	100.0
	25	Percentage of DCA	30.0	***45.0***	18.8	6.3	0.0	100.0
		Percentage of SCA	24.4	***32.6***	***30.2***	12.8	0.0	100.0
	30	Percentage of DCA	***29.3***	***50.7***	14.7	5.3	0.0	100.0
		Percentage of SCA	23.0	***44.6***	***29.7***	2.7	0.0	100.0
	35	Percentage of DCA	**42.4**	**42.4**	13.6	1.7	0.0	100.0
		Percentage of SCA	***35.6***	***32.2***	25.4	5.1	1.7	100.0
	40	Percentage of DCA	***39.3***	***57.1***	3.6	0.0	0.0	100.0
		Percentage of SCA	27.6	***55.2***	17.2	0.0	0.0	100.0
	45	Percentage of DCA	***28.6***	0.0	***71.4***	0.0	0.0	100.0
		Percentage of SCA	28.6	0.0	***71.4***	0.0	0.0	100.0
Total	Percentage of DCA		26.5	41.8	22.8	5.8	3.2	100.0
	Percentage of SCA		21.0	33.8	30.1	8.5	6.5	100.0

Source Same as Table 3. Besides, Maps of the villages have been taken from the Town and Village Directory of the Census of India (1991) and overlaying operation performed using GIS platform. N.B.: Column title marked as 1.00, 2.00, 3.00, 4.00 and 5.00 represent the percentage of double-/single-cropped area converted from a particular village from 1989. Figures 1, 2, 3, 4, and 5 stand for 10 % or less, 10–20, 20–30, 30–40 and 40 % or more respectively

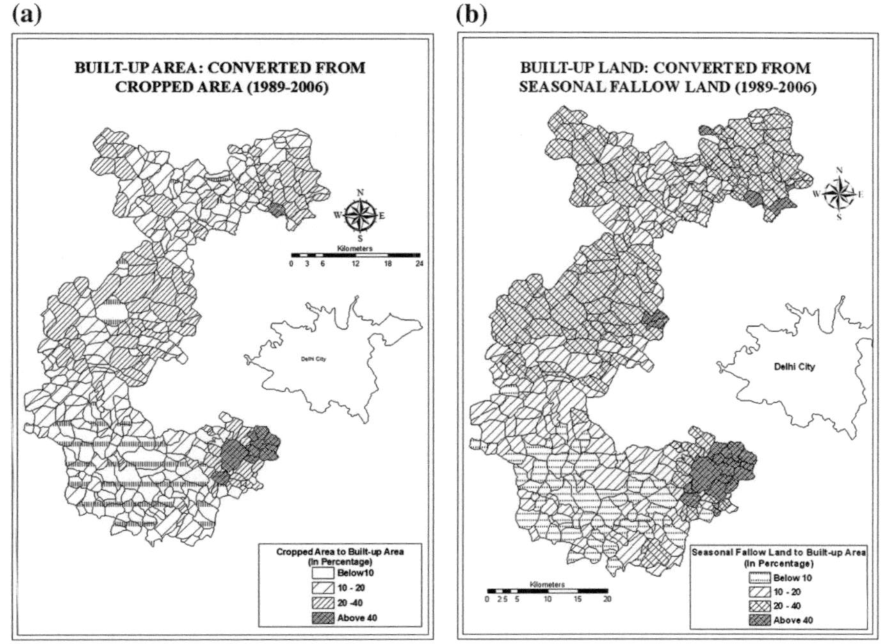

Fig. 7 **a** Percentage of cropped area converted into built-up area and **b** percentage of seasonal fallow converted into built-up area between 1989 and 2006

which were close to the urban centre or at a medium distance (20–35 km) from the urban centre. There is significant negative correlation between distance from the city centre and proportional conversion of fallow lands in the villages. However, proportion of single-cropped area converted to built-up area does not seem to be too high in the villages closer to the urban centre, and there exists a positive relationship with conversion of single-cropped area and distance from the city centre. In other words, number of villages that experienced conversion of higher proportion of double-cropped area increased with increasing distance from the urban centre. A similar kind of pattern has been seen between the conversion of wasteland and distance from the city centre. A significant positive correlation between these two phenomena exists. Figures 9a, b and 10 depicts all such phenomena clearly.

In Delhi, or for that matter in any other urban centre, land is acquired from the land-owners for any development-plan initiated by Government. In Delhi, Delhi Development Authority (DDA) is the public authority that is empowered to acquire land for different developmental purposes within the National Capital Territory (NCT). Record of DDA also shows that most of the acquisition of land took place in the north and north-westerly direction from the city centre.[9]

[9]Data collected on acquisition of land for DDA was collected from DDA Head Office, New Delhi in March, 2008.

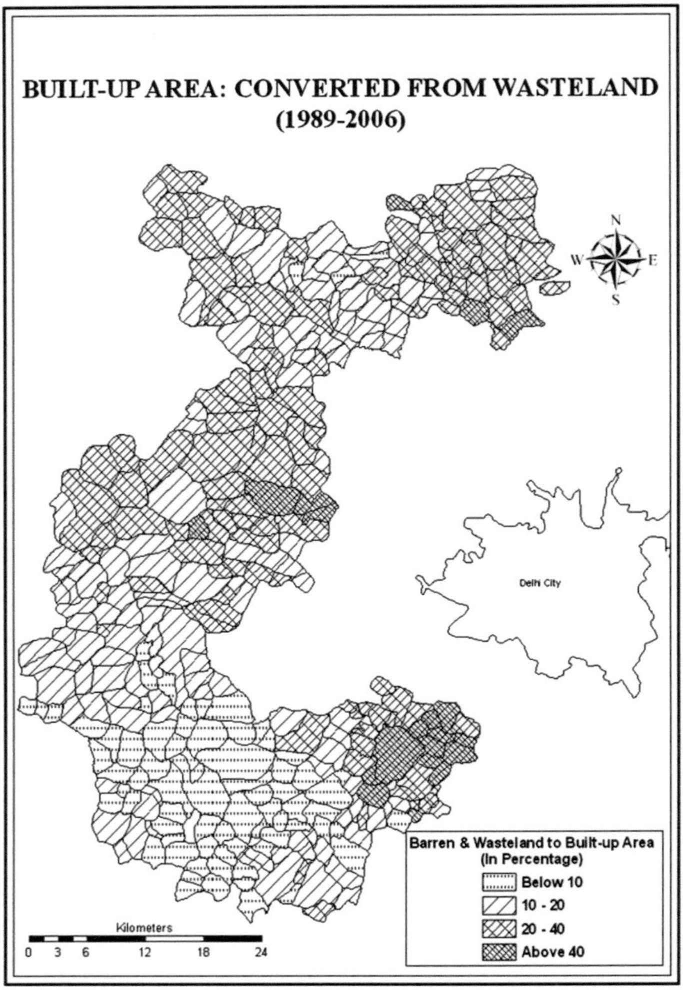

Fig. 8 Percentage of wasteland converted into Built-Up Area between 1989 and 2006

Two villages were selected in the periphery of Delhi for looking into the impact of expansion of built-up area around urban centre upon the livelihood of the farmers.[10] One of the study-villages *Rani Khera* is also located in the fast growing north-western region of Delhi. It was one among many other villages where over 10 % of village area was acquired in the post-reform period (post-1990). The second village that was selected for the study was *Manesar* village, located some 10 km away from Gurgaon city and located within Gurgaon CD Block. Over 95 % of total area of Manesar has been acquired for different projects (over 35 % in the

[10]The exploratory field-survey was conducted in the first-half of 2008.

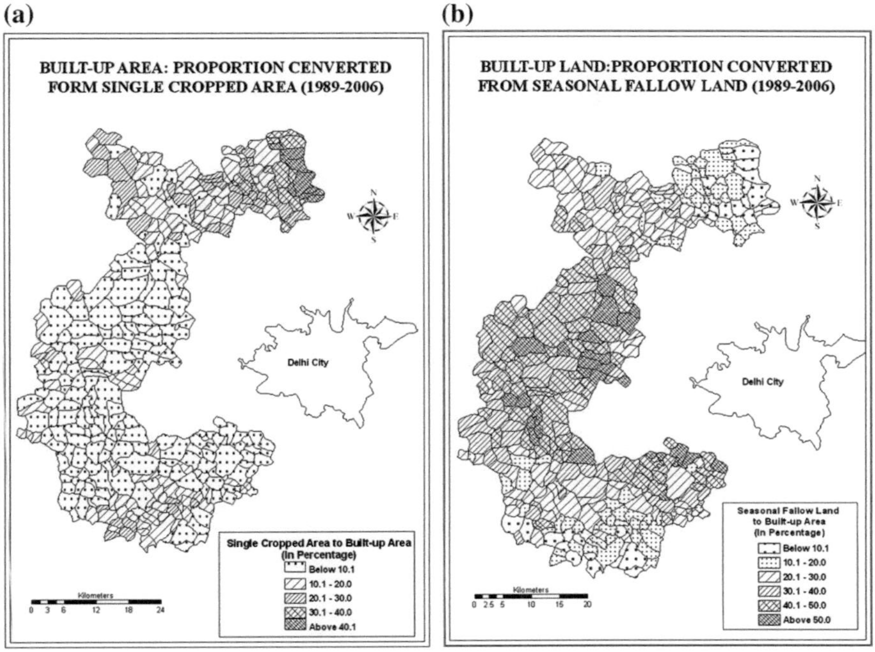

Fig. 9 **a** Proportion of single-cropped area and **b** proportion of fallow land contributed to built-up area

post-liberalization period), and acquired lands were mainly double-cropped land and barren lands.

Some observations can be brought out here as were found from the field study. First, there has been an increase in loss of cultivable land in the post-reform period, as is shown in the study based on secondary data, owing to the increased developmental activities. Second, the phenomenon of loss of cultivable land is largely found closer to the urban centre and as one move away from the centre, it becomes less persistent. Third, the growth of urban area over rural land has a clear spatial pattern; in Delhi, it has spread mainly towards the north-west and south. Fourth, although some wastelands have been converted, cultivated land was the category from which major outflows took place. With the acquisition of land, landless farmers have been affected more than the owner–farmers. In such a situation they are more desperate to find a job outside in contrast to the small owner–farmer who continued to lead a fair quality of living even after acquisition of portions of their farmlands. Lastly, there is dissatisfaction among the farmers over the whole process of acquisition and provided compensation. Lands are acquired and kept vacant for long and by the time it is put to use, the price of such land increases manifold in comparison to the actual amount paid to the farmers during acquisition. Hence, dissent amongst the affected farmers is evident. While they felt that though acquisition of land is almost inevitable, there is clearly some space for better policy so far as land acquisition and related compensation packages are concerned.

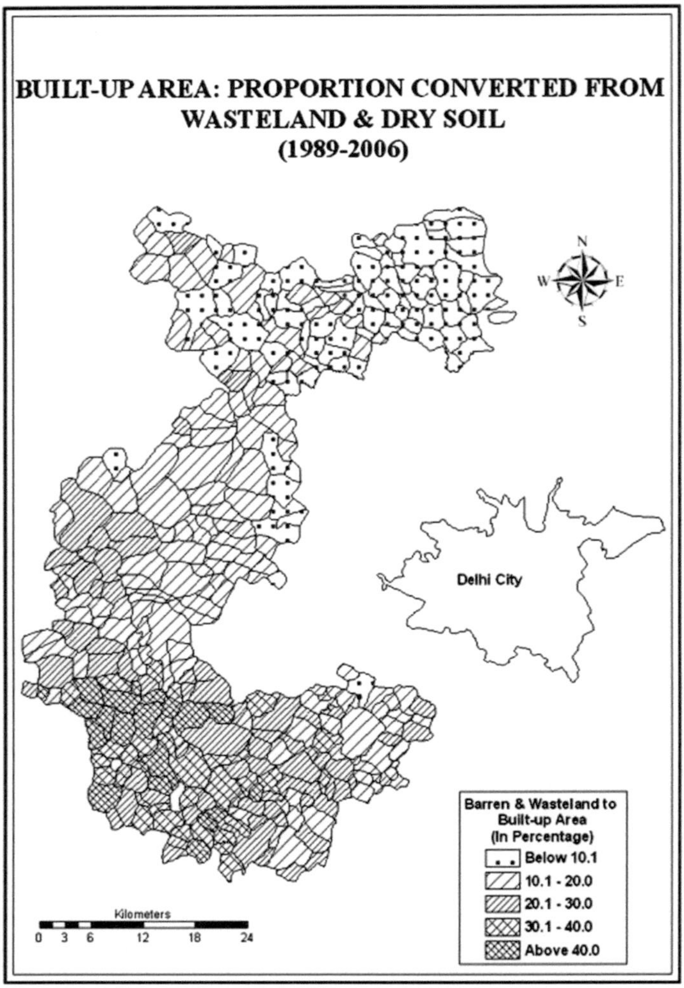

Fig. 10 Proportion of wastelands contributed to built-up area

Conclusion

In a nutshell, the complex dynamics of land utilization is quite evident around the large metropolitan cities of India. Though there are evidences that wastelands have also been used to a large extent, but the consumption of farmland is much higher and such a trend is also supported by the findings of the field work that was carried out around Delhi. The impact of conversion is more prominent on the fallow lands and single-cropped areas and closer to the urban centre of Delhi. There still remains scope for conversion of considerable amount of wastelands in the peripheral blocks of Delhi. In most of the cases government has carried out mass acquisition of farmlands for many developmental purposes. The present level of growth that the capital city is experiencing for the last two decades is posing a substantial threat to the farmlands surrounding it. This phenomenon is resulting in not only physical transfer of lands from one use to another, but also economic deprivation of the cultivators who were dependent on such land, in the long run.

References

Alig, R. J., & Healy, R. G. (1987). Urban and built-up land area changes in the united states: an empirical investigation of determinants. *Land Economics, 63*(3), 215–226.

Anderson, J. R. et al. (1976). A land use and land cover classification system for use with remote sensor data. *Geological Survey Professional Paper 964*, A Revision of the Land Use Classification System as presented in U.S. Geological Survey Circular 671, Washington, USA.

Blobaum, R. (1974). The Loss of Agricultural Land. *Citizen's advisory committee on environmental quality*, Washington D.C., Washington, USA.

Boserup, E. (1965). The conditions of agricultural growth: the economics of agrarian change and population pressure. London, UK: George Allen & Unwin Ltd.

Chadha et al. (2004) "Land Resources", 2nd Volume of the 27-volume Series 'State of the Indian Farmer: A Millennium Study'. Published in Association with Dept. of Agriculture, Government of India; Academic Foundation, New Delhi, India.

Coupin, P., & Bauer, M. (1996). Digital change detection in forest ecosystem with remote sensing imagery. *Remote Sensing Reviews, 13*, 207–234.

Fazal, S. (2000) Urban expansion and loss of agricultural land—a GIS based study of Saharanpur City, India. *Environment and Urbanization, 12*, 133–149. Retrieved from http://eau.sagepub.com

Gillies, J., & Mittlebach, F. (1958). Urban pressures on california land: a comment. *Land Economics, 34*(1), 80–83.

Goldar, B. (2007). Location of plants of foreign companies in India. Institute of Economic Growth: University of Delhi Enclave, Delhi, India.

Hart, J.F. (1976). Urban encroachment on rural areas. *Geographical Review, 66*(1), 1–17.

Harvey, R. O., & Clark, W. A. V. (1965). The nature and economics of urban sprawl. *Land Economics, 41*(1), 1–9.

Kydd, J. (2002). Agriculture and rural livelihoods: is globalization opening or blocking paths out of rural poverty? Network Paper No. 121, January 2002, Agricultural Extension and Research Network, London, UK.

Lal, T. (2001). Peri-urban land-use dynamics in the National Capital Territory of Delhi: A geographical analysis. Thesis submitted to JNU, New Delhi, India.

Lopez, E. et al. (2001). Predicting land-cover and land-use change in the urban fringe: A case in Mexico city, Mexico. *Landscape and Urban Planning, 55*(4), 271–285(15).

Pachauri, M. K. (1986). Suburbanization process in Delhi Metropolitan Region: A temporal and spatial Analysis. Thesis submitted to JNU, New Delhi, India.

Plaut, T. R. (1980). Urban expansion and the loss of farmland in the United States: Implications for the future. *American Journal of Agricultural Economics, 62*(3), 537–542.

Shaw, A. (2005). Peri-urban interface of Indian Cities: growth, governance and local initiatives. *Economic and Political Weekly*, 129–136.

Shaw, A. et. al. (2006). Metropolitan restructuring in post-liberalized India: Separating the global and the local; and their retrieval of data of CAPEX, CMIE (Centre for Monitoring the Indian Economy), February 2005.

Sridharan, N. (2006), Peri-Urban Dynamics: Case Studies in Chennai, Hyderabad and Mumbai. CHS Occasional paper, No.17, 2006, French Research Institutes in India, New Delhi, India.

Young, A. (1999). Is there really spare land? A critique of estimates of available cultivable land in developing countries. *Environment, Development and Sustainability, 1*, 3–18.

Zhao, S. X. B. et al. (2003). Globalization and the dominance of large cities in contemporary China. Retrieved 31 May, 2003, from http://linkinghub.elsevier.com/retrieve/ii/S0264275103000313

Urban Form and Regional Development of National Capital Region

Ankita Choudhary and Milap Punia

Abstract Urban form of a specific city is the result of a variety of influences, including site and topography, economic and demographic development and planning efforts in the past. Various scholars have explored the origins of differences in urban form through comparison with socio-economic developmental indicators and historical trajectories in urban development. Even in case of Delhi National Capital Region (NCR) some differences are expected in the urban form since the towns though belonging to the same region have gone through different histories in the past and the present pattern of growth is also different for different towns. In this paper, an attempt has been made to quantify spatial urban patterns from optical remote sensing datasets to describe forms, structures and changes in urban land use. Taking urban area as a spatial landscape unit, various landscape indices have been used to describe the urban form in the area. In order to test the effect of level of development on the urban form a correlation was run between different class metrics, socio-economic development and infrastructural development for different cities of NCR. The levels of development of the towns have been calculated using Principal Component Analysis Method. Towns of NCR have shown more or less similar pattern for the urban form, yet some differences are there mainly because of their different levels of economic development and location. Most of the towns have seen increase in built up along the national highway or state highway. Towns with the dominance of agricultural base have simpler form in comparison to the towns with industrial base and they grow in a uniform manner in all

A. Choudhary (✉) · M. Punia
Centre for the Study of Regional Development, School of Social Sciences, Jawaharlal Nehru University, New Delhi, India
e-mail: ankita.delhi@gmail.com

M. Punia
e-mail: milap.jnu@gmail.com

S.S. Acharya et al. (eds.), *Marginalization in Globalizing Delhi: Issues of Land, Livelihoods and Health*, DOI 10.1007/978-81-322-3583-5_3

the directions. The datasets used are based on the remote sensing images (Landsat TM, 1989, Landsat TM, 2000 and Landsat TM, 2011) of National Capital Region and statistical analysis of primary census abstract and town directory for the data pertaining to towns for their level of development.

Keywords Urban form · Regional development · Landscape metrix and indices · NCR

Introduction

Urbanization is the most drastic form of land use change affecting biodiversity and ecosystem functioning and services far beyond the limits of cities. To understand the process of urbanization itself as well as its ecological consequences, it is important to quantify the spatiotemporal patterns of urbanization (Wu et al. 2011). Urban form, like the density or compactness of a city, influences daily life and is an important factor for both quality of life and environmental impact. However, urban form itself is mainly referred to as a property of a city and therefore static for a given point in time, while urban growth is a dynamic process that alters urban structure. The land use characteristics in the NCR are influenced mainly by two factors: Line no 41. The first has been the continuous and rapid increase of the economic activities, particularly in the Delhi Urban Area (DUA) and the second is the consequential rise in population within the DUA mostly due to inflow of migrants who seek employment opportunities created by the economic activities. An analysis of urban form reveals the problems and challenges of urban development. From a policy point of view, it is necessary to identify areas with a high need of policy intervention and to determine the diversity of urban development (Schwarz 2010).

It has been felt that as Delhi will grow, its problem of land, housing, transportation and management of essential infrastructure like water supply and sewerage would become more acute. Thus, in 1985 with the enactment of the National Capital Region Planning Board Act by the Union Parliament, with the concurrence of the participating States of Haryana, Rajasthan and Uttar Pradesh, NCR Planning Board was constituted. It has been recognized that the planned growth of Delhi is possible only in a regional context. Because of this urban dynamics in and around Delhi, National Capital Region was proposed. Thus, there is a need to study the towns in NCR to see whether there is a holistic development in the region and how different they are from each other in terms of their urban forms.

Contextualizing relationship between form and development is quite complex. Discontinuous development in urban areas suggests sprawl; contiguous development suggests a more compact urban form, this sometimes also being referred to criterion for the smart cities. It may involve planning, keeping in urban form perspectives vis-a-vis energy efficiency, infrastructures, transport and climatic resilient urban areas. Weitz and Moore (1998), concluded that development inside urban boundaries tends to be contiguous to the urban core rather than dispersed, could be consistent with the envisioned policies for urban form, but the urban development patterns can be improved by applying additional urban growth management tools. These tools may involve, in Indian context, interventions like containing/regulating development of urban densities, preserving urban and peri-urban agriculture and protecting forest lands from encroachment. On the contrary the contemporary urban growth patterns suggest suburbanisation or developments in suburban localities and leapfrogging of activities beyond urban boundaries. For sustainable growth of the region one needs to look into the characteristics of the built up in the region. Here, the importance of urban form comes into picture. Thus, for NCR an attempt has been made to characterize urban form and find out its relation with the level of development.

In National Capital Region around 37.5 % population is urbanized and 62.5 % population is categorized as rural population. According to census 2011, there are three million plus cities in National Capital Region; Ghaziabad, Faridabad and Meerut, respectively. Out of these, Ghaziabad has highest population followed by Faridabad and Meerut. Apart from contiguous spread of NCT, one needs to explore the dynamics of other settlements in the region so that a holistic approach to plan the region could be applied. Further, there has been a growing interest in the role of small and medium towns in rural development.

Urban form of a specific city is the result of a variety of influences, including site and topography, economic and demographic development and planning efforts in the past. Various scholars have explored the origins of differences in urban form through comparison with socio-economic developmental indicators and historical trajectories in urban development. Even in case of National Capital Region (NCR) some differences are expected in the urban form since the towns though belonging to the same region have gone through different histories in the past, practice different economic activities and the present pattern of growth is also different for towns. In this paper, an attempt has been made to quantify spatial urban patterns from optical remote sensing datasets to describe structures and changes in urban land use. Taking urban area as a spatial landscape unit, various landscape indices have been used to describe the urban form in the area. In order to test the effect of level of development on the urban form, a correlation was run between different class metrics, socio-economic development and infrastructural development for different cities of NCR. The levels of development of the towns have been calculated using Principal Component Analysis Method.

The increasing agricultural land demand, changing consumption patterns, urbanization and economic development intensifies the human intervention on natural areas which ultimately result into changes in Land use/land cover (LULC) (Sharma et al. 2013). Population pressure coupled with immigration from different parts of the country in search of employment has put tremendous pressure on the natural resources—land, water and air—of Delhi and surrounding areas, known as the NCR (Kumar 2009). As from various studies it is explained that the hinterland of National Capital Region is shrinking due to land acquisition for built-up or industrial purpose. This land use land cover change due to urbanization of hinterland is causing social, cultural and economic changes. The datasets used for analysing some of the changes are based on the remote sensing images (Landsat TM 1989, Landsat TM 2000 and Landsat TM 2011) of National Capital Region and statistical analysis of primary census abstract and town directory for the data pertaining to towns for their level of development.

Study Area

The National Capital Region (NCR) is an interstate region comprising of the entire NCT of Delhi (Delhi sub-region), eight districts of Haryana (Haryana sub-region), one district of Rajasthan (Rajasthan sub-region) and five districts of Uttar Pradesh (Uttar Pradesh sub region). The Constituent Areas of the National Capital Region are as under:

(a) National Capital Territory of Delhi (1,483 km^2). This accounts for 4.41 % of the total area of NCR.
(b) Haryana Sub-region comprising of Faridabad, Gurgaon, Rohtak, Sonipat, Rewari, Jhajjar, Mewat and Panipat districts. This accounts for 30.33 % (13,413 km^2) of the area of the State and 39.95 % of the area of NCR.
(c) Rajasthan Sub-region comprises of Alwar district. The area is 2.29 % (7,829 km^2) of the total area of the State and 23.32 % of the area of NCR.
(d) Uttar Pradesh Sub-region comprising of five districts, namely Meerut, Ghaziabad, Gautam Buddha Nagar, Bulandshahr and Baghpat. This accounts for 4.50 % (10,853 km^2) of the area of the State and 32.32 % of the area of NCR. Thus, the total area of NCR is 33,578 km^2.

There has been a regular demand from various states regarding inclusion of more districts in NCR, namely Bharatpur, Jhunjhanu from Rajasthan, Jind, Mahendragarh, and Bhiwani from Haryana and Mujaffarnagar from Uttar Pradesh.

Methodology

Landscape metrics were developed by landscape ecologists to identify various landscape forms. Landscape metrics are indices that quantify specific spatial characteristics of patches, classes of patches, or entire landscape mosaics. It is the study of structure, function and change in a heterogeneous land area which contains interacting ecosystems, used spatial metric extensively in planning and managing forest landscape ecology (Forman and Godron 1986). Landscape ecology is concerned with the connections and interactions between forest stands across the landscape, and with the effects of both natural and human disturbances on the landscape. Because people have become one of the major biological forces on the planet, much of the activity in the field of landscape ecology focuses on interactions between people and the biosphere. Same fundamentals of spatial landscape indices could be applied to urban areas for analysing various patterns of urban forms in rapidly transforming National Capital Region. Thus, it quantifies spatial urban patterns from high-resolution optical remote sensing data to describe structures and changes in urban land use. Taking urban area as a spatial landscape various landscape indices have been used to describe the urban form in the area.

The study is based on selected 13 cities of NCR which have seen a very high level of growth both in terms of population as well as areal growth, namely Gurgaon, Ghaziabad, Faridabad, Bulandshahar, Noida, Meerut, Baghpat, Panipat, Sonipat, Rohtak, Jhajjar, Rewari and Alwar. As stated above, different towns have followed different trajectories in the course of their development and thus will have different types of urban forms. The landscape metrics have been calculated using FRAGSTAT software at two levels, namely

(1) **Class level** for each patch type (class) in the mosaic, and
(2) **Landscape level** for landscape mosaic as a whole.

Different indices have been taken for both the levels.

Lynch and Rodwin (1958), articulated about fundamentals of urban form and viewed the city as being made up of what they call 'adapted space' for the accommodation of human activities and 'flow systems' for handling flows of people and goods. Although they differentiate between activities and flows on the one hand and adapted space and flow systems on the other, so far they have devoted their main effort to the latter level of analysis which they equate with the study of urban form. In their conceptual framework they are concerned first with a system for analysing urban form along with interactions. They propose evaluating urban form by six analytical categories: element types, quantity, density, grain, focal organization and generalized spatial distribution.

Element types, is a category for differentiating qualitatively between basic types of spaces and flow systems; and, as might be expected, quantity, has to do with measure of the size of particular types of adapted spaces of flow systems. Density, expressed either as a single measure or as a range of measures, has to do with compaction (of people, facilities, vehicles) per unit of space or capacity of channel. Grain, is their term to indicate how various elements of urban form are differentiated and separated. Adapted spaces and flow systems may be fine-grained or coarse-grained according to the extent of compaction or separation in their internal components (houses, multi-storey, streets) and how sharp or blurred these form elements are at the edges where transition occurs from one element to another. Focal organization, is concerned with the spatial disposition and interrelations among key points in the city (density peaks, dominant building types, major breaks between forms of transportation). Generalized spatial distribution, is the patterned organization of space as it might be seen from the air at a high altitude. This six-part classification system is the basic analytical tool they propose for classifying urban form.

The Landsat datasets are used for three time periods. i.e. 1989, 2000 and 2011 to show the change in the urban form. The mosaic image of NCR has been classified by supervised classification method to arrive at two binary classes, namely **urban** and **non-urban**. Different towns have been extracted from the NCR imagery in the form of subset imagery-based area of interest (AOI). The images are converted into a format compatible with FRAGSTAT software. It computes landscape indices statistics for each patch and class (patch type) in the landscape and for the landscape as a whole. At the class and landscape level, some of the metrics quantify landscape composition, while others quantify landscape configuration. Class metrics measure the aggregate properties of the patches belonging to a single class or patch type. Landscape metrics measure the aggregate properties of the entire patch mosaic. Numbers of metrics have been calculated like *Radius of Gyration, Percentage of Landscape, Largest Patch Index, Total Edge, Total Area, Perimeter–Area Ratio, Fractal Dimension Index, Contiguity Index, Perimeter–Area Fractal Dimension, Number of Patches, Patch Density, Contagion Index, Aggregation Index, Patch Richness Density, Shannon's Diversity Index, Simpson's Diversity Index,* etc. Then a correlation was run for all these indices and the indices showing very high correlation were dropped from the analysis since they showed more or less similar thing. For example, number of patches and patch density shows similar things when the study area is constant and they show a very high correlation with each other. So, they have been removed from the analysis. On this basis only few metrics have been selected to describe the urban form of the towns. **Largest Patch Index**: *largest patch index* at the class level quantifies the percentage of total landscape area comprised by the largest patch. As such, it is a simple measure of dominance. **Fractal Dimension Index,** reflects the shape complexity across a range of spatial scales. **Contiguity Index**, assesses the spatial connectedness, or contiguity, of cells within a grid cell patch to provide an index on patch boundary configuration and thus patch shape. **Contagion Index** is inversely related to edge density, when edge density is very low, for example when a single class occupies a very large percentage of the landscape, contagion is high, and vice versa. **Radius of Gyration** is a measure of patch extent (i.e. how far-reaching it is). And **Shannon's diversity index** is a popular measure of diversity in community ecology, applied here to urban landscapes to understand heterogeneity or homogeneity of landscape units.

From the representation as shown in Fig. 1, one can see that national capital region has gone through major land use transformation in last two decades (1989–2011). The population of NCR was 19.8 million in 1981 and as per 2011 census, it was 46.04 million, so region witnessed two-and-a-half times increase from 1981 to 2011. In order to characterize the built environment, landscape metrics were calculated as shown in Table 1. These landscape metrics represents that how the landscape of NCR has changed over the time.

Largest Patch Index (LPI) has decreased over the decades reflects that the patch size of non-built up area has decreased or urban patch area has increased over the decades. The value for the *radius of gyration* which is a measure of patch extent has also declined showing that the patch extent of non-urban area has declined or in other sense the patch extent of urban area increased. The value of FRAC_AM has first decreased between 1989 and 2000 and then again increased in 2011. This

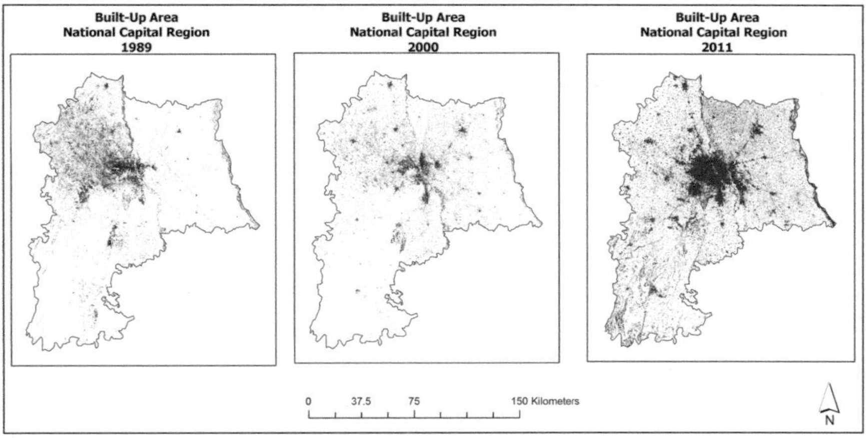

Fig. 1 Urban growth of national capital region 1989, 2000 and 2011 (Authors work)

Table 1 Landscape metrics of NCR 1989, 2000 and 2011 (Authors work)

NCR	1989	2000	2011
LPI	73.3323	49.2762	48.0327
GYRATE_AM	116089.95	92090.166	89101.65
FRAC_AM	1.2857	1.2346	1.2517
CONTIG_AM	0.9236	0.9439	0.9524
CONTAG	62.0131	60.1552	51.7202
SHDI	0.5907	0.7943	0.9194

LPI Largest patch index, *GYRATE_AM* Area weighted mean radius of gyration
FRAC_AM Area weighted mean fractal dimension index
CONTIG_AM Area weighted mean contiguity index
CONTAG Contagion index and *SHDI* Shannon's diversity index

shows that the shape became complex to simple and again back to complex form. The value of SHDI has also increased over time. SHDI increases as the number of different patch types (i.e. patch richness, PR) increases and/or the proportional distribution of area among patch types becomes more equitably distributed. The value of CONTIG_AM has first increased and then decreased. *Contiguity index* assesses the spatial connectedness, or contiguity of cells within a grid cell patch to provide an index on patch boundary configuration and thus patch shape. Thus it could be interpreted as an increase in spatial connectedness over the time. The value of CONTAG_AM has decreased over time, which shows that largely NCR region has disaggregated over the time.

The sub-regional analysis shows that there a is sharp variation in the level of urbanization in NCR. In 2011 there was an incredible growth of urban population in NCR. In 2011 in NCT Delhi the urbanization was 97.50 % while at national level it was just 31.16 %. There has been net addition of 2.9 million people in population of Delhi from 2001 to 2011. In 2011 the Ghaziabad district of Uttar Pradesh sub-region of NCR recorded 67.46 % urban population to total population which was highest in Uttar Pradesh sub-region. The level of urbanization in Meerut and Gautam Buddha Nagar was 51.13 % and 59.56 %, respectively, in 2011. In GTB Nagar the urban population was 37.39 % in 2001 which increased to 59.56 % in 2011, showing a significant increase in urbanization due to recent development of Okhla Industrial Area.

Meerut

Meerut became a metro city with 11.62 lakh population as per 2001 Census and has reached 34.47 lakh in 2011. It is located at a distance of about 60 km, on north east of National Capital, Delhi and is connected via NH 58. Meerut's advantageous geographical location and setting, nearness to the National Capital and rich agricultural and industrial activity in the surrounding region, the city presently acts as a major distribution centre for the diverse agriculture produce and industrial goods. Development of Meerut city can be seen mainly along Meerut-Delhi road, Meerut-Hapur road and Meerut-Mujhaffarnagar road. After Delhi Development Act of 1957, Government of UP also enacted the Uttar Pradesh Regulation of Build Operations Act in 1958 and later on, UP Urban Planning and Development Act in 1973. Thus Development plan was prepared and notified with the target year of 1991 which was further revised in 1997. The master plan provided for a balanced and integrated development of the city. Uttar Pradesh Awas Vikas Parishad (UPAVP), Uttar Pradesh State Industrial Development Corporation (UPSIDC) and Meerut Development Authority (MDA) started to develop new residential colonies and industrial projects in the suburbs of the city. Development started by these agencies was further accelerated through financial assistance by National Capital Region (NCR) Planning Board. Newly developed areas attracted the population from the main city as also from the other areas with the result that this city gradually grew to be a metropolitan city in the year 2001.

The spatial growth of Meerut has shown a finger shaped growth mainly along the major radial roads, according to some scholars, and can be seen from the representation in Fig. 2. The growth was restricted to the core city area till 70s but later it started spreading in all directions. The growth towards western side was mainly because of the Meerut bypass connectivity towards north and western side towards Trans Yamuna region, growth towards north was limited because of the presence of cantonment area.

An analysis of the landscape metrics shows that LPI has decreased over the decades showing that the patch size of non-built up area has decreased or one can say that the urban patch area has increased over the decades. The value for the *radius of gyration* which is a measure of patch extent has also declined showing that the patch extent of non-urban area has declined or in other sense the patch extent of urban area increased. The value of FRAC_AM has first decreased

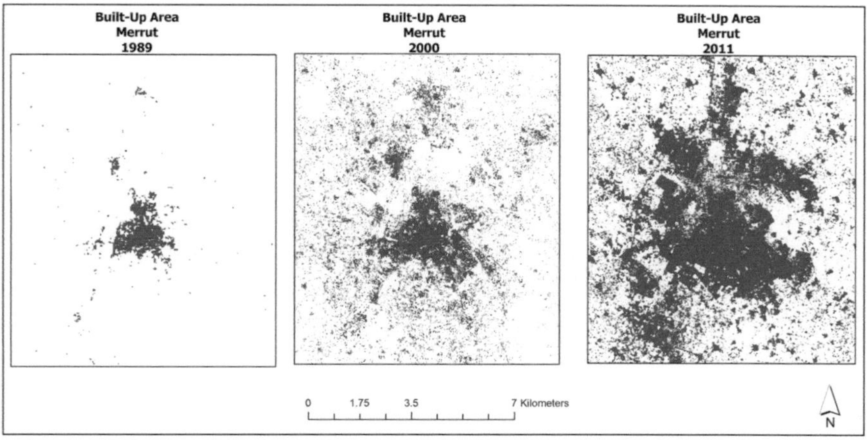

Fig. 2 Urban growth in Meerut 1989, 2000 and 2011 (Authors work)

between 1989 and 2000 and then again increased in 2011. This shows that the shape became complex to simple and again back to complex form. The value of SHDI has also increased over time. SHDI increases as the number of different patch types (i.e. patch richness, PR) increases and/or the proportional distribution of area among patch types becomes more equitable. This shows that the number built up patches have increased over time. The value of CONTIG_AM has first increased and then decreased. *Contiguity index* assesses the spatial connectedness, or contiguity, of cells within a grid cell patch to provide an index on patch boundary configuration and thus patch shape. Thus one can say that spatial connectedness has increased over the time. The value of CONTAG has decreased over time showing that the region has disaggregated over the time. From the maps, it is quite visible that all the built-up patches have increased in size and the number has also increased phenomenally over the time.

An analysis of class-level metrics has shown an increase in complexity with increasing value of *Fractal Dimension Index* and *Shannon's Diversity Index* over the period of time. Decreasing value of *Contagion Index* shows that a single class of built up has occupied a very large percentage of the landscape. Thus these indices show that both the extent and complexity has increased in the city of Meerut in terms of built-up area.

One of the reasons that could be attributed for such a land form is that the land acquisition in Meerut was not proper and was in excess to utlization/needs, along with further absence of regulations in terms of real estate and planning interventions at city level. Thus, city area experienced a transformation of residential use to commercial use and density resulted to rapid growth. Further increased rate of urbanization resulted in overstraining on urban infrastructure which is evident in the cluster analysis given later, where Meerut falls into a medium level of development level category.

Ghaziabad

According to the census 2011 the population of Ghaziabad district is 3.34 million and of Ghaziabad city 0.87 million. A net increase of around 10 lakh people can be seen in Ghaziabad district from 2001 to 2011. In the Ghaziabad district the decadal population growth rate is quite high (53.02 %). In the recent census data a declining trend of population growth is observed in Ghaziabad. Although, the population growth is declining but it is still very high. A number of industrial activities are activated in Ghaziabad city so this increase in population growth may be attributed mainly to the in-migration rather than natural increase (Fig. 3). Ghaziabad city is governed by Municipal Corporation which comes under Ghaziabad Urban Agglomeration. It was even featured in Newsweek international listed in the top 10 most dynamic cities of the world during the year 2006 (United Nations, 2011). Ghaziabad is part of the satellite area of Delhi. Ghaziabad is the most urbanized district of Uttar Pradesh sub-region in National Capital Region. According to census 2011, 82.34 % population of this district is urbanized. Rest only 17.66 % is rural population. While in 2001 only 68.54 % population was urbanized and rest 31.45 % was rural.

Ghaziabad has also seen an increase in the *largest patch index* which is higher in the decade 2000–2011 in comparison to 1989–2000. The complexity increased between 1989 and 2000 but again reduced during the decade 2000–2011. Other indices like *Radius of Gyration, Contiguity index*, Contagion have seen a decline showing a similar pattern for the town. Diversity has increased in the town landscape over the decades.

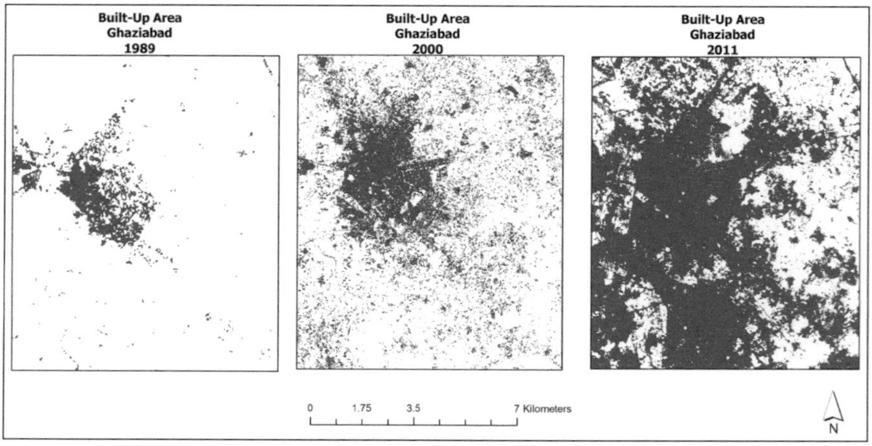

Fig. 3 Urban growth in Ghaziabad, 1989, 2000 and 2011 (Authors work)

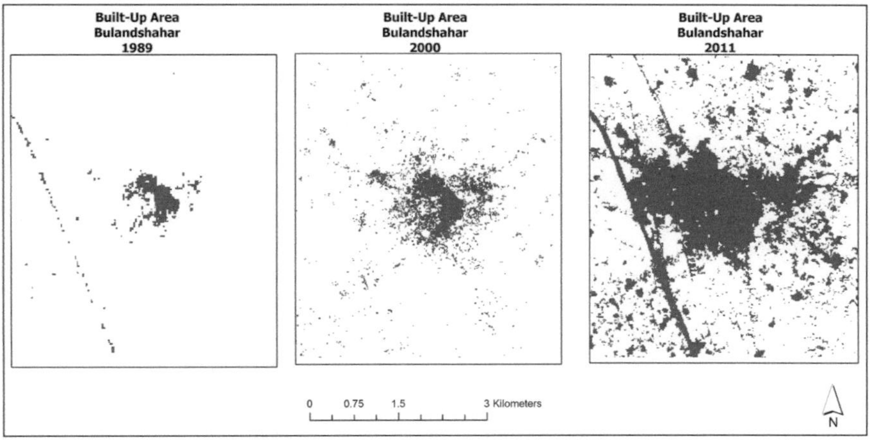

Fig. 4 Urban growth in Bulandshar, 1989, 2000 and 2011 (Authors work)

Bulandshahar

Being in the vicinity of the National Capital Region has resulted in rapid development of Bulandshahr and in the general improvement of the standard of its city life. As per provisional data of 2011 census, Bulandshahr urban agglomeration had a population of 0.23 million. The urban population was 19.34 % (1981) which increased to 24.8 % (2011), showing a very slow rate of urbanization. The built up has increased sharply in the decade 2000–2011 mainly along NH 91 which is clearly visible in the map. The *fractal dimension index* is close to 1 showing a simple geometrical shape for the town and it has increased over time showing that it has gained complexity. Bulandshahr is among one of the towns considered as priority town in NCR draft plan 2021 and will continue to grow like this in future (Fig. 4).

Baghpat

The city was previously as small town and had a small commercial centre known as the Mandi. From the Figure given below it is visible that a number of built-up patches have developed in the vicinity of the town. According to census 19.71 % urbanization was measured in 2001 which increased to 21.05 % in 2011. Baghpat is the least urbanized district of Uttar Pradesh sub-region in National Capital Region. For Baghpat most of the indicators show a similar pattern to that of Meerut as one can see from Table 2. But the decrease is much higher in case of Baghpat in comparison to Meerut showing a sharp change in the urban form. It has gone through much larger disaggregation. Here the value for *Shannon's Diversity index* has also seen a higher value and thus reflects a much larger diversification mainly due to the development of built up in the surrounding of the town rather within the town itself. Patch contiguity, or connectedness, has also increased and the increase is much higher in the decade 2000–2011 in comparison to 1989–2000. The *Area Weighted Mean Fractal Dimension Index* is close to 1 and thus indicates that Baghpat has a simple geometrical shape very similar to a rectangle.

Noida

The New Okhla Industrial Development Area, which is analogous to the Planning Area/Notified Area of Noida city falls within the district of Gautam Buddha Nagar. It covers 81 revenue villages and a total of about 20,316 ha of land. It is located in close proximity to the metropolitan city of Delhi and lies along the eastern and south eastern boundaries of the National Capital Territory of Delhi. It is bounded by the river Yamuna and the city of Delhi in the West and the South–West, National Highway 24 and the city of Ghaziabad in the North, river Hindon and Greater Noida Area in the East, and the confluence of rivers Yamuna and Hindon in the South. In last census decade the urban population of GTB Nagar almost doubled. The industrial and commercial activities in the GTB Nagar district have caused significant increase in urban population.

The value of SHDI for Noida increased over time. SHDI increases as the number of different patch types (i.e. patch richness, PR) increases and/or the proportional distribution of area among patch types becomes more equitable. This shows that the number built up patches have increased over time. The value of CONTIG_AM has first increased and then decreased. *Contiguity index* assesses the spatial connectedness, or contiguity, of cells within a grid cell patch to provide an index on patch boundary configuration and thus patch shape. Thus one can say that spatial connectedness has increased over the time. The value of CONTAG has decreased over time showing that the region has disaggregated over the time (Fig. 5).

Alwar

Alwar nestles in the foot hills of the Aravalli Ranges which traverse the town south-west. The town is easily accessible from Haryana as well as from Uttar Pradesh, the two adjoining States to Rajasthan. Because of its strategic location, Alwar was selected as a regional priority town in the National Capital Regional Plan of the Government of India. In Alwar for all the 3 years the value of FRAC_AM is close to 1 which shows that it has a simple geometry and the value has seen an increase over the time period showing departure from a simple shape towards convoluted shape, though the increase is negligible. The table 2 shows that Alwar was in maximally aggregated category in 1989 as most of the area was non-urban but later on disaggregation started happening because of increase in the urban patch. Disaggregation was

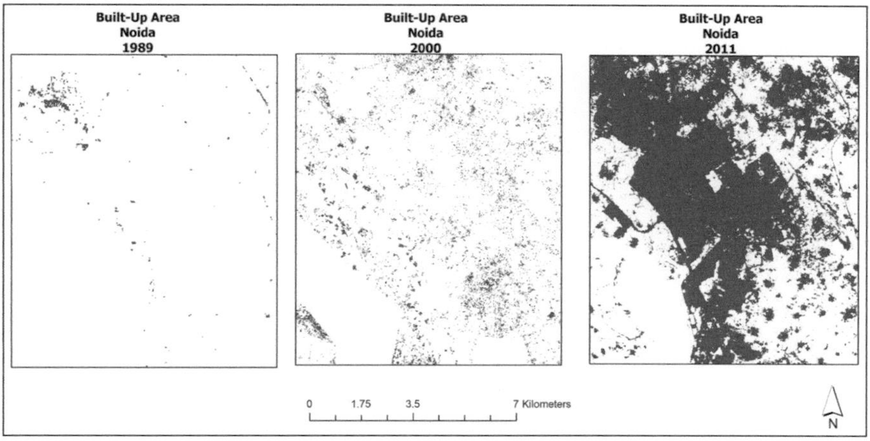

Fig. 5 Urban growth in Noida, 1989, 2000 and 2011 (Authors work)

at its maximum for the year 2011 showing higher rate of urbanization in the decade. The value for the SHDI has increased over the period reflecting that Alwar has seen an increase in diversity mainly due to urbanization and decrease in the non-urban area. One can say that Shannon's Diversity increased with urbanization largely due to the increasing uneven areal distribution of the land use types. The variation of the landscape metrics in Alwar have shown an increasing ratio of built-up zones within the total landscape area as well as increasing spatial disaggregation of the landscape. In the whole NCR in 2011 the lowest level of urbanization was recorded as 17.82 % which was in Alwar District of Rajasthan sub-region.

In 2011 around 39.4 % population of Haryana sub-region is urban population. In 2011 all district of Haryana sub-region has showed significant increase in the level of urbanization. In Faridabad district the level of urbanization has increased from 55.65 % (2001) to 79.44 % (2011), indicating a sharp 25 % increase in the urban population from 2001 to 2011. Gurgaon district has shown enormous increase in share of urban population to total population from 19.91 % in 1981 to 68.82 % in 2011. The urban population of Gurgaon district has increased around 46 % in the last census decade. In 2008 two new districts Palwal and Mewat have been carved out of Faridabad and Gurgaon districts respectively. In 2011 Palwal and Mewat districts registered, respectively, 25.39 and 11.38 % urbanization. Thus Mewat was the least urbanized district in NCR in 2011 (Fig. 6).

Rewari

Rewari is a city and a municipal council in Rewari district in the state of Haryana. It is located in south-west Haryana around 82 km from Delhi and 51 km from Gurgaon. Rewari is connected by three national highways: NH-8 (Delhi–Jaipur-Mumbai),

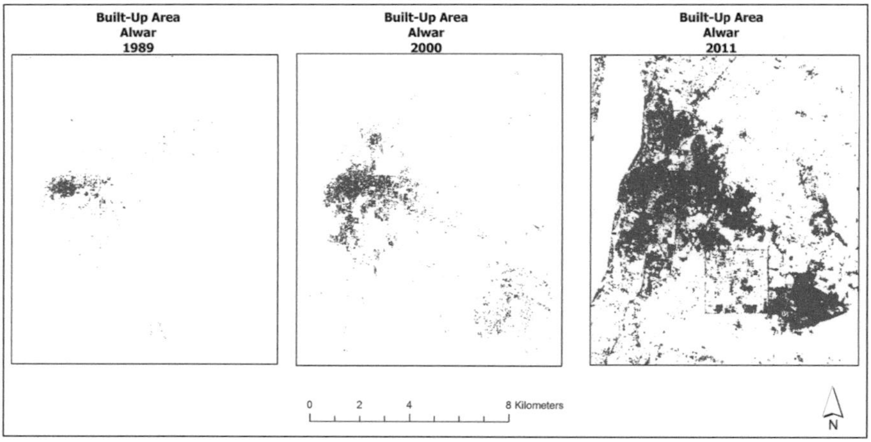

Fig. 6 Urban growth in Alwar 1989, 2000 and 2011 (Authors work)

NH-71 (Jalandhar-Rohtak-Jhajjar-Rewari) and NH-71B (Rewari-Dharuhera-Sohna-Palwal). Instead of these locational benefits this district has not urbanized as fast as Gurgaon and Faridabad districts of Haryana sub-region of NCR. In 2001 only 17.79 % population was urban which increased to 25.82 % in 2011, adding 95,237 more people to the urban population. In Rewari prominently three industrial areas have developed, which are Dharuhera industrial area, Rewari industrial area and Bawal industrial area.

In these industrial areas the products range is wide, such as, Motor Cycles, televisions, non-woven carpets floor tiles, beer, cotton and synthetic Yarn, metal cans, jelley filled, telephone cables, copper and brass sheets and circles, zippers, disposable syringes and heavy earth movers and a host of other consumer and industrial products. There are 56 large & medium scale and 2250 small scale and rural industries in the district (Fig. 7).

Jhajjar

Jhajjar is connected to Gurgaon, Rewari, Rohtak, Bahadurgarh, Delhi and other towns by roads. National Highway NH-71 from Jalandhar to Rewari passes through Jhajjar. Kundli-Manesar-Palwal Expressway (KMP Expressway), whose construction may be completed by 2017, will make access to the town easier. At present Jhajjar is developing at a great pace with the development of SEZs and power plant. In 2011 around 25.39 % population is urban. The *LPI index* shows that the patch size of non-built up area has decreased over the time period. The value of FRAC_AM shows that the urbanization is spreading in a complex manner. The decreasing CONTAG_AM value indicates the disaggregation in the region. The *Fractal Dimension Index* and *Shannon's Diversity Index* show that extent and complexity is increasing slowly in the region (Fig. 8).

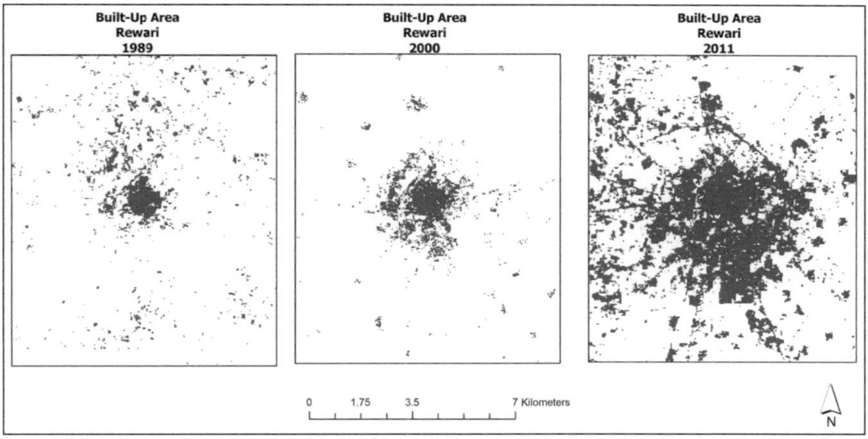

Fig. 7 Urban growth in Rewari 1989, 2000 and 2011 (Authors work)

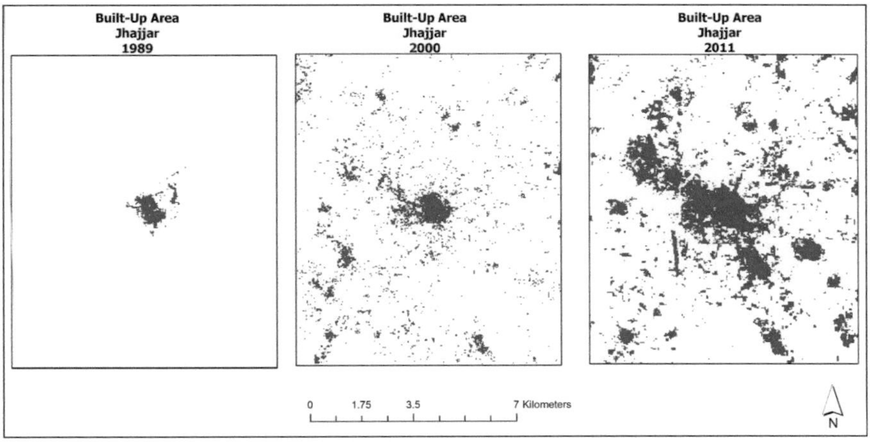

Fig. 8 Urban growth in Jhajjar 1989, 2000 and 2011 (Authors work)

Rohtak

Rohtak is one of the oldest cities in India. Rohtak is one of the eight priority towns (Regional Centres) of National Capital Region (NCR) Regional Plan 2001. It lies 70 km north–west from Delhi, the National Capital of India on National Highway No. 10, it spreads over 100.57 km^2.

A study has shown that urban sprawl is along the state and national highways. In fact there has been substantial road development, construction of over bridges on the entry and exit points of the city, widening of the roads within the city by removing encroachments. The outward expansion of the ring road system is found

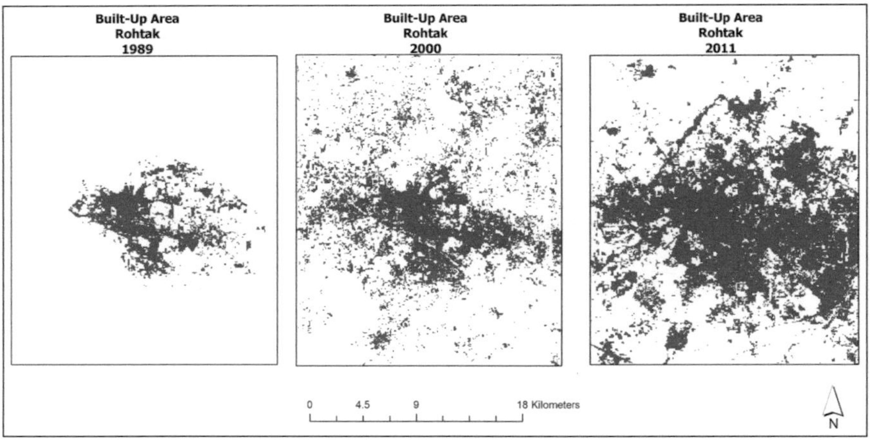

Fig. 9 Urban growth in Rohtak 1989, 2000 and 2011 (Authors work)

to be one of the most important driving forces explaining the temporal and spatial pattern of land use change (Singh and Kumar 2012). In 1981, 19.83 % population was urbanized which increased to 35.06 and 42.02 % respectively in 2001 and 2011. The data analysis shows changes in extent and complexity of the region from 1989 to 2000 but from 2000 to 2011, no change was observed (Fig. 9).

Gurgaon

Gurgaon has also seen a very steep increase in the built up area in the decade 2000–2011. The complexity of the shape has increased over the decades. The increase in the diversity of the region has been sharp in the decade 2000–2011 in comparison to 1989–2000. In case of Gurgaon district, the expansion of the city has altered patterns of rural natural resource use, created social, cultural and economic changes, and bred resentment among many peri-urban residents against urban authorities (Narain 2009).

From the table, one can see that LPI has decreased over the decades showing that the patch size of non-built up area has decreased or one can say that the urban patch area has increased over the decades. The value for the *radius of gyration* which is a measure of patch extent has also declined showing that the patch extent of non-urban area has declined or in other sense the patch extent of urban area increased. The value of FRAC_AM has firstly decreased between 1989 and 2000 and then again increased in 2011. This shows that the shape became complex to simple and again back to complex form. The value of SHDI has also increased over time. SHDI increases as the number of different patch types (i.e. patch richness, PR) increases and/or the proportional distribution of area among patch types becomes more equitable. This shows that the number built up patches

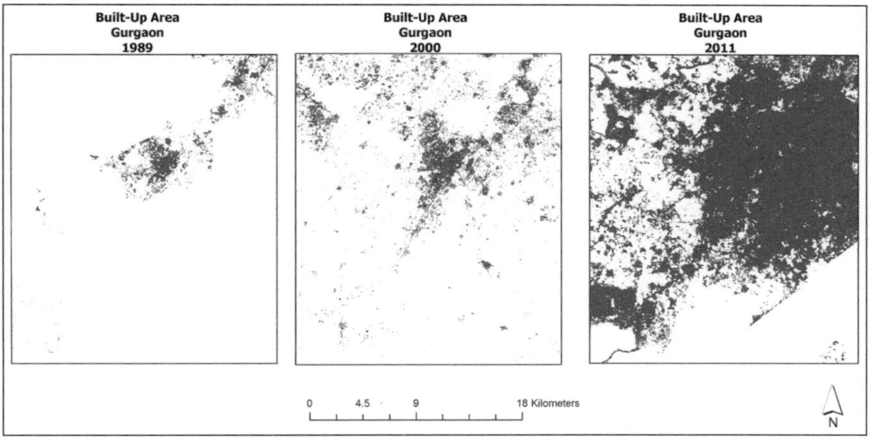

Fig. 10 Urban growth in Gurgaon 1989, 2000 and 2011 (Authors work)

have increased over time. The value of CONTIG_AM has first increased and then decreased. *Contiguity index* assesses the spatial connectedness, or contiguity, of cells within a grid cell patch to provide an index on patch boundary configuration and thus patch shape. Thus one can say that spatial connectedness has increased over the time. The value of CONTAG has decreased over time showing that the region has disaggregated over the time. From the map, it is quite visible that all the built up patches have increased in size and the number has also increased phenomenally over the time (Fig. 10).

Faridabad

Faridabad is an important constituent of NCR and is identified as a Central National Capital Region (CNCR) city. Also Faridabad is a notified Metropolitan area of Delhi and is part of NCR for which NCRPB is the primary planning agency. Faridabad city is the most populated and most industrialized in whole of Haryana. The district headquarter is situated in Faridabad city. Faridabad alone is generating about 60 % of the revenues of Haryana with its large number of industrial units. A 20-year Development Plan (For the Horizon 2011) was prepared by the Town & Country Planning Department of Haryana for the entire of Faridabad Controlled Area (FCA). The growth trends indicate spill into outer/peripheral areas (FCDP 2012).

Faridabad also shows a similar pattern to that of other towns in the region. An interesting feature is that the complexity increased between 1989 and 2000 but decreased between 2000 and 2011. Other indices like *Radius of Gyration, Contiguity index*, Contagion have seen a decline showing a similar pattern for the

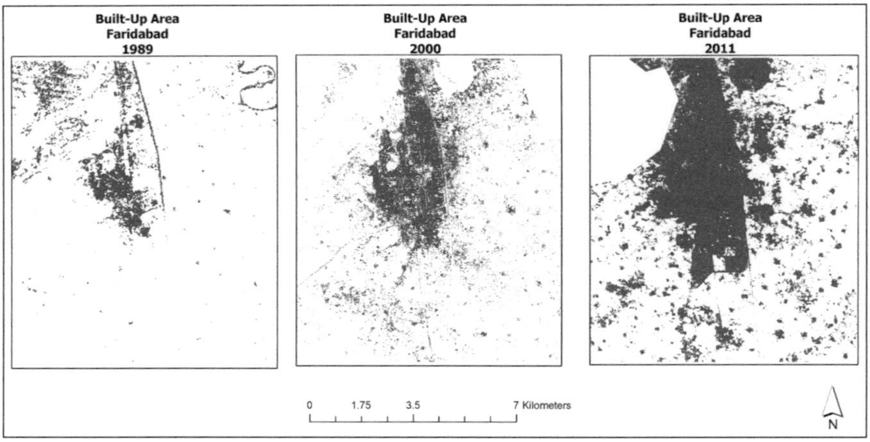

Fig. 11 Urban growth in Faridabad 1989, 2000 and 2011 (Authors work)

town. *Largest patch index* has also shown a decline but to lesser extent in comparison to other towns. SHDI value has increased showing increase in diversity for the region (Fig. 11).

Panipat

Panipat has population of 1.20 million as per 2011 census and is located on NH-1 leading to Amritsar. It is an ancient and historic city which is known for traditional handloom industry. In 1981, 31.34 % population was urbanized which increased to 40.53 and 45.97 %, respectively, in 2001 and 2011. In the analysis the value of Largest Patch Index (LPI) shows sharp decrease from 2000 to 2011. It indicates that the patch size of non-built up area is decreasing fastly. The value of FRAC_AM first increased from 1989 to 2000 then it decreased again from 2000 to 2011. So it may be said that the shape became complex to simple and again back to complex form. The decreasing CONTAG_AM value indicates that the non-built up is being changed into other land uses. The increase in the SHDI value shows that the number of built-up patches has increased. From Fig. 12 it is clearly visible that the built-up area has spread over the time.

Sonipat

From the table, one can see that LPI has decreased over the decades showing that the patch size of non-built up area has decreased or one can say that the urban patch area has increased over the decades. The value for the *radius of gyration*

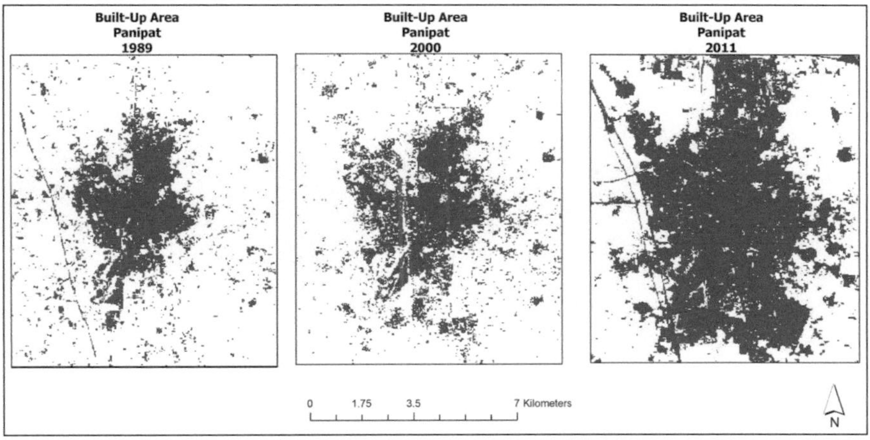

Fig. 12 Urban growth in Panipat 1989, 2000 and 2011 (Authors work)

which is a measure of patch extent has also declined showing that the patch extent of non-urban area has declined or in other sense the patch extent of urban area increased. The value of FRAC_AM has increased over the three decades which shows that there has been an increase in the complexity of the shape. The value of SHDI has also increased over time. SHDI increases as the number of different patch types (i.e. patch richness, PR) increases and/or the proportional distribution of area among patch types becomes more equitable. This shows that the number built-up patches have increased over time. The value of CONTIG_AM has decreased. *Contiguity index* assesses the spatial connectedness, or contiguity, of cells within a grid cell patch to provide an index on patch boundary configuration and thus patch shape. Thus one can say that spatial connectedness has decreased over the time. The value of CONTAG has decreased over time showing that the region has aggregated over the time. From the table 2, it is quite visible that all the built up patches have increased in size and the number has also increased phenomenally over the time. It has increased radially in all direction.

All the towns except Rohtak (no change in 2011) have seen an increase in diversity mainly because initially non-urban class dominated the landscape and now due to the increase in the built up the percentage of non-built up which is generally vegetation and agricultural land has decreased in absolute terms giving the landscape more diversity. And since the value has increased over the decades it shows that the landscape is getting dominated by the built up. For the decade 2011 maximum SHDI was shown by Ghaziabad, Panipat, Gurgaon, Noida, etc., while lowest was shown by Jhajjar, Rewari, Alwar. *Contagion index* has seen a decrease in the value for all the towns because the patch which was non-built up was now dominated by built-up leading to more disaggregation in the landscape, similar pattern is observed for all the towns (Table 2).

Table 2 Landscape metrics for major towns in National Capital Region 1989, 2000, and 2011 (Authors work)

City/town	Year	LPI	GYRATE_AM	FRAC_AM	CONTIG_AM	CONTAG	SHDI
Bulandshahar	1989	97.60	4038.6	1.09	0.98	92.20	0.13
Bulandshahar	2000	93.80	4003.2	1.21	0.96	82.95	0.24
Bulandshahar	2011	55.02	3031.1	1.28	0.90	58.92	**0.61**
Baghpat	1989	98.02	4503.3	1.11	0.98	93.15	0.10
Baghpat	2000	97.49	4486.3	1.13	0.98	91.71	0.12
Baghpat	2011	70.59	3477.4	1.33	0.82	52.28	**0.62**
Meerut	1989	97.34	8110.1	1.10	0.99	93.00	0.12
Meerut	2000	86.73	7543.8	1.33	0.90	70.39	0.39
Meerut	2011	62.15	7024.3	1.35	0.88	54.39	**0.66**
Noida	1989	99.04	12177.1	1.11	0.99	96.29	0.06
Noida	2000	95.00	11684.5	1.31	0.94	83.64	0.20
Noida	2011	32.30	8152.1	1.30	0.93	58.12	**0.68**
Ghaziabad	1989	94.96	7727.4	1.16	0.98	88.27	0.20
Ghaziabad	2000	80.56	6881.2	1.35	0.87	62.62	0.48
Ghaziabad	2011	53.94	5123.7	1.32	0.90	54.56	**0.69**
Alwar	1989	98.53	5747.4	1.08	0.99	94.35	0.09
Alwar	2000	95.98	5658.8	1.18	0.97	87.44	0.18
Alwar	2011	73.66	5079.6	1.28	0.92	62.20	0.58
Rohtak	1989	94.07	4487.7	1.16	0.97	85.24	0.23
Rohtak	2000	82.59	4197.7	1.30	0.89	65.67	0.46
Rohtak	2011	82.59	4197.7	1.30	0.89	65.67	**0.46**
Jhajjhar	1989	98.80	4518.0	1.04	0.99	95.52	0.07
Jhajjhar	2000	93.88	4316.5	1.24	0.94	81.37	0.25
Jhajhhar	2011	82.86	3988.3	1.27	0.92	67.52	**0.47**
Sonipat	1989	87.42	4415.3	1.21	0.95	76.17	0.37
Sonipat	2000	86.15	4279.2	1.28	0.91	70.80	0.40
Sonipat	2011	65.21	4024.4	1.29	0.90	56.93	**0.66**
Faridabad	1989	93.42	9394.4	1.22	0.97	85.16	0.24
Faridabad	2000	85.86	9308.2	1.31	0.93	72.66	0.39
Faridabad	2011	70.70	8812.5	1.28	0.95	64.41	**0.60**
Panipat	1989	85.77	4366.3	1.25	0.94	72.41	0.42
Panipat	2000	83.34	4340.8	1.27	0.92	69.42	0.45
Panipat	2011	31.41	2816.4	1.25	0.92	57.77	**0.68**
Gurgaon	1989	97.58	10644.6	1.17	0.98	92.19	0.12
Gurgaon	2000	93.90	10342.7	1.28	0.96	83.30	0.23
Gurgaon	2011	34.44	6479.2	1.29	0.93	58.04	**0.68**

LPI Largest patch index, *GYRATE_AM* Area weighted mean radius of gyration
FRAC_AM Area weighted mean fractal dimension index, *CONTIG_AM* Area weighted mean contiguity index
CONTAG Contagion index, *SHDI* Shannon's diversity index

Urban Form and Levels of Development

In order to test the effect of level of development on the urban form a correlation was run between different class metrics, socio-economic development and infrastructural development. The levels of development of the towns have been calculated using Principal Component Analysis Method. Different indicators used for the calculation of socio-economic development are: Adult sex ratio, sex ratio (0–6) age group, literacy rate, male literacy rate, female literacy rate and work participation rate. For the calculation of infrastructural development of towns following indicators were used: Electrification (Number of Connections) for domestic use per thousand populations, number of hospitals per thousand population, number of primary schools per thousand populations, number of cinema halls per thousand populations and number of banks per thousand populations. Though the correlation between socio-economic development and landscape metrics was not significant, it was significant in case of infrastructural development. *Percentage landscape index* was significantly correlated (0.837) with the infrastructural development. Other indices which showed significant correlation with infrastructural development are *largest patch index* and *fractal dimension index* and *radius of gyration.* With the increase in the level of infrastructural development, the complexity of the built-up also increases as shown by the *fractal dimension index.* These show that with increasing level of infrastructural development, urban landform becomes more complex and percentage of built up increases. NCR as a case study has shown that a planned development is the need of the hour so the land should be utilized judiciously and haphazard development must be checked. The analysis at more disaggregated level will be more helpful to represent the form and regional development of the city.

This signifies that with the level of infrastructural development the built up increases in size as depicted by *Percentage Landscape index* and *Largest Patch index.* The *fractal dimension index* shows that with increased level of infrastructural development the complexity of the built up also increases. The level of socio-economic development is positively correlated with these indices but the correlation is not significant. With density also none of the correlations are significant (Tables 3 and 4).

Cluster Analysis

All towns were clubbed into different groups based on their landscape metrics. Cluster analysis in SPSS 12.0, a widely used statistics package, has been used to extract characteristic patterns in urban form for assessment of their incidence by region. The cluster analysis employed a combination of hierarchical and k-means cluster methods to maximize the power of the results. First, hierarchical cluster analysis was used to obtain the rough number of classifications; then k-means

Table 3 Landscape metrics for various cities of National Capital Region (Authors work)

Towns	PLAND	LPI	GYRATE_AM	FRAC_AM	CONTIG_AM
Jhajjar	15.959	4.1314	496.2637	1.1822	0.7572
Baghpat	28.491	6.4237	472.3105	1.1882	0.6847
Rohtak	15.5561	8.4511	969.2115	1.2473	0.6723
Rewari	23.7496	13.15	1159.7676	1.2394	0.8041
Alwar	22.9433	14.417	1860.4165	1.268	0.8447
Bulandshahar	26.1704	17.3769	1490.9057	1.231	0.8195
Faridabad	27.6385	20.5667	3934.5108	1.2443	0.9069
Meerut	34.5071	24.7482	3588.3844	1.2947	0.8238
Sonipat	32.5551	25.5293	2289.1702	1.2732	0.8625
Panipat	35.9032	31.4109	2500.0453	1.2713	0.9009
Noida	39.7643	32.2998	7687.7925	1.3114	0.9124
Gurgaon	38.4554	34.4437	6859.4668	1.333	0.9096
Ghaziabad	57.9247	53.9394	6440.8942	1.3399	0.9111

Table 4 Different clusters of towns based on Class Metrics, 2000 (Authors work)

Towns	Cluster
Faridabad	1
Meerut	1
Panipat	1
Sonipat	1
Baghpat	2
Alwar	2
Bulandshahar	2
Jhajjar	2
Rewari	2
Rohtak	2
Ghaziabad	3
Gurgaon	3
Noida	3

cluster analysis, which utilized the number of groups extracted from the hierarchical analysis, was executed to make the classification. The k-means method had the advantage that it enabled the group centres to be adjusted iteratively.

From the cluster analysis three classes of towns have come up:

Cluster 1 It comprises of the cities Faridabad, Meerut, Panipat and Sonipat. These towns generally show a moderate level of growth. These have seen a high level of growth in recent years and could be clubbed with the Cluster 3 towns. But when one compares them with Cluster 3 towns then these towns have moderate values for all the indices. These towns have a mixture of both agricultural and industrial base.

Cluster 2 It comprises of the towns like Baghpat, Bulandshahr, Jhajjar, Rewari and Rohtak. These towns have experienced low values for all the indices. They have grown slowly in comparison to other towns mainly because of the dominance of agricultural economy and these towns are not very integrated with NCTs globalized economy. But of late these towns have seen a boost in terms of their growth and economy. Most of these towns are small in size and some of them like Baghpat come under Class III town. Thus size of the town is also related to the urban form of the landscape.

Cluster 3 It comprises of the cities of Ghaziabad, Gurgaon, and Noida. From the table below one can see that all these towns have seen overall higher values for all the indices. The complexity and disaggregation has seen a higher value in comparison to other towns. The main reason is their rapid rate of urbanization in the recent decade is growth of these satellite towns in National Capital Region.

Conclusion

It is found that towns vary in their urban form in national capital region, though differences arise mainly because of different settings or surroundings, level of infrastructure development and main mode of production. The cities with good connectivity and as part of NCT's contiguous spread have higher degree of complexity in the shape. These towns experienced greater expansion because of urban growth and benefits out of urban agglomeration economics. Similarly, towns with the dominance of agricultural base have simpler form in comparison to the towns with industrial base and they grow in a uniform manner representing simpler forms. Thus, spatial indices successfully helped to understand the relationship between urban form and development, though availability of information regarding infrastructure development at city level could have brought better insight. From an ecologists point of view the industrial and infrastructural changes in these cities raise our concern about the protection and enrichment of the natural habitat and environment of the city itself and surroundings also. An important future research work could be evaluation of different spatial metrics (spatial urban indices) to develop robust measurements for quantifying urban structures to study levels of development. Spatial measurements allow a very robust characterization of urban form and are useful for representing urban processes and functionality and contributing to urban models.

References

Forman, R. T. T., & Godron, M. (1986). *Landscape ecology* (p. 620). New York: Wiley.

Kumar, P. (2009). Assessment of economic drivers of land use change in urban ecosystems of Delhi, India. *Journal of the Human Environment, 38*(1), 35–39.

Lynch, K., & Rodwin, L. (1958). A theory of urban form. *Journal of the American Institute of Planners, 4*(4), 201–214.

Narain, V. (2009). Growing city, shrinking hinterland: Land acquisition, transition and conflict in peri-urban Gurgaon, India. *International Institute for Environment and Development (IIED), 21*(2), 501–512.

Sharma, M. P., Archana, Prawasi, R., & Hooda, R.S. (2013). Land use/land cover change detection in National Capital Region (NCR) Delhi: A case study of Gurgaon District. *International Journal of Remote Sensing & Geoscience, 2*(5), 42–45.

Schwarz, N. (2010). Urban form revisited: Selecting indicators for characterizing European cities. *Landscape and Urban Planning, 96*(1), 29–47.

Singh, N., & Kumar, J. (2012). Urban growth and its impact on cityscape: A geospatial analysis of Rohtak City, India. *Journal of Geographic Information, 4*(1), 12–19.

Weitz, J., & Moore, T. (1998). Development inside urban growth boundaries: Oregon's Empirical evidence of contiguous urban form. *Journal of the American Planning Association, 64*(4), 424–440.

Wu, J. G., Jenerette, J. D., Buyantuyev, A., & Redman, C. L. (2011). Quantifying spatiotemporal patterns of urbanization: The case of the two fastest growing metropolitan regions in the United States. *Ecological Complexity, 8*, 1–8.

Marginalization and Socio-ecological Transformation in New Urban Peripheries: A Case Study of Gurgaon

Milap Punia

Abstract Marginalization is a dynamic and multilayered concept with a large granularity in terms of intensity and its meaning. Societies can be marginalized at the global level whereas classes and communities can be marginalized from the dominant power structures of society and ethnic groups, families or individuals can be marginalized within our social milieu. Inequality, hierarchy and deprivation on the parochial basis are interwoven with the normative fabric of Indian society throughout the history. Metropolitan cities reflect expansion of existing urban and peri-urban areas with a significant socio-ecological transformation in terms of employment, education, and work force participation and land use changes. From the point of view of New Economic Geography Theory 2009, the growth dynamic of metros is influenced by their proximity and dependence to a metropolis and the probable spillover effect. To relate it further with agriculture land loss that was compensated for urban development, the entry point of discussion is the change in production of space in the post-globalization era. It order to understand how land got reappropriated by dispossessing farmers for urban development in Gurgaon, remote sensing datasets are used. Datasets of LISS-IV, IRS-P6 of 5.8 m spatial resolution for 2008 and 2013 is used along with Gurgaon Municipal Corporation's (GMC) ward boundary to represent sociopolitical meaning of this expansion and ways of life within the suburb. However, in recent times the economic forces of globalization have transformed the existing structures in all socio-economic spheres, this paper tries to examine marginalization with this backdrop. Marginalization here we are referring to a complex process rather than a static single parameter. Income could be one single parameter of marginalization, but

M. Punia (✉)
Centre for the Study of Regional Development,
School of Social Sciences, Jawaharlal Nehru University, New Delhi, India
e-mail: milap.jnu@gmail.com

S.S. Acharya et al. (eds.), *Marginalization in Globalizing Delhi: Issues of Land, Livelihoods and Health*, DOI 10.1007/978-81-322-3583-5_4

here we are looking into the multiple dimensions of marginalization, i.e. assets, education, work force participation, employment and land. Socio Economic Caste Census data (SECC) of 2011 used to articulate mentioned multiple dimensions of marginalization across spatial units varying from urban core to rural hinterland in north transact, across municipal ward number 34 in central Gurgaon; Harhi Harsaru, a new census town on periphery and Village Dhankot.

Keywords Socio-Ecological transformation · New urban peripheries · Marginalization

Introduction

Human interaction and its role in a society is understood as a dynamic and principle process of promoting belief, nurturing faith, fostering relations and strengthening institutions that enable people to participate in social, economic, cultural and political life. It is in this process where societies engage and endeavour to achieve a stable, safe and just environment. Though modern democratic societies strive to achieve diversity, pluralism, multiculturalism, equality of opportunity, tolerance, non-discrimination, non-violence, solidarity, and participation of all sections of the society including disadvantaged and vulnerable groups and individuals but an equalitarian just society remains utopian idea. The modern democratic societies are hierarchically organized, every society is fractured and stratified though it is a matter of degree, how much differently stratified one society is from the other. Societies exhibits their paradoxical character privileged, rich and '*haves*' at one end and disadvantaged, poor and '*have not's* at the other end makes the real fabric of society. Therefore, marginalization, social exclusion and relative deprivation are unwanted, but a real manifestation of a societal system. There are groups, individuals, places, spaces and cultures which are on margins, even in modern democratic societies. Now it is important to study societies living in these rapidly urbanizing regions to further understand marginalization and shrinking socio-economic spaces. The present work has adopted an inductive route of explanation. It generalizes the peri-urban space from selected spatial units of analysis. Its vantage point is the change in production of space in the post-globalization era. To assess the marginalization of places, groups, communities and individual beings Yadav and Punia (2014) studied socio-economic and ecological transformations of the peri-urban region of Gurgaon in south-west transact towards Mewat district, Haryana and found that there is hardly any trickle-down effect in the post-globalization era.

The increasing urban growth is an outcome of multiple urbanization processes and has some distinct characteristics. The affecting processes are mainly location factor and globalization while the main two characteristics can be recognized as increasing built-up expansion beyond existing city boundaries and the emergence of new centres of activity in the periphery of metro cities. The pattern and pace of land development in which the rate of land consumed for urban purposes exceeds the rate of population growth, and which results in an inefficient and consumptive use of land and its associated resources. As a consequence, urban and peri-urban areas are expanding with unplanned and uncontrolled urban growth leading to change in land use pattern along the highways, loss of open green spaces and surface water bodies, which is termed as urban sprawl (Sudhira et al. 2003; Cheng and Masser 2003; Rahman et al. 2011; Jiang et al. 2007; Punia and Singh 2012). However, all these studies have come up with different methodologies in quantifying urban spread but the common approach is to consider the behaviour of built-up areas and population density over the spatial and temporal changes taking place.

While, understanding informality and urban growth in suburbs, scholars like Roy (2009) argued that the dominant theorizations of global city regions are rooted in the western experience and are thus unable to analyze multiple forms of metropolitan modernities. The author, further articulated worlding of south Asian cities and production of space through informality. There is a tendency to imagine the ‘informal’ as a sphere of unregulated, even illegal activity, outside the scope of the state, a domain of survival by the poor and marginalized, often wiped out by gentrification and redevelopment. Informality lies within the scope of the state rather than outside it. It is often the power of the state that determines what is informal and what is not (Portes et al. 1989). And in many instances the state itself operates in informalized ways, thereby gaining a territorialized flexibility that it does not fully have with merely formal mechanisms of accumulation and legitimation. These too are, to borrow a term from Brenner (2004), ‘state spaces’. For example, the rapid peri-urbanization that is unfolding at the edges of the world’s largest cities is an informalized process, often in violation of or in absence of master plans and state norms but often informally sanctioned by the state (Roy 2003). This means that informality is not an unregulated domain, but rather is structured through various forms of extralegal, social, and discursive regulation. This exactly seems to be happening in peripheries of Delhi, especially in Gurgaon and thus this paper would make an attempt to understand social, economic and land transformations, where lot of informality is involved and possible interventions through city master plans. Socio Economic Caste Census data (SECC) of 2011 is used to articulate mentioned multiple dimensions of marginalization across spatial units varying from urban core to rural hinterland in north transact, across municipal ward number 34 in central Gurgaon, Harhi Harsaru, a new census town on periphery and Village Dhankot.

Study Area and Methodology

Spatial units of analysis are selected along transact in north direction of Gurgaon towards Jhajhar. It includes municipal ward number 34 part of city core of Gurgaon, Garhi Harsaru, a new town on periphery and village Dhankot in continuity. The study makes an attempt to understand marginalization and the spatiality of the selected indicators of socio-economic condition and their correlation.

Socio Economic Caste Census (SECC 2011) is data used to analyze occupation, education and informality and remote sensing datasets to decipher the land consumed for urban development. The Indian government has conducted a Socio Economic Caste Census (SECC 2011) survey of national population along with decennial population enumeration in 2011. The rural and urban socio-economic followed common enumeration approach and taken up entire nation concurrently, with the questionnaire in rural and urban being different. To understand marginalization and socio-economic processes across continuum in terms of employment, education, ownership, energy and household other characteristics, SECC data (2011) is used. Urban land use and land cover changes are linked to socio-economic activities (Lambin et al. 2003; Avelar et al. 2009). Therefore, it is essential to combine remote sensing data-derived parameters with socio-economic parameters to analyze the spatial–temporal changes of urban growth. Urban growth and land use change are related to globalization and have profound impact on global environmental change (Lambin and Meyfroidt 2011). To analyze leapfrogging of urban growth beyond municipal boundaries and to further understand the localities, where land transformations happened in last one decade, LISS-IV remote sensing datasets of 2008 and 2013 are used. The SECC data harmonized across continuum, 600 households selected from Gurgaon municipal ward number 34, around 624 households from town Garhi Harsaru and 229 households from village Dhankot. Gurgaon municipal corporation ward number 34 covers around 180 enumeration blocks. It includes Chakkerpur, Sikanderpur Ghosi villages, DLF Phase 1, DLF Phase 2, Global Business Park, DLF Phase 4, Mall road, Sector 27 and Sector 28. Chakkerpur village now represents a conflicting 'urban enclave' situated in the centre of Gurgaon, where former peasantry and migrant workers live next to each other.

Urbanization and Urban Growth in Haryana

The release of urbanization figures from the 2011 Census has evoked several reactions. For the first time, the absolute growth in urban population (91 million) in India is more than its rural counterpart (90.5 million). The urban growth rate, which fell in the last two decades, also rose in this census. But the major surprise came with the number of census towns (CTs) rising from 1,362 to 3,894. Bhagat (2011) estimates that 44 % of the urban growth between 2001 and 2011 is natural growth, and the remaining 56 % is due to net reclassification, expansion of boundaries and migration.

The state of Haryana has also been witnessing the high rate of urbanization owing to migration and rural push factors. The state has about 29 % urban populations in 2001 which is now increased to about 35 % in 2011 (Census of India 2011). During 1991–2001, the decennial urban growth rate was about 51 % while during 2001–2011 it decreased to 44 %. The most urbanized district is Faridabad having about 80 % population living in the urban area to the total population of the district. Gurgaon has taken the second place with 69 % urban population followed by

Panchkula (55 %), Panipat (46 %), Ambala (44 %) and Rohtak (42 %). During 2001–2011, the increase in urban population shows a different trend. Gurgaon district registered the highest percentage of increase in urban population (182 %), followed by Rewari district (70 %) during 2001–2011. According to 2011 census, around 52 new census towns (CTs) have been reported during the previous decade, i.e. 2001–2011 in Haryana. In most of the cases, the villages at the periphery of the towns have been converted and reclassified into towns. Three new CTs namely Badshapur, Bhondsi and Garhi Harsaru around Gurgaon have emerged in its periphery.

Land Use Change and Growth of Peri-urban Delhi (Gurgaon Suburb)

Pattern of urban development is one among many ways of describing the spatial structure and relationship of fixed activities in an urban region. Owens (1986) noted that different aspects of spatial structures become important as we move across various scales. At metropolitan scale, different aspects of spatial structure are form, density, grain and connectivity. The third element grain indicates the diversity of functional land use such as residential, commercial, industrial and institutional. To examine land use changes in Gurgaon Millennium city, remote sensing datasets of LISS-IV, onboard IRS-P6 of 5.8 m spatial resolution is examined for 2008 and 2013. The extracted built area, a proxy for urban settlements is representing land use class as an outcome for demand from commercial, industrial, housing and infrastructure footprints. For extracting information at administrative unit, Gurgaon Municipal Corporation's (GMC) boundary is considered along with 5 km of buffer to the GMC boundary (refer Fig. 1). The reported land use change for built-up area showed an increase of 89.7 km^2 from 2008 to 2013, while agricultural land decreased by 81.1 km^2. Majority of land transformed from agriculture to built-up was brought through various land acquisitions from farmers of neighbouring villages (38 villages are already part of current built-up area and about 63 are in transitory process). These transformations of land for urban uses and in rural fringes, beyond municipal boundaries are driven by the spillover of demands for land from metropolitan areas. It could be connectivity and proximity to major metropolitan region for deriving the decisions to locate new enterprises or a real estate project. Thus, transformation in the peripheries could suffice criteria for increase in business activities or for becoming a census town. If we visualize stated changes from systemic regional approach then it can explain the feedback mechanism of surrounding villages for socio-economic reasons (for marketing their products, education, health, banking, etc.). These feedback controls could be further explained like for instance, when new enterprises in a city multiply and diverse rapidly, the information feeds back in the form of crowding, inconvenience and increasing competition for the city space; it triggers off the appropriate correction: some enterprises move out of the city into the countryside, although still within reach of city services and markets they require.

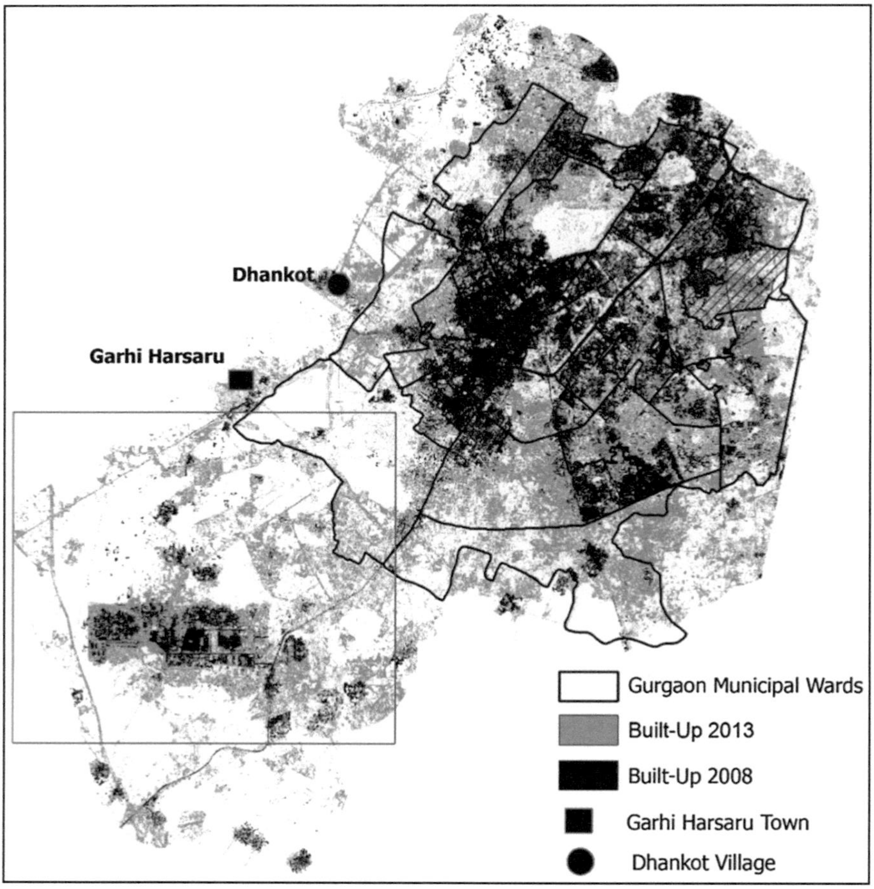

Fig. 1 Gurgaon land use change 2008–2013 (authors work). *Source* Analysis based on LISS-IV, IRSP6 remote sensing datasets of 2008 and 2013

Gurgaon is now expanding, beyond its municipal boundaries incorporating the industrial township of Manesar, 20 km along the NH-8 highway. Even now, the influence of Gurgaon penetrated up to distant towns, like Dharuheda, Bhiwadi (around 50 km) in south-west, to Sultanpur in north and Sohna in south. So, it is eminently possible that certain segments of Gurgaon's urbanization processes are autonomous and of independent of Delhi, but defiantly part of larger metropolitan system. Denis et al. (2012) on defining subaltern in terms of dependent or autonomous growth, explains that in a state where urbanization might occur at the periphery of metropolises, but it may not be dependent on them. Now, Gurgaon simply cannot be explained by its location or other given resources. Its existence as city and the sources of growth lie within itself, in the processes and growth system that go on within it. Maintaining the view that cities are not ordained; they are wholly existential. Thus, once the suburb city becomes mature, growth automatically spills over and harnesses the advantage of connectivity, proximity and available state policies for land regulation.

Interventions Through Master Plans

Land is very complex to understand in Indian context, since it is very densely knitted with society and its social milieu. Land is brought for residential, commercial and industrial use through notification of master plans. Delhi Lease and Finance limited was the first company in 1985 to own a 3000 acres (12.14 km^2) and started plotted development and therein no stopping for Gurgaon morphing into a chameleon as mentioned by Baudrillard (1986) regarding metropolis. In last 6 to 7 years, Department of Town and Country Planning (DTCP) has issued three notifications of three successive master plans for Gurgaon. State released first draft Master Plan (MP) 2021 on 1 July 2006 and finally notified on 05 February 2007; and reflected a shift from the draft plan with a land use change to facilitate the demand for housing. Within 4 years Master plan 2025 draft was released on 4 October 2010 and notified on 24 May 2011. Between MP 2021 and MP 2025, the state government converted few sectors of agricultural land to residential and commercial use. On 15 November 2012, the Master Plan 2031 draft was released that notified on 04 September 2012 after conversion of Special Economic Zone (SEZ) land into residential and commercial use. The box in Fig. 1 indicates the areas where major interventions were made through various master plans for land conversion and relaxation provided to real estate. This corroborates to Roy (2003) regarding informality in South Asia and explains that the rapid peri-urbanization that is unfolding at the edges of the world's largest cities (in this case Delhi) is an informalized process, often in violation of master plans and state norms but often informally sanctioned by the state. The State policy intervenes in land in two ways, viz. regulate land use and direct physical growth through the master planning process and invest in infrastructure. These actions affect the patterns of land development, as well as, the characteristics of real estate market. Since the mid-90s, the State's strategies for stimulating growth in and around cities included the creation of spatial enclaves and implementation of mega infrastructure projects especially transport corridors. The rural fringes adjoining metros are one of the sites for such interventions.

It is out of scope for this paper to attempt land transformation practices, but however work done by scholars (Roy 2003; Debroy and Bhandari 2009; Keivani and Mattingly 2007) articulated that land developers and highly connected people collude informally to assist, and allow land conversion through state's intervention in the name of urbanization and growth.

Marginalization and Shrinking Socio-Economic Space

Globalization is widely seen as a powerful engine that has the potential to promote growth and development. For many years, however, concerns have also been raised about the effects of globalization on society may be in terms of marginalization. There are number of issues regarding the sustainability of globalization from a social point of view. This study is limited in sense that it do not want to address the linkages between globalization and other indicators of marginalization like employment, education and question of land. However, it draws some conclusions from datasets that are being analyzed to study recent transformations along selected urban–rural transact.

Jacobs (1969) articulated that how work gets diversified and expanded is of essence in understanding cities because cities are places where adding new work to the older work proceeds vigorously. Indeed, any settlement where this happens becomes city. Because of this process city economics are more complicated and diverse. This argument supports the view that cities are primary necessity for economic development and expansion, including rural development. The core of all the processes of city growth is this root process that is adding new kinds of work to other kinds of older work or replacing imports by exports. Cities, as Brenner et al. (2012, pp 03) stated that "they are major basing points for the production, circulation and consumption of commodities, and their evolving internal socio-spatial organization, governance systems, and patterns of sociopolitical conflicts must be understood". These (built environment to land use systems, networks of production and exchange, and metropolitan-wide infrastructure arrangements) profit-oriented strategies of urban restructuring are intensely contested among dominant, subordinate and marginalized social forces. Chowdhury (2011) reported that there has been a marginal increase in urban employment mainly due to an increase in male employment, while female employment has come down. In total, there has been an increase in employment of less than a million people in the country between 2004–2005 and 2009–2010, a period in which the Indian economy was growing rapidly.

Gurgaon municipal ward number 34, small town on north Garhi Harsaru and Village Dhankot about 8 kms from Gurgaon is studied to investigate social and economic dynamics across urban–rural continuum using SECC data of 2011 (refer Fig. 1). The socio-economic data is analyzed both at household level and individual level. House ownership among households in ward number 34, Garhi Harsaru and Dhankot is 99.3, 94.1 and 86.5 %, respectively. Similarly, households in Gurgaon muncipal ward number 34 have more number of four and five rooms in their houses, thus it means households in inner part of city have better physical capital and have better access to good quality housing. Majority of households in Dhankot village have two or one rooms and is contrary to ward number 34. It could imply that people have rented houses or they own one and two room houses, since migrant worker cannot afford to pay more for housing. Proportion of household having refrigeration appliance is 88.3, 38.2 and 56.6 % across urban–rural continuum. Mobile communication penetration is 95, 69.1 and 98.3 % across households of Gurgaon municipal ward number 34, Garhi Harsaru town and Village Dhankot. In terms of urban amenities, 97, 99 and 74 % of households have access to electricity, toilets and washing machines across continuum.

Only 8 % of households have land ownership in Garhi Harsaru town in comparison to Dhankot village (14 %). In terms of farm-level assets, Dhankot households have water pumps to 5.7 % of total households, level of mechanization is 3.5 and 1 % households have access to kisan (farmers) credit card, whereas households in Garhi Harsaru have hardly any financial support towards farm activities. Sex ratio is lowest (763) in Dhankot village, followed by Garhi Harsaru (829) and Gurgaon municipal ward number 34 (831).

Marginalization is often conceptualized in terms of people, groups or communities getting marginalized but this work along with these dimensions also explore the marginalization in terms of space, and it seeks to explain how certain places or regions exhibits marginalization character differently. The educational processes have considerable influence on the way the inputs are transformed into output. There are evidences from the literature that education has a positive role over growth and development, but there are also studies that indicate disparity in male and female which is not a positive sign, i.e. development which is not gendered is endangered.

Status of education at graduation level (refer Table 1) is surprisingly high in Garhi Harsaru town (6.8 %) in comparison to Gurgaon city (6.0 %). Differences in education attainment are more striking at primary to secondary level between male and female.

Low rate of women workforce participation across all age groups indicate that women have simply withdrawn from the labour market in India, pointing towards social conservatism and existing gender discrimination. And it could be argued that more women are pursuing higher education resulting in a decline in women labour force participation rate, especially in 15–19 and 20–24 age groups. It is assumed that increased female labour force participation may hint towards the positive impacts of development. Among major reasons for the female labour force participation rate is women increased orientation towards combining

Table 1 Pattern of education across urban–rural continuum

	Garhi Harsaru	Dhankot	Gurgoan	Total	Garhi Harsaru	Dhankot	Gurgoan	Total
Graduate	134	28	49	211	6.8	5.7	6.0	6.5
Hr. Secondary	259	51	113	423	13.2	10.3	13.8	12.9
Secondary	263	74	152	489	13.4	15.0	18.6	15.0
Middle	424	64	183	671	21.7	13.0	22.3	20.5
Primary	502	112	180	794	25.6	22.7	22.0	24.3
Not literate	376	164	142	682	19.2	33.3	17.3	20.9
Total	1,958	493	819	3,270	100.0	100.0	100.0	100.0

Source Calculated from provisional SECC 2011

Table 2 Age groupwise workforce participation rate

	Garhi Harsaru town		Dhankot village		Gurgaon sector 34		Total	
Age group	Male	Female	Male	Female	Male	Female	Male	Female
15–19	6.83	3.92	0	0	9.09	0	6.25	2.61
20–24	58.40	0	46.15	5.88	32.60	0	50.27	1.09
25–29	84.48	3.03	92.68	3.44	84.61	0	86.22	2.36
30–34	94.44	1.85	95.83	0	86.48	7.14	92.48	3.19
35–39	96.87	9.33	100	0	86.20	5.26	94.11	7.03
40–44	92.75	3.57	100	0	96.87	3.12	94.78	3
45–49	92.85	8.69	100	0	87.5	0	92.63	5
50–54	92.30	9.75	71.42	0	72.72	0	85.18	6.15
55–59	79.31	5.12	100	0	100	0	87.5	3.63
60 and above	54.34	5.26	57.69	0	42.55	5.55	51.51	4.68
Total	69.10	4.43	68.84	1.85	63.06	2.38	67.53	3.54

Source Calculated from provisional SECC 2011

parenthood with away-from-home work. In addition to the sociological changes that accompany increasing female workforce participation rates, some major economic effects can be expected. Perhaps the single most important one could be increased household family income.

However, from Table 2, it seems that complete biasness exist in total workforce against women participation. But relatively Garhi Harsaru town in Gurgaon's periphery reported higher women workforce participation rate than municipal ward number 34. We expected higher female labour force participation rates in central part of the city, because of residences of higher income families and access to better infrastructure.

Table 2 reveals a wide gap in male–female educational attainment which obstruct the entry of the female in the work force and ultimately lead to marginalization of women from public sphere as it curtails their mobility and emancipation process. It is evident and widespread recognition that education is a major driver of economic competitiveness in an increasingly knowledge-driven global economy. The role of technological capacity in development is coming to be viewed as central to the industrializing effort and as the driving factor in shaping economic development (Mathews 2007).

Occupational structure manifest many other hidden intricacies of the social institutional structure of an economy, thus 14 classes of occupation are explored at municipal ward level as per SECC urban questionnaires. Helper is a broad category which includes shop worker/helper/staff in retail enterprise/waiter/distribution worker/attendant, hawker includes Street vendor/cobbler/hawker/other service provider working on streets, construction worker includes plumber/mason/labour/painter/welder/security guard/coolie and other head-load worker, cleaner includes

Table 3 Occupation in Gurgaon municipal ward 34

Income source	Freq.	%
Rag picker	1	0.12
Begging	2	0.24
Domestic worker	6	0.73
Hawker	8	0.97
Construction	33	4
Cleaning	20	2.43
Home based	8	0.97
Transport	15	1.82
Helper	21	2.55
Mechanic	5	0.61
Security guard	2	0.24
Other (formal jobs)	100	12.14
Renter	24	2.91
No income	579	70.27
Total	824	100

Source Calculated from provisional SECC 2011

sanitation worker/gardener and mechanic includes, electrician/assembler/repair worker (Table 3).

Out of total, 70 % belongs to no income category and it reflects dependents including housewives and school going children. 12.14 % manpower engaged in formal sector, while about 14.8 % belongs to people that engaged in small petty jobs including mechanic, domestic workers, cleaning and other casual works. In light of these patterns, it is important to further understand how cities could be repositioned within increasingly volatile, financialized circuits of capital accumulation. It points towards associated process of profit-driven urbanization, commodification and re-commodification of urban spaces.

It is evident from analysis of SECC data that bigger cities are more exclusionary in nature than smaller towns, as is the case of Garhi Harsaru town on Gurgaon's periphery. Garhi Harsaru is more preferable location to start new business enterprise, have relatively more private jobs, education attainment at various levels and higher female workforce participation rate than municipal ward number 34 at the centre of Gurgaon Millennium city. Thus towns on the periphery offer more opportunities apart from rent seeking approach that further propels the real estate developers to grab land at relatively lower prices than in metro peripheries to steer urban growth. This development seems to arise out of rapid transformation of rural settlements to urban areas and fundamental changes in spatial structures. In case of Gurgaon, urban planning after opening of economy in 1991 led to evolution of millennium city from a panchayat; the margins of the city now are more dominated by mass production of housing demand triggered by builders as well as extensive spread of institutions of business interests. Development gap is seen through set of indicators (amenities, land ownership, education & workforce participation) across municipal ward number 34 Gurgaon, small town Garhi Harsaru and village Dhankot using Socio Economic Caste Census 2011. Analysis of occupation in particular municipal ward revealed about various economic activities people are engaged and how city engine works? There is a high concentration in low paid jobs, increase in informalization and which clearly reflects marginalization through engagement in informal, elementary occupations, low female work participation and around 70 percent idling population. In meanwhile, the farmers are reduced to workers and landless labourers are pushed to margins of the society.

References

Avelar, S., Zah, R., & Tavares-Corrêa, C. (2009). Linking socioeconomic classes and land cover data in Lima, Peru: Assessment through the application of remote sensing and GIS. *International Journal of Applied Earth Observation and Geoinformation, 11*, 27–37.

Baudrillard, J. (1986). *America*. New York: Verso.

Bhagat, R. B. (2011). Emerging pattern of urbanisation in India. *Economic and Political Weekly, 46*(34), 10–13.

Brenner, N. (2004). *New state spaces: Urban governance and the rescaling of statehood*. New York: Oxford University Press.

Brenner, N., Marcuse, P. & Mayer, M. (Eds.) (2012). *Cities for People, Not for Profit: Critical Urban Theory and the Right to the City*. Routledge.

Census of India. (2011). *Provisional population totals paper 1 of 2011 India*. Retrieved December 12, 2013, from http://www.censusindia.gov.in/2011-prov-results/prov_results_paper1_india.html

Cheng, J., & Masser, I. (2003). Urban growth pattern modeling: a case study of Wuhan City, PR China. *Landscape Urban Planning, 62*(4), 199–217.

Chowdhury, S. (2011). Employment in India: What Does the Latest Data Show. *Economic and Political Weekly, 96*(32), 23–26.

Debroy, V., & Bhandari, L. (2009). Gurgaon and Faridabad—An exercise in contrasts, center on democracy, development, and the rule of law Freeman Spogli institute for international studies.

Denis, E., Mukhopadhyay, P., & Zerah, M. H. (2012). Subaltern urbanization in India. *Economic and Political Weekly, 96*(30), 52–62.

Jacobs, J. (1969). *The Economy of Cities*. New York: Vintage Books.

Jiang, J., Liu, S., Yuan, H., & Zhang, Q. (2007). Measuring Urban Sprawl in Beijing with Geo-spatial Indices. *Journal of Geographical Sciences, 17*(4), 469–478.

Keivani, R., & Mattingly, M. (2007). The interface of globalization and peripheral land in the cities of the south: Implications for urban governance and local economic development. *International Journal of Urban and Regional Research, 31*(2), 459–474.

Lambin, E. F., Geist, H. J., & Lepers, E. (2003). Dynamics of land-use and land-cover change in tropical regions. *Annual Review of Environment and Resources, 28*, 205–241.

Lambin, E. F., & Meyfroidt, P. (2011). Global land use change, economic globalization, and the looming land scarcity. *Proceedings of the National Academy of Sciences, 108*(9), 3465–3472.

Mathews, J. A. (2007). Catch-up strategies and the latecomer effect in Industrial development. *New Political Economy, 11*(3), 313–335.

Owens, S. (1986). *Energy*. U.K., Peon: Planning and Urban Form.

Portes, A., Castells, M., & Benton, L. (1989). *The Informal Economy*. Baltimore, MD: Johns Hopkins University Press.

Punia, M., & Singh, L. (2012). Entropy approach for assessment of urban growth: A case study of Jaipur, India. *Indian Society of Remote Sensing, 40*(2), 231–244.

Rahman, A., Aggarwal, S. P., Netzband, M., & Fazal, S. (2011). Monitoring urban sprawl using remote sensing and GIS techniques of a fast growing urban centre, India. *IEEE Journal of Selected Topics in Applied Earth Observations and Remote Sensing, 4*(1), 56–65.
Roy, A. (2003). City Requiem, Calcutta: Gender and the Politics of Poverty. Minneapolis: University of Minnesota Press.
Roy, A. (2009). The 21st-century metropolis: New geographies of theory. *Regional Studies, 43*(6), 819–830.
SECC. (2011). Socio-economic caste census. Retrieved February 15, 2013, from http://secc.gov.in/district
Sudhira, S., Ramachandra, T. V., & Jagadish, K. S. (2003). Urban sprawl: metrics, dynamics and modelling using GIS. *International Journal of Applied Earth Observation and Geoinformation, 5*, 29–39.
Yadav, A., & Punia, M. (2014). Socio-economic and ecological transformations of the peri-urban region of Gurgaon: An analysis of the trickle-down effect in the post globalization era. *International Archives of Photogrammramtry, Remote Sensing and Spatial Information Sciences, 40*(8), 1269–1276.

Ecosystem Services in NCT Delhi

Chandra Prakash Morya and Milap Punia

Abstract National Capital Region (NCR) is the fastest sprawling urban agglomeration in India. The growing demand for land due to increasing pressure of population is affecting the land use pattern in National Capital Territory (NCT) Delhi. It is comprehended that urban sprawl and resulting changes in land use land cover are significantly impacting ecosystem services and functions in NCT Delhi which are difficult to quantify and measure. The study area covers an area of 1504.42 km^2. The NCR Planning Board measures 9.02 % increase in built-up area and 7.52 % decrease in agriculture area in NCT Delhi from 1999 to 2012. The central objective is to quantify changes in land use/land cover and ecosystem services due to urban sprawl in NCT Delhi. The eight land use land cover categories were identified using data provided by European Space Agency for 1991, 2003, and 2010. In nineteen years time period, the major changes in land use/land cover has been observed in Built-up, Agricultural land and Forests. The Built-up, agricultural land and forest have changed, respectively, 14.9 %, −13.7 %, and 30.5 % from 1991 to 2010. Further, the coefficients published by Costanza et al. (Nature, 387:253–260, 1997) were used to quantify changes in ecosystem services delivered by each land use land cover category. The value of ecosystem services is estimated by multiplying the land area of each biome by the value coefficient of the equivalent biome which has been used as the proxy for that land use land cover category. The valuation of ecosystem services shows only a 0.62 % net decline in the total ecosystem services in the study area. If we assume a linear decrease in the ecosystem services, it shows a net cumulative

C.P. Morya (✉)
Department of Geography, University of Rajasthan, Jaipur, India
e-mail: Chandra.morya@gmail.com

M. Punia
Centre for the Study of Regional Development, School of Social Sciences, Jawaharlal Nehru University, New Delhi, India
e-mail: Milap.punia@gmail.com

S.S. Acharya et al. (eds.), *Marginalization in Globalizing Delhi: Issues of Land, Livelihoods and Health*, DOI 10.1007/978-81-322-3583-5_5

loss of US$ 5.54 million over the 19 years time period of the study. The decline is relatively small that could be attributed to the sharp decrease in the agricultural land utilization. When we assume the ±50 % shift in the value coefficient of river bed, the estimated annual ecosystem service values changed ±34.89 % (US$ 3.85 ha^{-1} per year) between 1991 and 2010. Further, the contribution of the various ecosystem functions was measured to the overall total value of the ecosystem services across all the time periods. The additional sensitivity analysis suggests that the estimated ecosystem value is inelastic with respect to that coefficient. It is concluded that the continued decrease in ecosystem services will lead to the lesser access of services at higher cost, especially to the poor, so further policy formation and land reclamation should be based on the study of environmental losses.

Keywords Ecosystem services · Biomes · Disturbance regulation · Sensitivity · NCT Delhi

Introduction

In the last three census decades (1981–2011), India has experienced a significant growth in urban population. The census reports 17.29 % urban population in 1951 which has increased to 31.16 % in 2011 in India. The decadal growth rate of population shows a declining trend 23.87, 21.54 and 17.64 % in 1981–1991, 1991–2001, and 2001–2011, respectively, but the population density has increased from 325 persons/km^2 in 2001 to 382 persons/km^2 in 2011 (Census 2011). The population in large cities is growing rapidly and the small cities are experiencing slower rate of urbanization (Kundu 2006; Kundu and Lompard 2012), as 42.6 % urban population of India is concentrated only in 53 metropolitan cities (NCRPB). Such increasing population pressure in big cities as well as its impact on peri-urban areas is expected to significantly affect the developmental processes if not maintained in scientific and environmental friendly way. According to census 2011 Mumbai, Delhi, Kolkata, and Chennai, the above-said four metropolitan cities together account 15.4 % urban population of India. Delhi is the most urbanized union territory of India having a density as high as 11,297 persons/km^2 in 2011. The population density in NCT Delhi in 1981 was 4194 persons/km^2 which has increased to 11,297 persons/km^2 in 2011. According to NCR planning board, this resulted into 9.02 % increase in built-up area and 7.52 % decrease in agriculture area from 1999 to 2012 in NCT Delhi. Although the population growth rate is declining, it has added 2.9 million persons during the last decade (2010–2011) in NCT Delhi. In last three census years (1991, 2001, and 2011), the population of NCT Delhi is measured 9.42 million, 13.85 million, and 16.75 million. The decadal growth rates are measured 47.03 and 20.93 % in 1991–2001 and 2001–2011, respectively. The contribution of net migrants in 2001 was 17.64 %. Meanwhile, the population density in National Capital Region has also doubled from 1981 to 2011. It reflects that urbanization in NCT Delhi has affected the surrounded regions also. According to NCR planning board, in whole NCR the urban population has increased from 50.2 % in 1991 to 62.5 % in 2011. This growth can be largely attributed to the in-migration and population growth in the study area.

The urban sprawl and increasing population density are direct driver and indirect driver, respectively, that cause change in the land use pattern of any area (Lambin et al. 2001; Mcdonald et al. 2013). This has resulted change in the land use/land cover in the National Capital Region of India. It is estimated that in NCT Delhi the built-up has increased 9.02 % while agricultural land has decreased 7.52 % from 1999 to 2012 (NCRPB). This increase in built-up and population density is expected to have impacted the natural environment, natural resources, and open spaces within NCT Delhi as well as in surrounding areas also (Mohan et al. 2011; Nagendra et al. 2014). This change in land use land cover ultimately affects the functioning of the ecosystems of that area. The functioning and interaction of the ecosystems within an area provides many benefits that are termed as ecosystem services (Costanza et al. 1997; MEA 2005). Ecosystem goods and services are the benefits that living organisms derive directly or indirectly from ecosystem functions that maintain the Earth's life support system (Zhao et al. 2004). The changes in functioning of ecosystems result into the changes in the availability of goods and services from those ecosystems (Vejre et al. 2010).

The land use/land cover changes are the direct drivers of changes in ecosystem services (Turner et al. 1994). In this paper, an attempt has been made to measure the changes in land use land cover as well as the changes in ecosystem services of NCT Delhi from 1991 to 2010. The ecosystem services are derived both directly and indirectly. When the land use land cover changes significantly affects the ecosystems, monitoring and projecting the changes in ecosystem services become difficult as the same services are derived indirectly (Kreuter et al. 2001). To measure the ecosystem services the approach suggested by Costanza et al. (1997) has been used. He has estimated the economic value of 17 ecosystem services for 16 biomes of the entire biosphere. The main objectives of the study were: (1) to measure the changes in land use/land cover of NCT Delhi from 1991 to 2010; (2) to find out the effectiveness of using generalized ecosystem services value coefficient suggested by Costanza et al. (1997); (3) and to suggest some policy recommendations for the sustainable land use/land cover changes.

Methods and Estimation Approach

Study Area and Database

The National Capital Territory of India, Delhi is located in northern India between the latitudes of 28° 24′ 17″ and 28° 53′ 00″ North and longitudes of 76° 50′ 24″ and 77° 20′ 37″ East. It is bordered by Rajasthan, Haryana, and Uttar Pradesh states of India. It comprises an area of 1483 km^2 but for analysis purpose 1504.42 km^2 is considered as study area. It is situated in the alluvial fertile land of Ganges river system having an average elevation of 216 meters from the sea level. The river Yamuna is the major stream which passes through its eastern part. The major portion of city extends on the right bank of the Yamuna River. The study area is generally flat except for a low ridge which extends from South–South west to North–North east part. It is the extension of the Aravalli hills of the Rajasthan state of India which reaches the height of 318 meters in the study area. It is the second largest metropolitan city of India after Mumbai having a population of 16.75 million (2011). It works as central node of industrial regions, tourism, transportation, etc., of Northern India.

The datasets have been taken from the secondary sources. The data used for analysis is for three time periods 1991, 2003, and 2010, respectively. The data related to be land use land cover has been taken from the study conducted by ESA on "Historical Assessment of Spatial Growth of Built-Ups in Metropolitan Areas of Delhi and Mumbai in India and Dhaka in Bangladesh" in the framework of the "*eoworld*" initiative supported by the European Space Agency (ESA). The data has been provided in various land use land cover categories that can be aggregated across various levels. Finally on the characteristics of the study area eight land use land cover categories were identified, namely Built-up, Urban Greenery, Agricultural Land, Forest, Other Natural and Semi-natural Areas including Wetlands, Bare Land (including fallow land), Water Bodies, and River Bed. Built-up includes residential, nonresidential built-up, industrial sites, airport, yards, landfill sites, etc. Urban Greenery includes urban parks, urban gardens, urban forests, tree cover along the roads and railway lines, zoological parks, commercial and industrial green belts, avenues and boulevards, etc. Agricultural land includes cultivated land, plantation and horticulture. The rocky, hilly tracts, gullied land, scrub land, saline land, water logged areas or wetlands, semi-arid pastures and rangelands have been included in the category 'Other Natural and Semi-natural Areas including Wetlands'. The Bare Land includes land which is not occupied by cultivation, built-up, scrub land, or any type of grass cover. The category Water Bodies includes flowing water bodies like river, canal, etc. and stagnant water bodies like ponds, lakes, etc., and associated surfaces.

Assignment of Ecosystem Service Values

The ecosystem service values for the eight land use land cover categories have been obtained through Costanza et al. (1997) approach. The LULC categories were compared with the 16 biomes identified by Costanza et al. (1997) in his ecosystem services valuation model. The land use land cover categories used by Costanza et al. (1997) was of different categorization. To resolve this problem and for local fit, for each land use/land cover category the most representative and similar biome was used as proxy. In the study area, the total estimated value of ecosystem services was calculated using the following formula:

$$\mathrm{ESV} = \sum (A_k x \ \mathrm{VC}_k)$$

where ESV is the total estimated ecosystem service value, A_k is the area (ha) and VC_k is the value coefficient (US$/ha/year) for land use category '*k*'.

Although the biomes used as proxy for land use/land cover category categories were not perfect matches, they represent particular land use/land cover

Table 1 Biome equivalents and corresponding ecosystem service coefficients (Costanza et al. 1997)

Land use land cover category	Equivalent biome	Ecosystem service coefficient (US$/ha/year)	
		1994	2014
Built-up	Urban	0	0
Urban greenery	Temperate/boreal forest	302	482.72
agricultural land	Cropland	92	147.05
Forest	Forests	969	1548.86
Other natural and semi-natural Areas including wetlands	Grass/rangelands	244	390.01
Bare land (including fallow land)	Cropland	92	147.05
Water bodies	Lakes/rivers	8498	13,583.34
River bed	Floodplains	19,581	31,298.57

category. As urban greenery is different from Costanza's temperate/boreal forest but urban greenery cannot be assigned value equal to the forest cover, so it has been assigned lower value than forests. Both the bare land (including fallow land) and agricultural land has been assigned value equal to the cropland because the bare land is also as much fertile as agricultural land. River bed was considered equivalent to the flood plain so it gains highest value from all other categories. The average global value of ecosystem services calculated by Costanza et al. (1997) were according 1994 US$ prices. To correctly value each land use land cover category according current prices the 1994 US$ prices were converted into 2014 US$ prices. Although the river bed was assigned the highest value there was no change in the area of that category, so results were not expected to be overwhelmed (Table 1).

The contribution of the 17 ecosystem functions was measured to the overall total value of the ecosystem services for all the time periods to find out the change in the contribution of each ecosystem functions in providing ecosystem services. For this, each ecosystem function was ranked according to their contribution in a particular year and an overall rank was given on their contribution from 1991 to 2010. The uncertainties of proxy values could affect the results, so I did sensitivity analysis using the standard economic concept of elasticity to determine the dependency of the ecosystem values on the applied coefficients. The following equation was used to calculate the coefficient of sensitivity:

$$CS = \frac{(\mathrm{ESV}_j - \mathrm{ESV}_i)/\mathrm{ESV}_i}{(\mathrm{VC}_{jk} - \mathrm{VC}_{ik})/\mathrm{VC}_{ik}}$$

where CS is the coefficient of sensitivity, VC is the value coefficient, ESV is the total estimated ecosystem service value, 'k' represents the land use category and 'i' and 'j' represent the initial and adjusted values, respectively. The ecosystem value coefficients were adjusted ±50 % for each land use/land cover category. The impact of adjustment with the coefficients on the estimates of the total ecosystem service values has been presented. The coefficient of sensitivity expresses the robustness of the results with respect to the coefficient. The ratio between percentage change in the estimated total ecosystem value and the percentage change in the adjusted valuation coefficient explains the robustness of total estimated ecosystem values.

Results

Land Use/Land Cover Changes

Land use changes associated with urbanization drive climate change and pollution, which alter properties of ecosystems at local, regional, and continental scales (Grimm et al. 2008). The interaction of human and ecosystems varies from place to place. It makes necessary to observe and estimate the land use changes with caution so that substantial general inferences can be drawn to examine changes in ecosystem services. The changes in the eight land use land cover categories are presented in the Fig. 1.

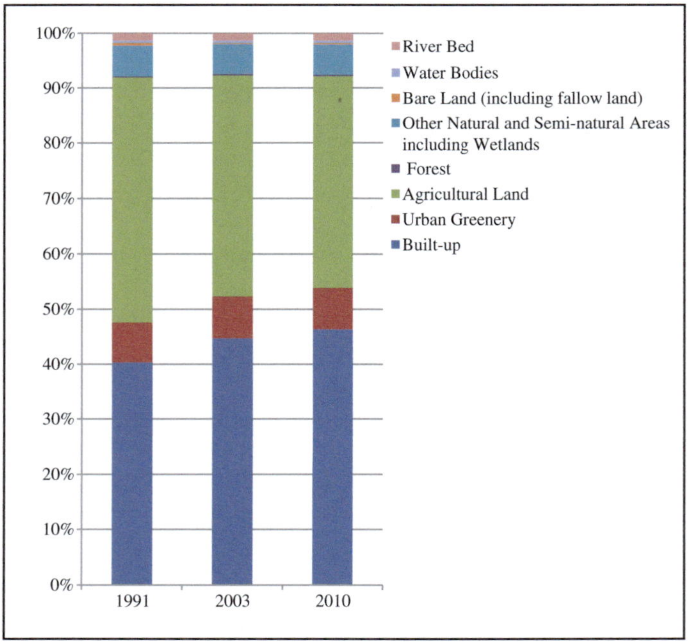

Fig. 1 Land use/land cover change in NCT Delhi, 1991–2010 (authors work)

In 1991, the agricultural land category dominated all other categories with 44.36 % area. It was followed by built-up category with 40.32 % area. Later in 2003 and 2010, the area under agricultural land category has decreased and remained 39.97 and 38.30 %, respectively. The area under agricultural land category decreased 9.9 and 4.2 % in 1991–2003 and 2003–2010, respectively. The overall decrease in agricultural land category was measured 14.2 % from 1991 to 2010. While the area under category built-up, by contrast, has increased and reached 44.67 and 46.31 % in 2003 and 2010, respectively. The built-up showed 10.8 and 3.7 % increase in 1991–2003 and 2003–2010, respectively. The NRSC reports that this increase in built-up is due to conversion of agricultural land into non-agricultural use. Around 14.9 % increase was measured in the area of built-up category from 1991 to 2003. Thus the built-up category dominated all other categories by area in 2003 and 2010. The forest cover has increased from 245.9 ha to 320.8 ha from 1991 to 2010. The forest cover measured 29.9 % increase from 1991 to 2003 while only 0.4 % increase was measured from 2003 to 2010. The NCR regional plan states although there has been increase in forest cover dense forest has decreased while open forest cover has increased (Table 2).

The area under urban greenery category was 7.25 % and shows a slight 3.8 % increase from 1991 to 2010. This increase in urban greenery can be attributed to the development of green buffers along transport networks in the city. The ESA data reveals no change in river bed throughout the 19 years time period but various reports indicate that significant part of river bed has been lost in last 20 years. In 1991, the category water bodies were 689.6 % which increased 5.6 % in 19 years and reached up to 727.9 ha in 2010. The category other natural and semi-natural areas including wetlands had 8428.6 ha area, covering 5.6 % area in 1991. Around 62 ha decrease was measured in category other natural and semi-natural areas including wetlands. The area covered by category bare land was 707.9 ha in 1991 which remained 221.7 ha and 339.7 ha in 2003 and 2010, respectively. Thus bare land including fallow land has decreased around 52 % from 1991 to 2010.

Estimation of Changes in Ecosystem Services

The land use/land change data and associated assigned ecosystem service value coefficient has been used to calculate total estimated ecosystem service value for all the three years, 1991, 2003, and 2010, respectively. The ecosystem service value calculated for 150,442 ha area reveals that there has been a 0.58 million per year (i.e., 0.62 % or US$ 4.12 ha^{-1} per year) net decline in ecosystem services from 1991 to 2010 (Table 3). If we assume a linear decrease from 1991 to 2010, it represents a cumulative loss of US$ 5.54 million in ecosystem services over the 19 years time period. The analysis shows that there was 0.36 % decline in ecosystem services from 1991 to 2003, higher than 0.27 % from 2003 to 2010. If we calculate the actual decrease by adding the decline of ecosystem service during these two time periods, we obtain a cumulative loss of US$ 5.19 million (shaded area in Fig. 2).

Table 2 Total area (ha) of each land use land cover category in Delhi, India and changes in LULC from 1991 to 2010 (ESA)

Land use land cover	Total area (ha)			1991–2003			2003–2010			1991–2010		
category	1991	2003	2010	ha	%	%/year	ha	%	%/year	ha	%	%/year
Built-up	60,655	67,208	69,676.9	6553	10.8	0.9	2469	3.7	0.5	9021.9	14.9	0.8
Urban greenery	10,900	11,483	11,313	583	5.3	0.4	−170	−1.5	−0.2	413	3.8	0.2
Agricultural land	66,733	60,138	57,615	−6595	−9.9	−0.8	−2523	−4.2	−0.6	−9118	−13.7	−0.7
Forest	245.9	319.4	320.8	73.5	29.9	2.5	1	0.4	0.1	74.9	30.5	1.6
Other natural and semi-natural Areas including wetlands	8428.6	8270.3	8366.6	−158.3	−1.9	−0.2	96	1.2	0.2	−62	−0.7	0
Bare land (including fallow land)	707.9	221.7	339.7	−486.2	−68.7	−5.7	118	53.2	7.6	−368.2	−52	−2.7
Water bodies	689.6	717.3	727.9	27.7	4	0.3	11	1.5	0.2	38.3	5.6	0.3
River bed	2082	2082	2082	0	0	0	0	0	0	0	0	0

Table 3 Total ecosystem service value (ESV in US$ × 10^6/year) estimated for each land use land cover category in the study area using Costanza et al. value coefficients, and overall change and the rate of change between 1991 and 2010 (authors work)

Land use land cover category	ESV (US$ × 10^6 per year)			1991–2003			2003–2010			1991–2010		
	1991	2003	2010	$ × 10^6	%	%/year	$ × 10^6	%	%/year	$ × 10^6	%	%/year
Built-up	0.00	0.00	0.00	0.00	0.00	0.00	0.00	0.00	0.00	0.00	0.00	0.00
Urban greenery	5.26	5.54	5.46	0.28	5.35	0.45	−0.08	−1.48	−0.21	0.20	3.79	0.20
Agricultural land	9.81	8.84	8.47	−0.97	−9.88	−0.82	−0.37	−4.20	−0.60	−1.34	−13.66	−0.72
Forest	0.38	0.49	0.50	0.11	29.89	2.49	0.00	0.44	0.06	0.12	30.46	1.60
Other natural and semi-natural Areas including wetlands	3.29	3.23	3.26	−0.06	−1.88	−0.16	0.04	1.16	0.17	−0.02	−0.74	−0.04
Bare land (including fallow land)	0.10	0.03	0.05	−0.07	−68.68	−5.72	0.02	53.23	7.60	−0.05	−52.01	−2.74
Water bodies	9.37	9.74	9.89	0.38	4.02	0.33	0.14	1.48	0.21	0.52	5.55	0.29
River bed	65.16	65.16	65.16	0.00	0.00	0.00	0.00	0.00	0.00	0.00	0.00	0.00
Total	93.38	93.05	92.79	−0.33	−0.36	–	−0.25	−0.27	–	−0.58	−0.62	–

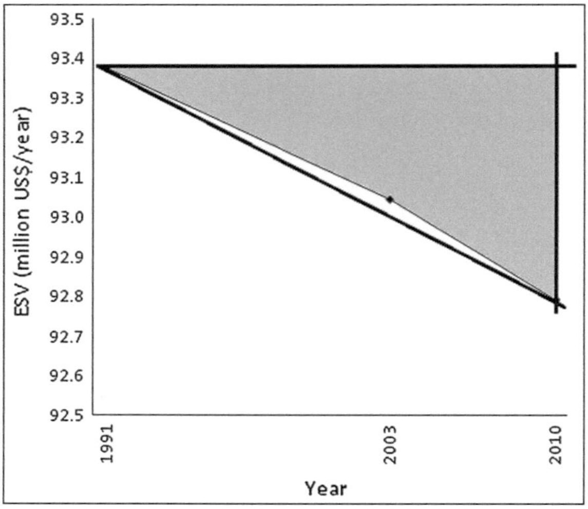

Fig. 2 Cumulative value by accessing a linear decrease in ecosystem services from 1991 to 2010 (authors work)

There is need to accurately measure the cumulative loss of ecosystem services, preferably annually if possible. Ecosystem services value was not assigned to the built-up, since conversion to built-up area is irreversible and there is hardly any contribution to ecosystem services. If a value is assigned to Built-up category it may have had a significant effect on our estimate or underestimate the ecosystem value of other land use/land cover categories. In summary, the net cumulative loss of US$ 5.19 million appeared to have resulted due to continuous conversion of agricultural land into non-agricultural uses.

Apart from calculating estimated land use/land cover change impacts on the total value of ecosystem services, we have also analyzed the impact of land use/ land cover change on the 17 ecosystem functions suggested by Costanza et al. The services provided by different ecosystem functions were calculated individually using the following formula:

$$\mathrm{ESV}_f = \sum \left(A_k x\ \mathrm{VC}_{fk}\right),$$

where ESV_f is the total estimated ecosystem value of the individual function 'f', A_k is the area in hectare for land use category 'k' and VC_{fk} is the value coefficient of individual function 'f' (US$ ha^{-1} per year) for land use category 'k' (Table 4).

We have ranked the contribution of ecosystem functions based on their estimated ESV_f to overall value of ecosystem services in each year 1991, 2003, and 2010. The overall rank was given on the basis of contribution of each ecosystem function across the three years of analysis. The tendency in Table 4 shows the shift in the contribution of ecosystem function to the total ecosystem services over the time period. The upward arrow signals positive contribution, downward arrow signals negative contribution, and a dash signals no change. The contribution of the ecosystem function 'water supply' has dominated followed by 'disturbance regulation' over the 19 years time period.

Table 4 Estimated annual value of ecosystem functions (ESV_f US$ × 10^6/year) (authors work)

Ecosystem function	1991			2003			2010			Overall rank	Tendency
	ESV_f	%	Rank	ESV_f	%	Rank	ESV_f	%	Rank		
Gas regulation	0.976	1.045	12	0.974	1.047	12	0.975	1.051	12	12	↓
Climate regulation	1.589	1.701	10	1.687	1.813	9	1.664	1.793	9	9	↑
Disturbance regulation	24.095	25.804	2	24.095	25.896	2	24.095	25.966	2	2	–
Water regulation	6.143	6.578	5	6.383	6.860	5	6.476	6.979	5	5	↑
Water supply	27.627	29.586	1	27.721	29.793	1	27.757	29.912	1	1	↑
Erosion control	0.428	0.459	14	0.432	0.465	14	0.437	0.471	14	14	↑
Soil formation	0.192	0.205	15	0.202	0.217	15	0.199	0.215	15	15	↑
Nutrient cycling	0.142	0.152	16	0.184	0.198	16	0.185	0.199	16	16	↑
Waste treatment	8.976	9.613	3	9.075	9.753	3	9.076	9.781	3	3	↑
Pollination	1.846	1.977	9	1.681	1.807	10	1.631	1.758	10	10	↓
Biological control	2.967	3.178	7	2.694	2.895	7	2.604	2.806	8	7	↓
Habitat/refugia	1.461	1.565	11	1.461	1.570	11	1.461	1.574	11	11	–
Food production	7.814	8.368	4	7.239	7.780	4	7.029	7.575	4	4	↓
Raw materials	0.653	0.699	13	0.692	0.744	13	0.686	0.739	13	13	↑
Genetic resources	0.006	0.007	17	0.008	0.009	17	0.008	0.009	17	17	↑
Recreation	2.568	2.750	8	2.619	2.814	8	2.613	2.816	7	8	↑
Cultural	5.896	6.314	6	5.898	6.339	6	5.898	6.356	6	6	↑
Total	93.378	100	–	93.046	100	–	92.794	100	–	–	–

There no change was observed in the supply of ecosystem services by the ecosystem functions 'disturbance regulation' and 'habitat/refugia'. The ecosystem function water supply contributes (29.9 %) highest followed by disturbance regulation (25.96 %) in 2010. The ecosystem functions, water supply, disturbance regulation, waste treatment, food production and cultural, each contributed more than 5 % to the value of total ecosystem services. The contribution of ecosystem functions, climate regulation, water regulation, water supply, erosion control, soil formation, nutrient cycling, waste management, raw materials, genetic resources, recreation, and cultural has increased over 19 years time period of the study. While the contribution of gas regulation, pollination, biological control, and food production has decreased substantially over the 19 years time period.

Ecosystem Services Sensitivity Analysis

An attempt was made to know that to what level total ecosystem services are affected due to change in any particular ecosystem value coefficient, so the alternative ecosystem value coefficient (±50 % change in the coefficient) were used to examine the changes in total ecosystem services value. The built-up category was assigned no value coefficient so sensitivity analysis could not be done for built-up. There was no change in the area of river bed category, so assigning a high value coefficient (31,298.57 US$/ha/year) to river bed has not affected the results over different time periods but has underestimated coefficients of other land use/land cover categories. The value coefficient assigned to river bed is almost, 213 times of agricultural land, 80 times of other natural and semi-natural areas including wetlands, 65 times of urban greenery and 20 times of forest (Table 1).

According to the ESA data, over the time periods no change was measured in the area of river bed. The alternative value coefficient for river bed caused ±34.89 % change in the actual total ecosystem services value. So the change in river bed could have significantly affected the value of ecosystem services. Nevertheless, there is scope for articulation around construction activities on 200 ha of riverbed (Temple and transport depo) and its socio-spatial configuration related to urban planning. (Follmann 2015) studied informality, flexibility, and exceptionality that is involved in managing Yamuna's riverbed. The ecosystem value coefficient assigned to agricultural land is low (147.05 US$/ha/year) but the area covered by agricultural land is very high (44.3 % in 1991 and 38.3 % in 2010), so the alternative value coefficient could affect the results significantly. The alternative value coefficients used for agricultural land and water bodies affect the actual total ecosystem services value ±4.54 and ±5.29 %, respectively (Table 5).

The coefficient of sensitivity expresses the robustness of the adjusted results with respect to the coefficient. It is the ratio between percentage change between the estimated total ecosystem value and the percentage change in the adjusted valuation coefficient. If the ratio is greater than one, then it explains that the estimated ecosystem service value is elastic with respect to that coefficient, but if the ratio is less than

Table 5 Total estimated ecosystem service value and percentage change in estimated total ecosystem service value and coefficient of sensitivity (CS) associated with adjustment of ecosystem valuation coefficients (VC) (authors work)

LULC category	ESV_f (US$ × 10^6)		1991–2010 change		Effect of changing CV from original value			
	1991	2010	$ × 10^6	% change	1991		2010	
					%	CS	%	CS
Urban greenery VC +50 %	96.01	95.52	0.48	0.50	2.82	0.056	2.92	0.059
Urban greenery VC −50 %	90.75	90.06	0.68	0.75	−2.82	−0.056	−2.92	−0.059
Agricultural land VC +50 %	98.28	97.03	1.25	1.28	5.25	0.105	4.54	0.091
Agricultural land VC −50 %	88.47	88.56	−0.09	−0.10	−5.25	−0.105	−4.54	−0.091
Forest VC +50 %	93.57	93.04	0.53	0.56	0.20	0.004	0.27	0.005
Forest VC −50 %	93.19	92.55	0.64	0.69	−0.20	−0.004	−0.27	−0.005
Other natural and semi-natural areas including wetlands VC +50 %	95.02	94.43	0.60	0.63	1.76	0.035	1.75	0.035
Other natural and semi-natural areas including Wetlands VC −50 %	91.73	91.16	0.57	0.62	−1.76	−0.035	−1.75	−0.035
Bare land (including fallow land) VC +50 %	93.43	92.82	0.61	0.65	0.06	0.001	0.03	0.001
Bare land (including fallow land) VC −50 %	93.33	92.77	0.56	0.60	−0.06	−0.001	−0.03	−0.001
Water bodies VC +50 %	98.06	97.74	0.32	0.33	5.02	0.100	5.29	0.107
Water bodies VC −50 %	88.69	87.85	0.84	0.95	−5.02	−0.100	−5.29	−0.107
River bed VC +50 %	125.96	125.38	0.58	0.46	34.89	0.698	34.89	0.702
River bed VC −50 %	60.80	60.21	0.58	0.96	−34.89	−0.698	−34.89	−0.702

one, then the estimated ecosystem services value is considered to be inelastic with respect to that coefficient. The sensitivity analysis reflects that the estimated ecosystem value for every land use/land cover category is inelastic or robust with respect to that coefficient. The coefficient of sensitivity resulted high for river bed; it may be due to the effect of assigning higher value coefficient to the river bed category. The results of alternative value coefficients and sensitivity analysis emphasis to obtain correct value coefficients for all land use/land cover categories, especially for dominant categories. It is strongly recommended to use correct and most equivalent value coefficients to quantify correctly the ecosystem services value.

Conclusion

In a country like India, people are more dependent on ecosystems, like agricultural areas and natural areas. These ecosystems are sources of direct benefits, providing food, fiber, fuel-wood, fodder and timber, etc. It is essentially necessary to improve these ecosystems instead of deteriorating them by unmanaged utilization. In the study area, the most important features having more ecological importance than other features are 'agricultural land' and 'other natural and semi-natural area including wetlands'. The process of urbanization in NCT Delhi reveals continuing urban sprawl and resultant pressure is causing shrinkage in land use/land covers that are very important for a balanced development of ecosystems. The LULC change results reveal that from 1991 to 2010 built-up has increased around 9021 ha vis-a-vis agricultural land has decreased 9118 ha within 19 years time period. It is considered that urban sprawl is responsible for most of the agricultural land change (Bolund and Hunhammar 1999). The large-scale land reclamation activities for non-agricultural uses are causing urban sprawl (Singh 2000). In recent decades, the urban sprawl is intensified due to real estate developers, urban affluence, high estate taxes for rural land owners and negative incentives of land developers to sustain rural land use with perspective of ecosystem development (Breuste et al. 2013).

We calculated the total ecosystem service value for eight land use/land cover categories using the (Costanza et al. 1997) coefficient as proxy value. Although the coefficients used are not perfect matches, we can know the relative situation of an area over different time periods. To obtain the absolute value coefficients for the specific land use/land cover category are very difficult but coefficients tend to affect estimates of the magnitude of ecosystem values more than the estimates of directional change at specific points in time (De Groot et al. 2012). We found that total ecosystem service value has declined 0.58 million per year (i.e., 0.62 % or US\$ 4.12 ha^{-1} per year). This decrease in ecosystem services value can be largely attributed to the conversion of agricultural land for non-agricultural uses (Jiang et al. 2013; Kumar 2009). Assuming a linear decrease, it represents a cumulative loss of US\$ 5.54 million in ecosystem services over the 19 years time period. The contribution of various ecosystem functions reveals that the contribution of climate regulation, water regulation, water supply, erosion control, soil formation, nutrient cycling, waste management, raw materials, genetic resources, recreation and cultural has increased while the contribution of gas regulation, pollination, biological control and food production has decreased substantially over the 19 years time period.

Although the value coefficients suggested by Costanza can be objected as they can be used for wide biomes which encompass several related ecosystems. These coefficients vary from place to place and are not perfect matches for microlevel studies but still these can present the picture of a region in different time periods. The advancement that can be done is to set up benchmark value coefficients for dominant ecosystem types for each biome, so that more accurate value coefficients can be applied at the local levels.

The ESA data reveals no change in river bed but various reports indicate that significant part of river bed has been lost in last 20 years. River bed helps in groundwater recharge, spread and passage of flood waters during the monsoon, regulating thermal currents in the city and habitat for numerous life forms which has been lost due to the various construction activities, like construction of Delhi metro Depot, Common wealth games village, railway bridges, construction of NH-24, etc. So it can be expected that the actual decrease in ecosystem services is much more. If we talk about forests only 32 % are dense forests; rests are open forests. The expected decrease in dense forests will further cause a decrease in availability of ecosystem services. It requires densification of forests which will enrich biodiversity as well as habitats of various life forms. The continuous encroachments over the agricultural land of Ganges alluvial system will decrease the availability of ecosystem services in the future. The services will be available but in less quantity, that will increase access cost of the ecosystem services. In NCT Delhi, it is expected that poor will be the most affected section of humanity because poor people has to access these ecosystem services and goods at higher cost on daily basis. For a sustainable development of ecosystems within the study area, it is necessary to clearly understand the factors that facilitate urban sprawl and the developer's incentives should be drawn towards protecting and enhancing ecosystems. To correctly quantify the ecosystem services loss, the more detailed study of the impacts of land use/land cover changes is necessary.

Acknowledgements We would like to thank European Space agency and World Bank for allowing public use of remote sensing services related to spatial growth of built-ups in Metropolitan areas of Delhi as a part of initiative for use of earth observation for development.

References

Bolund, P., & Hunhammar, S. (1999). Ecosystem services in urban areas. *Ecological Economics, 29*, 293–301.

Breuste, J., Dagmar Haase, D., & Elmqvist, T. (2013). Urban landscapes and ecosystem services. In S. Wratten, H. Sandhu, R. Cullen & R. Costanza (Eds.), *Ecosystem services in agricultural and urban landscapes* (pp. 83–104). John Wiley & Sons. Ltd.

Census of India. (2011). Final population data sheets.

Costanza, R., d'Arge, R., de Groot, R., Farber, S., Grasso, M., Hannon, B., ... van den Belt, M. (1997). The value of the world's ecosystem services and natural capital. *Nature, 387*, 253–260.

De Groot, R., Brander, L., van der Ploeg, S., Costanza, R., Bernard, F., Braat, L., ... van Beukering, P. (2012). Global estimates of the value of ecosystems and their services in monetary units. *Ecosystem Services, 1*, 50–61.

Follmann, A. (2015). Urban mega-projects for a 'world-class' riverfront—The interplay of informality, flexibility and exceptionality along the Yamuna in Delhi. *India. Habitat International, 45*(3), 213–222.

Grimm, N. B., Faeth, S. H., Golubiewski, N. E., Redman, C. L., Wu, J., Bai, X & Brigs, J. M. (2008). Global change and the ecology of cities. *Science, 319*, 756–760.

Jiang, L., Deng, X., & Seto, K. C. (2013). The impact of urban expansion on agricultural land use intensity in China. *Land Use Policy, 35*, 33–39.

Kreuter, U. P., Harris, H. G., Matlock, M. D., & Lacey, R. E. (2001). Change in ecosystem service values in the San Antonio area, Texas. *Ecological Economics, 39*, 333–346.

Kumar, P. (2009). Assessment of economic drivers of land use change in urban ecosystems of Delhi, India. *A Journal of the Human Environment, 38*(1), 35–39.

Kundu, A. (2006). Trends & patterns of urbanization and their economic implications. In *India Infrastructure Report* (pp. 28–41).

Kundu, A., & Lopamudra, R. S. (2012). Migration and exclusionary urbanisation in India. *Economic & Political Weekly, 47*(26/27), 219–227.

Lambin, E. F., Turner, B. L., Geist, H. J., Agbola, S. B., Angelsen, A., Bruce, J.W., ... Xu, J. (2001). The causes of land-use and land-cover change: Moving beyond the myths. *Global environmental Change, 11*, 261–269.

McDonald, R. I., Marcotullio, P. J. & Guneralp, B. (2013). *Chapter 3: Urbanization and global trends; urbanization, biodiversity and ecosystem services: Challenges and opportunities a global assessment a part of the cities and biodiversity outlook project* (pp. 31–52).

Millennium Ecosystem Assessment -MEA. (2005). *Ecosystems and human wellbeing: Synthesis*. Washington, DC: Island Press.

Mohan, M., Pathan, S. K., Narendrareddy, K., kandya, A., & Pandey, S. (2011). Dynamics of urbanization and its impact on land-use/land-cover: A case study of megacity Delhi. *Journal of Environmental Protection, 2*, 1274–1283.

Nagendra, H., Sudhira, H. S., Katti, M., Tengo, M., & Schewenius, M. (2014). Urbanization and its impacts on land use, biodiversity and ecosystems in India. *Interdisciplinia, 2*, 305–313.

Singh, R. B. (2000). Environmental consequences of agricultural development: A case study from the Green Revolution state of Haryana, India. *Agriculture, Ecosystems & Environment, 82*, 97–103.

Turner, B. L., Meyer, W. B., & Skole, D. L. (1994). global land-use/land-cover change: Towards an integrated program of study. *Ambio, 23*(1), 91–95.

Vejre, H., Jensen, F. S., & Thorsen, B. J. (2010). Demonstrating the importance of intangible ecosystem services from peri-urban landscapes. *Ecological Complexity, 7*, 338–348.

Zhao, B., Kreuter, U., Li, B., Ma, Z., Chen, J., & Nakagoshi, N. (2004). An ecosystem service value assessment of land-use change on Chongming Island, China. *Land Use Policy, 21*, 139–148.

Examining Equity in Spatial Distribution of Recreational and Social Infrastructure in Delhi

Talat Munshi, Zia-ul-Haque and Yogi Joseph

Abstract A significant indicator of marginalization in Indian cities is the mismatch between infrastructure demand and supply. Accessibility studies have demonstrated how different areas within the same city enjoy variable amounts of accessibility to social infrastructure like schools and parks. Core areas of Indian cities generally enjoy good levels of accessibility while newly developing peripheral areas suffer most from the lack of adequate social infrastructure. Planning processes have failed to keep pace with market-led development. Sub-optimal levels of accessibility to social infrastructure can have negative implications on human development leading to increased marginalization of communities. This paper examines the accessibility to parks enjoyed by residents of Delhi's Zone-E bordering Ghaziabad and Noida. It claims that the master plan mechanism in Delhi has failed to ensure equitable access to parks. More specifically, it argues that the master plan mechanism has failed to recognize that actual densities on ground are far higher than those used while planning for social infrastructure. Additionally, the presence of physical barriers like expressways exacerbates the lack of accessibility since they discourage crossing by pedestrians and cyclists. The paper concludes by suggesting ways to arrive at a more equitable distribution of social infrastructure through preparation of local accessibility plans using participatory methods.

T. Munshi (✉)
Urban and Regional Planning Program, Faculty of Planning,
CEPT University, Ahmedabad, India
e-mail: talat@cept.ac.in

Zia-ul-Haque
Regional Centre for Urban & Environmental Studies (MoUD GOI), Lucknow, India

Y. Joseph
Centre for Urban Equity, CEPT University, Ahmedabad, India

S.S. Acharya et al. (eds.), *Marginalization in Globalizing Delhi: Issues of Land, Livelihoods and Health*, DOI 10.1007/978-81-322-3583-5_6

Keywords Accessibility · Inequity · Marginalization · Delhi · Master plan · Local accessibility plans

Background

Urban planning in India is based on a 'predict and provide' model that depends excessively on centralized allocation of resources. Planners use mathematical methods to project future population based on existing trends. The population estimates are used to allocate infrastructure (physical and social) using guidelines such as the Urban Development Plan Formulation and Implementation (UDPFI) guidelines (Ministry of Urban Affairs and Employment 1996).[1] The efficacy of this approach based on population projections that are often off the mark is debatable. Diwan (2009) and Ilhamdaniah et al. (2005) show that the ineffectiveness of conventional planning processes has left parts of cities in chronic deficiency of social infrastructure. The use of static zones, poor understanding of externalities of transport costs and neglect of the effects of an ill-regulated urban land market on land development has led to a severely lopsided development in Indian cities like Delhi. Individuals who can afford higher rents and transport costs are able to live in a location that has better services. The poor and lower middle class can seldom afford formal housing in cities owing to their low levels of affordability and lack of adequate supply of low-income housing.

The influence of urban form on social sustainability is complex as it touches upon issues of quality of life and social equity. In the USA, Europe and Australia it is considered that higher densities and mixed use urban forms lead to a better quality of life owing to greater social interaction fostering community spirit and cultural vitality (Rudlin and Falk 2009). Curtis (2008) lists proximity to work, shops and basic social, educational and leisure facilities as reasons for an enhanced quality of life. Most Indian cities have historically had highly dense cores as well as a rich mix of land use (Munshi et al. 2014). They would thus be expected to rank high on quality of life and social equity which is far from the truth in most cases. The typical problems in Indian cities result from a weakness of land use development control, particularly in peripheral areas of the city. This is typically on account of the failures of master plans[2] that have not been able to control urban sprawl and speculative peripheral development often at densities inadequate to be sustainably served by physical and social infrastructure (Dimitriou 2006). The resulting growth pattern is often a combination of organic growth and planned

[1]In the case of physical infrastructure like water supply and sanitation, Central Public Health and Environmental Engineering Organization (CPHEEO) manuals are used.

[2]Alternatively known as development plan in several Indian cities. A master plan is a long term perspective plan for guiding the sustainable planned development of the city. This document lays down the planning guidelines, policies, development codes and space requirements for various socio-economic activities supporting the city population during the plan period.

growth (Batty and Longley 1994). This type of growth is responsible for increased spatial segregation, social polarization and spatial inequalities (Castells 1996). Latin American and North American literature highlights the high social and economic costs of segregated living (Matsuo 2011; Korsu and Wenglenski 2010; Matas et al. 2010).

Given the lopsided and inequitable manner in which our cities have grown, equity of access has become an important dimension to evaluate the availability of opportunities. Parks and recreation spaces are important public goods that all members of the community must have access to. In the case of the well-to-do, lack of accessibility to parks may not be a major issue as they have easy access to private spaces of recreation such as clubs and gymkhanas. The poor and the lower middle class, on the other hand, depend on public parks and *maidans* for their recreational needs. This paper, taking the specific case of Zone-E[3] in National Capital Territory (NCT) of Delhi, highlights the spatial inequity in accessibility to parks using network distance-based accessibility measures. In the following section, a quick review of literature related to accessibility and equity is presented. This is followed by a description of the master planning process as followed in Delhi. Finally, accessibility analysis is used to highlight the spatial variability in accessibility to parks for various parts within the same zone of the city.

Equity and Accessibility

Equity refers to the justness or fairness with which a certain resource has been distributed (Smith 1986 as quoted in Nicholls 2001). There are multiple perspectives on equity including equality, compensatory, demand and market. While it would be interesting to operationalize the last three, owing to lack of sufficient data, this paper looks at equity from the equality perspective. Within equity studies with regard to accessibility to social infrastructure, there are 'outcomes' as well as 'process' studies. 'Outcomes' studies deal with the distribution of various resources relative to the socio-economic characteristics of residents while 'process' studies are interested in the reasons that cause such distribution.

Accessibility can be defined as 'ease of reaching', and is concerned with increasing the ability with which people in different locations, and with differing availability of transport, can reach different services or opportunities, such as employment, shopping and leisure (Stantchev and Merat 2010). Traditionally, accessibility-related studies have looked at efficiency of distribution as key to good accessibility based on Weber's location theory. Planners have used many techniques in the provision of social infrastructure. The UDPFI norms, for example specify that a city

[3]An administrative zone out of the fifteen that the National Capital Territory (NCT) of Delhi is divided into. A detailed discussion is presented later.

must have 10–12 m^2 of recreational facilities per person (Ministry of Urban Affairs and Employment 1996). Depending upon the size of the town (small, medium, large and metro), an allocation of 1.2 ha to 1.6 ha of recreational open spaces is recommended per 1000 persons. There are similar standards for smaller units such as a neighbourhood or cluster. This ‘container’ approach has many limitations, the least of them being that it disregards the spatial distribution of people as well as opportunities.

Elsewhere, there are instances where planners have used buffers of a fixed radius based on their impressions of walkable or cycling distances. People whose residences fall within these circular buffers (with their centre being the facility) are said to be ‘covered’ by the facility. Despite its advantages over the ‘container’ approach, it must be said that this ‘radius’ method disregards the fact that people can hardly travel in straight lines. Interruptions like compound walls, rivers, railway lines, etc, force them to rationalize their choice of access path to a service they might want to use. To overcome the disadvantages of the previous two approaches, this paper proposes to use the ‘network analysis’ method where individuals are allowed to make rational choices based on the characteristics of the choices available to them to reach the facility from their place of residence. Information on attributes like length and congestion prevalent on a road help people make these choices. For this purpose, network analysis using tools like ArcGIS® and FlowMap® are used to find out the relative accessibilities enjoyed by people to a facility like parks. This paper shares its methodology with Talen and Anselin (1998) who argue for a socio-spatial measurement of accessibility and use both the ‘radius’ as well as ‘network analysis’ methods to highlight the need to use the right method for accessibility analysis. They go on to assess the degree of equity based on the levels of access. Given the lack of sufficient data required to carry out such detailed analysis, the latter part is beyond the purview of this paper.

The Case of Delhi

As of 2011, the NCT of Delhi had a population of 16.32 million which forms a subset of the National Capital Region (NCR) with a population of 45.2 million (Registrar General of India 2011). NCT of Delhi is highly urbanized with 93.18 % of its population living in urban areas as against the national average of 31.16 %. During 1991–2001, the urban population of Delhi increased at 3.87 % annual growth rate. This rate of growth of population stabilized to around 1.8 % in the next decade. The 2021 Master Plan for Delhi (2005) is currently in force. It was prepared by the Delhi Development Authority (DDA) under the provisions of the Delhi Development Act 1957. Prior to the current plan, three plans were prepared at various points of time (Fig. 1 and 2) in response to various historical incidents. The philosophy of public sector led growth and development process continued in general till the process of economic reforms was initiated in the early 90s (Nath 2007). A review of the planning processes in Delhi (Munshi et al. 2015) reveals that, land demand for various uses is calculated assuming a residential development density of around 150 persons per hectare and implemented through master plans and zonal plans. However, in reality, barring Lutyen's Delhi, where most government bungalows and land is located, the DDA has been able to enforce very little control, owing to the inadequacies of development control regulations as well as faulty monitoring mechanism. As a result, against the planned densities of around 150 persons per hectare, vast parts of Delhi have ended up with four or more times that figure. Figure 2 illustrates how the built area in Delhi has expanded over the years (Fig. 1).

The case for selection of Delhi as a candidate for research is based upon the fact that unlike some of the other Indian cities, Delhi has had a history of strict state control over land for a long time with DDA acquiring agricultural land, providing infrastructure and auctioning the land for development. This should ideally have translated into good availability of social infrastructure like parks. However, given that the pressure on land is very high owing to the status of Delhi as the national capital and an important economic centre of North India, there is severe stress on green and open spaces. As this paper illustrates later, this has resulted in reduced accessibility to parks for a significant number of people. Delhi is divided into 15 zones starting from A to P as shown in Fig. 3. Of these, zones A–H are located completely in the urban area of Delhi. The zones J to L, N and P form part of the urban extension. Zone O is located in the riverbed and no development is allowed in that zone. Table 1 shows the existing population and holding capacity of these zones as well as the urban extensions. As is evident, Zone-E accommodates a population of 2.8 million as against its holding capacity of 1.8 million

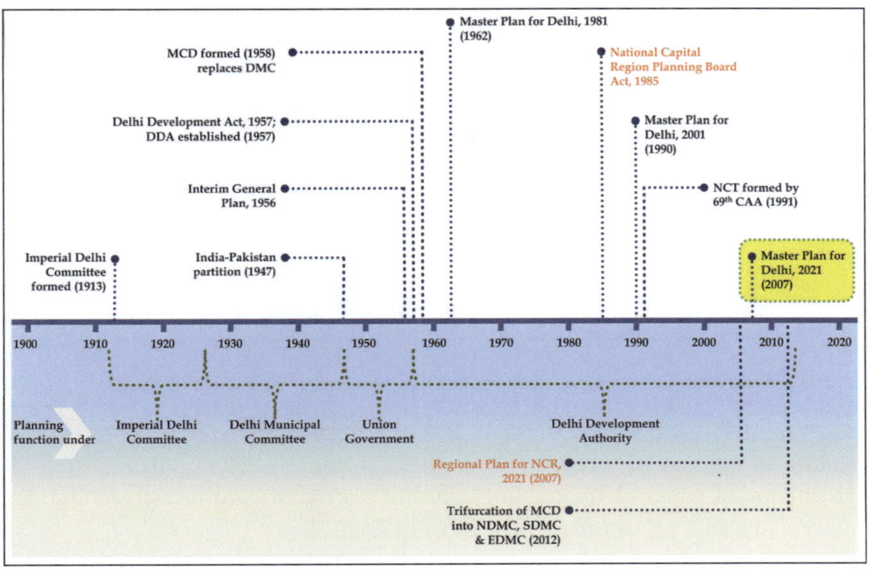

Fig. 1 Timeline of urban planning processes in Delhi in relation to historical incidents. *Source* Munshi et al. (2015)

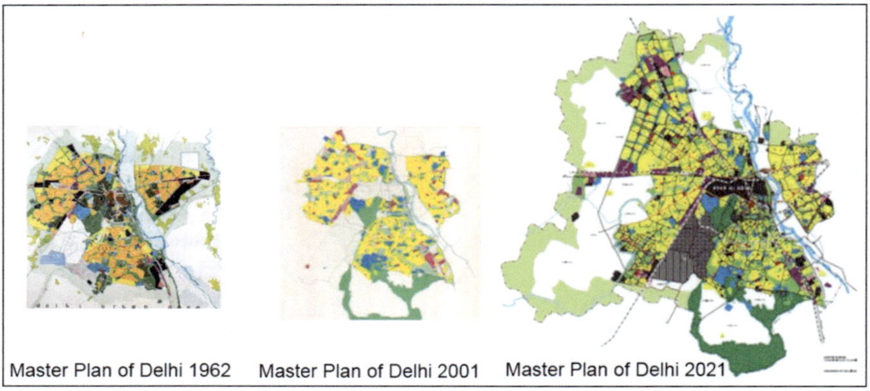

Fig. 2 Master plans for Delhi: Proposed land use. *Source* Delhi Development Authority (2005)

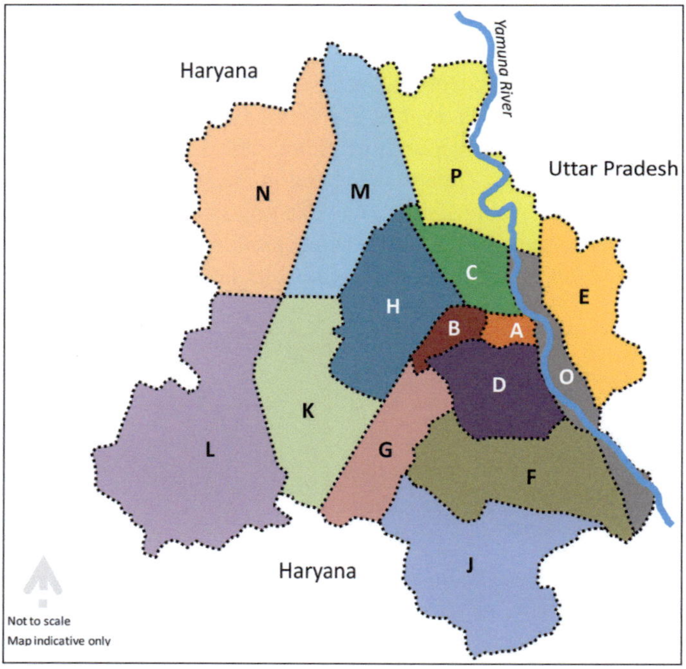

Fig. 3 Zones in NCT as per master plan for Delhi, 2021. *Source* Munshi et al. (2015)

resulting in a stress of around 156 % which is highest among other zones. The high amount of stress on the holding capacity motivates us to investigate the state of access to social infrastructure like parks in Zone-E.

Zone-E has a total area of around 88 km^2 which amounts to around 6 % of the total area of the NCT of Delhi. The 1962 Master Plan identified Zone-E for a balanced mix of land use. However, in the period between 1981 and 1992,

Table 1 Population in various zones in existing urban area of Delhi (2005)

Zone	Holding capacity '01	Existing population '01	Extent of stress (%)
A	4,20,000	5,70,000	136
B	6,30,000	6,24,000	99
C	7,51,000	6,79,000	90
D	7,55,000	5,87,000	78
E	17,89,000	27,98,000	**156**
F	12,78,000	17,17,000	134
G	14,90,000	16,29,000	109
H	18,65,000	12,26,000	66
Subtotal	89,78,000	98,30,000	109
Dwarka	32,22,000	10,70,000	33
Rohini-III			
Rohini-IV			
Narela			
Grand Total	1,22,00,000	1,09,00,000	89

Source Delhi Development Authority (2005)

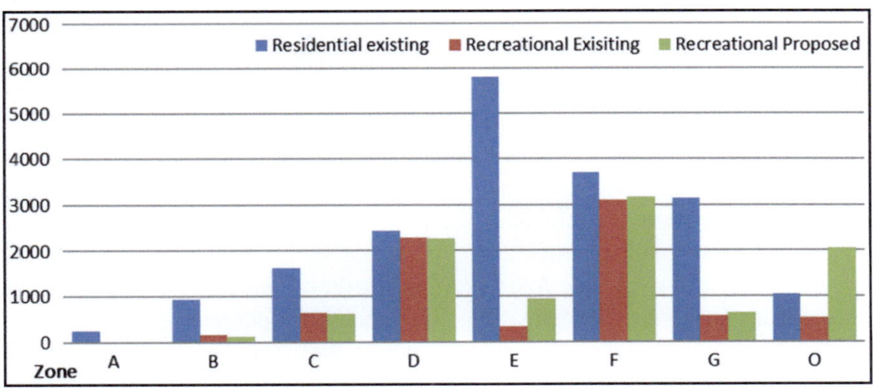

Fig. 4 Existing (2001) and proposed (2001) area (in hectares) under recreational use

the zone experienced exponential growth as its population increased from 0.75 million to around 2 million. The most visible repercussion of this development is felt on the area under recreational use and other social amenities. Figure 4 shows a comparison of existing and proposed recreational space. It is obvious that the existing recreational space is far below what was proposed. The proposed recreational space was to serve a population density of around 150 persons per hectare. As a result, a large section of the population living in the zone is not serviced. The case for other social infrastructure facilities is also likely to be similar.

Table 2 Land use break-up as per UDPFI guidelines

Land use	Size of the town			
	Small	Medium	Large	Metro
Residential	45–50 %	40–45 %	35–40 %	35–40 %
Commercial	2–3 %	3–4 %	4–5 %	4–5 %
Industrial	8–10 %	8–10 %	10–12 %	12–14 %
Public/semi-public	6–8 %	10–12 %	12–14 %	14–16 %
Recreational	12–14 %	18–20 %	18–20 %	20–25 %
Transport	10–12 %	12–14 %	12–14 %	15–18 %
Agri/water bodies	Balance	Balance	Balance	Balance

Source Ministry of Urban Affairs and Employment (1996)

Table 3 DDA-adopted norms for provision of parks

Category	Population per unit (lakhs)	Area provision (ha)	Proposed need (ha)
City park	10	3×100	300
District park	5	6×25	150
Community park	1	30×5	150
Historical monuments	–	–	600

Source Delhi Development Authority (2005)

The UDPFI guidelines (as shown in Table 2) prescribe that in metro towns the area under recreation space should be to the tune of 20–25 % and another 14–16 % of area should be reserved for public and semi-public spaces. These guidelines could also be questioned as they consider a fixed input density for all area proposed to be developed, which is around 150–160 persons per hectare. This in itself is much lower than the densities in most Indian cities. Second, the development control regulations are designed to decongest the city centre, thus the built up volumes are not very high. As a result, spill-over of commercial activities on to other spaces designated for recreation, public and semi-public uses are observed. The DDA has adopted population-based norms to assess area requirements for different categories of parks as shown in Table 3. It is clear that Zone-E requires about 600 ha of parks to serve the existing population. The proposal in the 2021 Master Plan (2005) is to earmark some land in Zone-O along the riverbed under this use. However, accessibility to these facilities is a function of the distance individuals have to travel to these locations. In the next section, we use network analysis methods to arrive at an assessment of locations that are serviced by the present provision of green spaces.

Accessibility to Recreational Facilities in Zone-E

Accessibility analysis is a useful tool for this purpose. Accessibility from the viewpoint of the user has been considered for the analysis. The impedance to people's travel has been taken as travel time, based on average speeds experienced on major roads. It must be noted that the average speed of Delhi roads is a function of the congestion experienced on these roads owing to various factors. The road network used for the analysis is complete to the level of neighbourhood level roads. It was digitized for the specific purpose of this research. Reasonable amount of accuracy can be claimed since the digitized network was observed to be fitting well on Google Earth® imagery. Zone-wise population data for Delhi was used to help distribute people spatially over land. The existing land-use map of Delhi came in handy in this process. The parks in the zone and around were identified from sources and marked according to their hierarchy.

Accessibility analysis requires the above data to be in machine-readable format. Since most of the above data is in raw format, it is required to convert the data to the above readable format for us to process the analysis. Since, ArcGIS® and FlowMap® software are used at various stages in this analysis; it was all the more essential to handle the collected data correctly. The residential area data is modelled in ArcGIS® software as origin locations. To this effect, Zone-E is tessellated into square blocks. Each tessellation is square in shape and measures one hectare in area with each side measuring 100 m. This size should ideally be as small as possible but depends largely on the capabilities of the machine on which this analysis is to be performed. The tessellations are then assigned with data on population and residential land-use component in that ward. Each centroid of the tessellation represents the origin of travel demand. Similarly, parks are located on the maps as destinations.

Roads have been considered to the order of local roads, thereby making the study as accurate as possible. People are modelled to take these travel paths to reach their parks from their residential locations. For roads not having relevant data, assumptions have been made on the average speeds experienced on roads of similar category in Delhi. Such assumptions are necessary in order to calculate the travel time taken for people to reach their destinations. The mode for travel used has been assumed to be either private or public modes. FlowMap® is used to perform accessibility analysis on the inputs generated in the previous step. For this purpose, a distance matrix was calculated which represented the travel distances between each of the centroids taken as origins and destinations, and using the network with its travel impedances. Potential accessibility (Geurs & van Wee 2006) from residence to parks was then measured based on destination-constrained accessibility model. Potential accessibility measures (also called gravity-based measures) have been widely used in urban and geographical studies since the late 1940s. The potential accessibility measure estimates the accessibility of opportunities in zone i to all other zones (n) in which smaller and/or more distant opportunities provide diminishing influences. The measure has the following form, assuming a negative exponential cost function:

$$A_i = \sum_{j=1}^{n} D_j \mathrm{e}^{-\beta c_{ij}}$$

where A_i is a measure of accessibility in zone i to all opportunities D in zone j, C_{ij} the costs of travel between i and j, and β the cost sensitivity parameter. In this case as it assumes that most individual will walk to the park the β is computed considering 500 m as the mean walking distance. Similarly, proximity analysis was done to find out the number of parks within a 10 min travel time from the residences. These provided us with the areas enjoying varying levels of accessibility.

The accessibility analysis reveals that 54 % of the residents are not able to access parks within a travel time of 10 min from their place of residence. This includes people who are not able to physically access a park within 10 min of travel time as well as those that are crowded out of parks. Figure 6 presents a map that shows the locations that do not enjoy access to parks within 10 min (Figs. 5, 7 and Table 4).

Table 5 shows that within the 46 % people that are able to access parks within 10 min, around 22 % people have access to only two parks and decreases progressively till only 1 % people have access to six parks (Fig. 8).

Table 6 shows that when the threshold is set to 5 min, the percentage of people who do not have access to parks increases to 75 %. Only 25 % people have access to at least one park. Only 4 % people have access to more than one park within 5 min (Fig. 9).

Table 7 reveals that only 16 % people need to travel more than ten minutes to access their nearest park. This may appear to be in contradiction to the 54 % people who have no access to parks. However, it must be considered that this is due to the capacity constraints. As Table 3 indicates, a community park is meant to cater to one lakh people. Given the paucity of parks in the neighbourhood, despite the parks being within reach, the quality of service is found to be low. Such parks appear crowded and are therefore not attractive to people (Fig. 7). This is vindicated by the catchment profile graphs as shown in Fig. 5 which indicates that when a threshold distance of 10 min is set, a majority of people are able to access parks

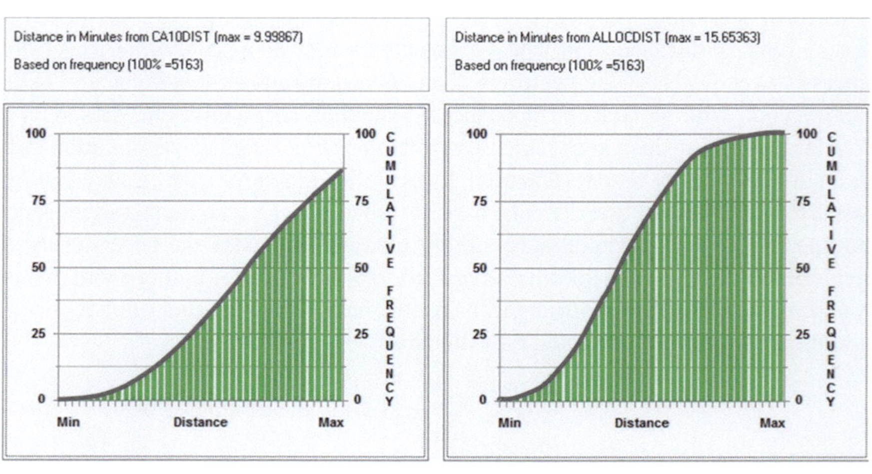

Fig. 5 Catchment profile display for allocation with 10 min threshold (*L*) and no threshold set (*R*)

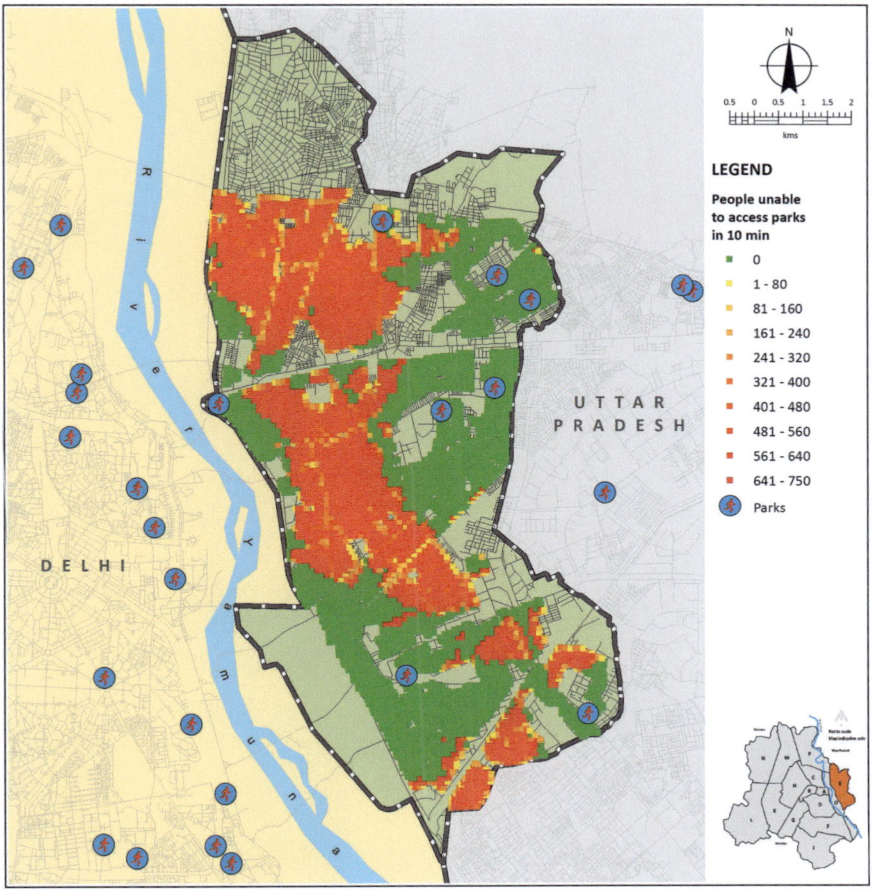

Fig. 6 Accessibility to parks within 10 min of travel time

only beyond 5 min. At the same time, when no thresholds are set, most people are able to access the parks. The concavity of the graph is higher when a threshold is set as opposed to when there are no thresholds.

Possible Interventions

Munshi (2016) illustrates the well-established relation between the built environment and mode choice. Land use policies must focus on accessibility and mixing of diverse uses, and transport supply will have to be location based to support non-motorized and public transport travel. As the accessibility analysis in the previous section demonstrates, a vast section of the residents of Zone-E is deprived of access to parks within walkable distances. Given the deprivation and

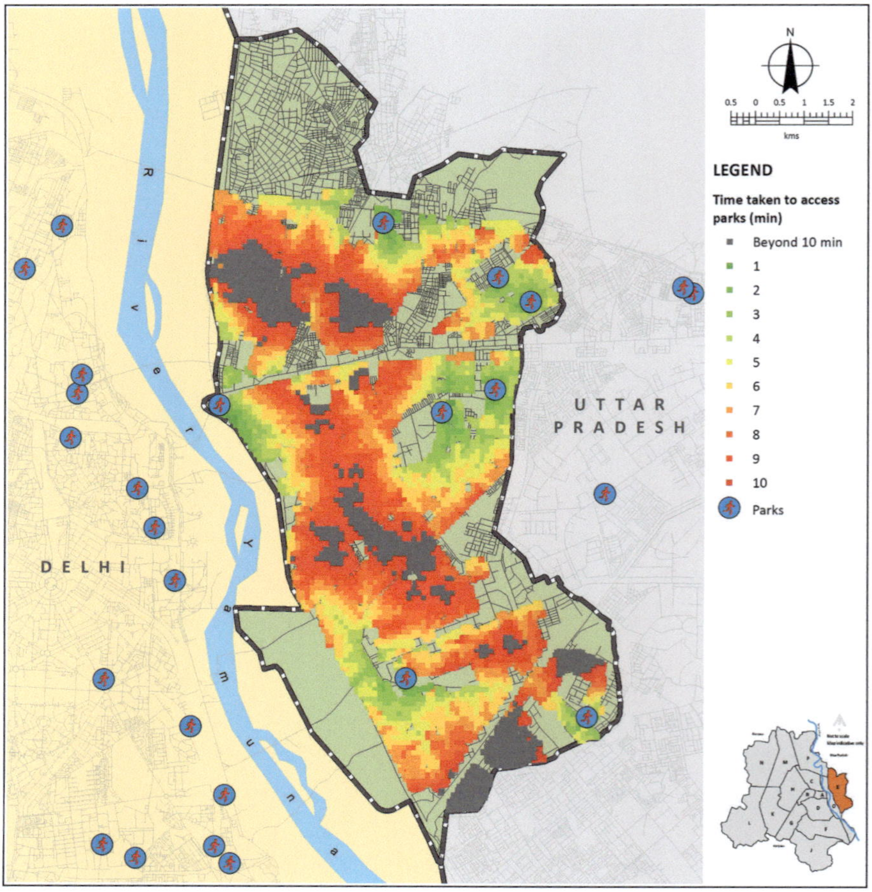

Fig. 7 Travel time taken to access the nearest park

Table 4 People served/not served by parks within 10 min of travel time

Particulars	Population	
	Sum	%
Served by parks	12,78,030	46
Not served by parks	15,19,970	54
Total	27,98,000	100

the previously documented effects of lack of access to recreational spaces, it is recommended that planners move towards addressing the issue. To start with, it is advisable to revise upwards the per capita requirement of recreational spaces. Our cities are only required to have only a quarter of recreational spaces per capita as compared to cities in the United States of America and United Kingdom. Also, the UDPFI standards and the proposed draft Urban and Regional Development Plan Formulation and Implementation (URDPFI) Guidelines (Ministry of Urban

Table 5 Number of parks in reach within 10 min of travel time

No. of parks	Population	
	Sum	%
0	7,620	0
1	15,13,517	54
2	6,02,107	22
3	4,77,654	17
4	1,25,760	4
5	50,290	2
6	21,052	1
Total	27,98,000	100

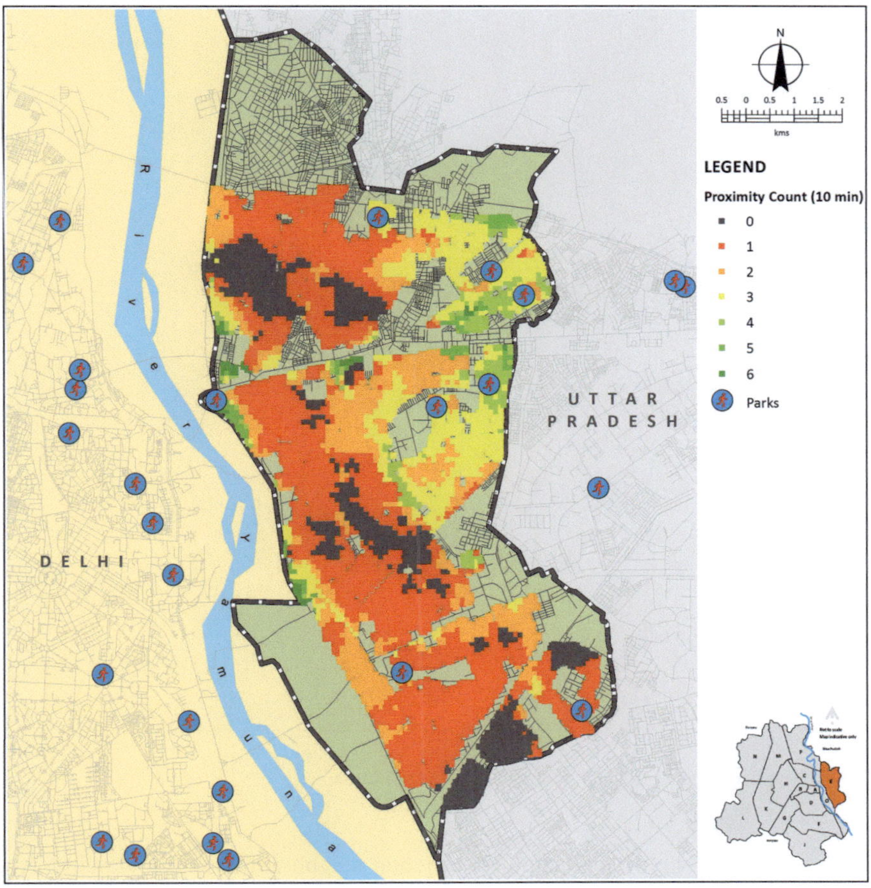

Fig. 8 Number of parks in reach within 10 min of travel time

Table 6 Number of parks in reach within 5 min of travel time

No. of parks	Population	
	Sum	%
0	21,06,506	75
1	5,74,086	21
2	1,16,812	4
3	596	0
Total	27,98,000	100

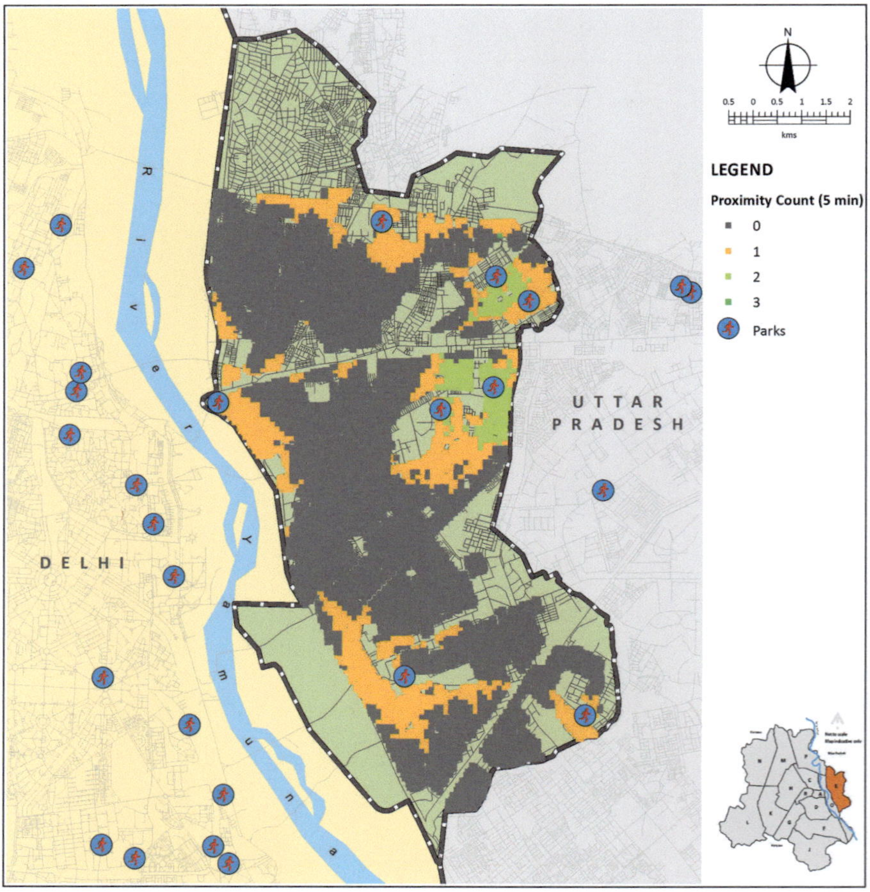

Fig. 9 Number of parks in reach within 5 min of travel time

Development 2014a, b) advocate only city and neighbourhood-level standards for provision of recreational spaces using the 'container' approach. The demerits of using such approaches are well documented in literature such as Nicholls (2001) and Talen and Anselin (1998). The inadequacy of recreational spaces in Indian cities bears witness to the ineffectiveness of the 'container' approach.

Table 7 Travel time taken to access the nearest park

Time threshold (min)	Population	
	Sum	%
Beyond 10	4,52,088	16
0–1	19,661	1
1–2	56,782	2
2–3	1,39,874	5
3–4	1,94,906	7
4–5	2,80,271	10
5–6	3,23,582	12
6–7	3,75,744	13
7–8	3,56,544	13
8–9	3,23,064	12
9–10	2,75,485	10
Total	27,98,000	100

Since acquiring land for public purposes is problematic in Indian cities, it is recommended that our cities consider using local accessibility planning in brownfield development. Joshi et al. (2013) demonstrate the need for such planning in the Indian context. Mahadevia et al. (2014a) present examples of how local accessibility planning has been used in international and Indian context. Mahadevia et al. (2014a) have developed and tested a methodology for local accessibility planning that uses participatory methods to prepare local are plans that are based on accessibility measures. When used in conjunction with town planning schemes[4] with appropriate legislative backup, the suggested local accessibility planning methodology can be effectively used to provide additional recreational spaces in brownfield environment. Since Delhi already has operational *mohalla* committees[5] for the past several years, they could be actively involved in the process.

Conclusion

This paper looks at Delhi's Zone-E and visualizes the levels of accessibility enjoyed by residents to various recreational spaces using network analysis methods as against the conventional 'container' or 'radius' approach. Additionally, it advocates the importance of accurately measuring distances from residences to

[4]For more on town planning schemes, please refer Ballaney (2013) who writes extensively on the development planning-town planning scheme mechanism that has proved to be a popular method of land development in Gujarat.

[5]It must be also mentioned that Lama-Rewal (2007) and Mahadevia et al. (2014b) warn about the problematic nature of residents welfare association led local governance mechanisms as they may sideline the voices of the marginalized.

destinations. The paucity of recreational spaces leads people to opt for alternatives. The well-to-do may access private clubs and recreation centres to get around the lack of access to public recreation spaces. They may also choose to relocate themselves to locations where there are enough avenues for recreation. The poor may resort to using streets and open plots for recreational spaces. People's cope-up mechanism in the event of lack of access to public spaces is a subject for further research. As also is the equity aspect of accessibility with specific regard to those sections of the society that are prone to marginalization. These groups may include less advantaged groups such as minorities and those whose housing characteristics indicate poverty. This paper concludes by suggesting interventions towards increasing the amount of recreational spaces in already existing neighbourhoods through participatory methods of local accessibility planning. These methods are a significant improvement over the current 'container' approach of arriving at social infrastructure requirements. It must be conceded, however, that the methods used in this paper do not differentiate between various recreational spaces on the basis of their quality or desirability among the residents. Finally, it is hoped that this paper highlights the spatial inequity in accessibility to parks in Zone-E of Delhi using network distance-based accessibility measures.

References

Ballaney, S., (2013). Supply of land for development: Land readjustment experience in Gujarat, India. In M. Permezel & V. Quinlan (Eds.), Nairobi: United Nations Human Settlements Programme.

Batty, M., & Longley, P. (1994). *Fractal cities: A geometry of form and function*. London: Academic Press.

Castells, M. (1996). *The rise of the network society: The information age: Economy, society and culture (Volume-1)*. New-Jersey: Wiley-Blackwell.

Curtis, C. (2008). Planning for sustainable accessibility: The implementation challenge. *Transport Policy, 15*(2), 104–112.

Delhi Development Authority. (2005). *Master plan for Delhi 2021*. New Delhi: Delhi Development Authority.

Dimitriou, H. T. (2006). Towards a generic sustainable urban transport strategy for middle-sized cities in Asia: Lessons from Ningbo. *Kanpur and Solo. Habitat International, 30*(4), 1082–1099.

Diwan, A., (2009). Planning for social infrastructure through accessibility for the city of Surat. Unpublished M. Plan Thesis, CEPT University Ahmedabad.

Geurs, K. T., & van Wee, B. (2006). Ex-post evaluation of thirty years of compact urban development in the Netherlands. *Urban Studies, 43*(1), 139–160.

Ilhamdaniah, Munshi, T., & Amer, S. (2005). Evaluating the planning of social infrastructures in Ahmedabad, India. In *Computers in Urban Planning and Urban Management (CUPUM) 2005 Conference* (pp. 1–11). London: University College London.

Joshi, R., Shah, K., Joseph, Y., Munshi, T., & Mahadevia, D. (2013). *A case for local accessibility planning in Indian cities*. Ahmedabad: Centre for Urban Equity, CEPT University.

Korsu, E., & Wenglenski, S. (2010). Job accessibility, residential segregation and risk of long-term unemployment in the Paris region. *Urban Studies, 47*(11), 2279–2324.

Lama-Rewal, S.T. (2007). Neighbourhood associations and local democracy: Delhi municipal elections 2007. *Economic & Political Weekly, XLII*(47), 51–60.

Mahadevia, D., Munshi, T., Joshi, R., Shah, K., Joseph, Y., & Advani, D. (2014a). *A methodology for local accessibility planning in Indian cities*. Ahmedabad: Centre for Urban Equity, CEPT University.

Mahadevia, D., Bhatia, N., & Bhatt, B. (2014b). *Resident welfare associations (RWAs) in BSUP sites of Ahmedabad: Experiences of mahila housing SEWA trust*. Ahmedabad: Centre for Urban Equity, CEPT University.

Matas, A., Raymond, J.-L., & Roig, J.-L. (2010). Job accessibility and female employment probability: The cases of Barcelona and Madrid. *Urban Studies, 47*(4), 769–787.

Matsuo, M. (2011). US metropolitan spatial structure and labour accessibility. *Urban Studies, 48*(11), 2283–2302.

Ministry of Urban Affairs and Employment. (1996). Urban Development Plans Formulation and Implementation (UDPFI) Guidelines, New Delhi: Centre for Research, Documentation & Training—Institute of Town Planners, India.

Ministry of Urban Development (2014a). *Urban and regional development plan formulation and implementation (URDPFI) Guidelines* (Vol. I). New Delhi: Ministry of Urban Development, Government of India.

Ministry of Urban Development. (2014b). Urban and regional development plan formulation and implementation (URDPFI) guidelines (Vols. II (A) and II (B)). New Delhi: Ministry of Urban Development, Government of India.

Munshi, T. (2016). Built environment and mode choice relationship for commute travel in the City of Rajkot, India. *Transportation Research Part D: Transport and Environment, 44*, 239–253.

Munshi, T., Joshi, R., Adhvaryu, B., Shah, K., Joseph, Y., Christian, P., et al. (2015). *Landuse transport integration for sustainable urbanism: Inputs for the development planning process*. Ahmedabad [Forthcoming]: Centre for Urban Land Policy, CEPT University.

Munshi, T., Zuidgeest, M., Brussel, M., & van Maarseveen, M. (2014). Logistic regression and cellular automata-based modelling of retail, commercial and residential development in the city of Ahmedabad, India. *Cities, 39*, 68–86.

Nath, V. (2007). *Urbanization, urban development, and metropolitan cities in India*. New Delhi: Concept Publishing Company.

Nicholls, S. (2001). Measuring the accessibility and equity of public parks: A case study using GIS. *Managing Leisure, 6*(4), 201–219.

Registrar General of India. (2011). Census of India: Population Enumeration Data (Final Population). Retrieved February 9, 2014, from http://www.censusindia.gov.in/2011census/population_enumeration.aspx

Rudlin, D., & Falk, N. (2009). *Sustainable urban neighbourhood: Building the 21st century home*. Burlington: Architectural Press.

Stantchev, D., & Merat, N. (2010). *Equity and accessibility: thematic research summary*. Delft: Transport Research Knowledge Centre.

Talen, E., & Anselin, L. (1998). Assessing spatial equity: An evaluation of measures of accessibility to public playgrounds. *Environment and Planning A, 30*(4), 595–613.

Land Acquisition Policy and Praxis: The Case of Peri-urban Delhi

Chinmoyee Mallik and Sucharita Sen

Abstract Until recently, land acquisition in India had been undertaken closely following the provisions laid down by the Land Acquisition Act of 1894 (i.e. during the time of this study) which was created by the colonial powers to seize private property in consonance with their imperialist motives. This Act has been amended several times by the State Governments. These amendments generally have pertained to the elaboration of compensation issues and have shrewdly retained the ambiguities to make way for corruption. The new land acquisition act has come to force only on 1 January 2014 and it has been referred to as "The Right to Fair Compensation and Transparency in Land Acquisition, Rehabilitation and Resettlement Act, 2013" (henceforth refereed to as the New Act). Although it marks a step forward in sensitively addressing some of the earlier concerns, it is not without a few loopholes that need to be questioned. This paper discusses the critical elements of the Land Acquisition Act of 1894 in comparison to the New Act, and through the case study of land acquisition in a village located in the urban fringe of Delhi, attempts to look into the nuances of the interlinkages between land dispossession and livelihood transformation. Specifically, this paper tries to assess the efficacy of the provisions laid down in the previous act in relation to the village study and attempts to comment upon implications of the livelihood outcomes of the farmers losing land to the state perpetrated land acquisition. This paper is composed of four sections. Section 1 contextualizes the study. Section 2 attempts

C. Mallik (✉)
Birati College, Kolkata, India
e-mail: chinmoyeemallik@gmail.com

S. Sen
Centre for the Study of Regional Development, School of Social Sciences,
Jawaharlal Nehru University, New Delhi, India
e-mail: ssen.jnu@gmail.com

S.S. Acharya et al. (eds.), *Marginalization in Globalizing Delhi: Issues of Land, Livelihoods and Health*, DOI 10.1007/978-81-322-3583-5_7

to critically discuss some of the provisions of the Land Acquisition Act 1894 and 2014 in relation to its implication to the land dispossessed. Section 3 elaborates upon the case study of land dispossession in a fringe village in Delhi with a view to highlight the drawbacks of the Land Acquisition framework in India. Section 4 attempts to conclude the discussion bringing out the concerns persisting in the current law with reference to the case study.

Keywords Land acquisition policy · Praxis · Disposation · Livelihood transformation · Peri-urban Delhi

The Context

Land, one of the most critical ingredients for any project, has emerged as the most contentious element, its acquisition being a sensitive matter of concern for the policy makers. Contemporary Global South in general and India in particular has been marked by processes of agricultural land grabs where land has been both a scarce resource and at the same time supports the livelihoods of majority of the population. In India, land, besides being a means of production, stands as a symbol of status of the households (Mearns 1999). Further, incidence of poverty is highly correlated with landlessness (Mearns 1999; Hanstad et al. 2004; Cotula et al. 2006). So, dispossession of land, which is central to rural livelihood, stands out as one of the most sensitive issues of concern.

Until recently, land acquisition in India had been undertaken closely following the provisions laid down by the Land Acquisition Act of 1894 (i.e. during the time of this study) which was created by the colonial powers to seize private property in consonance with their imperialist motives. This Act has been amended several times by the State Governments. These amendments generally have pertained to the elaboration of compensation issues and have shrewdly retained the ambiguities to make way for corruption. The new land acquisition act has come to force only on 1 January 2014 and it has been referred to as "The Right to Fair Compensation and Transparency in Land Acquisition, Rehabilitation and Resettlement Act, 2013" (henceforth refereed to as the New Act). Although it marks a step forward in sensitively addressing some of the earlier concerns, it is not without a few loopholes that needs to be questioned.

This paper very briefly discusses the critical elements of the Land Acquisition Act of 1894 in comparison to the New Act, and, through the case study of land acquisition in a village located in the urban fringe of Delhi, attempts to look into the nuances of the interlinkages between land dispossession and livelihood transformation. Specifically, this paper tries to assess the efficacy of the provisions laid down in the previous act in relation to the village study and attempts to comment upon implications of the livelihood outcomes of the farmers losing land to the state perpetrated land acquisition.

This paper is composed of four sections. Section 1 contextualizes the study. Section 2 attempts to critically discuss some of the provisions of the Land Acquisition Act 1894 and 2014 in relation to its implication to the land dispossessed. Section 3 elaborates upon the case study of land dispossession in a fringe village in Delhi with a view to highlight the drawbacks of the Land Acquisition framework in India. Section 4 attempts to conclude the discussion bringing out the concerns persisting in the current law with reference to the case study.

The Land Acquisition Framework in India: An Appraisal

> No statute in colonial India or independent India has been used against the interests of the poor in such a systematic and widespread manner, causing misery, as the Land Acquisition Act, 1894. From independence up to 1995, millions of persons were displaced from land due to a variety of reasons including forcible displacement for public projects. The judiciary has played a significant role in executing this statute without care for the effects of land acquisition on small and medium landholders and on agricultural labourers…

(Colin Gonsalves, senior advocate of the Supreme court of India and the executive director of Human Rights Law Network, India, 2010)

It has been evident that through the history of India's development trajectory that the "judiciary [has] remained oblivious to the suffering of the rural people" (Gonsalves 2010) and that there has been very crafty manipulation of the provisions in the Land Acquisition Act to ensure benefits to specific sections of the society. It is therefore worthwhile to take a critical overview of the specific provisions of the Land Acquisition Act of 1894 that have been commonly subjected to denigration. However, issues that are not directly relevant for the case study has not been elaborated in this paper.

(a) *Doctrine of Eminent Domain and Definition of 'Public Purpose'*

The origins of the term Eminent Domain can be traced to the legal treatise written by the Dutch jurist, Hugo Grotius in 1625, which proclaims the sovereign rights of the State to obtain private property for the public use and the reciprocal duty of the State to make good the loss thus negotiated by the owner. This doctrine has two precise components: first, the notions of compulsory and unquestionable stand of the state regarding acquisition of private property; second, the elaboration of the ambit of 'public purpose'.

The constitution of India considers the State as the sole owner of all property and extends supreme authority to take over any privately owned possession. This authority has been irrevocable and unquestionable. The clause of 'public purpose' institutionalizes and eventually justifies all encroachments of the State upon private property rights. This second component of what defines a 'public purpose'[1] has been perhaps the most treacherous element in association with the 'eminent domain' doctrine as it has the potential to engulf any fragment of the economy, if not clearly defined. This definition has undergone modifications several times, the most far reaching being that during the 1962 and in 1984 which allowed for acquisition for a private enterprise in addition to State enterprise, provided there has been a proclaimed 'public purpose'. The New Act has further widened the scope of "public purpose" by incorporating land acquisition by the Government for Public Private Partnership (PPP) projects. This leads to the next issue of concern, that is, Government acquisition for private company/PPP project.

(b) Gover*nment acquisition for private company/PPP*

The concern related to the sub-clause of government acquisition on behalf of any 'company' has been fallout of the broad definition of the purview of 'public purpose'. The exponents of government acquisition for private enterprise argue if any industrialist would have to obtain land directly from the farmers for any project, the hassles inherent to the process would potentially discourage any such initiatives. According to them, dominance of small and marginal land holdings, associated with unwarranted litigations flowing from poorly maintained land records are potential negative catalysts that can delay the commencement of any project (Morris and Pandey 2007). The eminent domain aspect of the state alone has been enabled to overcome this resistance. It is therefore convenient for the private entrepreneur if the state acquires land and makes it available to the capitalist. It follows logically that the relative capability of any state to make land available to the capitalist has emerged as the sole inducement to attract private investment into the state. Consequently, in the post-economic reform era, the states have been competing with each other, in a bid to succeed in a race to the bottom, to provide land at subsidized rates to the corporates to attract private investments and in turn squeezing the small agricultural land owners and those dependent on the land, leading to an unhealthy land ethics. In the neoliberal regime, with a pointed focus on urban-centric growth led by private investments, it is left to the states to create a 'favourable' business environment, often at the cost of their own electorates. Increasingly, a larger public acceptability of such processes is promoted through a new language that encourages states to create conditions for 'ease of doing business' through 'tax incentives' (as opposed to 'tax terrorism'), which undermines the basic principles of democracy. Thus, a political economy framework is necessary to appreciate the repositioning of the so-called 'democratic' state in the neo-liberal regime with respect to the corporate sector, and the fluid transition of the concept of 'public purpose' in these times.

[1]Public purpose of land acquisition generally refers to land requirements for the defence sector, infrastructure provisioning including government offices, hospitals, educational institutes, land for creating housing for the poor as well as project or natural calamity affected people and the like. In short, it encompasses all those endeavours that promise to extend benefits to the general public. It has been detailed under section 3 f of the 1894 Act and section 2 (1 & 2) of the New Act.

The other component of this discourse on government acquisition for corporations very deftly overlooks the basic issue of the unrealistic exposition of a 'benevolent capitalist' investing in public purpose and perpetually emphasizes the need for the state's eminent domain doctrine to overcome the resistances to industrialization. It indeed fails to question how a 'profit- minded' capitalist, who has come to set up an industry to enhance his gains, would strive for the cause of public or a social purpose and not really be committed to the cause of profit making (Basu 2007). It is surprising that an obvious fact that a capitalistic mode of production with an overt objective of profit maximization would fail to substantively address egalitarian issues as regional development or employment generation has bypassed the policy makers. Also, there is no political will to think through the ways in which such investors, that presumably represent 'public purposes' can be held accountable if they fail to achieve the above-mentioned objectives.

The New Act, besides smoothening the process of state acquisition for the corporate, has included some additional clauses (Clause 2 and 3 of Section 2) that are indeed significant, but their efficacy may be questionable. There are three basic inclusions—firstly, mandatory consent of 80 % of 'affected families' in case of state acquisition for private companies, and 70 % consent in case of public–private partnerships; secondly, the provision of the social impact assessment of the project-affected population; and thirdly, compulsive applicability of rehabilitation and resettlement in areas where land is obtained by private companies either through the Government or through direct negotiation. There are some concerns in relation to Clause 3 at least theoretically, to make the land acquisition law less authoritative and more participatory in case of its transfer to the private companies through the State. Given the political economy involved over the land issue, it may be problematic to rely too much upon the issue of "consent" of the "affected families". The process by which 'consent' would be sought is crucial as the process has been left to the discretion of the respective states and there are no universal guidelines provided in the New Act. It leaves the possibility open for the land broker to seek approval of the affected families through unfair means. Though the provision of social impact assessment, for the first time, consideres the landlesses' dependence on land, their identification is an extremely complex task and therefore, perhaps undermines its practical relevance.

(c) *Issue related to compensation*

Among the major issues related to compensation, here the two most significant components would be discussed

Computation of Compensation: The method commonly followed uses the average land price of all transactions taking place during the recent 3 years (obtained from land sale deeds) in the region selected for acquisition and a solatium of 30 % is added over the base price obtained in addition to the value of any other property that stands damaged due to the acquisition. The concerns arising out of this principle may be outlined as follows. First, the use of market price as the basis for evaluating the base land price in an economy that has been known for imperfect rural market has been unanimously acclaimed as the single most factor leading to undervaluation of the acquired land. Second, land transactions in India have been not only few, but also not well documented. Distress sale constitutes a considerable share of transactions and the full value is often concealed to escape stamp duty (Ghatak and Ghosh 2011). Third, the lack of clarity in land titles and inadequacies in the legal protection to private property operate actively as a further depressant of the market price of land (Morris and Pandey 2007). Thus, the choice of the prevailing market price obtained from land transaction documents seems to be inherently flawed.

The New Act, although have not shifted away from the previous theory and methodology of estimating the compensation value, it has amended some of its provisions. Market value determined through average sale price for similar type of land situated nearest to the village (for last 3 years) continues to be the basis for determining compensation[2] with all the drawbacks already discussed. However, there are three new additional subsections in the New Act. (i) some scope for negotiation in determining the compensation in case of state acquisition for private company, (ii) inclusion of a multiplier for the market value, which, however, is left to the discretion the State Government, and (iii) a solatium amount of 100 % imposed upon the estimated compensation value to arrive at the final award. Among these new inclusions, the factor of multiplier is slightly problematic as there are no standard guidelines outlined in the Act. For example, the multiplier, which can be a maximum of 4 times, till now ranges from 1.01 for Maharastra to 2 times in Rajasthan. Nonetheless, the New Act undoubtedly assures higher compensation to the affected families and somewhat addresses the earlier concerns regarding poor compensation. Also, the guideline in relation to the timeliness of disbursement of compensation is indeed appreciable.

Coverage of compensation net The other controversial aspect of the compensation issue concerns its coverage. Owing to improper documentation of property owned, often there has been problem in the identification of the real owner of landed property which has been notified for acquisition. Often, legal procedures entailing division of property among the heirs have not taken place that has frequently complicated both identification of the stakeholder as well as the disbursement of compensation.

The more sensitive concern centers round the question of inclusivity of all those who endure loss of livelihood rather than only those whose properties have been acquired. The Act of 1894 currently stipulates compensation entitlements to the land owners and registered bargadars[3] only. Clearly, in India, where the land reform has been far from being successful, an entitlement for the registered tenants is a farce in itself. Also, there had not been any effective legislation to compensate the agricultural labourers and other rural labour dependent upon the acquired plot of land in the 1894 Act.

---

[2]Detailed in section 26 of the New Act.

[3]The bargadars are entitled to receive 25 % of the compensation amount payable to the land owners according to 1894 Act.

The New Act has widened the definition of "affected families" to include the landless labourers as well as tenants (registered or usufruct rights), i.e. those whose livelihoods have been attached to the acquired land in addition to the land owners. The real challenge that has been associated with this well-intended amendment encircles around the problem of identification of "affected families" and the disbursement of compensation to each of them for livelihood loss. Additional compensation for multiple displacements is another addition that imparts a more humane facet to the compensation issue. Further, it has outlined an extensive resettlement and rehabilitation package in the form of employment guarantees, annuities, company shares, land-for-land, share of appreciated land value after resale, and replacement of lost homestead[4] and other such provisions which indeed marks a step forward all of which has been critiqued for not only promise increasing administrative costs but suffering from the gap of identification of stakeholder (Ghatak and Ghosh 2011; Chakraborty and Gupta 2012).

Land Dispossession and Livelihood Transformation in Peri-urban Delhi

The previous section discussed the critical elements of the Land Acquisition Act (1894) focusing upon the major areas of concern. This section presents a case study of land acquisition in a village lying in Northwest Delhi to look into the impact of land acquisition upon the livelihood status of the affected households. Delhi is expanding very rapidly, has possibilities of expansion in all directions, intruding into the states of both Haryana (Gurgaon and Faridabad districts) and Uttar Pradesh (Ghaziabad district). The city is thus guided by governance norms of both the states, and unlike most other large metropolitan cities in India, has experienced a multipolar growth, incorporating the cities in the adjoining districts, one of the most important one being Gurgaon. Particularly, in the post liberalization period, this expansion has been a landscape composed of modern residential buildings as well as for corporate houses and shopping malls, superimposed on the older landscape of villages and agricultural spaces. In most cases, the older settlements have remained intacts, with the agricultural land rapidly making way for new developments. This section attempts to trace the trajectory of livelihood transition of the land dispossessed with a view to assess the efficacy of the provisions laid down by the land Acquisition Act of 1894. The case study seeks to address the following questions: with some dependence on land, how land dispossession gets

[4]According to Ghatak and Ghosh (2011) although these provisions have introduced some amount of flexibility, these have not been secured against corrupt practices. For instance the employment guarantee option does not outline the conditions of job termination and allow the industrialist to sack the farmer who had been employed. Also, the partial payment of compensation in the form of company shares expose the farmers to the risks associated with it to add on to impending agony in relation to his incompetence in managing finance.

implicated in the emergent livelihoods? Who copes better with land loss and what is the role of the colonial land acquisition framework in determining the divergent shades of livelihood adjustments? A conjectural elaboration of remote interrelation is sought between the case study and the New Act, trying to speculate about implications for livelihood outcomes.

Rani Khera village located in Northwest Delhi where 19 % of agricultural land had been acquired through a notification in 2007 has been selected as the area of study. This village has been randomly selected from a group of villages having both relatively high share of acquired area after 1991 and persistence of agriculture. Rani Khera, falling within the NCR of Delhi has been exposed to urban influence for a considerable period. Yet, agriculture appears to be the predominant livelihood for the many people.

Methodological Issues and Data

This section is based on an exploratory field survey conducted during April 2008, where information was collected both at the households levels. The sample consists of 30 households (196 persons in total) selected purposively such that at least some of the family members of the household had been engaged in agricultural work prior to land acquisition. Questionnaire was canvassed at both household and individual level. Though the study is based upon small sample size and hence does not employ rigorous statistical analysis, it has been able to bring out significant issues that pave the pathway for further research.

Analysis and Results

i. **Change in Primary and Secondary Occupation**

Within the rural economy, owing to the seasonality of agricultural activity and uncertainty associated with it, farm households generally dwell upon multiplicity of activities. It often spans various types of activities associated with the farm-like crop cultivation along with livestock rearing and fishing. It may also comprise of a mix of farm and non-farm enterprise. In essence, such multiplicity of livelihood activities renders the household resilient to unforeseen perturbations that may potentially affect their sustenance. Hence, to effectively understand the working of the rural economy, it must look into at least the principal and subsidiary occupations of a household.[5]

Broadly it may be noted that following land acquisition, 15 out 36 persons who reported agriculture as their principal occupation have been displaced such that the

[5]Although the initial analysis discusses the trends of both principal and subsidiary occupations, the later part of the analysis pertains to the former only to focus on the major trends only.

Table 1 Change in the shares of the broad principal and subsidiary occupation categories (2007–2008)

Occupation categories	Occupations before land acquisition (2007)				Occupations after land acquisition (2008)			
	Primary occupations		Secondary occupations		Primary occupations		Secondary occupations	
	Count	Percent	Count	Percent	Count	Percent	Count	Percent
None	14	7.1	97	49.5	24	12.2	112	57.1
Agriculture	36	18.4	86	43.9	21	10.7	70	35.7
Non-agriculture	34	17.3	10	5.1	40	20.4	11	5.6
Students	55	28.1	2	1.0	55	28.1	2	1.0
Housewife	57	29.1	1	0.5	56	28.6	1	0.5
Total	196	100	196	100	196	100	196	100

Source Field Survey (2008)
Note Population above 5 years of age has been taken as often children are also engaged in agriculture as secondary occupation

share of workers having agriculture as principal occupation has declined from 18.4 to 10.7 % within just one year (Table 1). While a marginal increase in the share of workers in non-agriculture has been observed, there has been an increase in the share of non-workers from 7.1 to 12.2 % within 1 year. In terms of absolute numbers, out of the 15 people who were displaced from agriculture as principal occupation, only six of them have been able to secure alternative employment in the non-agricultural sector while the remaining nine have become jobless.

With respect to agriculture as subsidiary occupation, it has been observed that out of the 86 members who reported being in agriculture, 16 got displaced such that the share declined from 43.9 to 35.7 % within 1 year (Table 1). Out of the displaced agricultural workers, only one has been accommodated in non-agriculture while the remaining 15 persons have become unemployed with respect to subsidiary status work. So, the share of workers having no subsidiary occupation increased from 49.5 to 57.1 % (Table 1). The erosion of subsidiary activities has rendered households more vulnerable.

The displacement of the farmers and the virtual absence of their subsequent absorption into non-agricultural work highlights the incapability of the ensuing urban labour market to accommodate the additional labour released from agricultural sector. On the other hand, it also reflects the inability of the land dispossessed farmers to seize whatever opportunities exists. There is adequate evidence from earlier studies to insist upon the possibility of a stark mismatch between the stock of skill of the hitherto farmers and the human capital demand of the jobs available. The Act of 1894, in spite of its prevalence for now over a century, has not addressed this issue adequately. Although it mentions passingly that the land requiring body must impart skill to the "affected families" (by the 1894 Act it refers to the land owners and registered tenants only), it has rarely been effectively implemented. Also, by not including the most vulnerable group, that is the non-land owning but land dependent households, much of the relevance of this provision is self defeating.

ii. Occupational Shift and Category of Household

The land dispossessed households have been categorized into 'partially land lost' and 'completely land lost' for those who owned some land prior to land acquisition. There is a third category viz 'never owned land' that refers to the tenant farmers who have lost access to the tenanted holding following land acquisition by DDA. The first two categories of farmers are the ones who have received compensation by virtue of owning the acquired land. The latter group has been generally bypassed by the compensation net as the sampled households were unregistered tenants.

The nature of shift of workers who were in agriculture has been different for the different categories of households. While some of the agricultural workers from households affected by land acquisition have exhibited occupational shift, those hailing from the households that never lost any land are continuing with agriculture as primary and secondary occupations (Table 2). Such a phenomenon indicates that land continues to be a very significant source of livelihood and that urbanization has not offered enough opportunities which may act as a pull factor for shifting away from agriculture. Had there been any such pull factor operative, some of the member of the households unaffected by land acquisition would have shifted out of agriculture voluntarily.

For agriculture as principal occupation, worse affected have been the households who completely lost land and those who were tenant cultivators. A shift towards wage work from self cultivation as principal occupation is exhibited by members from these two categories of households (Table 2). Shift towards non-farm work

Table 2 Category of household and change in primary occupation (2007–2008)

Category of households		Change in primary occupation					Total
		Not applicable[a]	Cultivator to wage labourer	Agricultural worker to non-farm work	Agricultural worker to unemployed	Continuing with earlier agricultural occupation	
Never lost any land	Count	0	0	0	0	4	4
	Percentage	0.0	0.0	0.0	0.0	100	100.0
Partially lost land	Count	1	0	1	3	14	19
	Percentage	5.3	0.0	5.3	15.8	73.7	100.0
Completely lost land	Count	0	1	2	0	0	3
	Percentage	0.0	33.3	66.7	0.0	0.0	100.0
Never owned land	Count	1	2	3[b]	4	0	10
	Percentage	10.0	20.0	30.0	40.0	0.0	100.0
Total	Count	2	3	6	7	18	36
	Percentage	5.6	8.3	16.7	19.4	50.0	100.0

Source Field Survey, 2008

[a]This includes those individuals who left agriculture due to old age and has no relation to land dispossession

[b]Out of these three in non-farm, two are into petty non-farm work like vegetable vending and construction wage worker

has been more for the land-owning households than the tenants. It reiterates the proposition that even for diversification towards non-farm work, access to land plays a vital enabling role (Hanstad et al. 2004; Mearns 1999; Cotula et al. 2006). It has also been argued that land owners diversify their livelihoods to accumulate, while the landless and near landless diversify to survive (Ellis 1998). It is probable that access to land facilitate the land owning households' shift towards non-farm work, although induced by a push factor. For the landless households, this shift is principally towards petty non-farm work like vegetable vending. About one-fifth of the total land dispossessed population has become unemployed. About 40 % of the agricultural workers from landless households and 15.8 % of the partially land lost households that have become unemployed.

The preceding analysis reveals that the land-owning households have been relatively less affected by land dispossession because they already had alternative sources of income. Nonetheless, all the households suffering reduced access to land perceive deterioration in their livelihood. The different livelihood outcomes of the land-owning and landless tenant farmers emanate from their pre-existing differences in terms of education as well as economic status. In addition, the compensation receipt by land owners and its absence in case of the tenant farmers have furthered the differentiations sharpening the diverging livelihood outcomes.

Conclusion

The case study has pointed out the extreme vulnerability of the landless tenant farmers who do not own land but are considerably dependent on land. The study has revealed that although the villagers have been exposed to prolonged urban influences, land continues to be an integral part of their lives. Their proximity to urban area have not delinked their livelihoods from land-based activities. Asset ownership has emerged as a very significant enabling factor for diversification of livelihood towards high-return non-farm activities in response to land dispossession. The difference in the nature of occupational shift of the agricultural workers hailing from landed and landless households point towards the fact that access to land has played a very important role in determining the direction of occupational shift following land acquisition. This study has revealed that state perpetrated land acquisition and the compensation policies fail to take cognizance of the most disadvantaged groups comprising of the tenant cultivators and the agricultural labourers which is corroborated by the findings of other scholars. These two groups already lack asset ownership and through the land acquisition essentially lose their livelihoods. They are not compensated for their economic displacement. It also emphasizes the role of compensation in making good the loss of land at least partially. One of the major drawbacks of the earlier Act (1894) of not compensating the dependent on land other than the land owners has been substantively addressed in the New Act. The revision of the compensation provision in the New Act promises a significantly higher amount that is likely to trigger less unrest among the land losers. The New Act has includes the allowance of a provision of an increase in the compensation money upto four times to be implemented by the respective states. But as observed from experience, most states, like Maharastra and Rajasthan, have fixed the multiplier at half or less than the proposed benchmark. In an environment marked by an incessant competition among the states to make their territorries more attractive to public investment, it is unlikely that the other states would make this provision any higher than they have to. As mentioned above, the rates that apply for compensation are those of the revenue circles, and are much less than the actual market price of land. According to experts, a multiplier of 4 would be nearly equivalant to the actual market price in most places. On this count, the New Act has only partially fulfilled its objective to grant a 'fair' compensation to the farmers. But importantly, the inclusion of the consent clause and social impact assessment, in spite of problems associated with them, are the highlights of the New Act. These clauses, in their spirit, upholds the democratic principles on which the Nation State should act. The amendmends proposed in 2014 by the current Government, attempted to dilute precisely these principles, and hence faced justifiable opposition from a large number of political parties, civil society and farmers' groups that led to suspension of these amendments. In sum, it can be expected that the New Act, if implemented in its spirit, would not only reduce the injustice meted out to the affected population, but could create conditions for a broader consultative process with them that would be in agreement of the idea of social justice enshrined in the Constitution of the country.

References

Basu, P. K. (2007). Political economy of land grab. *Economic and Political Weekly*, 1281–1287.

Chakraborty, S., & Gupta A. (2012). Manabik Sarkar k Jomi Adhigrahan kortei hobe. *Anandabazar Patrika*, 7th February.

Cotula, L., Toulmin, C., & Quan, J. (2006). Policies and practices for securing and improving access to land. In *International Conference on Agrarian Reform and Rural Development (ICARRD)*, Issue Paper No. 1. Retrieved from http://www.icarrd.org/en/icard_doc_down/Issue_Paper1.pdf

Ellis, F. (1998). Household strategies and rural livelihood diversification. *Journal of Development Studies, 35*(1), 1–38.

Ghatak, M., & Gosh, P. (2011). The land acquisition bill: a critique and a proposal. Working Paper No. 204, Center for Development Economics, Department of Economics, Delhi School of Economics.

Gonsalves, C. (2010). Judicial failure on land acquisition for corporations. *Economic & Political Weekly, XLV*(32), 37–42.

Hanstad, T., Nielsen, R., & Brown, J. (2004). *Land and livelihoods: Making land rights real for* India's *rural poor*. Livelihood Support Programme, Working Paper 12, Rural Development Institute (RDI), USA. Retrieved from ftp://ftp.fao.org/docrep/fao/007/J2602E/J2602E00.pdf

Mearns, R. (1999). Access to land in rural India: Policy issues and options. World Bank Policy Research Working Paper No. 2123. Retrieved from http://papers.ssrn.com/sol3/papers.cfm?abstract_id=636208

Morris, S., & Pandey, A. (2007). Towards reform of land acquisition framework in India. *Economic & Political Weekly, 42*(22), 2083–2090.

Part II
Livelihoods and Vulnerability

Neo-Liberal Urbanization, Work Participation and Women: Comparing the Urban and Peri-urban Contexts of Delhi with Mumbai and Kolkata

Sucharita Sen

Abstract Urban spaces impacted by liberalization have not provided enough opportunities to work outside home for women. This paper compares the employment patterns of men and women in three cities both in urban cores, peri-urban areas and the residual parts of the respective states in which or adjacent to which three major metropolitan cities are located in. The paper concludes that though the urban locales of the peri-urban areas have been doing better in many respects vis-a-vis the residual states, these benefits are not distributed equally. Women are worse off in terms of work opportunities and unemployment rates in the peri-urban areas, and such conditions can be explained by the social and demographic changes that have taken place in the peri-urban areas around the large metropolitan cities. With a smaller household size and a lower working age-group sex ratio compared to the interior districts, the possible care burden on the adult women of the households could be a factor explaining their low work participation in these areas.

Keywords Urbanization · Core and Peri-Urban · Gender differences · Work and neo-liberal environment

In developing countries, a substantial and growing proportion lives in or around metropolitan areas and large cities, including the zone termed the 'peri-urban interface'. The interaction of the rural and the urban is often marked with contestations rather than smooth continuity of a transformation towards the urban.

S. Sen (✉)
Centre for the Study of Regional Development, School of Social Sciences, Jawaharlal Nehru University, New Delhi, India
e-mail: ssen.jnu@gmail.com

S.S. Acharya et al. (eds.), *Marginalization in Globalizing Delhi: Issues of Land, Livelihoods and Health*, DOI 10.1007/978-81-322-3583-5_8

The regions around the large metropolitan areas are often extremely vulnerable, particularly for those living in the margins of economic space, though they are in no way homogenous. They constitute the labourers, many of whom are migrants from adjoining rural areas and they have to undergo a transition in terms of entering the urban labour market, from agricultural land-based activities. In the current economic regime, the peri-urban areas around the large metropolitan regions have assumed a new dimension. The macro-growth process has become necessarily urban-centric, since the areas in and around the large cities, having better base infrastructure yield higher returns to investment. Since profits and related considerations drive the destination of the private investments, they have concentrated around the large cities in India in the post-reform period (Chakravorty 2000). Such investments entail massive changes in land-use and very often entail conversion of agricultural land to non-agricultural uses.

The transformations that take place in terms of land-use around the metropolitan cities in the post-globalization era are thus increasingly as a result of global or domestic private capital inflows. The new landscape includes large investment projects often involving "high-end" infrastructure, new industrial and service activities, the construction of new housing colonies and commercial ventures catering primarily to upper income groups. In a study that focuses on development around Hyderabad, it has been argued these are the outcome of a process of political assertion on the part of the regional government in the sphere of economic policy-making (Kennedy 2007). These policies have been successful in attracting investments from private firms, often by subdividing peri-urban spaces and increasing spatial differentiation (Kennedy 2007). The local decision-making processes, however, has weakened as a result of such larger policies and the space for a participatory and inclusive system in local urban issues have shrunk drastically. The peri-urban areas are even worse off, and are most often administratively outside the reach of the urban governance initiatives, though the land-use and resulting livelihood changes that are observed in these zones are almost entirely due to the urban-centric growth processes. In other words, the expansion of the city often alter patterns of rural natural resource use, that cause far-reaching social, cultural and economic changes for the people living in the peri-urban regions of large metropolitan cities (Narain 2009).

The work pattern changes are likely to have a gendered nature and women are expected to be impacted differently from men due to the selective nature of both cultural norms and economic opportunities. It is expected that with new and diversified opportunities for work in the urban areas that is characterized by a significant amount of flexibility in the production system of the post-Fordist era, women would find work opportunities suiting their comparatively restricted circumstances. India's experience, however, deviates significantly from the above pattern. Not only have women's work participation rates been historically far lower than that of men in the country, an additional matter of concern is that the overall rates have fallen consistently for the last quarter of a century (Abraham 2013; Chandrasekhar and Ghosh 2013). Explanations as prosperity-induced withdrawal driven by increases in real wage rates and education-related withdrawal for the younger age group have been offered as the primary reasons for such trends (IGAS 2012; Abraham 2009; Srivastava and Srivastava 2010; Himanshu 2011). Given the larger context of deceleration of women's work participation rates in the country, it is important to understand whether the workspaces in the peri-urban areas offer women specific opportunities emerging out of the process of urbanization, or they expose them to new vulnerabilities not observed in other regions. Also, since the women's burdens with their non-negotiable domestic responsibilities and care-giving role to the household is culturally rooted, on which the macroeconomic processes superimpose themselves, it is relevant to examine whether the work patterns with respect to them are more regionally embedded, or has a homogenized pattern due to the neo-liberal environment. *The paper specifically looks into the gendered work characteristics, in and around the three metropolitan cities of Delhi, Kolkata and Mumbai and specifically focus on work participation and wage rates vis-à-vis the states (residual) in which they are located over two period of time.*

Data and Concepts

Unit-level data of the employment-unemployment rounds (61st and 68th) of the National Sample Survey Organization would be used for the analysis. To analyze the effect of urban expansion on the peri-urban regions, the present study has grouped the analysis into three kinds of spaces—the metropolitan areas, districts adjoining the metropolitan cities (henceforth referred to District Around Metros or DAM) which represents the peri-urban areas, and the remaining district of the relevant states. The study area includes Delhi, Mumbai and Kolkata. Consequently, the study includes the following regions:

a. Delhi metropolitan area.
b. Districts around Delhi in Haryana that includes Gurgaon, Faridabad, Jhajjar and Sonipat. These together are taken to represent the peri-urban areas of Delhi due to data limitations. The districts adjoining Delhi in the east that falls in the state of Uttar Pradesh have not been included in the analysis.
c. Residual State (Delhi): The remaining districts of Haryana to provide a benchmark for the region outside of the peri-urban area.
d. Mumbai metropolitan area.
e. Districts around Mumbai and Greater Mumbai which includes Thane and Raigarh.
f. Residual State (Mumbai): Remaining districts of Maharastra.
g. Kolkata Metropolitan city.
h. Districts adjoining g, i.e. North and South 24 Parganas, Howrah and Hooghly.
i. Residual State (Kolkata): Remaining districts of West Bengal.

Most part of the study deals with the working age group, and hence the work patterns among children and the elderly is outside the scope of the study. To fulfil the broad aim of comparing access to livelihoods and livelihood status, two groups of variables have been used for the analysis.

1. Employment status by the usual activity status as defined by the National Sample Survey Organization in the Employment-unemployment rounds.[1] The analysis also includes categories of workers as *self-employed, regular wage/ salaried employee and casual wage labourer.*[2]
2. Wage rates comparison across the three spatial units.

---

[1]**Usual activity status:** As per the NSSO Employment-Unemployment rounds, the usual activity status relates to the activity status of a person during the reference period of 365 days preceding the date of survey. The activity status on which a person spent relatively longer time (major time criterion) during the 365 days preceding the date of survey is considered the *usual principal activity status* of the person. To decide the usual principal activity of a person, he/ she is first categorized as belonging to the labour force or not, during the reference period **on the basis of major time criterion**. Persons, thus, adjudged as not belonging to the labour force are assigned the broad activity status 'neither working nor available for work'. For the persons belonging to the labour force, the broad activity status of either 'working' or 'not working but seeking and/ or available for work' is then ascertained again on the basis of the relatively longer time spent in the labour force during the 365 days preceding the date of survey. Within the broad activity status so determined, the detailed activity status category of a person pursuing more than one such activity will be determined again on the basis of the relatively longer time spent.

[2]As per the Employment-Unemployment rounds, workers have been divided into the following categories: **Self-employed:** Persons who operate their own farm or non-farm enterprises or are engaged independently in a profession or trade on own-account or with one or a few partners are deemed to be self-employed in household enterprises. The essential feature of the self-employed is that they have *autonomy* (i.e., how, where and when to produce) and *economic independence* (i.e. market, scale of operation and money) for carrying out their operation. The remuneration of the self-employed consists of a non-separable combination of two parts: a reward for their labour and profit of their enterprise. The combined remuneration is given by the revenue from sale of output produced by self-employed persons *minus* the cost of purchased inputs in production.
The self-employed persons may again be categorized into the following three groups:
(i) **own-account workers:** They are the self-employed who operate their enterprises on their own-account or with one or a few partners and who during the reference period by and large, run their enterprise without hiring any labour. They may, however, have unpaid helpers to assist them in the activity of the enterprise.
(ii) **employers:** The self-employed persons who work on their own-account or with one or a few partners and by and large run their enterprise by hiring labour are the employers, and
(iii) **helpers in household enterprise:** The helpers are a category of self-employed persons mostly family members who keep themselves engaged in their household enterprises, working full or part time and do not receive any regular salary or wages in return for the work performed. They do not run the household enterprise on their own but assist the related person living in the same household in running the household enterprise.
Regular wage/salaried employee: Persons working in other's farm or non-farm enterprises (both household and non-household) and getting in return salary or wages on a regular basis (and not on the basis of daily or periodic renewal of work contract) are the regular wage/ salaried employees. *This category not only includes persons getting time wage but also persons receiving piece wage or salary and paid apprentices, both full time and part time.*
Casual wage labour: A person casually engaged in other's farm or non-farm enterprises (both household and non-household) and getting in return wage according to the terms of the daily or periodic work contract is a casual wage labour.

Comparing the Contexts of Peri-Urban Areas of the three Metropolitan Cities

Peri-urban areas of large metropolitan cities in existing literature have been considered to be potentially under both positive and negative influences of the processes of urbanization. It can be argued that the nature of influences that the metropolitan areas would have on their fringes would be dependent on the characteristics of the metropolitan area and the specific processes of growth that each of these centres are associated with. Though in the larger environment of globalization, they are expected to have a larger set of commonality, the consequences of these processes are likely to manifest differently given the local contexts.

Delhi is much larger compared to the other two cities under consideration. The satellite cities of Gurgaon, Faridabad and Noida, which are concentrated hubs of post-globalization industrial growth, constitute a continuum with Delhi Metropolitan Area. Mumbai and Kolkata, for different reasons, have little potential for areal expansion (Table 1). Thus Delhi is likely to interact directly, among other things, in terms of land transfers in its peri-urban area, compared to Mumbai and Kolkata. The rural areas around Delhi is highly developed agriculturally, which is not the case with the other two cities. Thus the peri-urban areas of Delhi is likely to be in a constant state of flux because of the physical transition that has become fast-paced particularly after the post 1991 regime of globalization and large city-centric growths. Also the rural peripheries are thus also likely to respond positively to increased urban demand of high-value agricultural commodities.

As a result of the above characteristic of Delhi, the rural component in terms of nature of livelihood in its the peri-urban fringe is much more pronounced, followed closely by Kolkata (Fig. 1). Mumbai's peri-urban area as defined by the study is much more urban in character than the other two metropolitan cities. The expansion of economic activities in the post-liberalization period is likely to be more functionally linked in the urban areas around Mumbai, and this may have resulted in increased spread of urbanization in the surrounding districts of Mumbai. Maharashtra agriculture, other than its sugarcane belt has been characterized by high instability due to its rain-fed characteristics. Its cotton belt has been particularly volatile and has been associated with farmers' distress resulting in a large number of suicides. Such vulnerabilities have been often associated with

Table 1 Comparison of selected parameters of three metropolitan cities

Parameters	Delhi	Mumbai	Kolkata
Area (km^2)	1483	157	185
Density (per km^2)***	9340	21190	24760
GDP in $ ID BN (2008)**	167	209	104
PWC rank**	37	29	61
MPCE *(in Rs)	2346	2342	3157
Spending Propensity*	60 %	54 %	65 %

Source ***Census of India 2011 **Price Water Cooper *NSSO 66th round

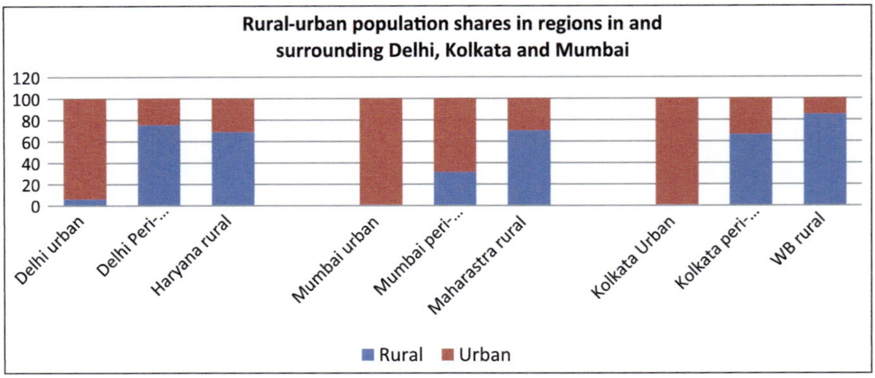

Fig. 1 Rural–urban population shares in regions in and surrounding Delhi, Kolkata and Mumbai

Table 2 Comparison of selected demographic characteristics in Urban core, Peri-Urban and residual districts

City	Variables		Urban core	Blocks around metro	residual districts
Delhi	Population Growth rate*	Urban	−2.07	7.00	−4.25
		Rural		−1.97	−3.50
	Household size		4.3	4.9	5.3
	Urban population share			56.1	13.1
Mumbai	Population Growth rate*	Urban	0.39	5.94	3.85
		Rural		0.96	0.77
	Household size		4.5	4.2	4.4
	Urban population share			89.3	51.0
Kolkata	Population Growth rate*	Urban	−0.17	8.95	3.00
		Rural		−1.52	0.19
	Household size		4.4	4.3	4.4
	Urban population share			38.0	38.9

Note *2001 over 2011
Source Census of India 2001 and 2011

diversion of resources to urban areas that fed into the non-primary sectors. This gets enhanced by the fact that the direct dependence on land as a means of livelihood is the maximum in the rural peri-urban areas of Mumbai compared to even its counterpart around Delhi (Table 2), where agriculture as a means of livelihood is significantly more profitable than Mumbai. Land as a means of livelihood is the least important in the districts around Kolkata (Table 2).

Though in terms of future potential to expansion into its immediate peripheries both Mumbai and Kolkata are restricted, there are significant differences between these two metropolitan cities (Table 1). Mumbai is the financial capital of India and in terms of its GDP, average income levels and in terms of its global ranking it is far ahead of Kolkata. In fact, in terms of most of these parameters, Delhi

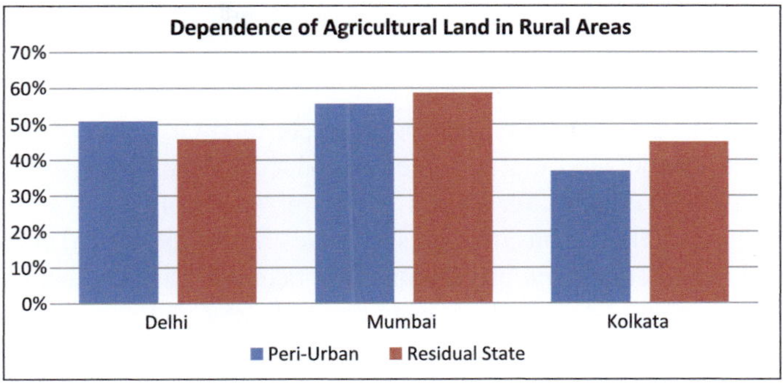

Fig. 2 Dependence of agricultural land in rural areas

is positioned in between the other two metropolises. Kolkata citizens spend a higher percentage of their income compared to its counterparts in both Mumbai and Delhi. The lower growth of Kolkata in terms of efficiency parameters could be rooted in the nature of development model followed by the West Bengal communist regime for many years in the past, notwithstanding the recent changes in this model that departed significantly in spirit from its slogan of 'land to the tiller'. Its past footprints could also result in lower inequality levels within and between the peri-urban areas and rural interiors (Fig. 2).

Impact of Urbanization on Demographic and Economic Parameters

In general, it has been observed that the post-reform growth in India, as in case of China has been associated with increased capital accumulation with an associated contribution of labour productivity to Total Factor Productivity (TFP) growth, with a major share of the growth coming from the services sector in case of India (Bosworth and Collins 2007). As mentioned before, much of this period has been associated with low employment generation in the non-agricultural sector, with the burden falling on the agricultural sector, characterized by far lower wage rates compared to the non-farm sector. Consequently, the shift of workers from agriculture to non-agricultural sector contributes to a very small percentage of the total growth in the economy. These trends have significance for the peri-urban context, where the demand for local economy to absorb agricultural worker to the non-agricultural fold is high due to the visible changes in land-use.

Social and Demographic Impacts of Urbanization Processes

The above-mentioned problem becomes more critical due to the current trends of urbanization that is visible in the peri-urban regions. In the past decade in India, there has been a clear stagnation of population in cores of the large metropolitan centres, accompanied a very rapid population growth in districts around the metropolitan cities, Bangalore being the only exception out of the metropolises (Kundu 2011). This trend gets explained by lower levels of rural to urban migration to these cities, a phenomenon that has been explained by the process of 'elite capture' of large cities, coming out from a policy of 'sanitizing' these cities (Kundu and Ray Saraswati 2012). Thus, though such cities have experienced an increase in income levels and better basic provisions, such benefits, have, in fact been exclusionary, through processes that have been contradictory and contentious, and not consensual, as some of the vision documents of the local bodies have projected (Kennedy and Zérah 2008; Kohli 2006). It has been noted from the experiences of Hyderabad and Mumbai that the city governance in both cases that are different in many other ways, have been narrowly defined as extending interface with the people and the Government through increased use of information and communication technology, rather than the more basic issue of agenda prioritizing (Kennedy and Zérah 2008). Such processes have given rise to not only the crowding of the hinterlands, but also what has been termed as 'degenerated peripheries', which have performed poorly in terms of basic services, and have been 'dark areas' with respect to urban municipal governance (Kennedy and Zérah 2008; Kundu 2009; Dupont 2007). Such processes would tend to have links with informalization of labour possibly leading to increased subsidiarization of work, along with some potential opportunities of getting higher wage rates emerging out of the expansion of non-agricultural activities for the households in the peri-urban areas.

The population growth rates in the peri-urban areas of the selected metropolises have been far higher not only compared to the city-cores and but also the residual states (Table 2). This does indicate migration from other parts of the state or outside in the last decade to the peri-urban areas. Additionally, the sex-ratio for the working age-group is mostly highest in the residual states, followed by the peri-urban regions, and the lowest in the core with the exception of Kolkata for the first comparative position (Fig. 3). It may be reasonable to conclude from the above

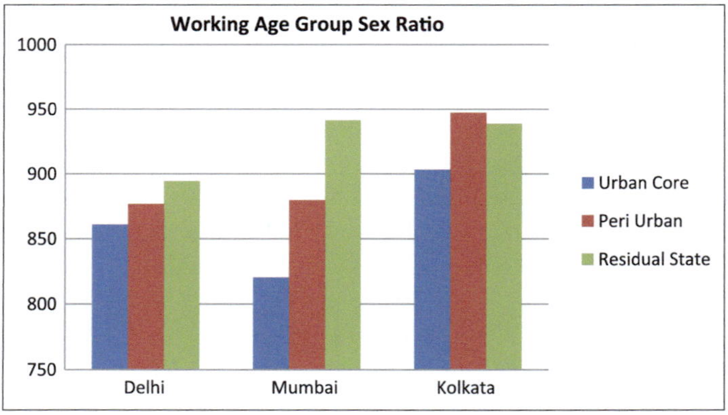

Fig. 3 Working age group sex ratio

that migration in the city-cores has typically been more male-selective, compared to that in the peri-urban areas, where more women have accompanied the male members of their families. The net land outflow from agriculture to non-agricultural activities is likely to impact the native population, particularly those living in the rural areas, and the households that were engaged in agriculture as well as those dependent primarily on agricultural wage work. It may be expected that the male members from both the migrant households as well as those affected by land outflows from agriculture are likely to be part of a transient working population, who may be engaged more than one short-term work or commuting to urban cores for work. This would have implications for the women of these households, who either may not be able to participate in the job markets or be able to take up only subsidiary and part-time occupations, having to handle the burden of the household in an alien environment without the social support of the extended family or being a part of a household where the earning members may be adjusting to new occupations, or both.

Economic Impacts of Urbanization and Rural Urban Differences

The linkages between the rural and urban areas are probably the most visible and inescapable in the peri-urban areas, particularly around the cities that are expanding fast. The distinctions between the rural and the urban, it has been argued, become less clear in these areas (Tacoli 1998).

Urbanization is seen to have positive externality effects on the rural peripheries too, along with negative ones. On the one hand, while it leads to a reduction of availability of land along with economic and social displacement in terms of rural livelihoods, there is evidence to believe that agriculture around the peripheries become more profitable either through intensification of land-use or a shift to high-value agriculture or both (Chadha et al. 2004). However, such high-value agriculture is unlikely to be able to compete in the long run for scarce land and labour resources, unless alternative production technologies for fruits, vegetables, flowers and the like become available (Midmore and Jansen 2003). Thus even the agriculture-dependent population who do not directly suffer land dispossession, are in a state of flux as they constantly compete with activities that are likely to overtake agriculture in terms of their ability to pay land rents.

Table 3 provides a rough comparison of the economic status of urban-core, peri-urban areas and the residual states. Some of these indicators are also an expression of rural–urban linkages. It may be observed that in urban areas both in terms of monthly per-capita consumption expenditure (MPCE) and the wage rates, there is a continuum from the urban core, peri-urban areas to the residual states taking these three spatial platforms in totality, a few city-wise differences notwithstanding. A higher MPCE may also reflect a higher cost of living, but taken considered in conjunction with a higher wage rate, this trend may be taken to indicate a more prosperous living. However, in rural areas, the overall peri-urban and residual state differences of the two variables under consideration are negligible.

Table 3 Economic continuum from Urban core to the residual states in Delhi, Mumbai and Kolkata

Sector	Cities	Geographical units	MPCE	Wage rate
Rural	Delhi	Peri-Urban	2137	349
		Residual state	1856	300
	Mumbai	Peri-Urban	1249	224
		Residual state	1498	224
	Kolkata	Peri-Urban	1353	197
		Residual state	1267	227
	All Metros	Peri-Urban	1473	235
		Residual state	1483	236
Urban	Delhi	Urban core	3389	596
		Peri-Urban	4050	796
		Residual state	2605	484
	Mumbai	Urban core	4003	497
		Peri-Urban	3479	460
		Residual state	2182	389
	Kolkata	Urban core	3042	413
		Peri-Urban	2329	376
		Residual state	1843	362
	All Metros	Urban core	3559	523
		Peri-Urban	3039	486
		Residual state	2160	397

Source Calculated from NSSO Employment-Unemployment Round (68th), 2011–12

Delhi's urban surroundings appear to have done better than both the city core and the residual area, both in terms of MPCE and wage rates in rural areas as well (Table 3). The urban foci of Gurgaon arguably lends itself to such patterns in urban areas, that can be termed as a strong 'intervening opportunity', stronger, in this case, than the urban core. The developed irrigated agriculture around Delhi leads to sharp differences in rural areas.

So far as share of non-workers is concerned, in the rural areas, the residual states in totality have a lower share compared to the peri-urban regions (Table 4). This could be due to a variety of reasons, including positive factors as greater share of children and youth attending educational institutions in the peri-urban regions. A matter that is of concern is that the share of workers on principal status,[3] a group that is better off than workers in the subsidiary status, is lower in the peri-urban regions, compared to the residual states for rural workers, and compared to the city core and by a smaller margin, the residual states in the urban

[3]A worker working only on the principal status is one that has round-the-year work or work for a major part of the year. The other workers are those who are working either only on subsidiary status, or on both principal and subsidiary status (two or more jobs) are ones who can be assumed to be in a greater amount of distress than the first group.

Table 4 Work participation rates across spatial units and gender in Delhi, Mumbai and Kolkata

		Male		Female		Female to male ratio of WPR	
		UPS[a] (%)	UPSS[b] (%)	UPS (%)	UPSS (%)	UPS	UPSS
Rural							
Delhi	Peri-Urban	77.7	78.2	9.8	27.1	0.13	0.35
	Residual	75.6	76.0	8.4	22.3	0.11	0.29
Mumbai	Peri-Urban	83.5	84.9	**18.8**	**56.8**	**0.22**	**0.67**
	Residual	79.9	80.8	46.1	56.4	0.58	**0.70**
Kolkata	Peri-Urban	**82.5**	**84.0**	**14.9**	29.1	0.18	0.35
	Residual	84.4	86.3	15.7	27.5	0.19	0.32
Total	Peri-Urban	81.8	83.0	**14.8**	**40.4**	0.18	0.49
	Residual	81.1	82.4	29.1	33.3	0.36	0.40
Urban							
Delhi	Urban Core	76.1	76.2	14.2	14.8	0.19	0.19
	Peri-Urban	**73.2**	**73.2**	14.5	***16.1***	***0.20***	***0.22***
	Residual	74.4	74.9	11.3	13.3	0.15	0.18
Mumbai	Urban Core	79.8	80.5	26.7	28.2	0.33	0.35
	Peri-Urban	78.0	78.7	**19.8**	**22.7**	0.25	0.29
	Residual	77.5	77.9	18.6	21.8	0.24	0.28
Kolkata	Urban Core	77.9	80.7	20.5	28.2	**0.26**	**0.35**
	Peri-Urban	***81.8***	***83.6***	**15.1**	**22.7**	**0.18**	**0.27**
	Residual	78.5	79.2	17.5	22.3	**0.22**	**0.28**
Total	Urban Core	78.0	78.8	20.7	22.9	**0.27**	0.29
	Peri-Urban	79.0	80.1	17.0	21.9	**0.21**	0.27
	Residual	77.3	77.8	17.5	20.9	**0.23**	0.27

Source Calculated from NSSO Employment-Unemployment Round (68th), 2011–12

[a]UPS or the Usual Principal Status is based on the principal work done by a person for the majority of the year

[b]UPSS or the Usual Principal and Subsidiary Status is based on the principal work as well as the shorter time work done by an individual. The difference in UPS and UPSS is the addition of the workers who are non-workers in the principal status, but working in the subsidiary status to the latter

areas. With this rider, the sectors that are associated with higher wage rate and security have a greater presence in the peri-urban areas. The share of worker in the peri-urban regions working in the non-farm sector as opposed to farm sector, and those in the organized enterprises as opposed to unorganized enterprises, is higher than in the residual states. The barriers to entry to the non-farm sectors are known to be higher in both the non-farm and organized sectors, as opposed to their respective counterparts, and the fact that more of the peri-urban population are engaged in such sectors is indicative of a set of higher levels of skill in these areas (Jatav and Sen 2013).

Though in terms of most of the parameters discussed above, most of the peri-urban areas seem to have gained from the opportunities typically associated with urbanization, there is empirical support to believe that women are often not able to access the opportunities with the same ease with men (Raju 2013; Paul and Raju 2014). Given the above evidences, there is a strong case to examine how the rapid economic changes that entail both opportunities and vulnerabilities impact the work characteristics of women as opposed to that of men in the peri-urban areas, and whether these characteristics are regionally embedded or dominated by the larger macro political economic considerations.

A Gendered Analysis of Employment Characteristics in Rural and Urban Peri-Urban Areas: A comparison of the Metropolitan Areas and Rural Interiors

It is important to look at employment stated through a gendered lens, as the context of peri-urban areas is likely to impact to women differently from men. Peri-urban areas could provide new employment opportunities, particularly in the urban parts, and these employment opportunities are likely to be skewed in favour of men rather than women. Such differences could result from limited access to skills and formal education among women and their relatively restricted physical mobility. In the rural sector, when men leave agriculture in favour of urban activities that fetch higher wage rates, women are usually left back in agriculture with added responsibilities.

The overall unemployment situation for the three metropolitan cities selected for the study is the highest in the peri-urban areas (Fig. 4). Also, the difference between males and females are extremely high (Fig. 4). This is explained by the trend in the urban parts of the three spaces that we have taken for the analysis. It is clear from Table 4 that the male female unemployment rate differences not only

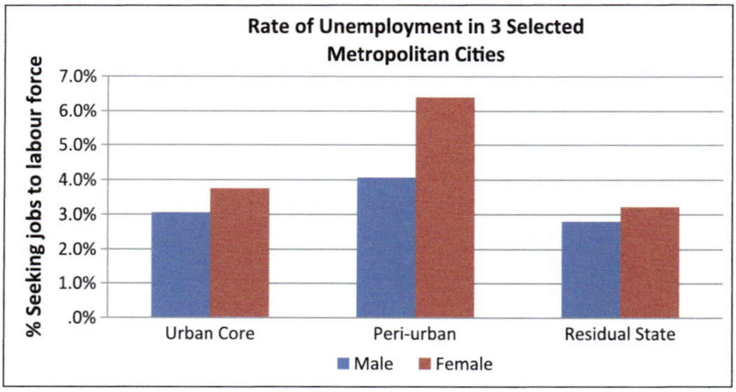

Fig. 4 Rate of unemployment in 3 selected metropolitan cities

become sharper, but it peaks more noticeably for women in the peri-urban areas in comparison to both the metropolitan areas and the interior districts under consideration. It is evident, therefore, that the urban opportunities that the peri-urban regions that may have to offer cannot be utilized by the women. This could be the necessities of higher travelling distances in such areas, and possibly due to specific nature of jobs that are coming up in such areas.

The gendered pattern of work reveals quite a few important patterns. First, while the male work participation rates (WPR) expectedly does not vary irrespective of the city location, the female WPR is culturally defined and is different each of the city locations. The WPRs are highest in Mumbai followed by Kolkata and then Delhi, conforming to the to the north-south gender differences. Second, the subsidiarization of work is very high among women in rural areas as observed from the differences in the UPS and UPSS WPRs, irrespective of the city. This is an expected pattern, and women typically due to care-giving responsibilities of family, is not able to join the labour market specifically in the rural areas, but do a lot of subsidiary work, one of the common ones being tending livestock. Subsidiarization among the women in urban areas is also high in and around Kolkata.

Further, Table 4 reveals that though the peri-urban space does not provide similar opportunity for women for the most part, around the city of Delhi, women in fact get more opportunities compared to even the city core. For men in Delhi, the situation is the reverse. Women may be taken in for the low-paid jobs that men are not willing to take up. The case of both Mumbai and Kolkata are just the reverse. The WPR is the lowest in the peri-urban areas compared to the other spatial counterparts and this is particularly observable in the rural areas around Mumbai. The causes of women working could be distress-driven or due to pull factors. Conversely, women holding back from work could be due to both positive and negative reasons. Among the younger in the working age group, a low work participation most often result due to them pursuing higher education. However, lack of mobility and restrictions due to patriarchal norms may not allow women to work or work only when a 'suitable' opportunity comes their way that suits their restricted mobility and the work conditions are acceptable within the norms of patriarchy. Thus, while the higher WPR of both men and women in the Delhi rural peri-urban areas is presumably due to high cropping intensity and developed agriculture, in urban peri-urban Delhi, female part-time work, possibly at a lower wage rate, may be taking over the men's jobs. So far as the quality of work is concerned, the spatial pattern for men are similar both in rural and urban areas. There is a continuum, as expected with respected to regular salaried jobs, when one moves away from the city core. In rural areas, Mumbai is an exception in the sense that the casualization is higher in the peri-urban areas. Other than this, both in rural and urban areas, casualization increases when one away from urban cores. Same is the pattern of male self-employed work in the urban areas.

The nature of work provides an insight into quality of work. Table 5 reveals some common characteristics. Unpaid family work reduces as one moves away from urban spaces. This can be understood both as wage opportunities provided

Table 5 Nature of work across spatial units in Delhi, Mumbai and Kolkata

	Urban centre	Spatial unit	Own-account worker (%)	Employer (%)	Unpaid family worker (%)	Regular salaried worker (%)	Casual wage labour (%)
Male							
Rural	Delhi	Peri-Urban	40.4	0.1	11.5	31.4	16.7
		Residual	38.2	1.3	18.2	13.2	29.1
	Mumbai	Peri-Urban	29.6	0.1	4.8	24.4	41.2
		Residual	37.1	0.5	14.6	13.4	34.3
	Kolkata	Peri-Urban	36.0	1.8	3.5	12.6	46.2
		Residual	33.4	1.6	6.4	7.4	51.1
	Total	Peri-Urban	35.8	1.2	5.0	17.6	40.4
		Residual	35.7	1.1	11.6	10.9	40.7
Urban	Delhi	Urban Core	25.3	5.2	4.2	61.5	3.8
		Peri-Urban	27.5	2.9	6.0	57.1	6.5
		Residual	28.7	6.4	9.3	40.4	15.2
	Mumbai	Urban Core	24.9	4.4	2.9	65.3	2.5
		Peri-Urban	23.9	4.0	4.5	63.4	4.2
		Residual	29.5	1.6	7.4	48.1	13.4
	Kolkata	Urban Core	31.3	8.8	7.3	44.7	7.8
		Peri-Urban	30.5	3.3	5.0	39.0	22.2
		Residual	42.5	1.6	4.8	32.6	18.4
	Total	Urban Core	26.2	5.5	4.2	60.1	4.0
		Peri-Urban	27.4	3.5	4.9	51.5	12.7
		Residual	32.0	2.1	7.1	44.1	14.6
Female							
Rural	Delhi	Peri-Urban	**37.4**	**0.0**	**10.9**	**6.0**	**45.7**
		Residual	**16.1**	**0.0**	**36.8**	**11.7**	**35.4**
	Mumbai	Peri-Urban	15.1	0.0	14.6	13.5	56.7
		Residual	6.7	0.0	42.2	4.0	47.0
	Kolkata	Peri-Urban	24.0	2.3	14.6	**15.8**	43.3
		Residual	29.5	0.1	13.1	**18.0**	39.3
	Total	Peri-Urban	23.4	1.6	14.3	14.4	46.3
		Residual	12.2	0.0	35.5	7.4	44.9
Urban	Delhi	Urban Core	15.0	0.7	6.5	77.6	0.2
		Peri-Urban	12.7	0.0	3.8	82.8	0.7
		Residual	12.8	0.2	8.5	71.8	6.7
	Mumbai	Urban Core	20.5	2.4	4.9	70.0	2.2
		Peri-Urban	21.4	0.0	4.5	71.9	2.2
		Residual	17.5	0.1	12.1	49.4	20.9
	Kolkata	Urban Core	**16.9**	**0.2**	**6.8**	**62.5**	**13.6**
		Peri-Urban	**34.3**	**0.0**	**3.8**	**46.3**	**15.6**
		Residual	**30.7**	**0.0**	**8.9**	**51.1**	**9.3**
	Total	Urban Core	18.4	1.5	5.7	70.7	3.7
		Peri-Urban	25.8	0.0	4.1	62.4	7.6
		Residual	19.8	0.1	11.2	51.4	17.6

Source Calculated from NSSO Employment-Unemployment Round (68th), 2011–12

by urbanization and increased monetization of the urban economies. Second, regular and salaried work shares are higher closer to urban spaces for men across the board. For women, the patterns are more irregular and city specific. Kolkata's peri-urban spaces do not fare well either in rural and urban locales in this respect. In urban Delhi and both rural and urban Mumbai, there is a higher incidence of regular and salaried jobs, compared to the other two spatial units in consideration. The shares of workers in regular and salaried jobs are low in the rural areas in general. The important question to ask with respect to urban areas is whether the women are occupying the low-paid salaried jobs in the peri-urban areas promoted by the fluid environment of these spaces. In other words, a large number of households are either migrant households or those who are facing land-loss in agriculture, are persuaded to seek urban options. The concentration of economic activities, characterized by a proliferation of informalization of work, both in the formal and informal sectors, provide options for men that may pay somewhat better, but are in no way regular. Women, due to restrictions of mobility and low access to education, may be filing up the niches of the jobs that offer regularity, but pay less. This aspect is analyzed in the section on wages.

The interpretation of self-employment and causalization are highly related in rural areas, as most often they indicate the allocation of workers in agriculture as cultivators and agricultural labourers. Rural areas in Haryana around Delhi practices a profitable rice–wheat cropping pattern, endowed with good infrastructure. The men hence hold on to the land more as cultivators, whereas this is not the case close to either Mumbai or Kolkata. The corresponding percentages of casual wage workers are lower in Delhi, and higher in Mumbai and Kolkata, compared to the self-employed cultivators. In both these cases, the casualization of rural workers is explained not only by wage work in agriculture but also substantially in the non-farm sector. The peri-urban areas of Delhi, and to a certain extent that in Kolkata, has better agricultural performances compared to the rest of the respective states. Hence, the share of self-employed cultivators is more in these spaces compared to the residual states. Some men do leave agriculture for urban opportunities in all the cities and this is indicated by higher women cultivators (self-employed in rural areas), compared to that in the residual states except in Kolkata. The incidence of casualization is higher among women in all the peri-urban spaces in rural areas. This indicates that a lot of women stay behind in agriculture in peri-urban areas and take up the men's work arena left by them to seek rural non-farm or urban opportunities both as cultivators and agricultural labourers.

While self-employment in rural areas primarily include cultivators, the same category indicate typically indicate tiny entrepreneurs in urban areas characterized by high amount of vulnerability. In the urban peri-urban spaces, incidence of women's participation in self-employed options, probably many of them home-based, is higher compared to that in the urban core and residual states. This pattern is not seen for men, whose engagement in self-employment in urban areas is the highest in the residual states, for the most part.

Gender Differences in Correlates of Participation in the Labour Market in and around Delhi Mumbai and Kolkata

The processes that explain participation in the labour market has been historically different for men and women, both socially and culturally. However, the efficiency norm with which the market functions in the neoliberal regime is expected to alter these social and cultural norms. Other than that, the peri-urban context offers us a manageable spatial platform to observe outcomes that are at work in the larger economy, in the sense of seeking merit in terms of employing labour. The social differences, in terms of gender should be minimized, under conditions of perfect competition, controlling for skill and experience.

The hypothesis that the processes at work in the market regime for men and women are governed by economic factors does not get validated by Table 6. There are significant differences for men and women, in fact, that indicate that the labour market functioning in the neo-liberal regime has not changed the patriarchal norms that dominated in the closed economy era. In fact, such differences probably have been retrenched in some ways.

Three sets of indicators have been used for the logit analysis to explain participation in labour market for men and women. The first is location-related indicators, which in this case are the three spatial units used for this study throughout, i.e. urban core, peri-urban areas and residual states. City and rural–urban locations are two more spatial elements that have been brought into this analysis. The second set of indicators relate to individual characteristics like employment, social group, marital status and age. Age is treated as a proxy for experience. The third set of indicators, i.e. the household characteristics, include the monthly per capita consumption expenditure (MPCE) and household size.

The logit analysis reveals that while urban cores offer more opportunities both for men and women compared to residual states, the peri-urban areas are not significantly different form the latter for easier entry into the labour market for men, and are in fact a more difficult space for women compared to the residual states. Thus the opportunities created by the urban processes are largely limited to the urban core for both genders in terms of entry to the labour market, and the space that is undergoing a change exclusively to cater to urban expansion, is infact, a restrictive space for women.

Rural location expectedly makes for easier entry to the labour market for both men and women. Delhi, has a more restrictive labour market compared to both Mumbai and Kolkata, for both men and women, much more for the latter compared to Mumbai. The fact that Delhi has experienced a higher degree of opening up to private investment and has benefitted in terms of higher growth from globalization processes compared to at least Kolkata, has made no difference to the situation portrayed above.

The individual characteristics work very differently in explaining the probability of being a worker for men and women. Men have a lower probability of being a worker if they are more educated, except that the probability declines somewhat

Table 6 Results of logit regression explaining probability of participating in the labour market

Variables	Male			Females		
	β	Exp(β)	Sig	B	Exp(β)	Sig
Categorical Variables						
Location (Reference: Residual States)						
Spatial location		–	0.00	–	–	0.00
Urban core	0.29	1.33	0.00	0.37	1.45	0.00
Peri-urban	0.08	1.08	0.17	−0.17	0.85	0.00
Cities (Reference: Delhi)						
Cities		–	0.00	–	–	0.00
Mumbai	0.50	1.65	0.00	1.26	3.53	0.00
Kolkata	0.27	1.31	0.00	0.28	1.33	0.00
Sector (Reference: Urban)						
Rural	0.15	1.16	0.00	0.49	1.64	0.00
Educational Attainment: Reference: High School and Above						
Educational attainment			0.00	–	–	0.00
Illiterate	0.68	1.98	0.00	0.26	1.29	0.00
Up to Primary	1.51	4.52	0.00	−0.07	0.93	0.19
Middle	0.59	1.80	0.00	−0.38	0.68	0.00
Secondary	0.04	1.04	0.45	−0.65	0.52	0.00
Social group(Reference: General Caste)						
Social group		–	0.06	–	–	0.00
Scheduled tribes	0.25	1.26	0.03	0.62	1.85	0.00
Scheduled castes	−0.07	0.95	0.37	0.19	1.21	0.00
Other backward Castes	0.12	1.05	0.33	0.01	1.01	0.87
Marital Status (Reference: Never Married)						
Marital status		–	0.00	–	–	0.00
Currently married	2.43	11.38	0.00	0.16	1.18	0.00
Divorced and Separated	−0.43	0.65	0.04	1.39	4.02	0.00
Continuous Variables						
Age	0.11	1.11	0.01	0.001	1.01	0.00
Household size	−0.02	0.98	0.07	−0.05	0.95	0.00
MPCE in Rs. '00	−0.01	0.99	0.00	0.00	1.00	0.11
Constant	−3.09	0.05	0.00	−2.73	0.07	0.00

Source Calculated from NSSO Employment-Unemployment Round (68th), 2011–12

from having a primary school attainment to being an illiterate. The norm of being the family breadwinner probably works for all men, but the choices are more numerous to people with higher education. For women, the probability of being a worker is the most for an illiterate, for the same reasons. But this apart, having a high school and above attainment facilitates entry into the labour market more than the lower educational attainments. The drop in probability is the maximum for the secondary level educational status, after the probability increases with subsequently lower educational levels, like the men. The social group identity does not make any major difference to the probability of being a worker for men, except that STs have a higher likelihood compared to the general category. For women, though, lower the caste group, higher the probability of entry to the job market, with the rider that STs, have an even higher probability than the SCs when compared to the general caste. It is well documented that though lower castes are generally disadvantaged in the social structure, paradoxically, the cultural barriers for women from such households to enter the job market is less marked compared to those upper caste women (Beteille 1991; Agarwal 1994). The cultural restrictions on the never married girls/women are high that prevent them from working, controlling for education and though the domestic and extra-domestic responsibilities that make it difficult for a married woman to work, the probability of the latter of being a worker is higher compared to the former. While the divorced and separated men have the lowest probability of working, their counterparts among women have the higher odds ratio of doing so, having no male support for earning their living. A higher age facilitates entry to the job market for both men and women, though to a lower extent in the case of latter.

Household size, expectedly, makes no difference to men in being a worker, whereas for women the chances that they can join work becomes less with a bigger household size, due to an increase in the care-giving responsibility. Finally, while a man from a poorer household have a higher probability of working, the economic background of the household does not make a significant difference for women.

Wage Differentials in Urban, Peri-Urban and Residual Interiors of 3 Selected Metropolitan Cities

There are enough evidences to believe that women find themselves clustered in the low wage sectors. Though a large amount of workers are in the self-employed category, their wage rates cannot be calculated.[4] Table 7 shows that without any exception, women get lower wage rates compared to men. The wage rate levels, expectedly, are higher among the regular salaried workers, but in the rural areas, women's wage rates are nearly 50 % lower than that of the men. In urban cores, the gender wage rate differential is the lowest among the regular salaried workers. However, this advantage drops significantly in the peri-urban areas, to a level a level slightly lower than the residual states. It may be recalled that though the share of the regular-salaried women were higher in two out of the three cities under consideration, they are paid around three fourth of their male counterparts.

Unlike the regular-salaried work, the wage rate differential is higher in the urban areas compared to the rural areas for casual work. The wage rates have gone

[4]City wise differences have not been estimated due to small samples in each category.

Table 7 Wage differentials among men and women in regular and casual work

Location	Spatial unit	Wages of regular and salaried workers (Rs.)			Wages of casual wage workers (Rs.)		
		Male	Female	Ratio	Male	Female	Ratio
Rural	Peri-Urban	379	203	0.54	146	109	0.74
	Residual	427	251	0.59	144	95	0.66
Urban	Urban Core	561	503	0.90	193	106	0.55
	Peri-Urban	594	435	0.73	152	99	0.65
	Residual	519	383	0.74	159	97	0.61

Source Calculated from NSSO Employment-Unemployment Round (68th), 2011–12

up recently in the rural areas due to National Rural Guarantee Schemes, and due to high women's participation in this scheme, their bargaining power has become better. In the urban areas, though, highest wage differentials are observed in the urban core, and it becomes relatively less in the peri-urban regions. In sum, for the better nature of jobs, i.e. peri-urban areas are relatively less favourable for women compared to the other two spatial units, whereas for daily wage work, it is more advantageous compared to men. This is particularly the case in rural areas, which men are leaving due to low profitability, and this is truer for the peri-urban areas than for the residual states, explaining the favourable wage rate differentials.

The informal sector has experienced high growth in many of the developing countries, with a rise in various forms of informality of employment. The Report on Conditions of Work and Promotion of Livelihoods in the Unorganized sector states that the unorganized workers consists

> of about 92 percent of the total workforce of about 457 million (as of 2004-05). For most of them, conditions of work are utterly deplorable and livelihood options extremely few. Such a sordid picture coexists uneasily with a shining India that has successfully confronted the challenge of globalization powered by increasing economic competition both within the country and across the world (GOI 2007, p. 1).

The informal sector does not capture all aspects of 'informalisation' of employment, since the formal sector is moving towards a greater informalization of work too. A part of the growing 'informalisation' of employment may be attributed to the globalization process of the economy. This is because enterprises tend to respond to competitive pressure in resorting to mixed-mode labour arrangements, in which observance of labour regulations for some workers is combined with the use of non-standard, atypical, alternative, irregular, precarious, etc., types of labour or various forms of subcontracting (Hussmanns 2004). Table 8 documents the high differences in the formal and informal employment as per the 68th round of NSSO Employment-Unemployment round. The advantages of being in formal employment is at least 3 times more wages for any of the location or sex. The urban-peri-urban areas hold higher advantages in formal employment vis-à-vis informal ones, which is even higher for women and translates into around 5 times higher wages. Such advantages are more in the residual states of rural areas, compared to the peri-urban areas, both for men and women. The incidence of

Table 8 Comparison of wage rates among formal and informal workers

Location	Sex		Informal	Formal	Ratio
Rural	Male	Peri-Urban	158	560	3.54
		Residual	159	613	3.84
	Female	Peri-Urban	112	344	3.06
		Residual	98	416	4.25
Urban	Male	Urban Core	286	954	3.34
		Peri-Urban	231	933	4.04
		Residual State	200	746	3.73
	Female	Urban Core	239	909	3.80
		Peri-Urban	160	771	4.83
		Residual State	124	663	5.37

Source Calculated from NSSO Employment-Unemployment Round (68th), 2011–12

informalization, however, is higher among women then men in rural areas (about 92 %), and is about the same as men in the urban areas (about 75 %).

Conclusion

Development theory and practice have focused on either "urban" or "rural" issues with little consideration of the interrelations between the two (Tacoli 1998). The economic landscapes around the large metropolitan cities are undergoing rapid changes in the post-globalization era becoming a space of opportunities and vulnerabilities, both due to processes of urban change. This paper attempts to understand some features of livelihoods in the peri-urban regions around three large metropolitan cities in India from a gendered lens.

The paper concludes that though market economy aiming for growth and efficiency aims at homogenizing spaces in terms of overriding economic considerations, the social and the cultural differences in the three spaces that we have taken for analysis plays out strongly in expressing differences of engagement with work among men and women. Thus though a few generalizations can be made about the fluid peri-urban areas, the differences across cities are stark, and also between men and women.

One of the generalizations that can be made is that by and large, the rural peri-urban areas are vulnerable in many cases, more than that of the interior districts. This is true of work participation, nature of work as well as wage differences. Delhi is better off in the rural peri-urban areas because of the high profitability of agriculture. However, this is also the reason why processes like land acquisition would impact the farmers more here than in other places, as the opportunity costs of losing agricultural land would particularly be high compared to the other two cities. Both Mumbai and Kolkata's peri-urban areas are worse off compared to the residual districts in the respective states, and this is despite the fact that the former has adopted a fast-paced globalization effort, having attained characteristics of a global city in many ways, and the latter which has had a slow start in terms of inviting private capital. What is clear from here is that opening up the economy to private investments is certainly not able to create adequate opportunities in the rural hinterland of large cities, which is where the intensity of capital flow is the most.

The urban locales of the peri-urban areas have been doing better, in fact in many respects vis-a-vis the urban cores. Better work opportunities, a greater share in more secure jobs, higher wage rates and lower gender differentials in wage rates have been found in case of both Delhi and Mumbai. However, these benefits are not distributed equally. Women are worse off in terms of work opportunities and unemployment rates in these areas, and such conditions can be explained by the social and demographic changes that have taken place in the peri-urban areas around the large metropolitan cities. With a smaller household size and a lower working age groups sex ratio compared to the interior districts (though lower than the urban core), the possible care burden on the adult women of the households could be a factor explaining their low WPR in these areas. A higher unemployment rate in these areas for women, exceeding that of men indicates that they are not able to fit into the opportunities that are available even in the urban part of the peri-urban areas. The traditional constraints of caste, marital status and number of family members they have to take care of operate as strongly, and the liberalized economic environment, in no way brings their way opportunities that suit their context. Thus the processes of urbanization at best, has created opportunities that are exclusive in nature and has not been able to make a dent in the patriarchy restricting women in participating in work.

Appendix I: District Around Metropolitan Cities

Metropolitan Centre	Districts representing peri-urban areas	
	2004–2005	2011–2012
Delhi	Gurgaon, Faridabad, Rohtak, Sonipat	Gurgaon, Faridabad, Rohtak, Sonipat Jhajjar
Mumbai	Thane, Raigarh	Thane, Raigarh
Kolkata	North 24 Parganas, South 24 Parganas, Haora, Hugli	North 24 Parganas, South 24 Parganas, Haora, Hugli

References

Abraham, V. (2009). Employment growth in rural India: Distress driven? *Economic and Political Weekly, 44*(16), 97–104.
Abraham, V. (2013). Missing labour or consistent "De-Feminisation". *Economic & Political Weekly, Xlviii*(31), 99–108.
Agarwal, B. (1994). *A Field of one's own: Gender and land rights in South Asia*. Cambridge, U.K.: Cambridge University Press.
Beteille, A. (1991). Society and politics in India: Essays in a comparative perspective. *London school of economics monographs on social anthropology*. New Delhi: Oxford University Press.
Bosworth, B., & Collins, S. M. (2007). *Accounting for growth: Comparing China and India* (No. w12943). National Bureau of Economic Research.
Chadha, G. K., Sen, S., & Sharma, H. R. (2004). *Land resources: State of Indian farmers*. New Delhi: Academic Foundation.
Chakravorty, S. (2000). How does structural reform affect regional development? Resolving contradictory theory with evidence from India*. *Economic Geography, 76*(4), 367–394.
Chandrasekhar, C. P., & Ghosh, J. (2013, November 11). Where have all the women workers gone? *Hindu Business Line*.
Dupont, V. (2007). Conflicting stakes and governance in the peripheries of large Indian metropolises–An introduction. *Cities, 24*(2), 89–94.
GOI. (2007). *Report on conditions of work and promotion of livelihoods in the unorganised sector*. New Delhi: National Commission for Enterprises in the Unorganised Sector, Government of India.
Himanshu, (2011). Employment trends in India: A Re-examination. *Economic and Political Weekly, 46*(37), 43–59.
Hussmanns, R. (2004). *Defining and measuring informal employment*. Geneva: Bureau of Statistics Paper, ILO.
Institute of Global and Area Studies (IGAS). (2012). Puzzling decline in rural women's labor force participation in India: A reexamination, No. 96. D. Neff, K. Sen, & V. Kling (Eds.), *GIGA Working paper*, Hamburg.
Jatav, M., & Sen, S. (2013). Drivers of non-farm employment in rural India. *Economic and Political Weekly, 48*(26–27).
Kennedy, L. (2007). Regional industrial policies driving peri-urban dynamics in Hyderabad, India. *Cities, 24*(2), 95–109.
Kennedy, L., & Zérah, M. H. (2008). The Shift to city-centric growth strategies: perspectives from Hyderabad and Mumbai. *Economic and Political Weekly*, 110–117.
Kohli, A. (2006). Politics of economic growth in India, 1980–2005: Part II: The 1990s and beyond. *Economic and Political Weekly*, 1361–1370.
Kundu, A. (2009). Exclusionary urbanisation in Asia: A macro overview. *Economic and Political weekly*, 48–58.
Kundu, A. (2011). Politics and economics of urban growth. *Economic and Political Weekly, 46*(20), 10–12.
Kundu, A., & Saraswati, L. R. (2012). Migration and exclusionary urbanisation in India. *Economic & Political Weekly, 47*(26), 219–227.
Midmore, D. J., & Jansen, H. G. (2003). Supplying vegetables to Asian cities: is there a case for peri-urban production? *Food Policy, 28*(1), 13–27.
Narain, V. (2009). Growing city, shrinking hinterland: land acquisition, transition and conflict in peri-urban Gurgaon, India. *Environment and Urbanization., 21*, 501–512.
Paul, T., & Raju, S. (2014). Gendered labour in India. *Economic & Political Weekly, 49*(29), 197.

Raju, S. (2013). Women in India's new generation jobs. *Economic & Political Weekly, 48*(36), 17.
Srivastava, N., & Srivastava, R. (2010). Women, work and employment outcomes in India. *Economic and Political Weekly, 48*(28), 49–63.
Tacoli, C. (1998). Rural-urban interactions; A guide to the literature. *Environment and Urbanization, 10*, 147–166.

Embedded or Liberated? An Exploration into the Social Milieu of Delhi

Pritha Chatterjee

Abstract Urban areas are long been seen as catalysts for social change not only in situ, but also in the surrounding rural areas. In general, cities are expected to rise above the regional constraints and behave independently as far as their social ambiences are concerned. They are essentially looked upon as socially modern entities allowing urbanites to escape from the shackles of traditional norms and customs. However, there are contrasting evidences and arguments suggesting that cities may not have universally applicable attributes and much depends upon their region-specific evolutionary trajectories. In India, for example, urbanization process has been quite different and is a result of historically evolved social, cultural and economic processes whereby the rural relations did not change radically enough to create an alienated uprooted peasantry that could occupy the cities. The close and dependent relation between cities and villages led to the formation of an internal organic relationship between the two entities, that is, they tend to follow the socio-cultural patterns of the social spaces in which they are situated rather than having distinct social characteristics. The present article tries to locate the cities in their regional context, with a special focus on Delhi. Delhi shares the boundary with two major states and in spite of its metropolitan culture is set in the north Indian socio-spatial space. In this sense, it is different from Kolkata and Chennai, which are more regionally rooted. In spite of sharing Delhi's metropolitan culture, Mumbai and Bangalore are part of a different socio-spatial context. The present analysis attempts to examine Delhi's socio-spatial embeddedness compared to those of the other metropolitan cities. The paper engages in detail with capital city of Delhi as a case for examining the social embeddedness.

P. Chatterjee (✉)
ActionAid India, New Delhi, India
e-mail: c.pritha@gmail.com

S.S. Acharya et al. (eds.), *Marginalization in Globalizing Delhi: Issues of Land, Livelihoods and Health*, DOI 10.1007/978-81-322-3583-5_9

Keywords Social space · Urbanization · Delhi · Socio-spatial embeddedness

> The city is, rather, a state of mind, a body of customs and traditions, and of the organized attitudes and sentiments that inhere in these customs and are transmitted with this tradition. The city is not, merely a physical mechanism and an artificial construction. It is involved in the vital processes of the people who compose it; it is a product of nature, and particularly of human nature (Park and Burgess 1925 cited in Massey et al. 1999).

Introduction

Cities have often been symbolically associated with modern values, lifestyles and ideas. They are seen as playing an important role in the conception and establishment of modernity. Within such urban spaces, the routinized day-to-day practices are not supposed to be bound by traditions as they are not embedded in the conventionally established socio-cultural practices. More contemporarily, the complex processes of global urbanization are supposed to render cities into all-embracing social spaces as the world and its ways pour into them, such that they are increasingly becoming the emblems of modern society (Amin and Thrift 2005; Kleniewski 2005). Cities are also portrayed as locus of social change having dominion over the surrounding countryside from where forces of social change would spread into surrounding rural areas (Gilbert and Gugler 1982; Potter and Evans 1998; Hubbard 2006).

While this can be true in the developed context, these propositions are highly debatable in the Indian context since the developmental trajectories of the cities here are significantly different from elsewhere. Given that most of the Indian cities have evolved from rural roots, rural–urban linkages continue to remain strong. It has often been argued that there are continuities of socio-cultural forms from rural to urban areas and posing the urban in stark contrast with the rural is a futile effort for the purposes of socio-cultural analysis especially in the Indian context (Lambert 1962; Olivieau 2005; Patel and Deb 2006).[1] There are contrasting evidence and arguments suggesting that cities may not have universally applicable attributes and much depends upon their region-specific evolutionary trajectories (Low 1996; Raju 2007, 2011).

In India, the rural relations did not change radically enough to create an alienated uprooted peasantry that could occupy the cities—unlike western cities. Instead, the close and dependent relation between cities and villages led to the formation of an internal organic relationship between the two entities (Lambert

[1]The overlap of rural and urban ways of life is greater in Indian cities than in the West. Prevalence of joint families, strong neighbourhood relations, rootedness in social and cultural attitudes are some of the strong sociological variables that supposedly differentiates Indian cities is from the cities of the West (Ramachandran 1989).

1962; Raju 1988; Mohan and Dasgupta 2005; Olivieau 2005; Patel and Deb 2006; Jayaram 2010). An implication of such a relationship is that cities sometimes do not stand as stark opposites to the rural hinterlands, but rather share similar characteristics with them. Low (1996, p. 399) termed Indian city as "traditional city" where conventional traditions and practices are still within urban spaces. Identities of caste, class, gender and ethnicity are strong markers shaping the urban spaces in India. In contrast, in economic sense, Indian cities are being locked in a conscious integration into the global political economy.

Located within this framework, the present study analyzes whether in spite of efforts of getting globally linked, Indian cities are socio-spatially embedded in their regional culture. It is further explored whether metropolitan cities of India, particularly Delhi, emerge as socially liberated spaces rather than embedded entities within their rural surrounding. The basic argument that runs through the analysis is that the spatial location of the cities becomes an influencing factor in determining their social characteristics. The metropolitan cities in the present analysis thus have been explored from two different aspects (i) as socially encrypted entities which are rooted in region-specific socio-cultural practices and customs, and (ii) essentially embedded within their rural hinterlands, thus not deviating in terms of social behaviour with their surrounding villages.

Concept of Embeddedness

The concept of embeddedness as propounded by Granovetter (1985) is crucial in the present analysis to understand whether urban centres of India are socially engrained in their respective regional spaces. Here, I follow Granovetter (1985) in his argument of embeddedness which says that behaviour and institutions are so constrained by ongoing social relations that to construe them as independent is a grievous misunderstanding. Social embeddedness is a complex construct quantification of which poses not only challenges but limitations as well. This concept is expressed here through women-centric indicators since the most stringent social norms that are persistent over time relate to women and how they are treated. As wives, daughters and mothers, women are the mediators, agents as well as the targets of social change. Often whether a society is modern or not is explained through changes in attitude towards women (Agarwal 1997).

Scholars have argued that such gendered norms are prevalent even in modern day global cities where women are seen as the 'home-makers', 'carriers of tradition', 'honour of the family' and so on. Such hegemonic cultural beliefs tend to get institutionalized in the norms and structures of public and private institutions like workplaces, families, etc. From the sex segregation of jobs to the differential role expectations from boys/men and girls/women—all indicate the prevalence of gender in all spheres of life. (Kolenda 1984; Basu 1999; Sen 2001; Bondi and Rose 2003; Raju 2011). The analysis is located within this frame of thought and initially explores the social characteristics of Class I cities of India (396 in numbers) to

Table 1 Selected wards and localities

Literacy zones	Name of wards	Ward number	Localities	Category of localities
Low literacy	Chattarpur	58	Arjangarh	E
	Rohini	33	Rohini colony	E
Medium literacy	Malviya nagar	11	Savitri nagar	D
	Gulomohar park	14	Gautam nagar	D
High literacy	Greater Kailash	9	Sheikh Sarai	D
	Pitampura north	32	Pitampura	D

Source Census of India 2001, MCD classification 2005–06

understand whether there emerges any regionally framed pattern, particularly along the famed north–south axis. The next section moves to mega cities in order to explore their relationships with their respective rural hinterlands.[2] The last section delves with the capital city of Delhi as a case for examining the social embeddedness, i.e. whether the city is socially engrained in its regional space.

Methodology

Choice of Indicators

To understand the notion of embeddedness of city space, several social attributes have been identified as proxy variables (Table 1) such as child sex ratio, female literacy and female work participation rates. These are attributes interconnected with lives of women in general since these are significantly conditioned by the location-specific societal norms and dictates. It is argued that social embeddedness as a phenomenon is best explained through the lives of women, since they are the mediators, agents as well as the targets of social change. (Sopher 1980a, b; Raju 1988, 2007).

Selection of Wards, Localities and Samples for Primary Survey

Female literacy was taken as the most important social indicator that has a bearing on many other factors (Kundu et al. 2002; Sen 2001) for identification of wards to be surveyed. The wards were ranked and grouped into three categories: high, medium and low. The average literacy levels were calculated individually for these three categories. Next, two wards whose literacy levels were closest to the average

[2]The villages were initially mapped around the respective cities and then grouped into different distance zones around the mega cities. The average values for child sex ratio, female literacy and work participation rates were plotted for the cities and the surrounding villages. The mean figures were then compared through the Test of Significance of Mean Values to find out whether the mean values differ significantly between the city and the respective rural hinterlands.

figure of that strata were chosen as the wards from where localities were selected for carrying out the fieldwork. Thus, in all six wards were identified, two from each literacy zones.

The Municipal Corporation of Delhi (MCD) divides the 2340 colonies spreading across 134 wards as per their payment of property tax. Once the wards were selected, the localities were identified. It was important that the localities have some homogeneity—for this the MCD zonations for tax purposes was used as a basis. The extreme ends of taxation zones were not included. It is to be noted that low literacy wards were invariably falling into category E which also occupied the lower wrung of the taxation hierarchy. The localities falling within the category D (Ward No. 11, 14, 9 and 32) and E (58 and 33) were chosen since they represented the middle income colonies (Map 1).

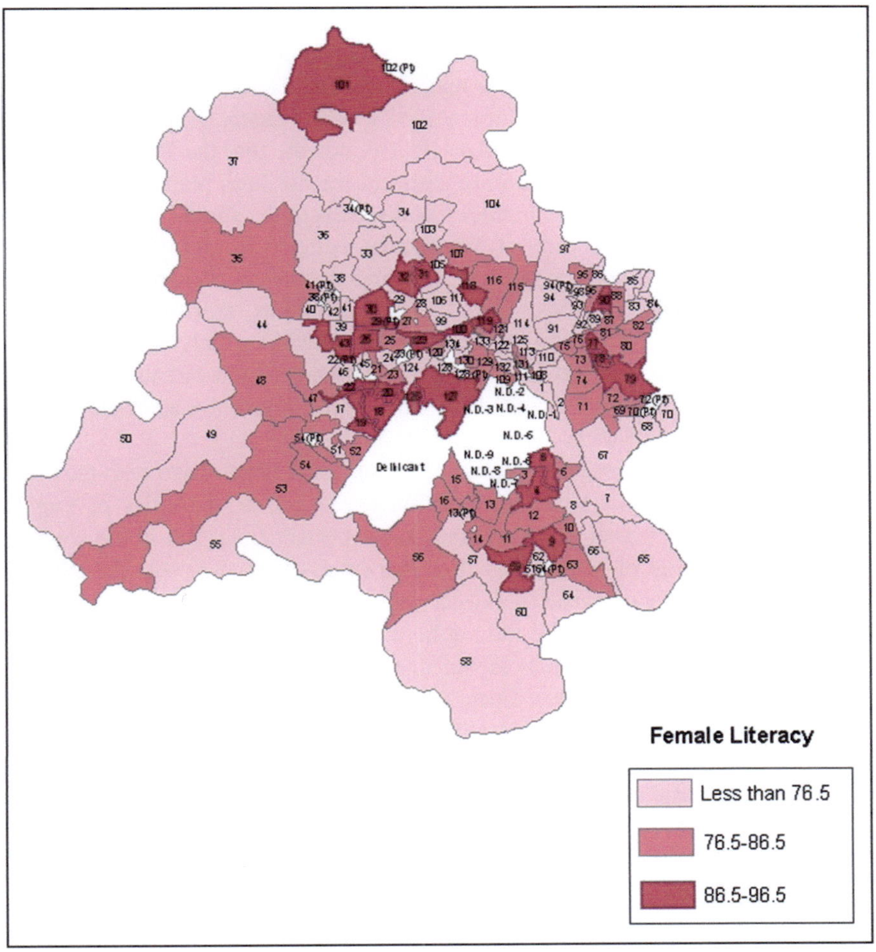

Map 1 Female literacy in Delhi

It was assumed that people who are staying in such localities also fall within the same economic group. It needs to be mentioned here, that high and medium literacy wards fell under the 'D' category, whereas low literacy wards fell under the 'E' category. From the chosen localities, 300 (50 from each locality) samples in total were collected. The respondents were chosen from amongst women between the age groups 22–45 years.

Indian Cities and Social Space

The Class I cities of India are an integral part of the Indian urban scene and are expected to be free from any regional socio-cultural biasness. This argument is based on an expectation that the basic level of services, motivations and provisions for diffusion of social well-being are uniformly available in the major urban centres (Haider 2000; Amin and Thrift 2005). In order to explore this proposition, the selected set of social indicators were mapped for the Class I cities to see if there exists the regional north–south differences in the social characteristics of the cities. The following maps (Maps. 2, 3 and 4) clearly indicate that the Indian cities follow a distinct regional pattern whereby cities in the northern plains exhibit social characteristics quite different from their counterparts in the south.[3] The Class I cities situated in the southern parts of the country registered high to very high child sex ratios as well as, female literacy rates and female work participation rates compared to the northern cities (Table 2).These attributes refer to women's position and the observed pattern is in conformity with widely researched and acknowledged divide that has long been the hallmark of the Indian social space (Dyson and Moore 1983; Agarwal 1994; Basu 1999; Jejeebhoy and Sathar 2001; Menon-Sen and Shiva Kumar 2001; Raju 2011).

There are certain zones in the northern social space which have extremely low sex ratios, extremely low work participation rates such as the cities of Punjab, Haryana and Uttar Pradesh but the literacy rates are moderate. But in the southern social space the zones of high to very high literacy rates coincide with the zones of high child sex ratio and female workforce participation rates. This is indicative of the fact that the Class I cities of the northern social space having high female literacy neither always ensure better labour market participation nor better child-survival rates whereas for the Class I cities of the South, the reverse conditions are true.

Table 2 further strengthens my argument that the cities located in their respective social spaces are socially different from each other as is evident from the low values of coefficient of variation. When the *t*-test is conducted to compare the

[3]In the course of analysis it emerged that cities falling in the central part i.e. Gujarat and Madhya Pradesh, and the extreme north eastern part of India do not clearly fall into any of the 'North' and 'South' categories of cities. Hence they have been kept out of the calculation that has been done in Table 2. Nevertheless, the cities of Madhya Pradesh and Gujarat have been plotted in the Maps. 2, 3 and 4.

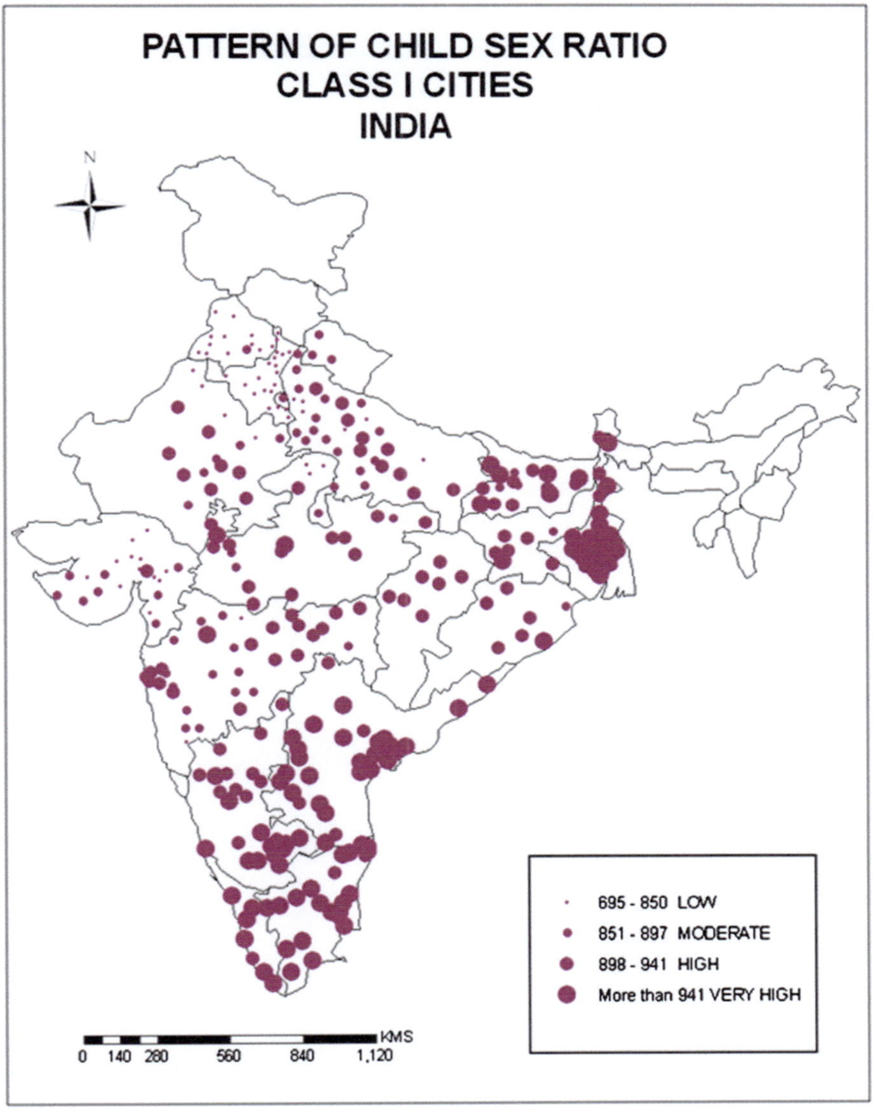

Map 2 Pattern of child sex ratio

means of each category, it emerges that the cities situated in the northern and the southern social spaces are significantly different from each other.

> Institutions mediate and shape ideological and metaphoric spaces in consonance with material realities and ecological specificities of the lay of the land (India), which has exciting potentials to decode the much discussed, but less explained, regionally gendered realm in India. Spatially embedded political, economic and social structures manifested through political and religious fundamentalism have been reclaiming women's subordination positions all over again although the language of subordinating forces may have changed (Raju 2011, p. 48).

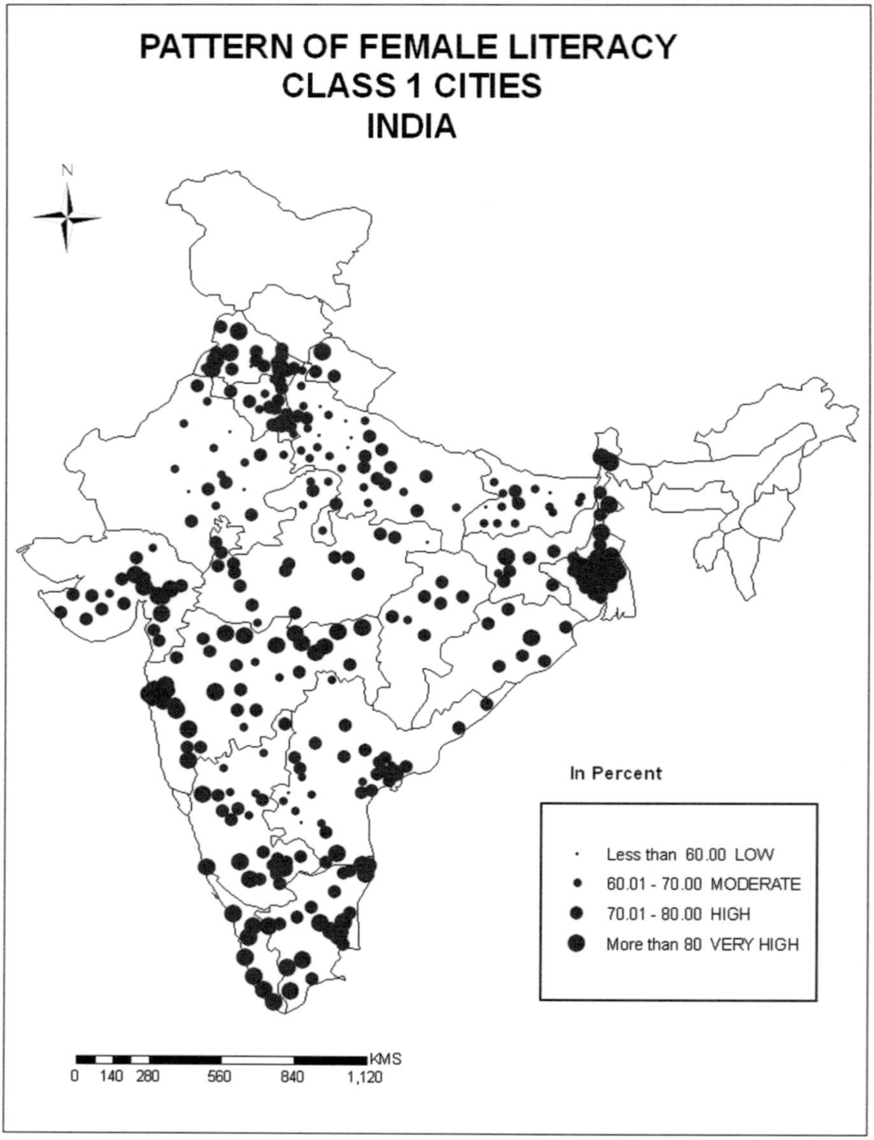

Map 3 Pattern of female literacy

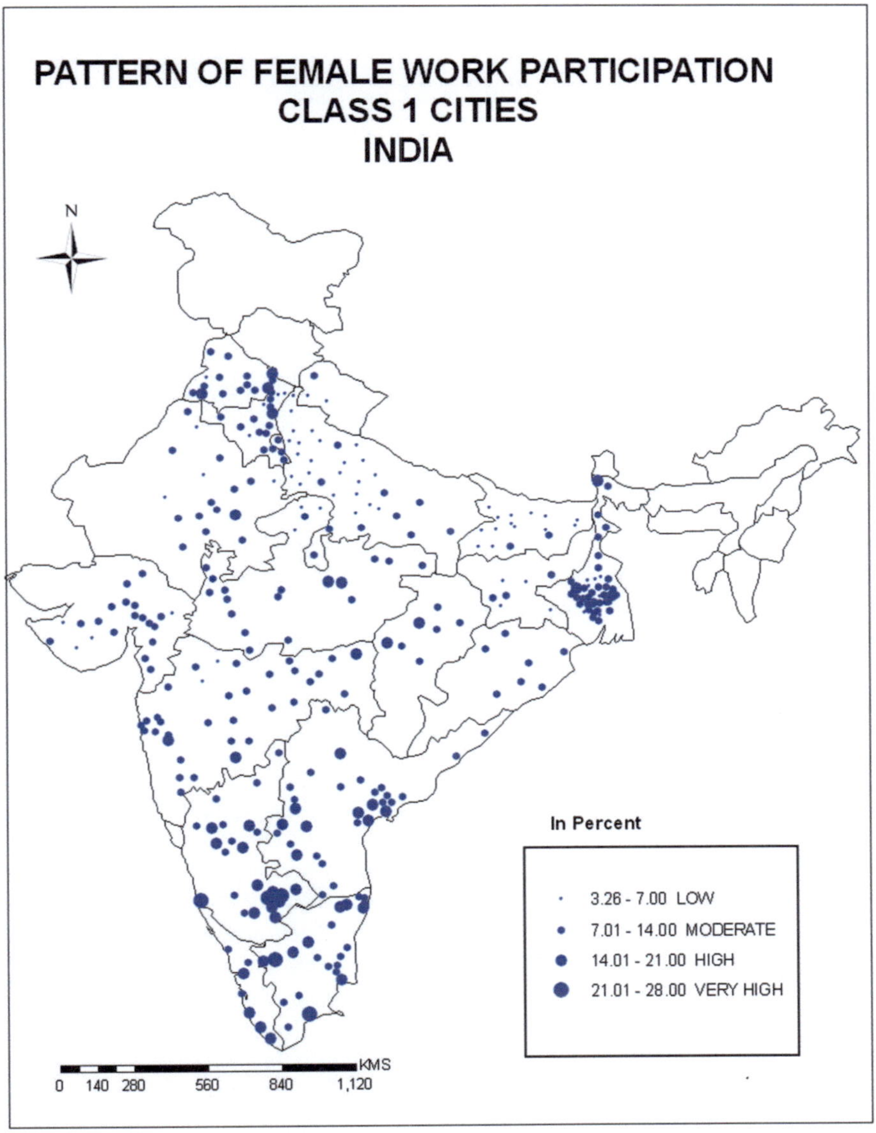

Map 4 Pattern of female work participation

Table 2 Social attributes of cities in India

	Mean		Standard deviations		Coefficient of variation		*t*-value
	North	South	North	South	North	South	
Child sex ratio	887	937	63.81	34.89	7.19	3.72	8.26
Female literacy	72.44	76.45	8.17	7.84	11.33	10.25	4.30
Female workforce Rate	8.49	12.94	3.08	3.78	36.29	29.19	10.53

Source Computed from Primary Census Abstract 2001

Mega Cities and Their Embeddedness

Having shown the embedded character of the Class I cities within the larger regional frame, this section now analyzes whether the mega cities of India are socially similar with their immediate rural surroundings. In order to interrogate this question, the villages have been grouped in different bands according to their distance from the centres of respective mega city. The same set of indicators as in the earlier attempt to locate the cities in the regional space has been taken for this analysis. The villages surrounding the respective cities were grouped within the concentric circles (from the city centres) of the six mega cities under observation.[4] The differences in indicators' values for each circle were statistically tested for significance, the details of which are provided below. It is argued that if cities were to show disconnect with the rural surroundings, these indicators would significantly differ between the two.

The intertwining of the individual cities with their rural hinterlands is seen through the variations in child sex ratio, literacy and workforce participation rates. The assumption is to look into the variation in these attributes in the cities and their surrounding villages under scrutiny. It is proposed that if the cities exhibit significant differences from the surroundings, they are independent of their regional entrenchment. In contrast, if they have social attributes in sync with the hinterland, they are deeply rooted in the local socio-cultural milieu. The following section draws a comparative analysis between Delhi and the five other mega cities by mapping the trajectories of social attributes across the rural surroundings.

In terms of child sex ratio (Fig. 1), the cities located in the south have relatively better counts than the cities elsewhere. They increasingly improve with the distance from the city in case of Kolkata, and Mumbai. However, for the cities of Chennai, Bangalore the patterns do not show much variation with increase in distance although there are a few aberrations in some distance zones.[5] For the city of Delhi, the trend of child sex ratio is rather dismal where it goes on decreasing as one moves away from the city into the surrounding rural hinterland.

It was expected that the female literacy rates (Fig. 2) would tend to go down as the distance from the city increases due to lack of infrastructure and educational facilities. Low levels of female literacy are not only indicative of poor infrastructure, but also other social deterrents. Here also the city of Delhi records a constant increase in the female literacy as one moves away from the city. Mumbai has a

[4]An attempt was made to delineate the area of the cities' influence on their surroundings. This proved to be a challenging task and must be acknowledged as such in terms of fixing the functional centres of the cities, which may not necessarily be the geographical ones.

[5]An important observation made by Kish around the metropolises of America that around the main city grows up residential suburbs. These areas are quite exclusive in nature and tend to have a high proportion of woman, a relatively small proportion of foreign born; while in the industrial suburbs the conditions are reversed.

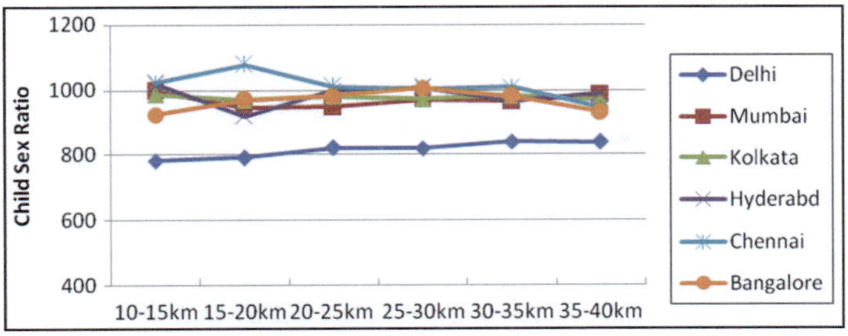

Fig. 1 Patterns of child sex ratio around the mega cities of India

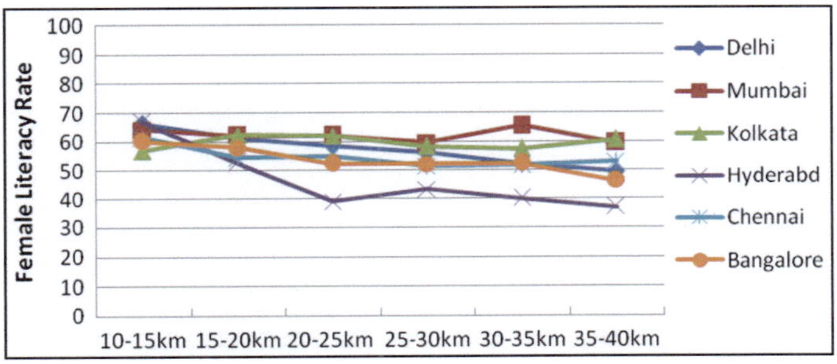

Fig. 2 Pattern of female literacy around the mega cities of India

similar trend where after a sharp drop in the areas adjoining the city there is an increase in the sex ratio. The particular social outlook where girls are looked upon as transient members of the family on their way to marriage and boys as permanent bread earners can be argued to have continued in these regions.

Female workforce participation rates are symptomatic of societal acceptance or reticence (Raju 2011). It is of interest to note that almost all villages from city outwards have lower female workforce participation with some fluctuations which is not surprising in itself (Fig. 3). However, Kolkata stands out in terms of distinctly lower proportion of women in the workforce. Mumbai and other metropolis share their pattern with the surroundings whereas Kolkata and its surroundings have uniformly low presence of their females in the workforce. Female work participation rate shows a fluctuating trend as one moves away from the cities. In the distance zones closer to the city there are initial upswings in the rates, but with increasing distance the rates go down. It is to be noted that, the city of Delhi does not show fluctuations in terms of female literacy rate and child sex ratio as one moves away from the city centre on to the periphery.

While it emerges that there is a decreasing trend in the social indicators concerned around the mega cities under consideration, whether the cities are uniquely placed amidst socially backward rural hinterlands is something that needs to be

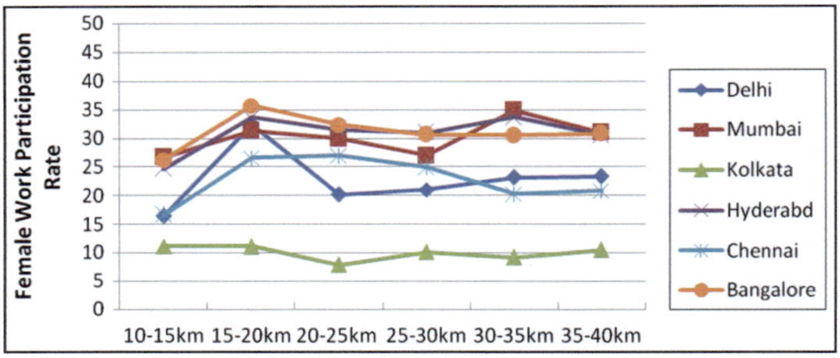

Fig. 3 Pattern of female work participation around the mega cities of India

further explored. In the light of the present study with a few exceptions (such as Bangalore and Mumbai in the south) the Indian mega cities do not stand as socially unique entities different from their surrounding backward rural hinterlands. Table 3 shows the comparison of the *t*-values from the comparison of mean figures in each category and it emerges that, the city and the surrounding villages do not emerge as significantly different social entities from each other.

Tracing back the origin of the cities of India and especially Delhi, it can be seen that they witnessed a gradual organic growth from the villages.[6] Scholars have argued that Indian cities are extensions of villages rather they are 'overgrown villages' and hence the social similarity (Shah 1988). The city and the village are the elements of the same civilization and the same social institutions such as caste, kinship and religion are found to exist in both villages and towns (Pocock 1960; Potter and Evans 1998).[7] Given such similarity between the social institutions and norms it is quite likely that the cities and adjoining villages would tend to be socially similar. Ramachandran (1989) argued that the rural migrants in spite of the freedom allowed by the city tend to become clannish. They belong more

[6]The mega cities of India are quite similar as far as their origin and growth is considered. The mega cities of today have evolved from earlier existing rural settlements. For example, Mumbai was originally a cluster of seven islands separated by tidal marshes. In less than 3 centuries of British patronage, Mumbai grew from an insignificant group of villages to the largest city in western India and a metropolis of national and international importance. Similarly Kolkata also evolved from three small villages namely Kalikata, Sutanuti, Gobindapur and rose to prominence during the British period. Delhi, Chennai have evolved to such major metropolises from small villages and hamlets.

[7]Pocock (1960) emphasizes on the similarity of institutions and argued that the term 'rural' and 'urban' is faulty to use to identify social categories. He is against both the concepts of rural–urban dichotomy as well as rural–urban continuum. But he nevertheless recognized certain differences between the village and the town where he stated that city was the most complete and abiding expression of the essential social values.

Table 3 The distance-decay between the mega cities and their surroundings

Distance code (km)	Child sex ratio	Female literacy	Female WPR
Delhi			
10–15	5.49	3.44	2.76
15–20	5.80	7.01	8.48
20–25	2.79	11.17	15.39
25–30	2.99	13.62	9.59
30–35	1.00	14.28	9.97
35–40	2.18	16.08	15.24
Mumbai			
10–15			
15–20	0.90	0.53	0.85
20–25	0.04	0.03	0.48
25–30	1	1.04	0.85
30–35	0.21	2.16	3.1
35–40	0.52	3.13	2.5
Kolkata			
10–15	1.92	9.78	1.48
15–20	2.72	12.50	2.74
20–25	4.32	15.24	9.73
25–30	4.53	18.56	5.24
30–35	5.52	18.48	6.58
35–40	4.92	18.64	5.02
Hyderabad			
10–15	1.78	2.80	5.00
15–20	1.75	4.76	7.67
20–25	1.53	2.94	9.68
25–30	3.70	23.99	24.71
30–35	1.20	23.55	13.12
35–40	2.25	33.11	19.99
Chennai			
10–15	0.56	2.61	0.55
15–20	1.67	9.73	4.78
20–25	1.32	14.25	6.19
25–30	2.09	12.00	5.12
30–35	0.67	6.17	1.27
35–40	0.68	10.50	4.72
Bangalore			
10–15	0.79	1.23	3.44
15–20	1.72	1.94	6.01
20–25	0.44	4.86	2.04
25–30	1.36	0.21	4.13
30–35	1.69	0.27	0.10
35–40	0.17	6.58	0.23

Source Computed from Census of India 2001, Primary Census Abstract 2001 and Village Directory 2001. The tabulated values are *t*-values computed by comparing zonal means of each indicator respectively closely to their social groups and the social practices (marriage rules, extended families) do not change in spite of their urban living.[8]

The parameters used in the analysis collectively represent the status of women in a particular societal context and hence are indicative of the existing societal norms and conditions. Since such parameters are not found to be differing amongst the cities and the rural surrounding, the cities can be said to be socially embedded within its regional space.

As shown by Maps (1, 2 and 3) Delhi seems to be more similar to its regional surrounding amidst the other metropolitan cities. Table 3 further supports this argument as is evident from the *t*-values.[9]

Delhi being a metropolitan and capital city, it was expected that it would be socially progressive when it comes to women's role in the society.[10] The following section based on primary data pertaining to women's work and aspirations, helps to substantiate preceding observations. Given that gender inequality is embedded in the history of India, especially in the northern regions, whether the social situatedness of the city has any bearing on its social behaviour has been taken up for further analysis.

---

[8]Studies of neighborhood patterns in Indian cities have shown that the cities have much common with the rural social patterns. The migrants coming from the adjacent rural areas tend to build up their own enclaves within the city, and retained enough of the rural base to serve as a "resting stage" in the process of adjustment to city life and the new migrant in the city tries to seek as associates only those who come from the same kinship group, village or province. The inhabitants of rural areas and cities move from one to the other and often use resources provided by these spaces by "keeping one foot in and one foot out" (Olivieau 2005, p. 14).

[9]In the secondary data analysis, the mean values of child sex ratio, female literacy and female work force participation rate have been compared with those of the villages in successive distance bands. Further, for some selected indicators, the inter-locality differences have been calculated all through the analysis. The difference is further tested for determining the significance levels using the formula: $X1 - X2/\sqrt{(\mathrm{SD}_1^2/n_1) + (\mathrm{SD}_2^2/n_2)}$. Here, $X1$ denotes mean of the first group, $X2$ denotes mean of the second group, SD_1 denotes standard deviation of first group, SD_2 denotes standard deviation of second group, n_1 denotes number of observations of the first group and n_2 denotes number of observations of the first group. The *t*-test, and any statistical test of this sort, consists of three steps—Define the null and alternate hypothesis, Calculate the *t*-statistic for the data, Compare t_{calc} to the tabulated *t*-value, for the appropriate significance level and degree of freedom. If $t_{\mathrm{calc}} > t_{\mathrm{tab}}$, we reject the null hypothesis and accept the alternate hypothesis. Otherwise, we accept the null hypothesis.

[10]Delhi is the capital city of India and is the central seat of all kinds of economic, administrative functions of the country. Delhi, as the capital city of India, is also the locus and hub of economic development and global investments. For instance, the city has the Indira Gandhi International (IGI) Airport is bigger than the airports of Mumbai, Hyderabad and Bangalore put together with the Terminal 3 being the eighth largest terminal in the world. The airport is connected to the heart of the city by a high speed airport Express Metro. Further, the per capita income of Delhi is amongst the highest in the country estimated to be about Rs. 2.1 lakh in 2011–12 and it is predicted that it would be amongst the richest cities in the country. Delhi, over the years has developed as a major centre of service sector including information technology, offering large number of employment opportunities than Noida and Gurgaon.

As already elaborated, the study has been conducted across three selected wards of Delhi which were chosen on the basis of female literacy rates. From these selected wards, six localities were chosen, two from each for further investigation. It should be mentioned here that only women were chosen as respondents between the age group 21–45 years. It is argued here that embeddedness as a social phenomenon is best exhibited through the perception and behaviour of women since social norms tend to constrain their attitude most compared to men.[11]

Embedded Notion of Women's Work: What It Means

The intersection of spatiality with gendered construction is often exhibited in the way in which women's choices and aspirations of work differ remarkably between the northern and southern regions of India.[12]. This spatial binary coinciding with the traditional role of men as breadwinners and women as homemakers is particularly strong in India. Such role ideologies rigidly confine women to the home and often eliminate their opportunities for paid work and make them accept lower wages (Reskin 1993; Joshi and Sastry 1995; Kellet and Tipple 2000; Rege 2007). It is in this context that women's work in India becomes a socially meaningful category and has been used as a proxy for social embeddedness since it is shaped by the structures of patriarchal family, gender role ideology and labour market segregation practices (Miller 1982; Agarwal 1994; Jose 2005). Here, women's work is treated as a social indicator rather than an economic one. As Raju observes

> Public' and 'private' are not just about space organization per se in terms of relations of power within which these spheres are constituted, these spheres get constituted and experienced differently in different places, depending upon how patriarchy constitutes and gets constituted spatially. That is patriarchal structure even as a common referral domain for understanding overall gender relations gets intercepted by spatial contexts (Raju 2011, p. 40).

Whether social constructs have any bearing on the perceptions of urban Delhi has been explored in the subsequent sections through interrogating the following aspects—whether women should work or not, if at all she should, what should be

---

[11]Ideally men should have been interviewed but when it comes to embeddedness it can be argued that Embeddedness gets best articulated through women's viewpoints and perceptions. However, one can argue that men can give architected views; hence only women respondents were selected.

[12]The perceptions and attitude towards vary greatly across the regions of India. Girls studying in science institutes located in eastern region felt that there is a respectful attitude towards women, and that higher education among girls is considered desirable. Girls from the north reported a greater degree of conservatism in society (Gupta and Sharma 2003). The skilled women workers in the garment and electronic industries of Delhi and Chennai inspite of being located within the domestic sphere experienced gender friendly environs in Chennai as compared to Delhi which is more patriarchal.

her considerations, etc. Respondents were asked to rank the five reasons (already provided) in the order of importance (giving rank five to the reason they consider more important and rank 1 to the least). The ranking was to be done as per the respondents' perception. Thus, different reasons could get the same ranking.

To the initial question that whether women should take up paid job, 63 % of respondents said that women should work. Supporting oneself during emergencies seemed to be most important reason for a woman to work followed by gaining self-esteem and confidence. Ensuring economic returns of education and supporting family were seen as less important reasons to take up paid work which is not surprising because the internalization of socially architected constructs which assigns specific role of homemakers to women. The propositions get reaffirmed as according to the respondents, sharing responsibility after marriage is definitely important, but that should not dominate the decision of women to have a career since it is also their responsibility to take care of their families and children (Table 4).

> *When I got married, I was not working. But, nowadays due to this inflation and rising prices it is impossible to maintain a decent standard of living with only one person's income. Given a choice now, I would want to discontinue my job as it is difficult for me to take care of my daughter as well as manage office. I do not want my daughter to be brought up by our hired-help* (28 year old working woman in Locality II)

> *Often women are placed in situations of emergency such as taking care of her parents, mishaps and sometimes divorces. If you have a job, you feel confident and handle things better without depending on anybody else* (31 year old home-maker in Locality III).

In the Table 4, the *t*-values show the difference of means in responses across localities. The computed *t*-values show that the respondents do not differ much in their responses and hence their perceptions.

Table 4 Reasons important for a woman to work

Major reasons	Localities	Mean	*t*-value	Sig. (2 tailed)
To be independent	I	2.2	5.4	0.00
	II	2.1	9.5	0.00
	III	2.1		
To support herself during emergencies	I	3.9	7.6	0.00
	II	4.5	7.2	0.00
	III	4.1		
For self-esteem and confidence	I	2.5	3.6	0.00
	II	3.0	9.3	0.00
	III	3.0		
To support her husband after marriage	I	3.3	0.74	0.45
	II	3.7	4.4	0.00
	III	3.9		
To ensure economic returns after education	I	2.2	4.5	0.00
	II	2.1	6.2	0.00
	III	2.0		

Source Field Work—April/November 2011 in selected localities of Delhi

Table 5 Preferred Occupations for Women

First preference	% of respondents	Second preference	% of respondents	Third preference	% of respondents
Teaching/ academics	58	Home-based work	54	Teaching/ academics	34
Government service	28	Teaching/ academics	32	Home-based work	44
Health	12	Banking	8	Banking	14
MNCs	2	Government service	2	Others	8
Others	1	Health sector	2	–	–
Total	100	Total	100	Total	100

Source Field Work—April/November 2011 in selected localities of Delhi

Choice of Occupations

The segregation of women and men into distinctly different occupations is an important determinant of women's position in the formal labour market, which is not at par with men's. Respondents were asked about what kind of occupations women should take up keeping constant the statement that women should take up paid work. They were asked to state three suitable jobs for women in order of their preference. Table 5 summarizes the responses. 58 % of the respondents found academics or teaching as the most preferred profession for women, followed by 54 % of women favouring home-based work.

Respondents opined that these are the professions where it is easy for women to balance both family life and professional life given that such jobs have flexible working hours and decent working environment. Small scale business or home-based business options are also lucrative and suitable for women since they can take care of their domestic responsibilities efficiently. Jobs such as teaching, banking and government services were seen as 'safe' jobs for women as compared to ITES and media services which involved free mixing with men and unrestricted work schedules. Thus, they were less preferred by the respondents in spite of having high pay structures. Respondents felt that such work profiles often led to 'free mixing with men', 'late night schedules', 'irregular work hours' which is not good for girls from middle-class families.[13]

> A gender-typed occupation or job is one that is seen to require distinctly feminine or distinctly masculine characteristics. Examples of gender typed occupations are everywhere. When asked to describe the qualifications for being a nurse many would list characteristics assumed to be much more typical of women than men, such as nurturance and caretaking ability. Similarly many would say that jobs presumed to require aggression and competitiveness such as prosecutor are more appropriate for men than women (Wharton 2012, p. 182).

[13]Women working in call centers for example are considered less respectable in the urban middle-class imagination. Call centre workers are consistently perceived as less educated, less family oriented and thus unable to uphold the ideals of Indian womanhood.

Most of the working woman (43 %) in the present sample seemed to agree that they might have to quit job in the face of balancing their responsibility at home. Women's work outside the home is often an extension of their work in the family. In the present sample, on an average women work as kindergarten and primary school teachers (28 %) or nurses (17 %) and into home-based small business (33 %).[14] Especially, for women, the choice of part-time versus full-time work is likely to be based on a concern for balancing work and family responsibilities. In the present sample, 38 % of the women are into part-time work. Non-availability of any other helping hand and lack of cooperation from other family members has led to the women taking up part-time work.

The Framing of Women and Work

The rigidity of sexual division of labour, the tendencies to undercount and devaluate women's skills and contribution to the economy and the resultant differences in their economic positions vis-a-vis men is due to the overarching effect of patriarchy and its varied manifestations. Gendered notion of work is to a significant extent the result of prejudices and discrimination practised by the employers, fellow workers and the family. As a result of this, on one hand women's entry into labour market gets restricted due to lower qualifications and experiences and further they are handicapped by their relative immobility and the taboos they have to observe in their choice of jobs (Siltanen 1994; Banerjee 1998; Kantor 2003).

> At one extreme stands the ideal of good homemaker. Mother and wife, and at the other extreme is the image of the 'independent' employee, outward looking and assertive, at least in relative terms. The burden of simultaneous performance of these roles is the unique province of women. Once this is understood, the reasons why women's work continues to be determined more by such considerations as distance from the workplace and work timings rather than by education and skill becomes easier to understand (Joshi and Sastry 1995, p. 228).

Given such a context, the respondents were asked to rank their preference for a set of factors that they would consider before taking up a job. Among the various factors that influence the decision of women before taking up a job are varied-high remuneration, workplace closer to home, flexible working hours, location of

---

[14]Occupations such as government service and banking carry enormous social prestige for women. Mid range occupations such as teaching and secretarial work are often deemed acceptable occupations for women but other occupations such as market work and sales are often very low status occupations and are taken up out of sheer necessity. Gender based patterns are evident with women dominating fields such as food and nutrition, nursing, teaching and accountancy. In contrast, men are found in large numbers in engineering and technology, law firms and architecture. Further, in medicine women tend to specialize in 'soft' fields like paediatrics, gyanaecology while men go into surgery and other 'tough' fields.

workplace in 'safe' parts of the city and environment at the workplace. They were asked to rank 1 to the least and rank 5 to the most important factor. For each factor, the mean ranks were compared across the localities and then compared with the help of Test of Significance of means (*t*-values in Table 6).

On an average, the Fig. 4 shows that workplaces closer to home and jobs which had flexible working hours were most preferred by women. Income and job stability may be the prime job attributes considered by men, but job hours and locational convenience are likely to hold more importance for women. Because women are more likely than men to bear the main responsibility for home and children nonwage aspects of jobs are more important to women that they are to men (Thompson and Walker 1989, p. 851; Hanson and Pratt 1991).

Hanson and Pratt (1991) opined that female-centric occupations are available on a part-time basis, or offer convenient hours. Women shift their time and investment back and forth between paid and family work so that family life is sustained.

Table 6 Factors important for taking up a job

Major reasons	Localities	Mean	Std. dev	*t*-value	Sig. (2 tailed)
High Pay	I	3.98	1.09	0.964	0.336
	II	2.08	0.96	7.97	0.000
	III	2.88	2.88		
Closer to home	I	3.68	0.86	6.67	0.000
	II	3.64	1.14	5.08	0.000
	III	3.44	1.22		
Flexible or shorter working hours	I	3.36	0.92	4.56	0.000
	II	3.35	1.7	5.88	0.000
	III	3.39	1.18		
Location of workplace in safe part of city	I	2.82	0.99	6.07	0.000
	II	3.76	1.18	1.84	0.067
	III	3.49	0.87		
Environment in workplace	I	2.52	1.1	1.53	0.066
	II	2.10	1.2	5.91	0.000
	III	2.91	1.6		

Source Field Work—April/November 2011 in selected localities of Delhi

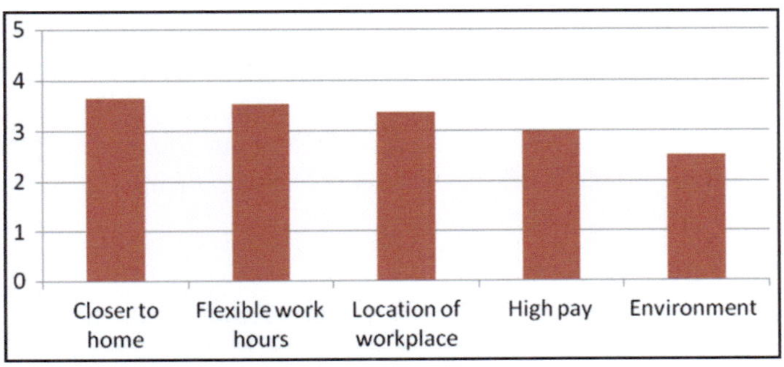

Fig. 4 Factors affecting women's work

Married working women usually do not want to change their jobs and negotiates lower positions in jobs which are near their homes.[15] Similar observations emerged from the present study.

It emerges from Table 6 that except for the consideration for environment at workplace, there is no significant difference in the responses across localities for the other factors as is evident from the *t*-values. The probable reason for such a difference might be due to the fact that most women in Locality I are less accustomed to a formal workplace and are mostly engaged into home-based work.

City's Socio-Spatial Situatedness and Perceptions of Work

In traditional patri-focal structure of the northern India, women are primarily associated with private sphere and a preoccupation with female chastity led social practices. This leads to the effective control of women through modes of seclusion, segregation, early marriage and rigid notions of 'male' and 'female' work spheres. Chanana (2007) rightly points out that the image of the ideal Hindu woman dominates and coexists with other images even now in an Indian woman's life. Fear of daughters travelling alone across towns, odd hours, long periods of study and fear of not finding a suitable match constitute barriers to women's access to education and employment opportunities (Nambissan 2004; Rustagi 2004). Similar perceptions seem to dominate the mind-sets of the respondents in the present sample where women seem to prioritize their roles as 'women' and 'mothers' first rather than individuals who can freely choose and pursue a career.

Further to assess whether such traditional ideas govern the lives of women, a set of five statements were constructed that implied prioritizing marriage and family as compared to career and job aspirations. Table 7 details out the statements. A score of 1 was assigned if the respondents strongly agreed to the statement and correspondingly a score of 5 if she strongly disagreed. This exercise was carried across all localities. Further, a *t*-test was carried out to understand whether there emerges any difference in the perception of women across the localities.

For women it is marriage which should be prioritized over career options. 65 % women strongly agreed that they would not wait for till they find a job for getting married. They put their marriage on a priority as compared to their own career and job. Specially by treating women's participation in paid work as something aberrant to what is being considered as appropriate and ideal for womanhood, social norms actively discourage and devalue women's labour force participation. Such notions are still persistent in urban Delhi as is evident when 52 % of respondents

[15]Kelkar also suggested that women's lower mobility has influenced recruitment policies in the IT industry. Human resource managers reported that they preferred to hire women rather than men, as women are more dedicated are likely to remain longer in job.

Table 7 Perception on Women's work Aspiration vis-a-vis Social Role

Major reasons	Localities	Mean	Std. dev	*t*-value	Sig. (2 tailed)
Job then marry	I	2.84	1.88	0.695	0.488
	II	3.02	1.76	3.32	0.000
	III	3.26	1.44		
Not take up job	I	3.80	1.47	5.58	0.000
	II	3.06	1.71	4.17	0.000
	III	2.34	1.48		
Not think about career	I	4.86	0.349	1.94	0.053
	II	4.67	0.911	4.50	0.000
	III	4.36	0.835		
Equal division of chores	I	2.79	1.84	1.99	0.047
	II	3.29	1.69	3.91	0.000
	III	3.41	1.47		
Working woman not suitable for taking care of children	I	2.76	1.80	4.05	0.000
	II	2.02	1.69	3.88	0.000
	III	2.17	1.38		

Source Field Work—April/November 2011 in selected localities of Delhi

strongly agree that married woman should not be take up work and girls should not be encouraged to pursue a career.

The 'working' status of women and their engagement in the public sphere is often seen as a direct threat to the family's honour especially in northern region of India. The definite roles of men and women as provider and caregiver and the extent of their rigidity have an implication on women's work status and career. Such notions not only restrict women from participating in the labour market but also families acknowledging that their women have to work to support families (Mukhopadhay and Seymour 1994; Raju 2011). Further, the complex relationships between traditional Indian social institutions—the joint family, arranged marriage, dowry, and *purdah,* or sexual segregation have their impacts of girls' schooling, education and job aspirations. The present study shows that the respondents in Delhi still are bound by such traditional thoughts and hence behaves in a conservative manner as far as women's work aspirations are concerned.

Feminists argue that even in contemporary times, the ideology of home and domestic space getting linked to womanhood and femininity is prevalent. Ensuring good childhoods has become the primary task of the mother, secondarily the task of the families and to a lesser extent the responsibility of the social institutions (Moen and Sweet 2003; Donner 2008; McDowell 1999; Reskin 1993). Similar is the case with the lives of middle-class women in Delhi as can be seen from Table 7 where respondents agree that working women cannot take care of their children when compared with mothers staying at home. Thus, it emerges that the education of the women, their marriages and their professional careers are arranged and represented in relation to their role of a mother. Thus, it is reaffirmed that the behaviour of the selected respondents in the city of Delhi greatly conform to the patriarchal notions prevalent in the northern regions of India within which the city is situated.

Spatial Hold on Social Behaviour and Perceptions

The influence of spatial hold and social locations has been the main core of explanation accounting for the observed perceptions in the city of Delhi as well.[16] The overarching effect of the regional hold is evident in the way respondents have a gendered notion about women's work. Such social behaviour is essentially the visible effects of patriarchy resulting in the low economic worth of women which is so strong in the northern regions of India. Stricter gender regimes in the north actually restrict the actual participation of women in the labour market and also their recognition as workers. The perceiving of girls as the family honour was very much obvious from the informal conversation during the interviews which placed less importance to their economic roles and discouraged taking up jobs outside home unless absolutely necessary for financial support to families. The gender relations in the northern region are articulated and mediated through particular codes of conduct set for women which restricts her access to employment and denies her ability to make choices for herself (Bhat and Zavier 2003; Dyson and Moore 1983).

Raju (2011) argued that woman's participation in the labour market has a distinct regional pattern-relatively low in northern states vis-a-vis the southern one. Such a marked regional variation cannot be always explained by economic factors but rather the influence of region-specific socio-cultural norms which are stringent in the north as compared to the south. Sopher (1980a, b, p. 188) argued that the extent to which women in India can enter the public sphere by acquiring education is an indication of the influence of modernization which however gets intersected by the traditional culture. Arguing within the same context, it can be said that the city of Delhi in spite of its urban location is greatly influenced by the dominant culture of the north Indian region which discourages the participation of women in paid job.

> It is not women's participation in economically productive activities that makes a qualitative difference to their lives and increases their worth. It is the worth, that is, the recognition that society inherently places on women that lies at the core of rejection/denial or permission to women to enter the public domain, paid work being one such manifestation (Raju 2011, p. 39).

---

[16]Dreze and Sen (2002, p. 234) showed, how female literacy and employment has a positive bearing in reducing child mortality inspite of having regional contrasts. They note that "regional contrasts in the extent of gender bias in chid survival are far more striking than the contrast relating to religious identity". The southern regions of India have gender-egalitarian environment as compared to the north which leads to the higher status of women in the south. In their study, the contrasts were captured through some dummy variables used for regional location. These dummy variables compress "information about a whole range of inter-related norms and practices related to marriage, mobility and inheritance which make up gender relations (Kabeer 2000 as cited in Raju 2011, p. 39).

Table 8 Social Embeddedness and Interruptions

Variables	B-value	Sig level	Exp (B)
Work status—working (rc)			
Non-working	1.07		2.91
Part-time working	−2.80	0.645	0.06
Family type—nuclear families (rc)			
Joint families	−0.15	0.377	0.85
Marital status—unmarried (rc)			
Married	0.56	0.466	1.75
Age—less than 25 years (rc)			
25–35 years	−0.60	0.239	0.54
35–45 years	−0.15	0.112	0.85
Education Level—Graduation (rc)			
Less than graduation	0.77	0.337	0.67
Up to secondary	−0.57	0.214	0.75
Constant	0.60		

Source Field Work—April/November 2011 in selected localities of Delhi; *rc* Reference Category, Negelkerke = 0.0412 2 log likelihood = 246.882; $n = 300$

Interruptions to Embeddedness

Social behaviour and perceptions are often influenced by a number of socio-demographic factors such as marital status, work status, age, type of family, etc. The net influence of such factors on women and their perceptions is ascertained by the following binary logistic regression analysis. Table 8 presents the likelihood of holding more traditional perceptions which is the dependent variable with five responses strongly agree, agree, partially agree, disagree and strongly disagree.

Table 8 shows that housewives/non-working women are more likely to be conservative compared to working women. Married woman are more likely to be conservative than unmarried woman. Apart from such factors, there are no conspicuous factors that explain the difference in perceptions of the respondents. It should be mentioned here that through the course of interviews as well, women who were engaged in some sort of paid work seemed to be less inclined to agree to the given statements. The respondents seem to abide by the conventional norms and practices and do not seem to question or doubt the dominant societal notions.

Conclusion

One of the major debates in urban theory is the evolving social identity of the city—whether cities produce a cosmopolitan culture and represents modernity or are they still reflective of the social processes affecting them.[17] It has been commonly argued by scholars that cities and villages are often dichotomous entities, with rural areas as the repository of 'folk' culture and cities as emblems of modernity. Situated within this framework of debate, the Indian metropolis with focus on Delhi were looked at to question whether urban spaces are spaces of modernity or are they socially embedded entities. It emerges from the analysis that Class I cities of India follow the trend of the respective regional spaces within which they are situated rather than having unique social characteristics. Cities in the northern social space show less gender-egalitarian patterns as compared to their southern counterparts in terms the selected social indicators such as child sex ratio, female literacy and female workforce participation rate. I argue here that the socio-cultural rootedness of the cities in their respective social spaces influences the cities to develop certain region-specific social characteristics rather than having unique social identities.

Further, social embeddedness of the city of Delhi is explored through choices and aspirations of women in economically productive activities, the argument being women's work participation is an important indicator of their worth in society. The analysis brings forth that patriarchally produced social relations between men and women, very typical of the northern social space, shape the perceptions of the women respondents of Delhi. Though 63 % of respondents agree that woman should work, such aspirations get framed within a "so far and no further" paradigm. Women are still seen as secondary earning member. Traditional occupations are preferred such as academics, government services rather than non-traditional occupations such as corporate sector, sales and media. Work preferences get shaped by working hours, locations closer to home rather than wage aspects. All such perceptions and role identities seem to emerge from the perception that the respondents identify with women's roles as mothers and primary bearer of household duties.

Thus, it is argued here that cities which are supposedly to be the carriers of modernity and social change in turn are marked by hegemonic gendered constructs that get institutionalised in the norms and structures of the society. It is noteworthy here that even in a city like Delhi which is aspiring to be a 'global city', women continue to remain the repository of such normative constructs. It seems that the

[17]Modernity or modernization is seen as a process for a total transformation of a traditional or pre-modern society with associated social organization that characterize the advanced, economically prosperous and relatively politically stable nations of the world. Pathak looks at modernity, as related to the spirit of freedom. This freedom is rooted in the critical consciousness that it generates. It means that one should not take things for granted but rather question it, verify it and subject everything to scrutiny.

social rootedness of the cities in general, and Delhi in particular is pulling them back into their age-old social customs and practices that are not quite at par with their international economic interconnectedness. The complex interplay of tradition, culture and gender constituting the urban social fabric thus imparts the city with an embedded social identity.

Acknowledgments I wish to acknowledge my supervisor Prof. Saraswati Raju for helping me conceptualize the Indian cities from a socio-spatial perspective, and integrate the concept of gender with geography.

References

Agarwal, B. (1997). "Bargaining and Gender Relations: Within and Beyond Household", *Feminist Economist*, *3*(1):1–51

Agarwal, B. (1994). *A Field of one's own: Gender and land rights in South Asia*. Cambridge: Cambridge University Press.

Amin, A., & Nigel, T. (2005). *Cities: Reimagining the Urban*. Cambridge: Polity Press.

Banerjee, N. (1998). Household dynamics and women in a changing economy. In M. Krishnaraj, R. Sudarshan & A. Shariff (Eds.), *Gender, Population & Development* (pp. 245–266). New Delhi: Oxford University Press.

Basu, A. M. (1999). Fertility decline and increasing gender imbalances in India. *Including A Possible South Indian Turnaround, Development and Changes, 30*, 237–263.

Bhat, M. P. N., & Zavier, A. J. F. (2003). Fertility decline and gender bias in Northern India. *Demography, 40*(4), 637–657.

Bondi, L., & Rose, D. (2003). Constructing gender, constructing the Urban: A review of Anglo-American feminist urban geography. *Gender Place and Culture, 10*(3), 229–245.

Chanana, K. (2007). Female sexuality and education of Hindu girls in India. In R. Sharmila (Ed.), *Sociology of gender the challenge of feminist sociological knowledge* (pp. 287–317). New Delhi:Sage Publications.

Donner, H. (2008). *Domestic Goddess: maternity, globalization, and middle class identity in contemporary India*. Ashgate Publishing Company.

Dreze, J., & Sen, A. (2002). *India: Development and participation*. Oxford: Oxford University Press.

Dyson, T., & Moore, M. (1983). On Kinship Structure, Female Autonomy, and Demographic Behavior in India. *Population and Development Review*, *9*(1): 35–60.

Gilbert, A., & Josef, G. (1982). Cities, Poverty and Development: Urbanization in the Third World, London: Oxford University Press.

Granovetter, M. (1985). Economic action and social structure: The problem of embeddedness. *Am. J. Social*, *91*(3):481–510.

Haider, S. (2000). Migrant women and urban experience in a squatter settlement. In V. Dupont, E. Tarlo & D. Vidal (Eds.), *Delhi urban space and human destinies* (pp. 29–50). Delhi: Manohar Publishers.

Hanson, S., & Pratt, G. (1991). Job search and the occupational segregation of women. *Annals of the Association of American Geographers, 81*(2), 229–253.

Hubbard, P. (2006). *City Key Ideas in Geography*, USA: Routledge.

Jayaram, T. (2010). Revisiting the city: The relevance of urban sociology today. *Economic and Political Weekly, 45*(35), 50–57.

Jejeebhoy, J., & Sathar, Z. A. (2001). Women's autonmoy in India and Pakistan: The influence of religion and region. *Population and Development Review, 27*(4), 687–712.

Jose, S. (2005). Women, paid work and empowerment in India: A review of evidence and issues, Occassional Paper 48:CWDS, Delhi. Retrieved from www.cwds.ac.in/ocpaper/womenpaid-work-sunny-ocpaper.pdf.

Joshi, A., & Sastry, N. (1995). Work and family: Conflict and its resolution. *Indian Journal of Gender Studies, 2*(2), 227–241.

Kantor, P. (2003). Women's Empowerment through Home-Based Work : Evidence from India, *Development and Change, 34*(3):425–445.

Kellett, P., & Tipple, A.G. (2000). The Home as Workplace: A Study of Income-generating Activities within the Domestic Setting. *Environment and Urbanisation, 12*(1): 203–213.

Kleniewski, N. (Ed.). (2005). *Cities and Society*. Australia: Blackwell Publishing.

Kolenda, P. (1984). Women as tribute. Woman as a flower: Images of "women" in weddings in North and South India. *American Ethnologist, 11*(1), 8–107.

Kundu, A., Pradhan, B. K., & Subramanian, A. (2002). Dichotomy or continuum analysis of impact of urban centres on their periphery. *Economic and Political Weekly, 37*(50), 5039–5046.

Lambert, R. (1962). The impact of urban society upon village life. In R. Turner (Ed.), *India's urban future* (pp. 94–116). Bombay: Oxford University Press.

Low Setha, M. (1996). The anthropology of cities: Imagining and theorizing the city. *Annual Review of Anthropology, 25*, 383–409.

Massey, D. B., Allen, J., & Pile, S. (Ed.). (1999). *City Worlds*. London: Routledge.

McDowell, L. (1999). Gender, Identity and Place, United States: Polity Press in association with Blackwell Publishers Limited.

Menon-Sen, K., & Shiva Kumar, A. K. (2001). *Women in India: How free? how equal?*. New Delhi: UNDP.

Miller, B. D. (1982). Female labor participation and female seclusion in rural India: A regional view. *Economic Development and Cultural Change, 30*(4), 777–794.

Mohan, R., & Dasgupta, S. (2005). The 21st century: Asia becomes urban. *Economic and Political Weekly, 40*(3), 213–223.

Moen, P., & Sweet, S. (2003). Time clocks: Work-hour strategies. In P. Moen (ed.), It's about time: Couples and Careers . Ithaca, NY: Cornell University Press, pp. 18–34.

Mukhopadhyay, C. C., & Seymour, S. (1994). *Women, Education and Family Structure in India*. Boulder: Westview Press. National Science Foundation (NSF).

Nambissan, G. B. (2004). Integrating gender concerns. Retrieved July 18, 2012 from http://www.india-seminar.com/2004/536/536geethab.nambissan.htm.

Olivieau, S. (2005). Peri-urbanisation in Tamil Nadu: A quantitative approach. CSH Occasional Paper No 15, Publication of the French Research Institutes in India, New Delhi: Rajdhani Art Press.

Park, R. E. and Burgess, E. W. (1925). The City, Chicago and London: The University of Chicago Press, pp 1-46.

Patel, S., & Deb, K. (2006). *Urban Studies*. New Delhi: Oxford University Press.

Pocock, D. D. (1960). Sociologies: Urban and rural. In M.S.A. Rao (Ed.), *Urban sociology in India* (pp. 97–120). New Delhi: Concept Publishing House.

Potter, R. B., & Evans, S. L. (1998). *The city in the developing world*. UK: Addison Longman Limited.

Raju, S., & Kuntala Lahiri Dutt (2011). *Doing Gender, Doing Geography Emerging Research*. New Delhi: Routledge.

Raju, S. (Ed.). (2011). *Gendered geographies space and place in South Asia*. New Delhi: Oxford University Press.

Raju, S. (2007). Sticky floors, high ceilings: skilled and 'gendered' workforce-learnings from Chennai and Delhi firms. *Social Change, 37*(4), 91–109.

Raju, S. (1988). Female literacy in India: The urban dimension. *Economic and Political Weekly, 23*(44), WS57–64.

Ramachandran, R. (1989). *Urbanization and urban systems in India*. New Delhi: Oxford University Press.

Rege, S. (2007). *Sociology of Gender*. New Delhi:Sage Publications.

Reskin, B. (1993). Sex segregation in the workplace. *Annual Review of Sociology, 19*(1), 241–270.

Rustagi, P. (2004). Significance of Gender-related Development Indicators: An Analysis of Indian States. *Indian Journal of Gender Studies*, *11*(3): 291–343.

Sen, A. (2001). Population and gender equity. *Journal of Public Health Policy, 22*(2), 169–174.

Shah, A. M. (1988). The rural-urban networks in India. *South Asia: Journal of South Asian Studies, 11*(2), 1–27.

Siltanen, J. (1994). *Locating Gender: Occupational Segregation, Wages and Domestic Responsibilities*, London: UCL Press Ltd.

Sopher, D. E. (1980a). Sex disparity in Literacy. In D.E. Sopher (Ed.), *An explanation of India: Geographic perspective on society and culture* (pp. 26–35). New York: Cornell University Press.

Sopher, D. E. (1980b). The geographical patterning of culture. In D.E. Sopher (Ed.), *An explanation of India: Geographic perspective on society and culture* (pp. 26–35). New York: Cornell University Press.

Thompson, L., & Walker, A. J. (1989). Gender in families: Women and men in marriage, work and parenthood. *Journal of Marriage and Family, 51*(4), 845–871.

Wharton, A. S. (2012). *The sociology of gender*. UK: Wiley Blackwell Publishing.

Gender Violence in Delhi: Perceptions and Experience

Sunita Reddy and Sanghmitra S. Acharya

Abstract Post Nirbaya case, a gruesome gang rape and murder of a girl, Delhi saw a huge public outrage, protests and demand for justice. As a result a new law 'Sexual Harassment of Women at Work Place Act' (2013) was passed. Despite the new law and other measures of increased surveillance, the sexual crimes against women continue and have increased. This paper is based on a larger study carried out in Delhi, among the school and college students and also slum locality to understand their perceptions and experiences of safe and unsafe spaces in the city. There are differential experiences of the respondents depending on the geographical location, and the class they belong to. For majority sexual violence in some form is very common in their everyday life experience and for some definitely in memory. Patriarchal norms and misogynist culture makes a woman risk violence every day from harassment of eve-teasing to extreme forms of violence, like acid throwing and rape. Mere infrastructural changes and additional surveillance will only restrict women further, however, change in the mindset of the men, sensitivity towards gender equality and right to the urban spaces are pre-requisite for safer environment for the women.

Keywords Sexual violence · Delhi · Safe and unsafe urban spaces · Patriarchy · Rape

S. Reddy (✉) · S.S. Acharya
Center of Social Medicine and Community Health, School of Social Sciences, Jawaharlal Nehru University, New Delhi, India
e-mail: sunitareddyjnu@gmail.com

S.S. Acharya et al. (eds.), *Marginalization in Globalizing Delhi: Issues of Land, Livelihoods and Health*, DOI 10.1007/978-81-322-3583-5_10

Introduction

The United Nations defines the concept "violence against women" as "any act of gender-based violence that results in, or is likely to result in, physical, sexual or psychological harm or suffering to women, including threats of such acts, coercion or arbitrary deprivation of liberty, whether occurring in public or in private life". Considering gravity of the matter, the UN adopted a 'Declaration on the Elimination of Violence against Women'. According to this declaration (Article 2) the violence against women encompasses (but not be limited to)

> any physical, sexual and psychological violence occurring in the family, including battering, sexual abuse of female children in the household, dowry-related violence, marital rape, female genital mutilation and other traditional practices harmful to women, non-spousal violence and violence related to exploitation.
>
> or
>
> ….any physical, sexual and psychological violence occurring within the general community, including rape, sexual abuse, sexual harassment and intimidation at work, in educational institutions and elsewhere, trafficking in women and forced prostitution
>
> or
>
> ….any Physical, sexual and psychological violence perpetrated or condoned by the State, wherever it occurs.

In the light of this UN declaration, there are a numbers of international agreements on harassment and discrimination against women. The CEDAW Convention[1] defines discrimination against women as "…any distinction, exclusion or restriction made on the basis of sex which has the effect or purpose of impairing or nullifying the recognition, enjoyment or exercise by women, irrespective of their marital status, on a basis of equality of men and women, of human rights and fundamental freedoms in the political, economic, social, cultural, civil or any other field."

Perspective to Understand Gender Violence

The patriarchal perspective on rape can be understood by taking into account Rubin's arguments of woman being the most primary commodity of exchange and her chastity and virginity becomes extremely important for patriarchy to operate. Also women's primary function as reproducers, their chastity becomes important for maintaining the purity of line of descent, when traced along male lines. Therefore, the worth of a woman in the society is directly tied to her chastity (Rubin 1975). Women are not thought of as independent beings but properties attached to men and therefore raping a woman is violation of her owner, the

[1]The Convention on the Elimination of All Forms of Discrimination against Women (CEDAW), adopted in 1979 by the UN General Assembly, is often described as an international bill of rights for women.

man, and of the family or the community at large. Rape is seen as devaluation of the woman as a property either waiting to be exchanged or already exchanged. Therefore, to prevent rape or sexual harassment greater regulation of women is prescribed. The onus of not getting raped or harassed is put on women themselves.

The issue of gender violence then boils down to mindset of men and even women in the patriarchal and misogynist society. Rape is seen as unacceptable both by men and women across all social strata and yet it continues. Nivedita Menon argues that from the most robust patriarch to the most passionate feminist, everyone shouts rape to be unacceptable but calls for a separate feminist analysis of rape or sexual violence at large. While for patriarchal forces rape is unacceptable because "…it is a crime against the honour of the family, while feminists denounce rape because it is a crime against the autonomy and bodily integrity of the woman." This distinction becomes important in a scenario when the politics of ending gender-based sexual violence faces the threat of being co-opted by the conservative forces to serve the ends of a very different politics (Menon 2012, p. 115).

Locating Gender-Based Violence in Context of Smart and Safe City

A 'smart city' is an urban region that is highly advanced in terms of overall infrastructure, sustainable real estate, communications and market viability. This idea is being promoted by the government. A smart city is expected to be equipped with basic infrastructure to provide good quality of life, a clean and sustainable environment. It is also supposed to assure water and electricity supply, sanitation and solid waste management, efficient urban mobility and public transport, robust IT connectivity, e-governance and citizen participation, safety and security of citizens (Larrdis 2014). Delhi has been a smart city from before. However, the success of such a city depends on residents, entrepreneurs and visitors becoming actively involved in energy saving and implementation of new technologies (TOI 2014). There are many ways to make residential, commercial and public spaces sustainable by ways of technology. Such cities take years to develop. Delhi has come to a point in history where it can become smart, but safety issues are still to be organized. Public safety has emerged as an important function for governments across the world. It involves the duty and function of the state to ensure the safety of its citizens, organizations and institutions against threats to their well-being as well as the traditional functions of law and order (UN Habitat II 1996). With more than half the global population living in urban areas, safe city is essential in ensuring secure living and prosperity. The basic principles of good governance must be concerned with urban safety strategy; and aim at reducing and preventing common problems of crime, violence, especially against women, and insecurity. Therefore, it is important that the notion of Smart City being promoted by the government should take into cognizance the elements of Safe City and converge towards providing the conducive environment which is safe and violence free for all citizens,

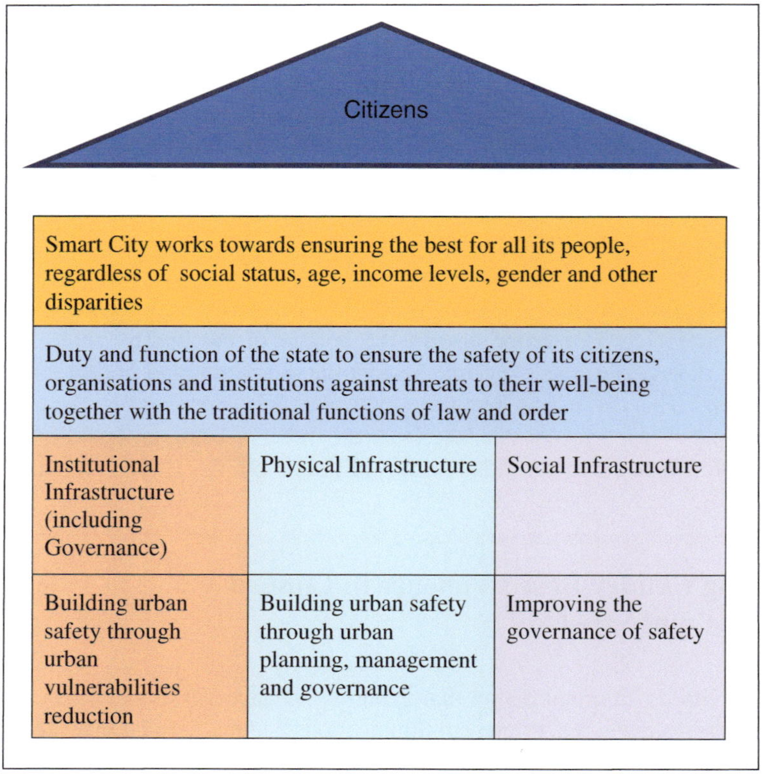

Fig. 1 Pillars of safe and smart city

particularly girls and women (Safe- Cities- the- India-Story 2014). Essentially, its Institutional Infrastructure (including Governance), Physical Infrastructure and Social Infrastructure constitute the three pillars on which a city rests. The centre of attention for each of these pillars is the citizen. In other words, a Smart City works towards ensuring the best for all its people, regardless of social status, age, income levels, gender and other disparities (Fig. 1).

Thus, it is pertinent to see the issue of sexual violence from feminist perspective, by respecting women's autonomy and bodily integrity. This can be achieved more by changing the mindset of men and even women, rather than mere law, infrastructural changes and having surveillance, which are still inadequate.

This paper first gives the data on the increased rape cases in Delhi in the past 6 years based on the crime records, and second based on the empirical research in selected schools, colleges and slum communities in South Delhi, analyzes the perception and experience of crime against women in everyday life.

Despite huge public protest and the new law 'Sexual Harassment of Women at Work Place Act' (2013), there has been increase in rape cases in Delhi. Figure 2, shows the increasing rape cases registered in Delhi in last 6 years along with the number of worked out cases, where the accused has been arrested. It contains the cases registered of both major and minor. There is clearly fivefold increase in the last 6 years.

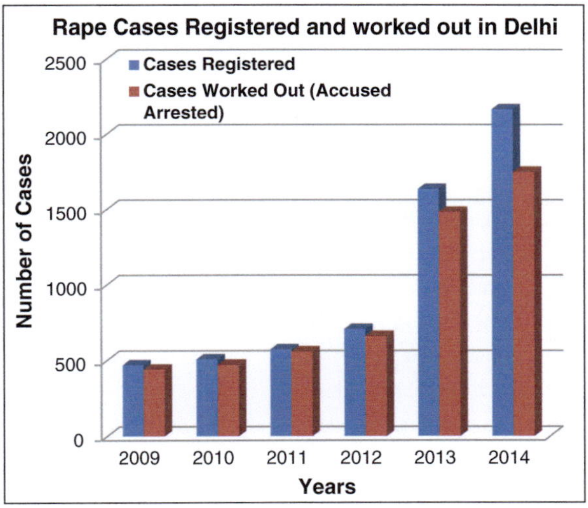

Fig. 2 Rape cases registered in Delhi. *Source* Deputy Commissioner of Police, Crime and Railways, Police Headquarters, New Delhi, the rape cases registered have gone up from 2009 to 2014

If we look at figures between the year 2012 and 2013, the cases more than doubled, after Nirbhaya case on 16 December. 2012. This case had led to a mass mobilization and protest against the system. The increase in the reporting can be also attributed to public protest and the new law gave courage to speak out, thus, even the old cases have been registered thereafter.

The data from the above source also showed the type of rape cases. Table 1 shows that rape is generally done by persons known or acquaintance and less by strangers. Only from 2013, additional factors have been analyzed like 'Live-in-relationship', 'refusal of marriage', pretext of providing job, 'Incestuous cases', 'acquaintance' 'stranger's rape', which were not categorized before.

In Table 1, Indicator 'live-in relationships' and 'refusal of marriage' are not mutually exclusive, because in many cases when a couple is in live-in relationship the reason for lodging FIR also is due to the refusal of marriage. The main concern, which arises out of it, is that, in most of the cases rapists were known to the victim. Very less number of cases falls under the category of stranger's rape cases.

Table 1 Types of the rape cases

		2009	2010	2011	2012	2013	2014
	Cases registered	469	507	572	706	1636	2166
1	Elopement cases	84	40	49	62	261	123
2	Live-in relationship					43	84
3	Refusal of marriage					232	529
4	Pretext of providing job					5	9
5	Incestuous cases					175	335
6	Acquaintances rape					1403	1745
7	Strangers rape case					58	86

Source Deputy Commissioner of Police, Crime and Railways, Police Headquarters, New Delhi, the rape cases registered have gone up from 2009 to 2014

Table 2 Place of crime

		2009	2010	2011	2012	2013	2014
	Cases registered	469	507	572	706	1636	2166
1	House/premises	276	382	498	633	1371	1801
2	Jhuggi cluster	26	22	26	23	43	47
3	Vehicle	4	12	13	19	33	45
4	Park/jungle/bushes						65
5	Shop/offices						25
6	Clinic/hospital/nursing home						8
7	Factory/go down/workshop						16
8	Subway/toilet						1
9	Hotel/Restaurant/Dhaba						70
10	School/college/educational institution						16
11	In train/platform		1	2	2	1	2
12	Other					188	40
	Total					1636	2166

Source Deputy Commissioner of Police, Crime and Railways, Police Headquarters, New Delhi, the rape cases registered have gone up from 2009 to 2014

Table 2 below shows the place of crime. Largest number of rape cases happened in home premises than the public spaces, institutions and work place. Thus, the new Act is also limited to only spaces where the crime is less frequent comparatively. This calls for urgent laws pertaining to reducing crime against women in their home premises. While in the patriarchal society, largely the mindset is that women should not venture out in late hours and pre-supposes home as safe haven.

Next section explores the perception of gender violence, and experiences of the respondents from selected school, colleges and slums of South Delhi. Part of the results are presented here, which is the part of a larger study, carried out by the authors under the auspices of SATAT, supported by Indian Council for Social Science Research.

Socio-Demographic Profile of the Respondents

Under this study, a total of 444 interviews were conducted in two schools and two colleges of the city of South Delhi. Of the total 444 samples, 49 % of the respondents were school students and 51 % respondents were college students. Interview was done in two schools—one high standard school (HSS) and other mid range school (MRS). Similarly, interview of college students was done in two colleges—one high standard college (HSC) and other mid-range college (MRC). Of the total school interviews, 15 % were from HSS, 34 % were from MRS similarly of the total college interviews, 26 % were from HSC and 25 % were from MRC.

The age profile of the total 444 samples was almost similar as of the total respondents, 49 % were from under 18 age groups constituted by school boys and girls, and 51 % were from 18 to 24 age groups largely represented by college boys and girls.

The social-category-wise composition of the respondents was dominated by the students of upper caste with 68, 17 % were from OBC category, 13 % from SC and 2 % from ST category. Religion wise 92 % were from Hindu religious, 4 % from Muslim community, 2.5 % Sikh, 1 % Christian and 0.5 % from Jain community.

Perception of Violence

Figure 3 indicates the perception about occurrence of violence against girls and women. Majority of them (76 %) felt that it is common or very common. The incidence of crimes against women happening all around and the media reporting of the same also fed into this perception. However, 13 % feel it is very rare.

Majority of our respondents especially women mentioned sexual harassment as an everyday experience, as common and very common (79.6 %), followed by boys (61.8 %). The important point to note here is how women internalize these occurrences as a part of their lives.

If we go further deep into the gender composition Fig. 4, the girls (>18 age and 18–24 age group) were more concerned about the issue and almost 100 % of them were sensitized with the same in comparison with the boys, 42 % of the girls stated it a very common problem, however, 37 % identified it as a common problem. There were 5 % girls who responded as a rare problem but 14 % of them responded it as very rare problem. A probable reason for this may be that they belong to the higher echelons of the society

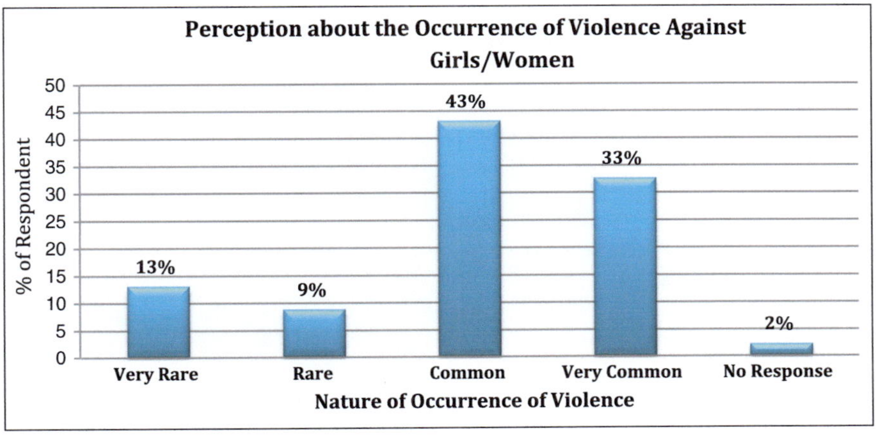

Fig. 3 Perception about the occurrence of violence against girls/women. *Source* Authors work

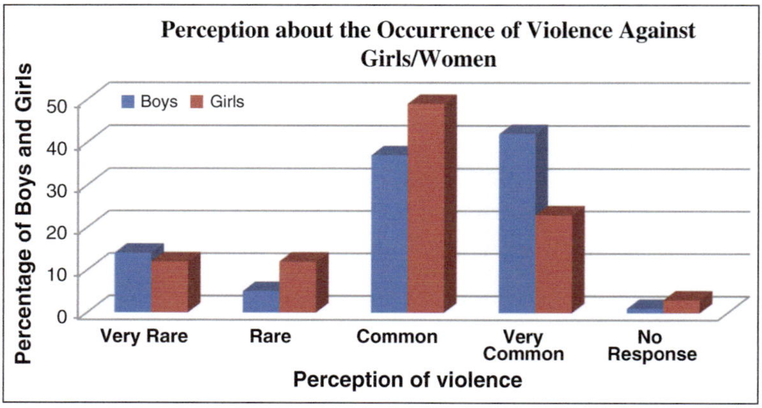

Fig. 4 Perception about the occurrence of violence against girls/women. *Source* Authors work

Sexual Behaviour Categorized as Violence and Harassment

Figure 5 shows various kinds of behaviour, which were listed to know the response of the participants to categorize them as either harassment or violence depending on the gravity of the behaviour. It was seen that most of the behaviour which does not involve physical contact like lewd cheesy comments, whistling, stalking were seen more as harassment than violence. However, showing pornography was more or less seen equally, as violence and harassment. There were no significant variation among boys and girls in categorizing.

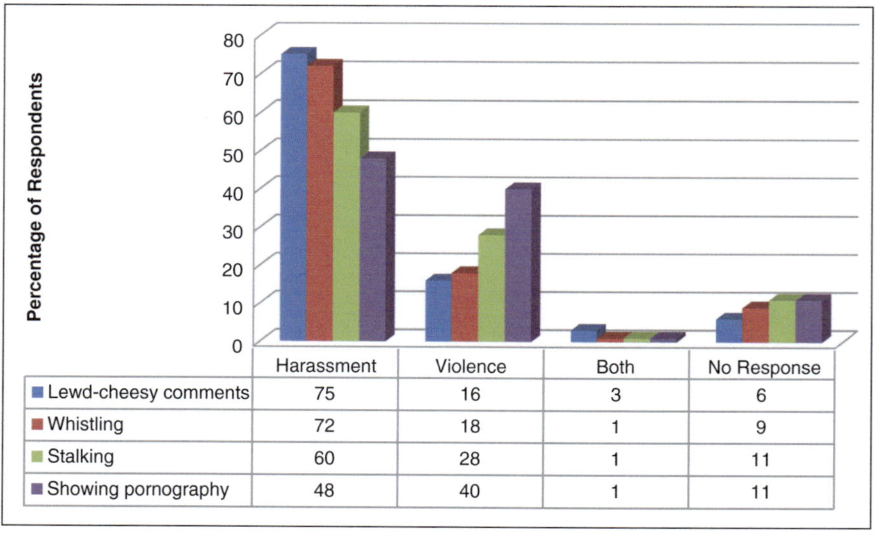

	Harassment	Violence	Both	No Response
Lewd-cheesy comments	75	16	3	6
Whistling	72	18	1	9
Stalking	60	28	1	11
Showing pornography	48	40	1	11

Fig. 5 Kind of behaviour (with physical contact) reported as violence and harassment with gender disparity. *Source* Authors work

When we analyzed the data about perception of respondents, regarding these offensive behaviours, both men and women were of the similar opinion. Of total persons interviewed, 75 % felt lewd cheesy comments as a kind of harassment, 16 % as violence, 3 % find them both harassment and violence and only 6 % were not able to give a satisfactory answer. Similarly, 72 % felt whistling was an act of harassment and 18 % felt it was violence. Regarding stalking, 60 % felt as an act of harassment, 28 % violence. Finally, regarding showing pornography, 48 % felt it was an act of harassment and 40 % felt it was violence.

Behaviour involving physical contact and their perception about the harassment and violence in Fig. 6 shows that majority of them felt they are violent behaviour and comparatively less percentage of the respondents saw it as harassment. Acid attack/blade cutting and physical attack were seen as more violent. Majority of the women categorized deliberate brushing against body, rubbing private parts, stroking and flashing as both harassment and violence.

All the behaviours which involved physical contact were invariably seemed by majority as violent. Figure 6 clearly indicates and also the nature of violence like physical attack and acid attack are seen as violent by majority. Though stoking, flashing and public masturbation does not involve physical contact, however, is seen as violent and repulsive.

Deliberate brushing against the body is a common kind of behaviour women generally face while travelling in public transport and at public places. Mostly it happens in the public transport systems like DTC buses, shared auto rickshaw, at bus stops, etc. 50 % of the respondents said that it is violence, 39 % said that it is a kind of harassment. Rubbing private parts against the other person's body was considered as violent by majority of the respondents nearly 56 %.

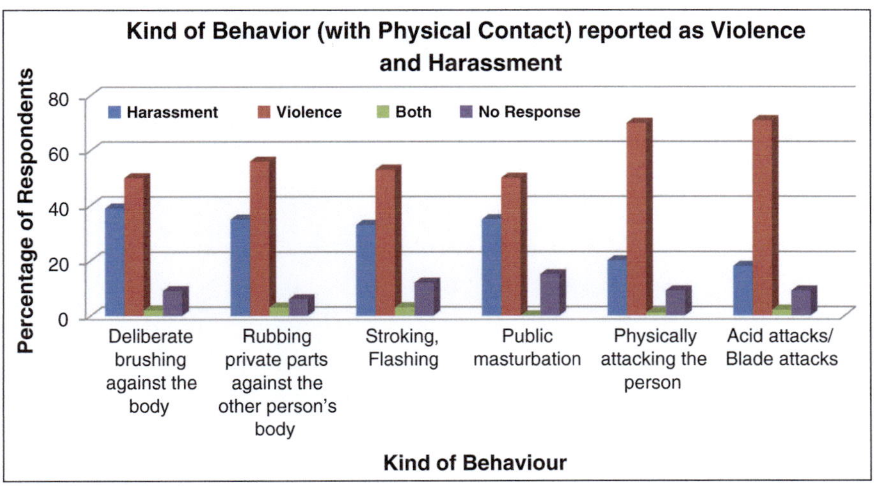

Fig. 6 Kind of behaviour (with physical contact) reported as violence and harassment. *Source* Authors work

Physically attacking the person is a serious violence opined by majority (70 %) of the respondents and similarly, acid attacks/blade attacks were obviously opined as violence by the majority (71 %) of the respondents. All the respondents agreed to the fact that such incidents happen in full public glare at crowded places like inside bus or at bus stops. Sometimes men deliberately brush their bodies against that of women and girls in the pretext of being in a congested space. Similarly, rubbing private parts against the other person's body, stroking, flashing, etc. were also reported as happening in public transports or at crowded places. While interacting with the respondents, some interesting facts came to light. For example, youngsters were among most notorious people identified for passing lewd cheesy comments; on the other hand in majority of the cases, elders or aged people were identified as culprits for touching the body or private parts of women and girls.

The important point to note here is how women experience these occurrences as a part of their daily lives. Women in Srinisvaspuri mentioned seeing men itch their private parts in public, pass of lewd cheesy comments, aiming things at their private parts or men trying to touch them, as part of their everyday experiences of negotiating the public space. Other women from the slums mentioned public masturbation, showing pornography, pinching, acid attacks and blade attacks among other things that they experienced in their daily lives. Interesting to note is that women in all these cases have internalized the experience of sexual harassment and it continues to inform their negotiations with the public space.

In the nature of crime, molestation is milder as compared to rape of various categories, either rape per se, or marital rape and custodial rape are of serious nature. Though marital rape is still being debated today in India, and not much of data is available on custodial rape. Figure 7 shows that the respondents however, see rape as violence and few of them see as harassment. Though the results are perplexing as still few of the respondents see it as harassment, it

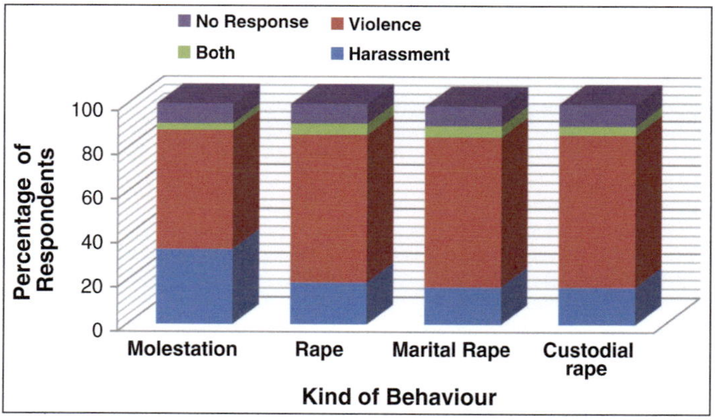

Fig. 7 Kind of behaviour (outrageous) perception of seriousness. *Source* Authors work

could be either because the age group around 16–18 are not so mature enough to understand the gravity of the crime like physical and acid attack in the previous table and rape.

For cases of molestation, 54 % respondents said that it is violence, 34 % said that it is a kind of harassment. The act of rape was considered as violence by 67 % of the respondents, 5 % said that it is both violence and harassment. Marital rape was opined as violence by 68 % of the respondents.

Safe and Unsafe Public Spaces

Entertainment Spaces and Eating Joints

In all our interviews, male and female respondents were able to identify certain spaces a more unsafe than the others and vice versa. Classifying public spaces under common categories, the entertainment and eating joints were listed as safe or unsafe. Figure 8 shows the categorization of safe and unsafe spaces with regards to pubs, cinema halls, discotheques and other places of entertainment that are the usual suspects.

Figure 8 shows that the pubs as very unsafe followed by cinema halls and hotels. Comparatively restaurants are seen as safe only by 50 % respondents. Combining unsafe and very unsafe, however, all three pubs, cinema halls and hotels are high on the scale.

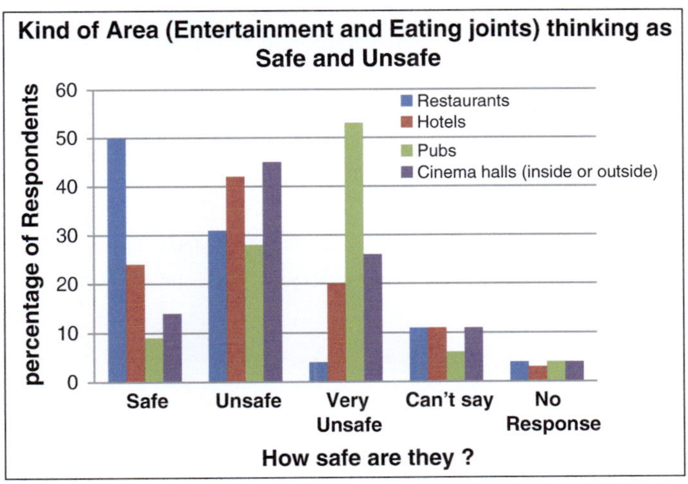

Fig. 8 Kind of area (entertainment and eating joints) thinking as safe and unsafe. *Source* Authors work

Civic Amenities and Social Facilities

Regarding the notions of safety and unsafe for the civic amenities and social facilities in public spaces, in Delhi, Table 3 shows that the public toilets were very unsafe, followed by parks as unsafe. Other buildings like auditoriums and monuments are also seen as unsafe. Even the police stations and hospitals were seen as unsafe though to a lesser extent.

Almost 79 % of the respondents feel that public toilets are unsafe. Numerically, for parks, 67 % replied unsafe and very unsafe. 45 % said gymnasiums are either unsafe or very unsafe and only 34 % respondents said they are safe.

Even police stations were considered as unsafe and very unsafe by 49 % of the respondents, which shows that the images of the police stations which are the protecting agencies too are negative. Even hospitals are seen as unsafe. Surprisingly, 45 % of the respondents replied that they are equally unsafe and very unsafe for women and girls. Public buildings were also considered as the unsafe places of Delhi as high as 55 % respondents considered them as unsafe and even very unsafe.

Thus, it shows that more or less all the public spaces with civic amenities are seen as unsafe. After gathering views of the respondents, one important perception which came out was that "women and girls are nowhere safe". Violence can happen anywhere, be it inside home or outside home, whether it is secluded area or a crowded area in the heart of the city, whether it is public place or private place.

Some of the respondents said that the secluded areas are dangerous for women and girls to walk alone but more than double the number of respondents said that they experienced sexual harassment at public places and people dare to do this in the pretext of crowd. They deliberately brush their body or private part or tease inside a crowded bus. One person was spotted putting off his pant in front of a women's college gate whenever he saw some girls crossing.

Many of the respondents drew our attention to the aftermath of any harassment/violence, and how the victims have to face further problems due to insensitive institutions. It was told that the personnel working in these institutions are not gender sensitive and also not trained to handle such issues with care and compassion, often blaming the girl/women in question.

Table 3 Kind of area (civic amenities and social facilities) perception as safe and unsafe

S.N	Kind of area (civic amenities and social facilities)	Safe	Unsafe	Very unsafe	Cannot say	No response
1	Parks	20	54	13	11	2
2	Gymnasium	34	32	10	18	6
3	Public toilets	6	43	36	11	4
4	Police station	31	37	12	15	5
5	Hospitals	41	33	12	11	3
6	Public buildings	27	42	13	14	4

Source Authors work

Table 4 Kind of area (educational and working place) thinking as safe and unsafe

S. N	Kind of area (educational and working place)	Safe	Unsafe	Very unsafe	Cannot say	No response
1	College premise	27	46	10	13	4
2	School premise	52	32	8	5	3
3	Your workplace	36	33	9	11	11
4	BPOs	13	44	20	14	9

Source Authors work

Reporting of the perception of safe and unsafe educational and workplace, Table 4 shows that school premises are seen as safe and BPOs as unsafe and most unsafe. The college premises are also seen as unsafe.

We tried to seek answers about "how safe are the educational institutes of Delhi"? The answers were not very different. The BPOs were considered as most unsafe place, on the other hand school premises were considered as most safe place by the entire respondents. A total of 64 % people were of the opinion that BPOs are either unsafe or very unsafe (44 + 20). College premises were second in the order in terms of recognized as unsafe place as 46 % respondents said that it is unsafe and 10 % said that they are very unsafe. Though, nearly 27 % respondents said that they are safe. About workplaces, around 45 % said they are either safe or very safe. Among all these places school premises were considered by 52 % as the safest place however, 32 % said that they are also unsafe place.

Some students said that college premises were safe but it became unsafe the moment they stepped out. Some girls confessed that in the college campus some of them are forced by boys to talk to them. It is interesting to note here that during special occasions like college festivals, college authorities separated the dancing areas of boys and girls to avoid unwanted incidents pointing out to the fear lurking everywhere and even the institutions tacit acceptance to it.

One of the students shared the experience of harassment by boys belonging to particular state and showing muscle strength,

> When I was talking to my friend in college some Haryanavi student came and passed some cheesy comment at us. They are very strong that's why I didn't react at that time but I feel very bad.

This also reveals the stereotyping of the boys from particular state as eve-teasers and further because of their muscle strength, they did not take any action, even though they felt, the harassment.

In a group discussion with the girls between the age group of 16–20 years, in KTJC shared,

> Outside the school, guys keep circling around us on their bikes. Not inside the school but outside. They also sit on the terrace of the school building and pass comments at girls.

Figure 9 shows the shopping and recreation centres as safe and unsafe. Markets were seen as most unsafe both by male and female respondents and malls are seen

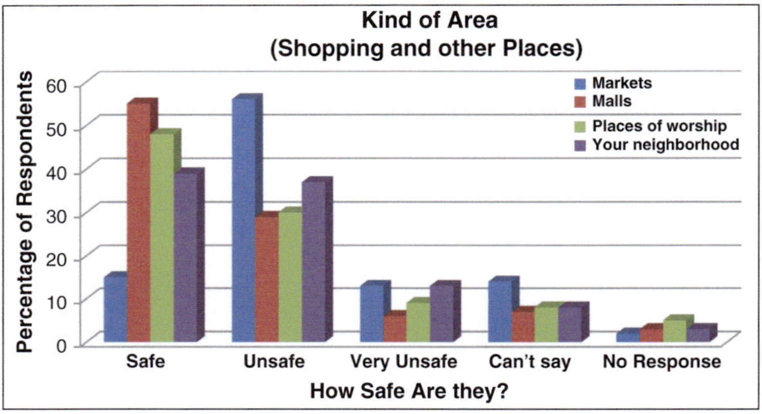

Fig. 9 Kind of area (shopping and other places). *Source* Authors work

as safer places. Neighbourhoods were seen as equally safe and unsafe by both. Some of them also felt the places of worship to be unsafe.

Public places like markets, malls, places of worship and even the neighbourhood are also very vulnerable places in Delhi. Among these places, markets were considered as most vulnerable place for occurrence of any violence against women however, malls were considered as safest place among all these places. Markets were opined unsafe by 56 % and very unsafe by 13 of the respondents. 50 % of the respondents were of the opinion that neighbourhood is also very much prone to occurrence of crime and violence as 37 % said that they are unsafe and 13 % said that they are very unsafe. 30 % of the respondents said that places of worships are also unsafe whereas 9 % people even stressed that they are very unsafe.

Market places came out to be the most unsafe place in our study. Many said people take advantage of the crowd and indulge in unwanted touching in the market places. One of the respondents said that she saw girls being harassed at Nehru Place. Other reported a man trying to kiss a girl at Nehru place. Many mentioned pushing and unwanted touching to be a common phenomenon in markets like that at Sarojini Nagar. A resident of Gandhi Camp narrated her experience of being in the market place in the following words,

They say things like, "'Where are you going?' 'You're looking good' and use dirty words while talking to us. In the market they hit you with onions at your rear. One day I went to the mandi one person said, 'you're very good looking very good, come with us'. Then one person aimed onions at my aunt's rear. When I protested some other men joined and started making dirty comments".

Two students from a private school in Delhi, narrated incidents of harassment in a temple and in their neighbourhood, respectively. The first recounted,

> In the Kalkaji Mandir in one of the festival days, when it was very crowded someone touched my friend's butt in the queue. She thought it was a mistake and must have happened because it was so crowded. She looked back and the guy moved back. Next when

> her parents and her brother moved ahead this time someone grabbed her by her breasts. She could not identify who it was as he disappeared in the crowd. She shouted, but no one heard her and no one took any actions. She could not tell the incident to her parents or her brother because of shame but also because it was a pious place and she thought describing such an incident would be inappropriate in that atmosphere.

Harassment and molestation at religious places can be quite common, however, may not be reported due because of being a place of worship. Further, the culture of silence and parents not having a free chat on these issues with children.

These experiences of the girls show the fear and anxiety in their everyday lives as they move out of their homes into the public spaces. The violence is even more serious in the context of slums, given the porous nature of the settlements.

A girl from Gandhi camp reported the following while talking about her neighbourhood,

> An incident happened in our neighbourhood. There was a Muslim girl. Her mother was out for work and she was alone in the home and a Muslim man came and started harassing her. He unzipped himself and started making dirty gestures. She started shouting but nobody could hear her. After this the guy warned her not to tell anybody about this and left.

Women in the slums reported feeling most unsafe in their neighbourhood. In one of the group discussions, a woman recounted the incident of a girl being raped in the camp itself by a resident of the same camp.

Respondents from schools and colleges identified family parties, malls and other gated spaces to be safest places where one could wear what one would like, not really bothered with the dress codes.

Violence and Modes of Transport

Means of transport were another major threat. One of the respondents mentioned being stared at by a man in the metro especially at her lower parts, despite expressing resentment through cold stares the man continued and it was in no way a deterrent that a man with whom she was romantically involved was present with her. Again another respondent mentioned that one day when he was in a Noida metro station some boys teased a girl and people who were standing around did not do anything to stop them including those in the authority. A group of students in a college mentioned Central Secretariat metro station to be one of the most unsafe places.

Another respondent mentioned her friend having a narrow escape from being molested by an auto driver. In yet another case a school student mentioned,

> Once I was out with a friend who was wearing shorts. Some men started staring at her. They even came and held on to the auto rickshaw. They were those Bihari 'Tapori' men who wear their collars high. When I tried protesting they slapped me. Some people from nearby came and saved us but the incident scarred my friend for her life. Now she never wears shorts. Even when she comes to play badminton she wears full length paijamas.

Experiences such as these can mark the psyche of the girl permanently, curtailing her freedom. While in the earlier case, the bystanders did not intervene, in the above case, their intervention helped to avert a major molestation. Again there is stereotyping of regional background of men who are seen as molesters.

Another respondent said that while travelling in an auto once an elderly person, who was her co-passenger, put his arms around her and refused to take note of her discomfort and removed only when she rebuked. In another incident, the respondent mentioned once while travelling in an auto with her friend the auto driver took them to an unknown place and she had to make fake phone calls and threaten him indirectly to be able to go back.

Many mentioned being harassed (unwanted touching, rubbing of private parts, etc.) in the bus and especially by elderly men in case of young girls who took advantage of the crowd and misbehaved. One of the respondents mentioned that "once she was standing in a bus and someone came and started touching a lady from behind, when rebuked he said a sorry but kept doing it again and again and she could not do anything". Another respondent mentioned that someone had pressed her hand on her first day of college while she was travelling in a bus. Later when she raised an alarm that person was asked to get off the bus.

In yet another incident a student noted,

> In January 2013, when I was coming to college from Sangam Vihar, the bus was very crowded and some girls didn't get a seat and were standing, some people were just behind them and when driver used the brakes, those peoples started touching these girls.

Yet another student said how people are not cooperative, as it delays the journey if the girl raises an alarm,

> I have many a times seen men stroking and molesting girls in the buses and if girls try to protest the bystanders do not help her to protest and raise voice against the perpetrators, infact, shout at the girls, as it delays the journey.

Another middle age professor of a college mentioned hitting men some ten times in the buses in Delhi to stop them from harassing. In a similar vein a college goer mentioned,

> Now-a-days people are always in a rush. If some incident of harassment happens in the bus nobody is ready to spend some time in redressing it like closing the doors and calling the police or trying to punish the harasser. They just try to ignore it.

One of the elder women respondents, now a faculty in a college while narrating her experience of her college days said,

> This has been the case since we were students. Today just reporting has increased. Those days even buses were less in number. We could not afford other vehicles. We suffered. Public transport and DTC buses were so unsafe. We were safe once we sat down. But the man in the next seat would try putting his arms around someone or the other. We would just see. I felt like saying 'Bhaiya just move ahead a little and stand.

The experience of women travelling in public vehicles is best summarized in the following words of a respondent.

> It's not an experience, it's a matter of day to day life, we girls have to face all these things while travelling, in buses people take benefit of the crowd and start touching the private parts of girls, and also in autos that run on shared basis.

Local trains were no exempt from this menace either. Bus terminals, auto stands were also mentioned as unsafe spaces where women mentioned experiencing lewd comments, unwanted gestures and stares. A woman from the camps summed up the experience of being at a railway station saying, "koi bhi, kahin bhi haath laga deta hai."

Main roads however were equally unsafe to some like the area around Nehru Nagar Bridge. The respondents from the slums reported having observed public masturbation along main roads. One of the students from a college mentioned being harassed by senior secondary students on their way from school in the past.

Some reported that a woman is not safe even when travelling in a private vehicle alone. Another student mentioned that one day when she and her sister were travelling in a Scooty, some boys came and hit her sister, who was at the back, on her chest and they could not do anything about it. Another student mentioned that some guys had tried to stop her car while she was driving one day and finally she had to call the police to get them out of her way.

The incidents shows rampant, stalking, eve-teasing, harassment in everyday life, most of the time the girls kept quiet, however, in few cases, they did call the police or shouted back and that made the harasser stop.

Time as a Factor for Violence

Generally it is understood that days are safer than nights and often, going out late in the evenings and coming late in the night is perceived as unsafe and meant to invite trouble.

The general perception about unsafe time is similarly perceived by the respondents in the study population. Figure 10 shows the opinions were also sought about

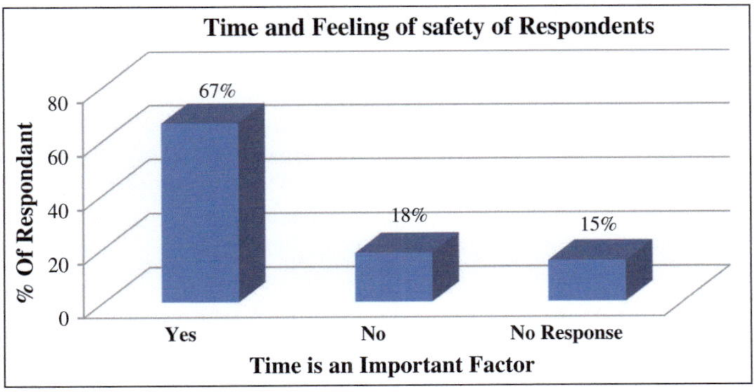

Fig. 10 Time and feeling of safety of respondents. *Source* Authors work

the time factor in the occurrence of violence. Time as a matter of fact was strongly supported by 67 % of the respondents. However, there were 18 % respondents feel, irrespective of time violence can be occur any point of time.

Table 5 gives further disaggregation on what time is most unsafe, early morning, day time, evening, after dark or time is not important, violence can happen any time. As understood, largely night time is most unsafe.

While enquiring about peopled perception about timing of violence the most unsafe time opined by all was ‘after dark’ which was responded by 80 % of the respondents followed by ‘evening’ which was chosen as most unsafe time by 44 % respondents. There were a significant number 25 % of the respondents who were of the opinion that occurrence of violence has no any specific time rather, it could happen at any point of time (Table 5).

Women in the slums mentioned that drunken people roam about in the night adding to their fears. Women expressing their fear of the night said,

This area is like that. A girl never feels safe when she steps out, neither during the day nor at night. It’s especially dangerous after dark. The slum area is particularly unsafe. You can’t go out after dark. The public toilets are very unsafe. In one of the instances, a girl in the slum was attacked and when she shouted, she was stabbed. Nothing was done on that case (Table 6).

Table 5 Perception about the time of occurrence of violence

S.N	Time Schedule	Most unsafe (perception) experiences (%)			
		Yes	No	Sometimes	No response
1	Early morning	23	40	29	8
2	Daytime	19	37	36	8
3	Evening	44	17	31	8
4	After dark	80	11	4	5
5	No specific time	25	7	22	47

Source Authors work

Table 6 Design considerations for safe cities

Type of alerts: real time or reactive or pro active	Type of cameras and sensors to be installed	Standardized systems for future integration and compatibility	Overall connectivity: dedicated or MPLS or multicast etc.
Design considerations for safe city	Integration with different agencies for inputs and consultation	Architecture to be adopted: centralized or decentralized or hybrid	Areas to be covered and hot spot identification
Integration of existing surveillance systems	Establishment of a command and control center	Reactive Analysis: Video forensics for legal evidence verification	Data center establishment and capacity Building

Source UN-Habitat Safer Cities Programme. Habitat Agenda on Human Settlements (Habitat II, 1996)

Age and Proneness to Sexual Violence

Age group is also an important aspect of this study because there is clear distinction amongst age groups as some of the age groups are perceived to be highly vulnerable for occurrence of violence and some are relatively less. However, a number of respondents said

> …..there is no age category for victims of sexual harassment she could be a 5 year old baby or a 70 year old lady. Incidents of sexual harassment apply equally to women and girls of all age groups.

Most Vulnerable Age Group

The study reveals that the young adults and teenagers/adolescent were found very high vulnerable whereas elders and infants were found as very low vulnerable. 45 % of the respondents said that vulnerability of young adults is 'very high' and 35 % said that 'high'. About teenagers and adolescent, 45 % said that their vulnerability is 'very high' and 32 % respondents said 'high'. Adults are considered as moderately vulnerable by maximum number respondents (37 %) but some of the respondents, nearly 23 % said that their vulnerability is also high and 17 % said that they are even very high vulnerable. Younger adolescents believed age group of 15–25 to be most vulnerable.

In our FGDs in the slums (Gandhi camp) adolescents were identified as most vulnerable by women between the age (15–25). One mentioned that two school going girls were abducted from outside their school when they went out for lunch break. Another in the same FGD mentioned a young adolescent Muslim girl being raped in the recent past. Another young woman mentioned numerous incidents of harassment herself. Another mentioned a school going Muslim girl being harassed on her way to school.

The elderly people were considered as very less vulnerable by 43 % of the respondents, 31 % said that they are less vulnerable. In the same way 57 % of the respondents were of the opinion that infants and children are very low and low vulnerable.

> One of the male students from a college told us that, 'When boys attain puberty they get attracted to the opposite sex. In this stage boys start teasing girls and sometimes cross the boundaries. As a young boy I have done it and I am ashamed of it and would and to apologize for that.'

Once again a student mentioned a girl being teased by her classmate in school. Some mentioned adolescents between 13 and 16 years of age as being most vulnerable. One narrated the experience of being stalked when she was thirteen. Another mentioned being stalked at while going to school and being whistled at inside a bus. Another school student said,

> A few boys from my school tried to touch my private parts. It went on for three days and then I reported it to our Senior Head Mistress.

One mentioned that age did not determine vulnerability because it was well possible for an 18-year-old man to rape a middle-aged woman. Another two echoed the same saying whether an infant or a seventy- or ninety-year-old, a woman always remains vulnerable. However, others identified children, adolescents and young women as most vulnerable. One of the students in FGD in a college also mentioned that 'even children are not spared'.

One of the respondents told us that aged women are also vulnerable because men think that they are physically weak and would not be able to resist. In another FGD, a college student mentioned seeing an elderly woman being harassed in a bus. In another discussion, in the same place with women over 25 years of age one mentioned a girl of five being kidnapped by a man of 30–35 in the railway station.

Women over 25 years of age in the slums said "ladki paanch saal ki hui nahi ki daar lagna shuru ho jata hai." but, she considered the adolescent girls of 15–16 years of age as most vulnerable. Even in our FDGs in the slums women mentioned that anyone could be raped at any time and she could be of any age.

In the group discussion, among the male of age group 18–30 years old at Karpuri Thakur Janjeevan Camp (KTJC), expressed "… Why men become violent? They thought the incidents of violence against women are common place, women often invited or caused their own violation. They pointed out that often sexual harassment was an outcome of revenge for when girls left their partners for 'greener meadows' or a logical response to the irresponsible westernized behaviour of women. Often boys confessed that were unable to control their urge to harass women and saw their behaviour as 'naturally triggered'. Often it involved 'acting like a man". This kind of understanding reiterates the patriarchal notions of controlling women and also giving biological reasons for their sexual violence.

Many women confessed that men sexually harassed women just for fun or to prove their machismo or to become popular amongst friends. One of the respondents, a woman professor from a college, expresses how 'male gaze' can be so penetrative, and leave an impact on the minds of women, in Delhi said,

> While sitting here also I can see a lot of violence happening. The "male gaze". It rips you apart. Even rape your soul. Not always rape needs to be physical, it can be merely through the gaze. That can be violative. And yes, it is unwanted. But sometimes one may just endure it. There are a lot of equations at work. So the system which grants power to some and let them abuse it also makes some others vulnerable.

Another professor around the age of 45, holding lawlessness to be the reason for feeling unsafe and insecure added,

> I think of myself as a brave woman. I am usually not afraid when out. But even then when I have to go out after 9.30 pm, I am scared 'aadhi ho jati hoon' meaning I reduce to half. Why? Because of the lawlessness. I am usually not afraid I can kill anyone if need be. But sometimes when it's necessary, I have to go out then I feel extremely scared. I am almost not able to recognise myself. Because there is no support system. There are many places and times, where I feel very scared. I can no longer relate to myself in such situations. It's not about wearing vulgar short dresses. I am not concerned about that. That comes much after. My fear is of a different kind.

This narrative gives a clear indication of how women irrespective of age group feels extremely vulnerable and fearful of the violence in the open spaces, owing to the increase in crime against women and the culprits going scot-free and judiciary taking very long time to book them and bring them to justice.

She further questions the name given to the victim 'Nirbhaya' which is so ironical, continued,

> ...(A) small point which did not come to me on my own but only after reading a blog. This was a blog about Nirbhaya. It questioned this name 'Nirbahaya' itself. What is this name- a woman who is fearless who would not break down who is bold and brave. But she had gone through the worst form of violence. There was so much abuse and yet her figure was glorified. But this was sheer helplessness.

The case of Nirbhaya also highlights the glorification of an individual who suffered so much and succumbed to extreme forms of brutality and sex crimes, further giving a name which is exactly opposite to the reality. Further, the case brought public outrage and protests to streets and coming up with new Act, giving hope that the situation would improve. However, post 2013, the situation has worsened, with increase in reporting of cases of sexual violence. The answers are not clear, is it due to increase in awareness and faith in judiciary that more and more women are coming forward to report, rather than silently enduring it. Or whether the crime has really gone up?

What was endured by Nirbhaya has a connect with the elements of safe cities program (UN Habitat 1996) which addresses the following

- Building urban safety through urban vulnerabilities reduction: Paying special attention to urban vulnerabilities and violence shall reduce the probability of crime and ensure a secure and safe city environment.
- Building urban safety through urban planning, management and governance: Sustainable urbanization by emphasizing inclusive and participatory urban planning, and local development practices, incorporates policy-making and strategy development.
- Improving the governance of safety: Enhancing urban safety and social cohesion are issues of good urban governance. They intend to create a city where safety is improved for its citizens and neighbourhoods, where there is fearless interaction among people and groups.

These aspects of good governance will create an enabling environment for the inhabitants of the city, allowing improved quality of life and fostering economic development. Therefore the design considerations which need to be explored for safe city.

Conclusion

In this section, we also covered question regarding safety issues, trying to gauge how far the city is perceived to be safe for women and girls. The answers were astonishing as there is no place/area which is supposedly safe for women.

Violence can occur outside home as well as inside her home; similarly violence can occur at secluded areas as well as in crowded areas. The only difference is degree of occurrence, home is perceived to be less prone to violence than outside as compared to crowded areas and secluded areas. Thus a major question is, can home be called safe? However, this study is not addressing this question. Women and girls are more prone to violence in public places. People dare to exhibit such offensive behaviours in the pretext of crowd in public transport system. Especially, the DTC buses are the most notorious places as identified by majority of the respondents. In the same way, there is no time span in the day when violence does not occur. The only thing is, it more frequent after the dark and odd times and in the day time probability of violence is probably comparatively less.

Thus, we see that women by the very fact that they are women are taken to be inherently rapable. Rape and sexual violence have been understood in a number of ways—as an act of power or an effect of socialization. Our study confirms both that it is an effect of re-establishing male power in a scenario when it is being challenged through new roles of women which give them parity with men and it also confirms sexual violence as an effect of socialization where women learn to live in the fear of violation. However, both these understandings are inadequate to understand sexual violence in totality. It must be understood that sexual violence is essentially understood as a sexual crime against women. The fear of sexual violence sets apart women from men and the women learn to regulate their lives in constant fear of facing sexual violence. It came up from our interviews that being a woman itself is enough to provoke sexual violence. Thus, gender violence is a way of systematically subordinating women and restricting their progress thus it just not mere difference of experiences between men and women but a way to maintain the inequality between men and women. Again, it is also the result of unequal status between and women where women are thought of as men's property or sexual objects for use by men and are humiliated in the home and outside for being women. Thus, sexual violence cannot be understood as a single aberrant act, a single interaction gone wrong or a law and order issue. The roots have to be located deeper in the forms of structural inequalities present in the society. It is something done to women by men to keep them in checks. Women on the other hand learn to live with the fear of being violated as part of their lives. Women even if they do not face sexual harassment directly always live in the fear of sexually harassed. They either derive this memory from the media or through socialization by family and friends. For MacKinnon, thus in order to develop an understanding of rape it is important to understand that rape and sexual violence is a part of complex that sets apart women as objects of sexual appropriation of the other sex and constructs the female gender as such. Further, the dichotomy between 'normal' sexual intercourse and sexual violence needs to be broken down and they need to be understood as a part of the same complex system. And third, sexual violence needs to be understood as a form of gender inequality rather than being dismissed just as a form of difference of experiences between the genders (Kennedy 2003).

It is thus important to realize that men who commit sexual violence are not psychologically different from other men and the possibility of sexual violence inheres from the hierarchical relation between men and women, i.e. it is a form of structural violence and not an aberrant phenomenon. This would also mean that the woman who is raped is no different from the woman who is not. A woman for being a woman is supposed to validate a man by satisfying a man's desire and if she denies such validation a man by virtue of the unequal relations in the society is entitled to use force obtain validation hence normalising rape and sexual violence

Then it can be argued that sexual violence is a way in which certain individuals are gendered as women (Kennedy 2003). In fact, then sexual violence becomes a way of defining and disciplining bodies by constructing them as violable. Also, this kind of reasoning is used when simply because someone is gendered as woman is held responsible for her own violation (Butler 1994). Going back to Mackinnon, the category woman is created as the object of the other's desire—so in principle, she is unrapable and yet if she is raped it is her own responsibility because she was supposed to protect herself. One of the most important ways of protecting herself would be to be at home, the arena where she belongs, being the domestic property of the man she is attached to and going out of home itself is inviting rape. Rape is nothing but such appropriation taking place on the street. "…a logic, that implies that rape is to marriage as the streets are to home, that "rape" is street marriage, a marriage without a home, a marriage for homeless girls, and that marriage that is domesticated rape, then rape is the logical consequence of enactment of her sex and sexuality outside domesticity" (Butler 1994, p. 53). Thus, we see through our study that whenever women veer out into the public arena they became targets of harassment and rape. This is everywhere from public transport to roads to travelling in personal vehicles, or being in the market place, religious places, public institutions or any other public place.

Interesting to note is that often this goes under reported. Women often try their best to prove their innocence before claiming their status as victims and often do not report such cases due to fear of public humiliation. The, debates around sexual violence are probably the starkest area where the division between the misogyny of classifying women into good and bad become the starkest. It is however common knowledge that these categories of the good woman/bad woman, *susheel aurat* and *baazaru aurat*, or Maddona and whore are not stable. Women live their lives with the constant fear of falling from grace and the impossibility of recovering the lost grace. A simple gesture, movement gesture or dress anything has the possibility of earning disrepute. Therefore, whenever a woman is raped for being what she is, it should be thoroughly questioned (Menon 2012).

Women in our interviews have often seen harassment as milder and mainly including behaviour that is without physical contact. Such behaviour is often termed as eve-teasing and needs to be given proper attention. Sunder Rajan defines, "Eve- teasing is the harassment of a woman in public- verbally, physically or both, a form of taunting with varying degrees of seriousness; the eve-teaser might act alone or in a group of like—minded men while the victim is usually single… the quaint term eve-teasing in India carries similar connotations of simultaneous gallantry and "harmless" male mischief and has passed into accepted usage.." (Sunder Rajan 2000, p. 341) She adds that 'eve-teasing' in the Indian context is marked by two major ambivalences—first, even though is it condemned socially, morally and legally it is also justified as a punishment to the brazen woman. Second, it reveals men's anxieties about female sexuality, superior social status or social mobility or all of these. Often such crimes are blamed on modernity—modernity is often made out to be a villain which has disturbed the existing social fabric and has created new anxieties leading to the violation of women. The entrenched misogyny of tradition is often discounted in such a narrative. It is often forgotten that women's rights are an important component of modernity and it is often forgotten that modernity brings women out into the public arena for the first time. Sunder Rajan in a thought provoking way urges her readers to go beyond the perpetrator and the victim and understand the act from the actions of the bystander. The non-interference, apathy or active complicity with the criminals exhibited by the bystanders according to her is important entry points to the issue. This is evident from our study where a large number of respondents have agreed that despite such instances happening in full public glare are seldom objected to or protested. Women have also internalized these happenings as a part of their everyday lives and as price to be paid for their entry into the public sphere. Moreover, the reaction of the law as experienced through its enforcing officers, according Sunder Rajan, are extensions of the same phenomenon. It is within the frame work of prevalent social attitudes that the act of sexual harassment, the reaction of the bystanders and by extension that of the law keepers are to be viewed. Only when viewed in this light we understand that eve-teasing becomes a new instrument in the post colonial scenario to keep women under control when women's entry into the public sphere becomes inevitable because of the so called 'modernisation project.' However, it is presented as one of those inherent risks that women must be brave if they have to and choose to enter the public sphere. Consequently, women are often blamed for being present in the wrong place aim the wrong time or dressing wrongly—urging them to correct themselves (Sunder Rajan 2000).

However, this exclusion of women from the public sphere through use of violence cannot be understood minus this politics to exclude those did not fit a particular vision of the city. This is evident from our responses where repeatedly certain categories of men are blamed for making the city unsafe for women. Safety, it is her claim and is directly related to the amount of claim one feels one has over a space. It is not as much protection from violence as the belief that if one is violated one's presence in that place will be seen as legitimate. Therefore, only the legitimate right to public space as citizens according to her can transform women's relation to the public. Phadke argues that since talking of safety of working class women in public spaces would actually mean also taking of safety of working class in general, a discourse that only focuses on the unmarked category of women focuses only on middle class women and rather serves to reinforce the boundaries of class and gender in access to public spaces (Phadke 2007). This is brought out through our interviews where we get to see that often the women residing in the slums face a greater threat of sexual violence than women in comparatively better off backgrounds though women in general in the city are unsafe. However, often in the discourse of providing safety to women these women come to be ignored and working class men are seen as the major threats to the upper class middle class women.

Another aspect of the problem is the lack of societal and infrastructural support for women.

Phadke argues that in present relation of women to the public space there is easy slippage between risks women choose and those that are imposed on her. The risk of accessing the public space might be actively chosen by the woman but the additional risk of putting up with lack of adequate infrastructure that it involves is not actively chosen but has to be included in one's calculations. Another risk that she points out is the risk of reputation that women have to face, including women who venture into the public space respectfully (obeying patriarchal norms of conduct) and purposefully (for purposes of education, employment, consumption). The onus to prove one-self respectable and virtuous over and over again to demand protection from and redressal of the violence faced is a risk that is not necessarily chosen (Phadke 2007).

Thus, women's empowerment cannot take a narrow view. If the city is to be made safer for women exclusions of men who are marginal in the city and often blamed for harassment have to be taken into consideration. The way of protecting women through more and more gated spaces which are private spaces but masquerade as public spaces (such as malls) seems to be faulty because the other class of women who cannot enter such spaces become targets of increased violence and adoption of a certain life style is only justified for a handful of women (ibid).

Thus, increasing women's right to the city includes projecting more and more the right of women to be present in the public space as an important right. It should not be exclusive to a group of women but all women in the city. It also means making situations conducive in the city for better access of women to the public space through improvement of infrastructural facilities like roads, public toilets, providing better lighting, opening up of helplines, making women aware of their rights through posters, hoardings, etc. However, this should not come to mean an ever increasing surveillance where by women's mobility is hampered and codes of morality are imposed ever more strictly on her. Also, a purely legalistic view to this problem would prove to be inadequate. There is a need to change the patriarchal thought structures and it is important for women to learn to not to be submissive and fight back instances of violence.

References

Butler, J. (1994). Contingent foundations: Feminism and the question of "postmodernism". *The postmodern turn: New perspectives on social theory* (pp. 153–170).

Kennedy, E. (2003). Feminist Responses to the Politics of Rape: Identifying the Women's Perspectives, Available from http://chrestomathy.cofc.edu/documents/vol2/kennedy.pdf(12 July, 2015)

Larrdis. (2014). Lok Sabha secretariat parliament library and reference, research, documentation and information service (Larrdis) members' reference service reference note. No. 28/RN/Ref./November/2014 For the use of Members of Parliament Not for Publication SMART CITIES.

Menon, N. (2012). *Seeing like a feminist*. Penguin UK.
Phadke, S. (2007). Dangerous liaisons: Women and men: Risk and reputation in Mumbai. *Economic and Political Weekly,* 1510–1518.
Rajan, R. S. (2000). The story of Draupadi's disrobing. *Mapping Histories: Essays Presented to Ravinder Kumar* 39.
Rubin, G. (1975). The political economy of sex. *Feminist Anthropology: A Reader* 87*.
Safe Cities in India Story. (2014). Retrieved July 2, 2015, from https://www.pwc.in/en_in/in/assets/pdfs/industries/government/safe-cities-the-india-story.pdf
TOI. (2015). What is 'Smart City' and How it work'. The Times of India. Retrieved May, 02, 2015, from http://timesofindia.indiatimes.com/What-is-a-smart-city-and-how-it-will-work/listshow/47128930.cms
UN-Habitat Safer Cities Programme. (1996). Habitat agenda on human settlements (Habitat II).

Migrant Women Workers in Construction and Domestic Work: Issues and Challenges

Sanghmitra S. Acharya and Sunita Reddy

Abstract Rural to urban migration in search of better working and living conditions is more like a mirage. The life is often harsh, pathetic, deplorable in place of destination like the Capital City Delhi, yet migration continues, as the place of origin is even more appalling where even survival is not secured. This is the story of 1010 migrant women workers in 9 districts of Delhi engaged in construction and domestic work. Largely hailing from the neighbouring states of Uttar Pradesh, Madhya Pradesh, Bihar, Orissa and West Bengal, they have migrated during the past 40 years. About 80 % of them are Scheduled Caste, landless agricultural labourers find it difficult to survive back home and therefore migrated to Delhi with lots of dreams and aspirations. Most of them live in JJ colonies and slums. Except for acquiring a few assets, their life in Delhi is as challenging as in the place of origin, with many women working hard to meet the ends. This paper analyzes 501 construction workers, 99 % of whom are into non-mechanical work, largely head loaders, and labourers, getting paid around 150 rupees per day, much less than the minimum wages and also unequal wages, more than 52 % reporting of injustice to payments. About 71 % are living in *kaccha* (semi permanent) house, single-room accommodation. Only 26 % have separate toilets. 86 % are not having any crèche facility, and 76 % with no place to rest. Few of them reported to have been injured and met with serious accidents and not been compensated and laid off thereby shifting to domestic work. There is urgency to provide the basic minimum facilities and better living conditions for those who form the backbone of the economic growth, be it the

S.S. Acharya (✉) · S. Reddy
Center of Social Medicine and Community Health, School of Social Sciences, Jawaharlal Nehru University, New Delhi, India
e-mail: sanghmitra.acharya@gmail.com

S.S. Acharya
Indian Institute of Dalit Studies, New Delhi, India

S.S. Acharya et al. (eds.), *Marginalization in Globalizing Delhi: Issues of Land, Livelihoods and Health*, DOI 10.1007/978-81-322-3583-5_11

construction sites or domestic workers. The vast informal and heterogeneous characteristics of the women workforce in India with growing informalization of employment, lack of visibility and voice of such workers call for improvement in the quality of employability and growth and extension of social protection to the unreached. This action research by the authors, further continues to provide skill building and placement for the domestic workers in collaboration with other organizations and also provide the social protection by facilitating the construction workers to register and get the benefits under the provisions of 'The building and other construction of workers Act, 1996' and 'The building and other construction workers welfare Cess Act, 1996' where hundreds of *crores* of rupees are stocked for their welfare, but no commitment and sensitivity so far to use this funds for the workers welfare.

Keywords Migrant women workers · Domestic workers · Construction workers · Delhi · Migration

Introduction and Background Literature

Globalization and liberalization have made migration across the world a common phenomenon. Rapid urbanization and development in the service sector have encouraged labour movement from rural to urban areas. Migration process includes movement of people from one place to another. There are number of causes which are responsible for migration. The causes that force to out-migrate are called *Push Factors*. These are under development of a region, unemployment, bad economic condition, unskilled and uneducated population, landlessness, and unavailability of health and education facilities, low level of urbanization and industrialization and social problems. All these factors lead to movement of people from one place to another in search of facilities and opportunities. On the other hand, the causes, which act as magnetic force or attract people inwards for in-migration are called *Pull Factors*. These are urbanization and industrialization of a region, leading to employment opportunities, availability of basic health and education facilities and social security. All these factors attract people for immigration towards the areas where these facilities are available. On the eve of discussion on international migration and development, convened by the UN General Assembly in New York on 3 and 4 October 2013, the experts said—"Migrants are human beings with human rights, not simply agents for economic development". It was observed that the migrants suffer abuse, exploitation and violence despite the legal human rights framework in place, which protects migrants as human beings, regardless of their administrative status or situation. International Convention on the Rights of Migrant Workers and their Families (ICRMW) takes into account the core human rights of the migrants but this treaty does not give migrant workers special treatment. It does not create new rights nor establish additional rights specifically for migrant workers. It, however, gives specific form to standards that protect all human beings so that they are meaningful within the context of migration. India is a signatory of the Convention on the Elimination of All Forms of Discrimination against Women (CEDAW). General

Recommendation No. 26 on Women Migrant Workers (2008) remains largely unimplemented. It suggests to respect, protect and fulfil the human rights of women migrant workers, against sex- and gender-based discrimination.

The present paper rests its argument from the derivation of Lee (1966), Zelinsky (1971), Stark (1991), Taylor (1999) on theorization of migration process. Apart from the personal factors, which are assumed to play an important role in determining migration decisions, different 'push' and 'pull' factors also play in the place of origin and place of destination, respectively. The New Economics of Labour Migration (NELM) assists in recognizing that a migration decision—who goes where and for how long, and to do what are joint decisions taken by the household, and differently for different members of the household. Labour migration within India is crucial for economic growth and contributes to improving the socio-economic condition of people. Migration can help, for example, to improve income, skill development and provide greater access to services like healthcare and education. Women constitute an overwhelming majority of migrants. Female migrants are less represented in regular jobs and more likely to be self-employed than non-migrant women. Domestic work has emerged as an important occupation for migrant women and girls. A gender perspective on migration is imperative since women have significantly different migration motivations, patterns, options and obstacles from men.

Another important fact under which this study is based is the fact that the women workers in 'construction' and 'domestic' work come from a lower socio-economic background with no literacy and skills fall in the unorganized sector. National Commission for Enterprise in the Unorganized sector (NCEUS) calculates 86 % in unorganized sector, and among the women it is 94 % employed in agriculture and allied activities, construction, transport, mining, manufacturing, small and medium enterprises and as contract labour. The other service, which demands women worker at a growing rate, is of domestic worker in urban areas.

It is well established through the literature, that most migrant workers experience distress in the places of origin and exploitation at places of destination (Griffin and Soskolne 2003; Iredale et al. 2003). The processes of migration and health are inextricably linked in complex ways, with migration impacting on the mental and physical health of individuals and communities. Health itself can be a motivation for moving or a reason for staying, and migration can have implications on the health of those who move, those who are left behind, and the communities that receive migrants (Jatrana et al. 2006). The challenge is that migrants usually form a class of invisible workers. They work in poor conditions, with no access to government services and schemes, which are usually available to other workers. There are different risks in source and destination areas. Needs of family members, including infants, children, adolescents and elderly who accompany migrant workers who are left behind in source areas also need to be addressed. Therefore, it is important to understand the factors contributing to exploitation and distress, related illnesses; and means to empower them through evolving strategies. Thus, in the empowerment framework and rights-based approach, the present paper will examine job opportunities, working conditions and social and economic security of women engaged in construction and domestic work.

The vulnerability of women worker especially in construction and domestic work is not addressed adequately. Some important studies on construction workers are carried out by Thadani and Todaro (1984), Kaveri (1993), Unni (2000), Mukta (2001), Chauhan and Sharma (2003) and more recent studies by Ghosh (2009), Geetika et al. (2011), Chawada et al. (2012), Singh (2012), Barara et al. (2012).

Gender differentials in these two different work spheres, construction and domestic vary substantially. In the construction sector, women do majorly unskilled labour involving carrying load; and in the domestic sector, unskilled and semi-skilled work restricted to homemaking. The construction women workers are fewer than the domestic women workers. However, the two different sectors have different demands and challenges for these women.

This paper is based on the study 'Migrant Women Workers in Construction and Domestic Spaces in Delhi Metropolitan Area: An Analytical Study of Empowerment and Challenges' sponsored by the Ministry of Women and Child Development. It undertakes a comparative analysis to understand the similarities and differences in the nature of work, among the women migrant workers in domestic and construction spheres. The challenges which the city poses to them and the risks which they are exposed to are the major concerns of the present paper. The metropolis that is Delhi, offers numerous opportunities for livelihoods which are also unorganized in nature. Delhi, as a metropolitan city, draws migrant population from various neighbouring states. Urban growth and industrialization in the city have attracted more migrants in recent decades. Rural to urban as well as urban to urban migration streams have broadened over last two to three decades. While urban sprawl has led to the engagement of migrant with the construction industry; increase in work participation rate among women in professional and skilled sector and nuclearization of families have generated demand for domestic workers. Fast-growing infrastructure development in the capital and surrounding regions draws huge migration by creating work opportunities in construction sector, as well as at homes for domestic helps. Some of the questions, thus posed through this paper are

- Who are these women? Why do they have to migrate? What are the push and the pull factors?
- Are there any state and social mechanisms which help them adapt to this change from the place of origin to the destination?
- Can there be measures to make their transition better and useful?
- Can the issues of abuse, exploitation and violence be addressed and how?
- What is the legal human rights framework which protects migrants as human beings, regardless of their administrative status or situation?

The specific objectives of the present paper are

- Understanding the 'pull and push factors' of migration, implications of migration on basic necessities and entitlements of the migrant women like, education, food security, medical facilities, housing, water and sanitation.
- To examine the existing conditions of work contract, forms of exploitation and abuse at construction sites and employers households.

- To understand the implications of working conditions on their health and wellbeing, child bearing and child care.

Study Design and Methods

This paper is based on the cross-sectional study which was carried out in the nine districts of National Capital Territory (NCT) of Delhi. The study sites were extracted on the basis of the sampling strategy based on the linear selection. Delhi Metro Rail routes were selected, and the closest construction site and the slum area to the identified Metro station were purposively selected, in each district, for the conduct of the study. Thus nine sites, one from each of the nine districts was selected to extract the construction sites so as to select the construction workers (Table 1). The study included both qualitative and quantitative methods of data collection. Quantitative method was employed by the use of structured questionnaire schedule canvassed to 501 construction and 509 domestic workers. The respondents selected were migrant women aged of 14–60 years, who worked at construction sites; and lived in the slums close by. Qualitative methods were geared towards capturing lived experiences. The life history methods were used along with the use of narratives in selected case studies. Selected employees at the construction sites/contractors/personnel's in placement agencies were also interviewed through semi-structured schedules. The fieldwork was conducted during October 2012 till July 2013. The women workers were randomly selected at construction site and in the slums. They were explained the purpose of the study and a verbal consent was taken. Anonymity of the respondents was ensured. Permission was also taken to photograph them and use them in publication of the research. Establishing rapport with the respondents to initiate the conduct of the study and getting permission to interview workers at the construction site was a major challenge.

Table 1 Sampling design for survey work

SN	District	Pop-2011	Percent of pop.	Samples (construction + domestic)	Sites
1	North West	3,651,261	21.79	55 + 55	1 + 1
2	North	883,418	5.27	57 + 56	1 + 1
3	North East	2,240,749	13.38	57 + 57	1 + 1
4	East	1,707,725	10.19	56 + 56	1 + 1
5	New Delhi	133,713	0.80	55 + 56	1 + 1
6	Central	578,671	3.45	55 + 56	1 + 2
7	West	2,531,583	15.11	56 + 58	1 + 1
8	South West	2,292,363	13.68	55 + 60	1 + 2
9	South	2,733,752	16.32	55 + 55	1 + 1
10	Delhi	16,753,235	100.00	501 + 509 = 1010	9 + 11

Source Authors work

Major Findings

Nearly one-third of India's population is migrant population. Half of this population has migrated from rural areas to cities in search of work. Lack of alternate livelihoods and skill development in source areas, locations from where migration originates, are the primary causes of migration from rural areas. Workers migrate seasonally, temporarily, or for a longer period, either within a state or across states. More often than not, they are vulnerable, exploited and work in conditions where their rights are not protected. Age of the migrant women is the one of the most important factor for out-migration from place of origin to destination. Most often it is the women of reproductive and productive age group between 15 and 45 years who migrate to follow the husband, or with family or for work. About 80 % of the study respondents were between the age group of 15–45 years. The religious composition shows that majority of the migrant women workers follow Hindu religion (89 %), followed by about 11 % Muslim women. Christian constitute only 0.5 %.

Majority of them (74 %) are Scheduled Castes, 11 % OBC and 5 % Scheduled Tribes (Fig. 1). About 86 % are married and about 8 % were widowed. About 61 % of the total migrant women got married before the legal age of 18 years. Majority of women (87 %) are illiterate, and are therefore left with no choice but to do unskilled jobs (Fig. 1)

The economic background of these women shows that 51 % of them earned less than $1.25 per day also called below poverty line (BPL). The Above Poverty Line Population has been classified into three categories. The above poverty line (APL-I) is with 40 % who are earning between ($1.25–2.50) per day; 7 % (APL-II) earn ($2.50–$3.25) and 2 % (APL-III) above $3.25 per day. Thus, more than half of the women workers are from the BPL families and rest from just above the poverty line.[1] This was also because most of them were illiterate (Fig. 2).

The migration pattern shows that 90 % of the migrant workers are coming from Northern India, and is mostly rural to urban migration. More than 90 % migration flow is from rural areas. The place of origin of the migrant women workers are from Uttar Pradesh (around 42 % in construction and 45 % in domestic work), followed by Madhya Pradesh in construction (23 %) and Bihar in domestic work (16 %). Chhattisgarh and Jharkhand are also contributing about 2–3 % of the migrant women workers in Delhi (Fig. 3).

The causes of out-migration or the push factors, functional at the place of origin, for 59 % construction worker, is largely unemployment and poor economic

[1]The conversion rate of the wages has been computed on the basis of the Dollar-Rupee rates at the two time points-beginning and the end of the field work during October 2012–July 2013. The value of dollar in October 2012 was $1 = Rs. 52.45 and in July 2013 it was $1 = Rs. 60.77. The average value, $1 = Rs. 56.59 is used for the computation. ($1.25 = Rs. 70.74; $2.50 = Rs. 141.48; $3.25 = Rs. 183.92). The values have been taken from the following websites http://www.exchange-rates.org/Rate/USD/INR/10-1-2012, http://www.tititudorancea.comz/usd_to_inr_exchange_rates_dollar_indian_rupee_nyfed.htm.

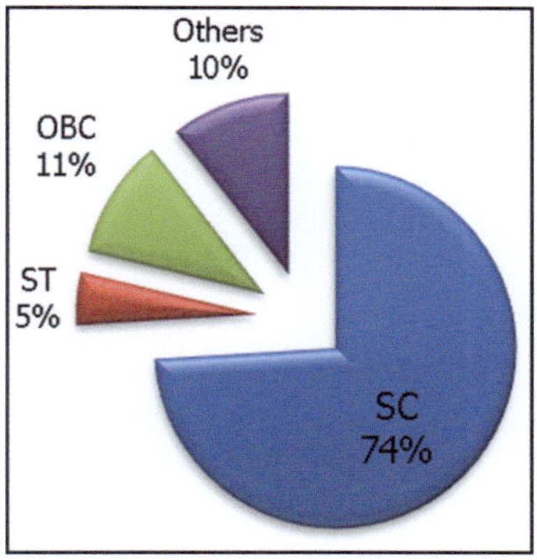

Fig. 1 Social composition of migrant women worker. *Source* Authors work

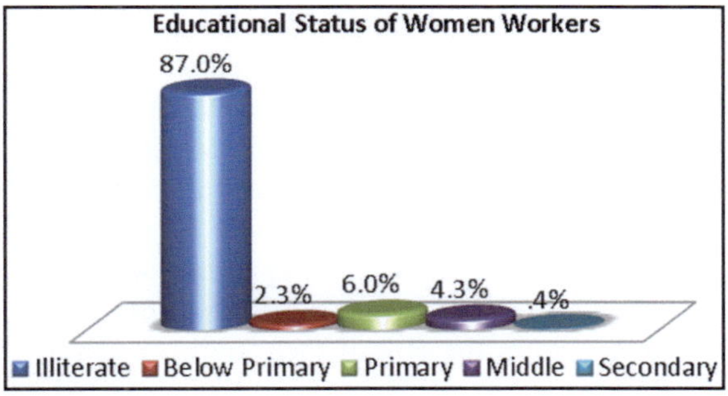

Fig. 2 Educational status of women workers. *Source* Authors work

condition of the family. Most of them were landless agricultural labourers who were forced to migrate due to poverty and lack of employment opportunities (See Box 1).

Box 1—The Push Factors…

Forty-two-year-old Balmuni belongs to a village, Buidummara Chakardarpur, Ranchi, Jharkhand. She comes from a family of landless, illiterate, unskilled, agricultural labourer with no source of income except their labour. She has four children—one boy and three girls. She had migrated to Delhi along with her husband *'some time in the winters'* of 2012 '*to take care of him'* who has migrated in search of employment. Later, as the hardships multiplied, she started working as a daily wage construction labourer along with her husband. She earns Rs. 145 per day and lives in a small *jhuggi* near the construction site. There is no provision of water, electricity, toilet facility. She narrated-

'Garibi ke karan mujhe kaam karna pad raha hai. Bina paani, bijli aur 'baher jane ki jagah (toilet) *ke rehte hai. Gaon mein to kam se kam*

naddi-talab to tha. Majoor bhi mil jati thi. Lekin pura nahin parda tha. Kabhi kabhi kaam ke paise bhi nahin milte thay... Bahut pareshani thi... isiliye socha ki marad ke saath rahenge to shayad kuch theek thak kam mil jaye'.

In other words, Balumuni was living without any facilities. But the hope to make it big in the 'city of better opportunities' gave her and her husband the strength to struggle for the living

This narratives point out that it was a struggle to even survive at the place of origin; they moved to Delhi, looking for employment opportunities. Delhi is considered to be a place of better opportunities by 57 % respondents, thereby choosing National Capital over other cities. The rest 33 % respondents migrated because their husband or family members were already living in Delhi.

In case of domestic workers, more than half of them (52.5 %) chose Delhi as their destination, because of the perceived employment opportunities. For 37 %, their family members or spouse were already in Delhi, which acted as a major pull factor. While 65 % construction workers chose Delhi for employment opportunities; the corresponding share among the domestic workers was 53 %. Most women also agreed that there were other opportunities like market, school and hospital also available in the city of their choice and was also a driver in selecting it. It is noteworthy that while 57 % women engaged in construction reported this as a reason, many more 70 % engaged in domestic work reported it as such. While the former was most likely to enter the city with anticipation to work, the latter got into work after observing for some time and then taking the plunge (Table 2). The

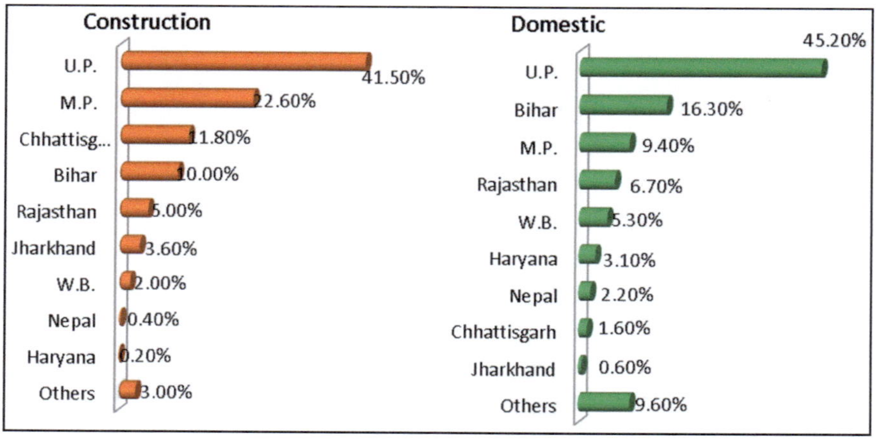

Fig. 3 Migrant women in construction and domestic sectors. *Source* Authors work

Table 2 Reasons for migration among migrant women workers

Reason	Construction (%)	Domestic (%)
Unemployment and poor economic condition	59	62
Employment opportunity	65	53
Better opportunity	57	70
Family/spouse in Delhi from before	33	60
Moved with family	13	35

Source Authors work

initial stay in Delhi for most (96 %) construction women workers was with their close family members or relatives.

Almost all women reported to have chosen to work in order to supplement the family income. Among those engaged in construction work, more than 65 %; and 59 % of those who chose to work as domestic help, reported poor income and bad economic conditions of the family as the factors to engaging in their respective works. About 53 % construction workers and 64 % of domestic workers reported that lack of skills and illiteracy disables them in taking up any other work. Since most of these workers either came with or followed their husband to Delhi, there were hardly any opportunities to develop their skills. There is also a perception that there is no skill needed for becoming a *'head-loader'* in the construction site or in doing the domestic chores as a help in others' houses. Thus the desire to learn is minimal and there is hardly any effort from the employers to build their capacities. There is a need to generate awareness about the need for training in both sectors, among this level of workers. While construction workers work for long days stretching often beyond the stipulated 8 h, domestic workers can either opt for full-time or part-time work schedules.

Nature of Work

Works in which construction workers engage are more arduous as compared to the domestic workers. There are two types of work, mechanized and non-mechanized in the construction industry. Almost all women workers (99 %) are engaged in non-mechanized work in construction industry. Regarding the nature of work done by women at construction site, around 35 % were carrying loads and climbing stairs, whereas rest were involved in some or the other labour work related to construction work. None of them were involved in any skilled work, the reason being illiteracy and no opportunity for learning any additional skills. However the working hours were reported to be in accordance with the Guidelines of the Labour Commission—8 h per day, which was reported to be followed by them (Fig. 4).

However, the domestic help work hours range from 2–3 h as part time to 24 × 7 as a live-in help. Domestic workers working full time only in one house were 17 %. They did cleaning, dusting, housekeeping and cooking. Large majority

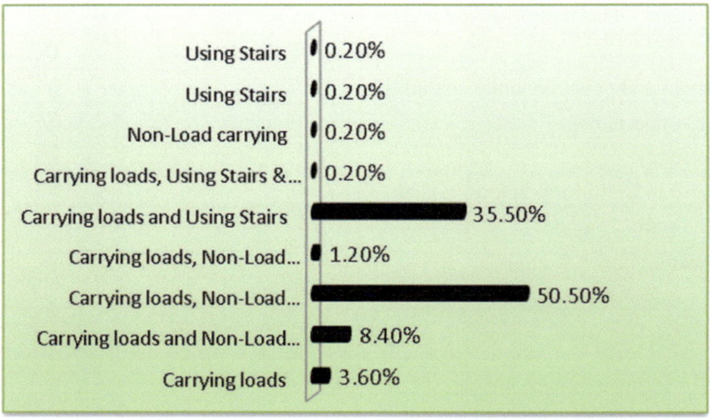

Fig. 4 Types of work done by construction workers. *Source* Authors work

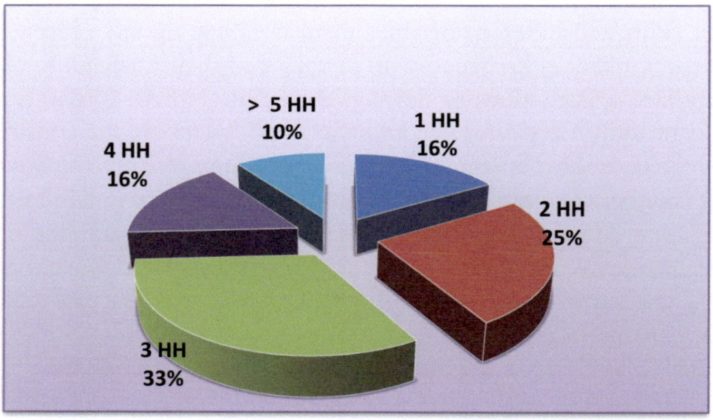

Fig. 5 Number of houses attended per day by domestic worker. *Source* Authors work

of women worked in three houses (33 %) followed by two houses (25 %). There are number of women who work in more than four houses (16 %), and there are as many 10 % who worked in five houses (Fig. 5). It was reported that they work in different houses every day and come back and work in their own houses. In some cases their elders' daughters or daughters-in-law took care of the homes.

Majority of the respondents, who are working part time in various houses, tend to clean the house, dust and clean the utensils. Thus, they are able to cover between two and five houses. Very rarely they are doing single job like cooking, caring for old and children; most of them are doing multiple jobs such as cleaning the floor, dusting, washing the clothes, caring for the children and the elderly (Fig. 6). The remuneration for their work also depend on various locality; the rates of different work are fixed in different areas. The salary either depends on each work or number of persons per households and the size of the house/number of rooms.

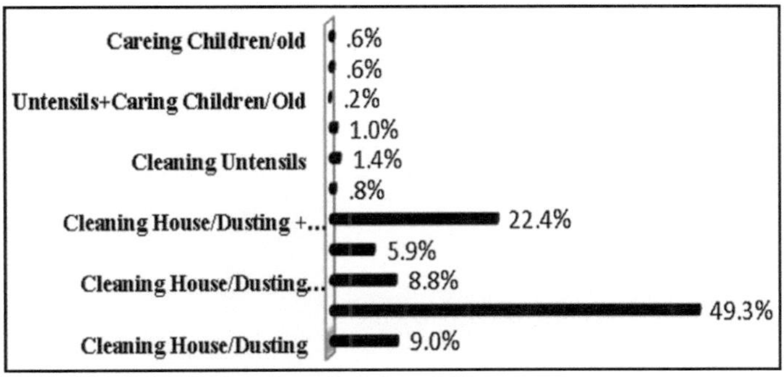

Fig. 6 Nature of jobs. *Source* Authors work

Income Earned

Wages per day is an important indicator to show the income levels, living conditions and economic status of the workers. The minimum rate of wages under the Minimum Wage Act 1948, in the Government of NCT Delhi (Office of the Labour Commissioner) wide notification no. 12 (142)/11/MW/Lab/2023-47 dated 26.07.2011, the minimum wage for unskilled is Rs. 297 per day and Rs. 7722 per month and for semi-skilled it is Rs. 328 per day and Rs. 8528 per month.[2] However, none of them are getting minimum wages as notified by the Delhi Government. About 40 % get only Rs. 150 per day, 22 % receive even less, Rs. 140 per day. However, about a quarter, 23 % receive Rs. 200 per day. Thus majority of the total construction women workers are getting wages between Rs. 140–200 per day, much less than the prescribed minimum wages (Fig. 7). The working conditions for these two sectors, construction and domestic are entirely different with different challenges.

Over and above getting lesser than the prescribed minimum wage constituted by the state, women worker also get less than men workers. About 25 % of the total construction women workers get Rs. 10–50 less than men workers, 6 % gets less than Rs. 50–100 than men workers and for 2 % the difference is more than 100 rupees. Thus, about one-third of the total construction women workers receive unequal wages as compared to men workers.

Wages of the domestic workers depends on two factors. Majority of them, 71 % reported that they receive their salary according to per household, while on the other hand 28 % reported that they get their salary according to per person in each household. In case of earning money per month per households, Fig. 8 shows that majority of them gets less than Rs. 1000 per month; it largely constitutes those who are doing a set of cleaning jobs. This amount is quite low given they work for around 2 h a day in each household. Calculating their wages for their work hourly

[2]http://www.phdcci.in/admin/admin_logged/banner_images/1367229054.pdf. Accessed on 2 Jan 2014.

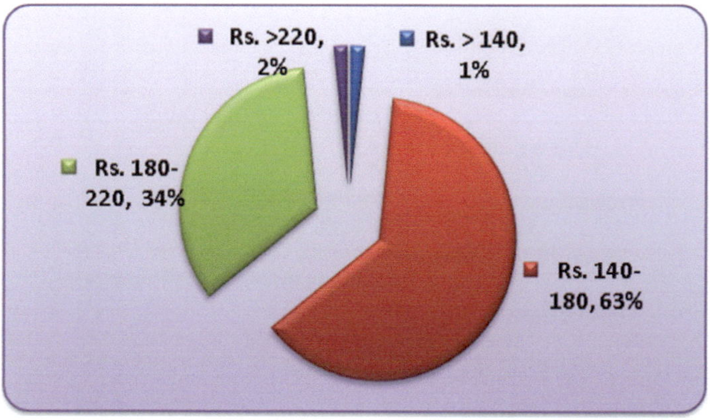

Fig. 7 Rate of wages per day for construction workers

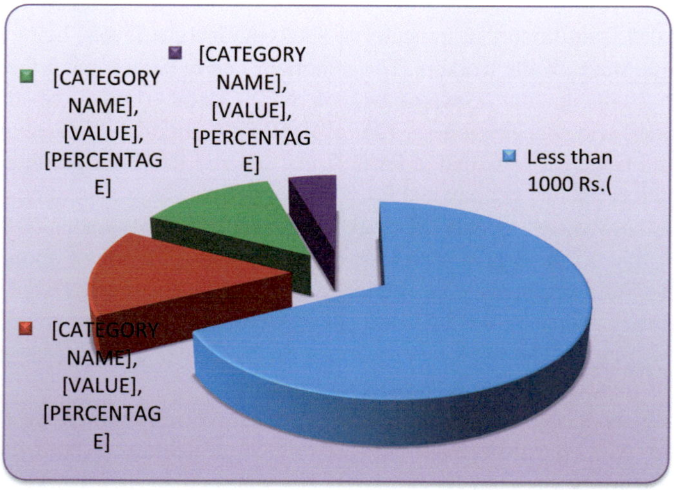

Fig. 8 Income per month per household. *Source* Authors work

becomes difficult so the wage is fixed for a month. If they are working in four houses, they earn Rs. 4000 per month. However, there are 15 % of them who earn between 1000 and 2000 rupees and very few (4 %) earn more than three thousand rupees (Fig. 8).

Living Conditions

The comparison of living conditions of construction workers and domestic workers between the places of origin, mostly rural to that of place of destination Delhi was done with the variables like ownership, type of house and living space. Other facilities like water supply, electricity, toilets, cooking fuel and ownership of assets were assessed. An attempt has been made to understand the changes in their socio-economic and living conditions of these women after migrating from their place of origin to place of destination.

The findings shows that the living conditions of these women have deteriorated accept for owning few assets. There is a sharp decline in the ownership of their own houses/*jhuggies* from the place of origin (97.40 %) to the place of destination (37.70 %), a drop by 59.7 %. Nearly half 45.30 % of the construction women workers live at the construction sites, in a tent or dilapidated temporary shelters. Space-wise distribution shows that back home in their villages, they had more space and nearly 45.30 % lived in two-room accommodations, which sharply fell and only 6 % live in two-room accommodation in Delhi. A large majority (94 %) are constrained for space and live in single-room accommodation, most of them having larger families, having children ranging from 3 to 7 in number with complete lack of privacy. With no proper water, electricity and toilet facilities, majority of them, around 74 %, still go for open defecation in the slums and at the construction sites (Fig. 9).

Thus, it can be assessed that there is a marginal improvement in owning assets however; the living conditions are pathetic with crowded spaces and lack of clean drinking water and sanitation facility. The availability of working opportunities is the pull factors and push factors being landlessness, lack of working opportunities and poverty. Other studies too have pointed out that the condition of migrant women workers in Delhi is not very hospitable and the very fact is proved true in the light of primary data collected in this study in terms of socio-economic condition and accessibility of housing facilities, assets and employment.

More than half of the workers, i.e. 58 % of the total respondents reported of cheating by construction authorities in one or the other ways. Wages differ between men and women. Only 67 % reported to get equal wages, while one-fourth of them reported a different of Rs. 50–100 in the wages of men and women (Fig. 10). Almost around 14 % are not sure of what should be the wages (Fig. 11). This is also likely to impact on living conditions.

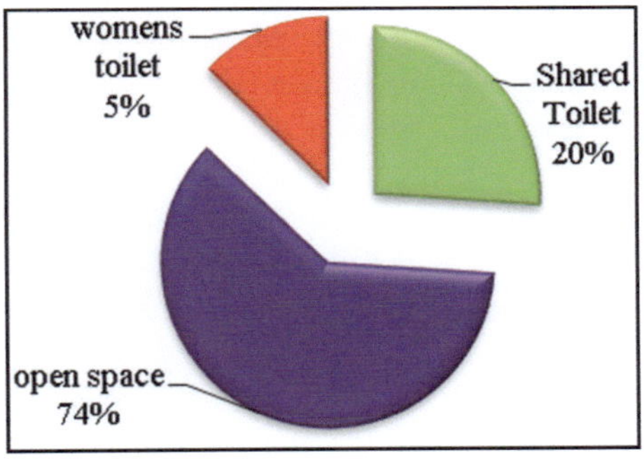

Fig. 9 Toilet facility at working sites. *Source* Authors work

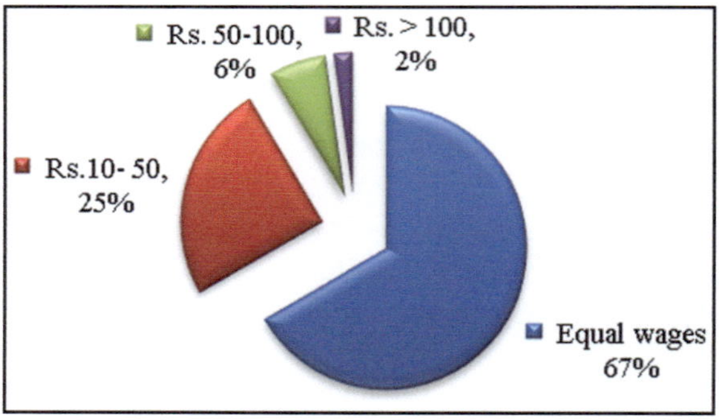

Fig. 10 Wage differs between men-women. *Source* Authors work

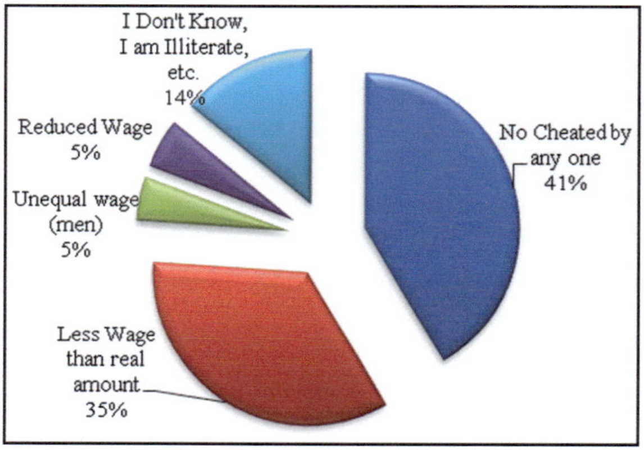

Fig. 11 Injustice in payments. *Source* Authors work

Health Condition

Being healthy not only depends on the food intake, safe drinking water and clean air, but also on the injuries and accidents that may occur in the work place. About 38 % of the total women construction workers have reported of injuries at work site. 51 % of them reported of no first aid arrangements at the working site. In few cases, the women who fell ill or felt weak switched to other work, majorly into domestic work.

As regards to health, 52 % of the women workers reported to have one or the other problem. In few cases, the problems are quite complex, where the women are single handedly managing both home and outside due to their widowhood, or missing husband or ailing husband. As a result of this in many cases, the children are not getting education, left alone at home, vulnerable to abuse and assault, they are barely able to get food on time. 86 % construction workers reported to have lack of crèche facility. Almost all of them who reported to have suffered major ill health (see Box 2) are in debts and had to borrow money from the local money-lenders, or their relatives.

Regarding the utilization of various public health services and entitlements, maximum utilization of service is for the pulse polio drops with 91 %, followed by

56 % availing reproductive child health services. However, the utilization of other services is comparatively low, which is a concern, like, free education for children 55 %, mid-day meal for 52 %, with nearly half of them not availing these essential services. Around 41 % utilized ration card, 38 % got uniform in school. Around 30 % got the services of the free health camp. The least access is to the services of ICDS/*Anganwadi* with 11 %, widow pension for 4 %, Janani SurakshaYojana for 3 %. Out of 4.4 % of migrant women who are above the age of 60 years, only 2.3 % are getting old age pension and only around 1 % for Indira Awas Yojana.

Box 2—Experiencing the Danger of Construction Work-Story of Kamala

Kamla is from Timarpur, 55 years old, belonging to caste Pathar migrated from Moradabad, UP. After migration, she lost her husband in a serious attack of brain fever. She started working in the construction industry as a daily wage labourer at the construction site near SanjoyBasti, Timarpur. She earned Rs. 150 per day. One day she met with a dangerous accident at construction site. She fell down from stairs with loaded bricks on her head and was injured severely on her head, backbone and whole body was afflicted by wounds. Consequently, she went into coma for two weeks. She got only first aid and was removed from work just after accident. After that she was admitted in a hospital, she spent three months in a hospital and had to borrow approximately Rs. 35,000 from her relatives, neighbours and co-workers. After being released from hospital she faced frequent spells of unconsciousness, body pain, lack of blood and weakness for six months. After the recovery and improvement in her health, she started working as a domestic help because she was removed from work by her employer due to her illness related absence.

It is evident, thus, that majority of the migrant women workers are deprived from the benefits of the schemes except Pulse Polio drops program, 65 % of the children are left alone unattended in the slums. They are alone at home in the *juggies,* which also indicate the high vulnerability of the children prone to all kinds of violence and abuse as being reported every day in Delhi. Since the houses in slums are not concrete and are often porous, the children are at risk for physical and sexual abuse. Further, the figures show only 2 % avail crèche facility, indicating lack of enough crèche facilities in the slum localities.

Domestic work is invisible and is seen as unskilled job. Most of the migrant population finds easy to get into domestic work. In the urban setting where both the couples are working, a domestic help becomes necessary to run the house. The daily chores in the households like cleaning, washing clothes and utensils, cooking and housekeeping, which are monotonous and repetitive and are seen as unskilled work by most people. For these everyday chores, domestic helps are hired, either full time or part time; most of them are women and girls. Though they work in the households, the home environment is equally unfavourable if the employers ill-treat them. There are cases of violence, mistreatment, sexual harassment, caste-based discrimination at the work place for the domestic workers. Under the right to privacy, within the four walls of the house, the laws cannot protect them. Thus, the situation of women workers in Delhi is a matter of grave concern. The women workers are engaged in different types of domestic works, building houses, roads, bridges, hospitals, schools and other facilities and are living in extremely difficult conditions. Irrespective of whether women workers are employed by the agency of large contractors or petty contractors or the public sectors, women workers face numerous problems such as unregulated employment, denial of legal minimum wages, insecure working conditions, risk of accidents, lack of crèche facilities, resting place, added to this is high inflation and expensive living. They are barely able to survive on daily basis, by having two square meals, which was not even possible back home in the villages. They are unable to support their children's education.

It can be thus, said, that the government has fallen short in creating an environment, where majority of these migrant women workers can get economic, social, cultural and physical security. In the migratory journey, women are often at a disadvantage than their counterpart men, and have to cope up numerous problems and offences based on gender, age, religion and caste. Migrants are the victim of urban pollution and insanitation. They live in areas where the living conditions are even worse than what they left behind in their native homes. The quality of life is miserable. In the case of construction workers, there were no permanent dwellings. The houses are temporary, tent like structures mostly of plastic sheets near or inside the site area.

The Support System

For the welfare of the construction workers, which falls in unorganized sector, 'The building and other construction workers (regulation of employment and conditions of service) Act, 1996' was passed. The Act is comprehensive and takes care of health, welfare and safety of the construction workers. This Act also has Welfare Cess Act 1996 and Cess Rules 1998 which lays down the procedures for labour administrators for realization of labour Cess as per the main Act 1996. Since the registration is required to be renewed annually, the live members with Delhi board are 92,817 workers who have renewed their registration with the construction board and they are entitled for various welfare schemes. Only register workers can avail the benefits of mandated welfare schemes. The building and other construction of workers (BOCW) Act 1996 provides registration and passbooks/identity cards, issued to them as token of registration with the board, which entitles them to avail 18 welfare schemes notified by 'The Building And Other Construction Workers' Welfare Cess Act, 1996 'like scholarships for children, retirement and family pension, health benefits, loan and advance for tools, housing loans, maternity benefit, RSBY, death and injury compensation. National Skill Mission was created for conceiving formulating, and implementing skills to various types of workers primarily engaged in unorganized workers. The Cess amount collected by different states varies. If this Cess amount is properly utilized and implemented 31 million people's life can be improved. If they are creating 200,000 million assets and contributing to the GDP to the tune of 1,965,550 million (NCEUS 2006; Srivastava 2013) it is criminal to not even provide basic amenities to them and their families.

While certain safeguards are in place for the workers in the construction industry, virtually no such measures are evident for the women in the domestic works. Their vulnerability as migrants is doubled when they seek work or work in the absence of safety nets. The Bill for domestic workers is in its nascent stage and has practical difficulties of defined work place in case of domestic work.

Challenges in Implementation of Safeguards

It has been observed that the workers are often not aware of schemes and programs addressing their interests. The employers do not take the responsibility of informing them. If at all there is any information given, the cumbersome procedures to fill the relevant forms and getting the benefits of a scheme is difficult. A large numbers of women migrant workers are without education and remain unskilled. Therefore, along with improving education and skills, providing help in filling the forms for different schemes may also be also considered as a programmatic input for their welfare.

Women in construction work do not get minimum wages, and get lesser wages than men. They are not aware of their entitled wages. Among the domestic workers, there is no stipulation of wage and therefore they have to fend for themselves to strike and balance wage vis-à-vis the work they are expected to do. Lack of childcare facilities, crèche, school and ICDS Centres should be addressed by the employers and monitored by State agencies. The other entitlements related to health and accident during work need to be brought under the purview of the efforts through which information can be disseminated and taken forward by filling relevant forms, etc. If adherence to the rules and regulations and rendering responsibilities by the employers, contractors are ensured, dignity of labour of these women toiling to achieve better lives will happen. Employers must be responsible for ensuring equal wages paid on time; providing medical and accident benefits; education allowances to workers and dependents; housing and weekly holiday to the workers in both the sectors

Summing Up

Suggestions to promote decent work for migrant workers in India include: developing a policy framework that gives priority to migrants, creates linkages between state and central policies on healthcare, education and social security and facilitating convergence of state and central resources. In this light, establishing institutional mechanisms for interstate coordination, especially for labour being brought to the cities by contractors is important. Improving enforcement of labour laws needs to be taken up on priority basis. Adopting a four-pronged approach for better protection of rights of workers that defines the roles and responsibilities of the state, employers, workers/trade unions/civil society organizations and emphasizes the use of social dialogue and collective bargaining for promoting the rights of migrant workers needs to be considered. Ensuring access and portability of social security schemes, for example, access to housing, water and sanitation, public distribution network/subsidized ratio in destination areas is important towards meeting this goal. Providing identity documents to migrants, which enables them to open bank accounts and enrol for welfare schemes can be the starting point. Universal registration of workers on a national platform and developing comprehensive databases; strengthening and/or setting up district facilitation centres, migrant information centres and gender resource centres is likely to affect positively. Strengthening the role of panchayats in registering workers; and that of vigilance committees to guard against bonded labour and child labour is yet another aspect. Registering workers by organizing enrolment camps on the construction sites and in the residential colonies; providing education and health services at the worksites or seasonal hostels; providing skills training, in particular for adolescents and young workers; and establishing a universal helpline for migrant work across the city will instil a sense of security and impact on work as well as the wellbeing.

Way Forward

In order to ensure the good living conditions and livelihoods, it is imperative, therefore to adhere to the norms that all the government schemes should be made facilitated to the workers at the construction site. Working hours and required medical leave should be given. Identity cards and other cards like Aadhar, BPL, voter I-card, should be made for them. An external redressal committee should be set up to enquire into the cases of wage exploitation, non-medical benefits, sexual exploitation and other forms of physical violence against the workers by the authorities. Labour department numbers/helplines should be provided at every working site.

As regards basic amenities, there need to be provision of safe drinking water facilities; toilets and enclosed bathing space separately for men and women;

provision of resting place separately for men and women at the construction site; providing shelters, which are safe and secure for all the workers. Implementation of RSBY should be more effectively implemented. Full coverage for treatment in case of injury and compensation in case of death to the kin of the person; and job placement to the eligible person in the family in case of death; providing expenses to carry proper death rites and rituals.

For the purpose of child care, under CSR the company should sponsor children's education in the nearby government schools. Their enrolment in school should be transferable to all the government schools in case of shifting from one place to another. There should be crèche facility in the vicinity of the work sites for women in both the sector, but more so for those in construction.

In case of the construction workers, it is the responsibility of employer or the contractor under Contract Labour (Regulation and Abolition) Act 1970 and BOCW Act 1996 that the crèche facility should be provided by the contractor. Women who are feeding should be given adequate breaks to feed the children at work site. Pregnant women should be given maternity leave for 6 months. For continuing the education of the children of construction workers, they should be enrolled in government schools and a provision to get transfer to nearby school, whenever their parents move for work. Under the corporate social responsibility (CSR), which is now mandatory to spend 2 % of their profits on social cause, the construction companies can take this as an opportunity to work for the welfare of the construction workers: their health, education for their children and basic minimum standards of living. Similar activities can be done by resident Welfare Associations, for example, for the domestic workers. Instead of seeing this as welfare, these should be seen as rights of the workers. Their hard work and contribution is immense in the urban infrastructural development and growth of economy. The labour of one woman enables other to contribute to the larger economy through the urban processes of a city feeding into the dynamics of growth and development.

References

Bharara, K., Sandhu, P., & Sidhu, M. (2012). Issues of occupational health and injuries among unskilled female labourers in construction industry: A scenario of Punjab State. *Studies in Home Computer Science, 6*(1), 1–6.

Chauhan, K., & Sharma, P. (2003). Physical problems suffered by Asian women workers involved in construction industry. In *Proceedings of Home Science Association of India XXV Biennial Conf*erence, HSAI Vol. 25 Biennial Conference, Nagpur.

Chawada, et al. (2012). Plight of female construction workers of Surat city. *Indian Journal of Community Health, 24*(1).

Geetika, Gupta, A., & Singh, T. (2011). Women working in informal sector in India: a saga of lopsided utilization of human capital. In *2011 International Conference on Economics and Finance Research IPEDR* (Vol. 4). Singapore: IACSIT Press.

Ghosh. (2009). India: Playing games with the construction workers. Retrieved 24 April, 2013, from http://www.macroscan.org/cur/aug09/cur050809Construction_Workers.htm

Griffin, J., & Varda, S. (2003). Psychological distress among Thai migrant workers in Israel. *Social Science and Medicine, 57*(5), 769–774.
Iredale, Robyn, R., Charles, H., & Stephen, C. (eds.) (2003). *Migration in the Asia Pacific: Population, settlement and citizenship issues*. Edward Elgar Publishing.
Jatrana, S., Mika, T., Brenda, S. A. Y. (eds.) (2006). *Migration and health in Asia*. Routledge.
Kaveri, M. S. (1993). Construction workers, unionization and gender: Women, work and inequity. In J. Cherian & K. V. Eswara Prasad (Eds.), The reality of gender. National Labour Institute.
Lee, S. E. (1966). A theory of Migration. Demography, Vol. 3, No. 1. pp. 47–5.
Mukta. (2001). *Role of women in the 21th Century*. New Delhi, Anmol Publication Private Limited (p. 3).
National Commission for Enterprises in the Unorganized Sector (NCEUS). (2006). Social Security for Unorganized Workers, Government of India, New Delhi, New Delhi.
Singh, S. (2012). The employment economic condition of construction workers and their level of satisfaction in Ahmedabad City: An empirical study. *European Journal of Social Sciences, 29*(4).
Srivastava, R. S. (2013). 'A Social Protection Floor for India' International Labour Officer, ILO DWT for South Asia and ILO country office for India. New Delhi. ILO.
Stark, O. (1991). *The migration of labor* (p. 237). Cambridge, MA: Basil Blackwell.
Taylor, E. J. (1999). The new economics of labour migration and the role of remittances in the migration process. *International Migration, 37*(1), 63–88.
Thadani, V. N., & Michael, P. T. (1984). Female migration: a conceptual framework'. In Women in the Cities of Asia: Migration and Urban Adaptation, James T.
Unni, J. (2000). Urban informal sector: size & income generation processes in Gujarat. SEWA-GIDR-ISST-NCAER. Report no. 2, New Delhi, National Council of Applied Economic Research.
Zelinsky, W. (1971). The hypothesis of the mobility transition. *Geographical Review*, 219–249.

Revealing the Vulnerabilities of Population and Places at Risk in Delhi

Tarun Prakash Meena and Milap Punia

Abstract India is witnessing upsurge in events of natural hazards, risk and increase in extreme climatic events almost every year. This may be accounted due to change in global climate, however, increasing population pressure on land and lack of regulations related to construction activities on river bed exaggerated the quantum of loss and damage. Thus, this study is an attempt to focus on the assessment of population at risk and to study how effectively assessment can be made about the spatial locations, which can help to reduce the impact and mobilize the resources at the earliest in adversity of hazard. As per 2011 census, 16.7 million people residing in Delhi NCT, out of which 1.49 million (11.64 %) are living in those areas which are highly prone to floods. An attempt has been made at disaggregated municipal ward level to assess the population at risk during 2010 floods adjoining to Yamuna river bed. Adopted methodology is based on remote sensing and geographic information system (GIS) based approaches to extract information for absolute population and density using LandScan data from Oak Ridge National Laboratory (ORNL). These estimated figures are validated with information from census for their further applicability. Results indicate that there is need for noticeable change in policy, with emphasis on loss and damage reduction through mitigation and preparedness. There is also strong need to study further spatial interactions with vulnerable populations in terms of their socio-economic constraints.

T.P. Meena (✉) · M. Punia
Centre for the Study of Regional Development, School of Social Sciences, Jawaharlal Nehru University, New Delhi, India
e-mail: tarun26005@gmail.com

M. Punia
e-mail: punia@mail.jnu.ac.in

S.S. Acharya et al. (eds.), *Marginalization in Globalizing Delhi: Issues of Land, Livelihoods and Health*, DOI 10.1007/978-81-322-3583-5_12

Keywords Population · Spatial · Mitigation · Risk · Delhi · Landscan · Vulnerabilities

Introduction

The population growth and climate is experiencing rapid change which leads to receiving increasing attention, not only from the scientists but also from policy-makers. They are growing in area, population and at the same time they are acquiring a new character as their people perform new tasks in the physical environment that increasingly reflect the use of new technology (Allefsen 1962). As research progresses, it is becoming clear that large-scale changes of the global climate system would seriously affect large numbers of people in various ways. Fundamental for the estimation of the extent of such impacts is population forecasts and predictions of changes in human habitation patterns. Demographic changes are also of prime concern for studies of human impacts on their local environments. The impact of large-scale climatic changes on humans (Sea level Change) and the impact of humans on the local and regional hydrology (Flood). Population changes, including the spatial distribution of people, are therefore essential for assessments of future water resources, in addition to climatic and hydrological parameters (Bengtsson et al. 2006).

According to census 2011 the average density of India is 382 persons/km^2. On an average, 57 more people inhibit every square kilometre in the country as compared to a decade ago (Census of India 2011). Population maps have a long history, but the recent development of powerful computers and software in combination with the increasing availability of various kinds of remote sensing data has led to a growing research activity in this area. In the last few decades several efforts to generate grid maps of population have thus been seen. On the global scale, Dobson et al. (2000), developed a global population dataset in 30 arc-seconds resolution (LandScan). The LandScan dataset is made by adopting an empirical model, which distributes sub-national census data to grids by using various remote sensing and ancillary data. In recent years it has been found that remote sensing is a cost-effective, technologically sound and an increasingly used technique for the analysis of population growth (Yeh et al. 2001). In light of above research, attention is being directed to the mapping and assessment of population growth using remote sensing and geographical Information system techniques. Using LandScan data it is easy to identify spatial changes of population which have occurred over the city landscape.

The scholars developed number of techniques for mapping globally variations of parameters within countries. As these techniques have become more sophisticated, and the capacity of computers to handle very large datasets with great speed has increased, the interest in developing methods for distributing population data to the grid cells of GIS maps has also increased. Initially, GIS specialists tended to direct their efforts towards establishing the coordinates of coastlines and country boundaries, and generating georeferenced datasets for physical and environmental variables that could be derived from high-resolution aerial photography and satellite imagery. Less effort was directed towards the development of georeferenced socio-economic datasets, mainly because such data is collected by censuses and surveys and compiled for political or administrative units, and direct interpolation techniques to estimate the spatial distribution of socio-economic variables are still lacking (Clark and Rhind 1992). Despite these limitations, improvements in the quality and accessibility of georeferenced environmental data have generated growing demand for more accurate and up-to-date spatial information about the global distribution of population variables. This demand has been driven by two different concerns within the development community. One relates to the interest of demographers, sociologists and urban planners in mapping urbanization processes and defining the location and socio-economic characteristics of population growth and population at hazard risk with more accuracy (Jeffrey and Tschirley 2005).

India has an area and population equal to that of Europe (excluding USSR) or that of agricultural China. According to the census 2011 India shares 17.5 % population of the world. The population of India is almost equal to the combined population of U.S.A., Brazil, Indonesia, Pakistan, Bangladesh and Japan put together (Census 2011). However, the moist alluvial soil regions of India have highest densities of population in the world (Hoffman 1948). Accuracy assessment of large-scale population datasets is always challenging due to the use of all geographically specific datasets to produce the population dataset, leaving little independent data for testing. However, simple comparison tests with existing gridded population datasets were undertaken. The 2008 version of LandScan is the most widely used population datasets, and was acquired and compared to the enumerated census datasets, 2011. To make the comparisons possible, population datasets were adjusted to the same year, after calculating exponential growth rate. Different methods were used to compare the Census population and LandScan datasets (Linard et al. 2010).

Scholars have produced a set of maps and represented hazard exposures that spatially delimit the populations that are at risk from various natural hazards (cyclones, tornadoes, earthquakes, floods, drought, volcanoes and landslides) (Dilley et al. 2005). Some of these, maps use LandScan to calculate disaster risk at the sub-national level in order to contribute to development planning and disaster prevention. Some populations are at multiple risks and thus their overall exposure to natural hazards is additive. This type of a vulnerability analysis requires the existence of sub-national population attribute data and hazard data for areas of interest, whether at a county level (Cutter and Emrich 2006), city level (Pelling 2003) or for a small island nation (Pelling and Uitto 2002).

Methodology

This study attempts to assess the relevance of raster population datasets in the events of natural hazards and compare patterns relating to urban agglomerations and population densities. For doing so, LandScan, 2008 raster population datasets from Oak Ridge Laboratory is used along with census datasets. It is useful to investigate and to assess the strengths and weaknesses of existing census data, methods (e.g., gaps in spatial and thematic coverage, counting individuals, proxy measures such as those derivable from Earth observations), and tools for estimating population living under risk conditions. It is imperative for decision-makers for identifying populations at risk categories, that are susceptible to the impact of natural or human-induced disasters, thus there are three critical elements of the data, each of which is a scale issue: spatial scale (how far below the national level can estimates be derived?); temporal scale (for how recent a time period can estimates be made?); and risk scale (how detailed are the available population characteristics of living, place of accommodation and shelter?) (Comenetz 2007). Since, Landscan data only reflects population number and density, thus for satisfying third element, more ground survey is required to understand household characteristics. Thus, only aspect of population captured by these approaches is total population size. No other demographic information that could identify risk (beyond being on the footprint of a Hazard), such as age, gender, or race or ethnicity, is currently available in these data collections. Nonetheless, one further do dasymetric modelling to integrate both datasets to have considerable utility and to be used for purposes including emergency planning and hazard management. To have confidence in Landscan data and its applicability, evaluation was carried out across various scales, namely state, districts and municipal wards. Later, application and estimation of vulnerable population across various municipal wards along Yamuna flood plain in Delhi was carried out (Fig. 1).

First, predicted population totals per state (district level for costal districts of India) were compared to the Census population adjusted estimates for the year 2008. The LandScan dataset was unsurprisingly nearly perfect, as the population data were matched approximately to Census population estimates in the modelling

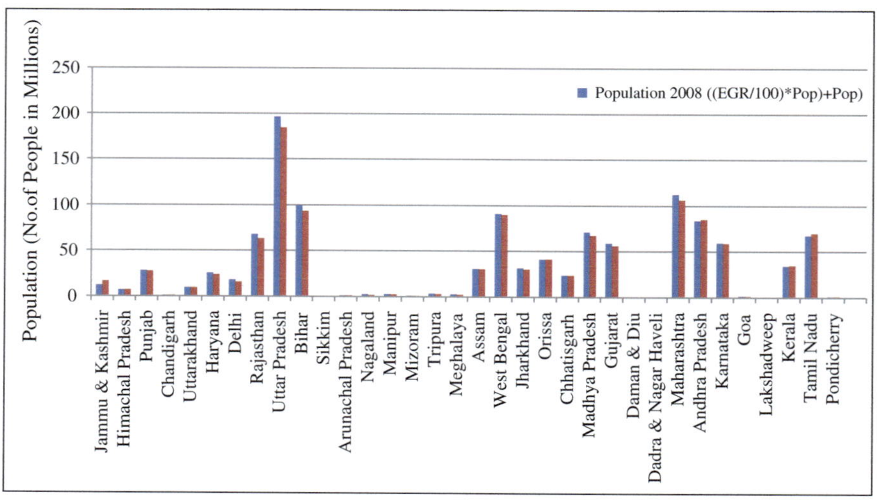

Fig. 1 Population comparison between census of India population (2008) and landscan 2008 (Authors work)

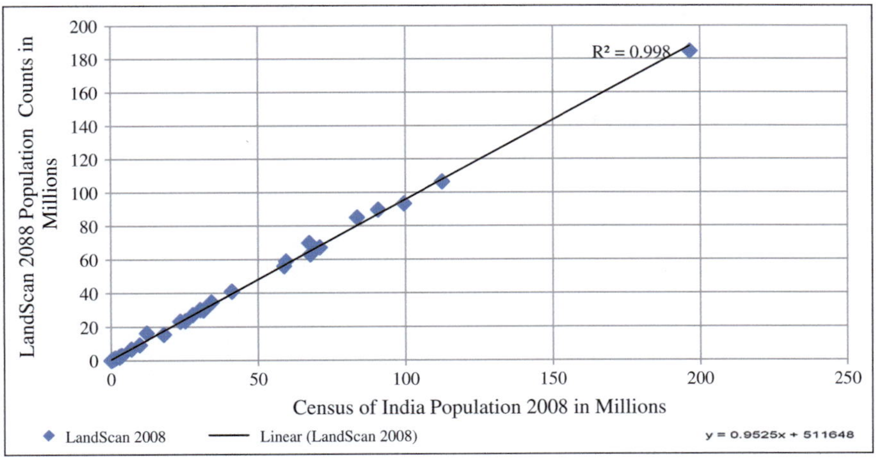

Fig. 2 Population comparison between census of India population (2008) and landscan 2008 (Authors work)

procedure. However, the aim is to observe how far away the LandScan datasets is from these most contemporary estimates. R^2 (0.999) were extracted and differences in population estimates per state/district were mapped.

Second, grid-based differences between datasets were measured. Unit-level absolute differences were mapped and plotted to explore tendencies in these differences. Third, the numbers of people predicted in towns and settlements with known population size have been compared. In order to allow the calculation of population predicted in small settlements (smaller than 1 km), the LandScan datasets were used for comparison (Fig. 2). (R^2) between predicted and observed population in towns and settlements were extracted. The impact of the choice of population dataset on estimates of the population at risk was tested for flood event in Delhi before common wealth games in 2010.

Comparison Between Census and LandScan Population Counts

Population densities are higher around the larger cities and along the Northern belt (Gangatic plain) of India. Analysis reflects that highest population density is in lower Gangatic plain, mainly concentrated in two major states of India, i.e. Bihar (1102 persons/km^2) and West Bengal (1029 persons/km^2). Grid-based difference measures led to interesting insights on where the differences between datasets are the most significant. Analysis shows that, for the large majority of pixels, the absolute difference between LandScan and Census is lower than 4 persons per 1 × 1 km grid square (Bengtsson et al. 2006). For these pixels with very low differences, the human population density is generally close to zero. However, the absolute differences can be much higher in more densely and extreme sparsely populated places.

In the LandScan dataset, the construction methodology means that populations are clustered around roads and less concentrated in towns, but more diffuse in rural areas. The total population per district predicted by the LandScan dataset is closer to the Census estimates than the any other dataset, though overall R^2s values are relatively high in LandScan. In this case value is near perfect positive correlation which shows that LandScan data at the state level sufficient for comparison purpose refer Fig. 1.

Delhi is one of the most ancient and historic cities of India. From British times to the present date, it has undergone several administrative changes due to its special characters as the National Capital. Delhi, which is more clearly depicted as Delhi region consisting various towns of nearby districts of several states. Expansion of Delhi to nearby regions also expands the boundaries of vulnerability. The built-up area in the National Capital Region, which includes residential, non-residential, landfill sites, etc., has increased by 34.6 % from 1999 to 2012 as per the figures in the Draft Revised Regional Plan-2021. The built-up area in the NCR has gone up from 2,76,566 to 3,72,370 ha showing an increase of 95,803 ha or 34.6 %. While the area under agriculture use has reduced marginally from 26,65,622 to 26,45,022 ha, green areas and water bodies have decreased substantially. Particularly, the Yamuna river bed has been lost due to the various construction activities, like construction of Delhi metro Depot, Common wealth Games Village, railway bridges, and construction of NH-24, etc. As per provisions of Sect. 3 and 5 of the Delhi Municipal Corporation Act, 1957 (as amended till date), the powers of the Central Government for delimitation of wards in MCD were delegated to the Lt. Governor of Delhi. Accordingly, the first delimitation of wards subsequent to the creation of the State Election Commission for Delhi, took place in 1993 on the basis of provisional census figures for 1991 (as final figures of population were not available at that time). At the time of the 2001 Census, there were 134 municipal wards in the MCD. However after Delimitation in 2007, the MCD area is presently divided into 272 wards and Delhi Municipal Corporation is divided into three corporations, namely north, south and east Delhi. Connotation of vulnerability is more social, than natural. But here it is used to highlight the vulnerability of population, which got effected because of flooding, thus spatial vulnerability assessment of Delhi can be productive for Hazard planning of the region (Fig. 3).

During common wealth games major infrastructure development took place with a large number of bridges, flyovers and the metro project under construction. After severe floods, the transport infrastructure is generally vulnerable. Major projects require special studies on seismic design criteria. Moreover, the Indian seismic codal provisions on bridges as these exist today are obsolete and inadequate (Jain et al. 1999). Flood risk in Delhi has the potential to go well beyond the statistics of deaths and injuries. Such a disaster in the country's capital, which also happens to be a major commercial and residential centre, will have huge economic and political implications which will affect the entire country and not just the population of Delhi. This adds an extra dimension to the flooding problem for Delhi.

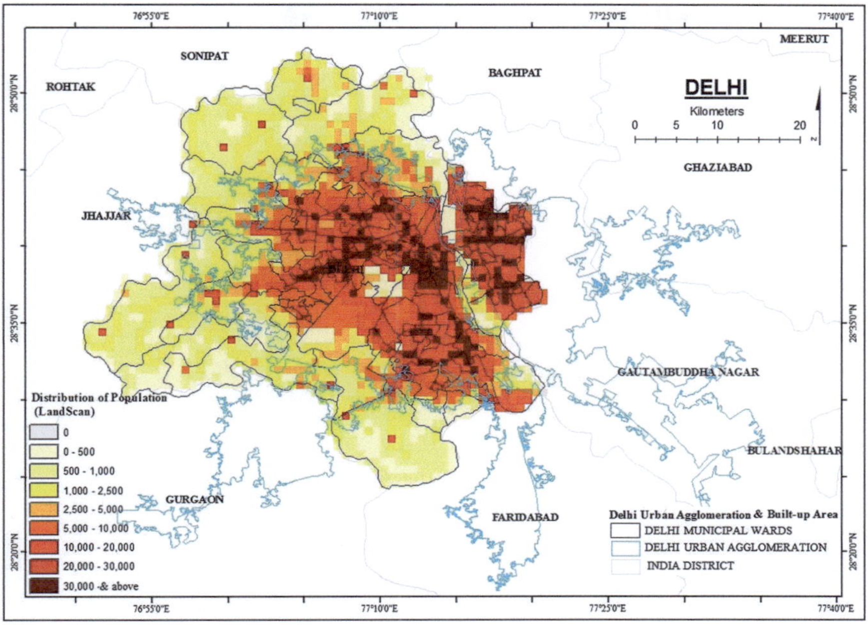

Fig. 3 Delhi Urban Agglomeration and built-up area

Delhi Floods 2010

The Delhi Flood Control Order mentions the division of National Capital Territory Delhi into four Flood Sectors, namely Shahadra, Wazirabad—Babrapur, Alipur and Nangloi—Najafgarh sectors. The unprotected flood prone area is about 1.7 % or 25 km towards the southeast and 5 % or 74 km^2 in the north-eastern parts, which is protected by earthen embankments, since every year water level rises in Yamuna above danger level and large population needs be evacuated to the top of the bunds or Delhi roads. Rise in water levels also cause back flows in the connecting drains and have effect on the city drain network causing overflow and causes of many monsoon related diseases. River Yamuna crossed its danger level (fixed at 204.83 m) 25 times during the last 33 years. Since 1900, Delhi has experienced six major floods in the years 1924, 1947, 1976, 1978, 1988, 1995, 2010 and 2013 when peak level of Yamuna River was one metre or more above danger level of 204.49 m at old rail bridge (2.66 m above the danger level) on sixth September 1978. The second record peak of 206.92 m was on 27 September 1988. In 1977, Najafgarh drain experienced heavy floods due to discharge from the Sahibi River. The drain breached at six places between Dhansa and Karkraula, marooning a number of villages in Najafgarh block. This resulted in huge loss and damages to life and property.

In September, 1978, River Yamuna experienced a devastating flood. Widespread breaches occurred in rural embankments, submerging 43 km^2 of

Table 1 Flood vulnerability around Yamuna river bed in Delhi (Authors work)

Population at risk: Delhi flood 2010			
Delhi ward no.	Population at risk	Population 2001	Percentage share of wards
2	9629	142,413	6.76
7	11,404	203,492	5.60
65	1682	170,792	0.98
71	58,577	120,882	48.46
74	13,225	145,540	9.09
75	21,570	97,127	22.21
91	10,403	154,666	6.73
94	23,102	145,276	15.90
102	5964	41,120	14.50
104	17,704	133,526	13.26
115	164	135,222	0.12
Delhi	*173,424*	*1,490,056*	*11.64*

agricultural land under 2 m of water, causing total loss of the kharif crop. In addition to this, colonies of north Delhi, namely Model town, Mukherjee Nagar, Nirankari Colony, etc., suffered heavy flood inundation, causing extensive damage to property. The total damage to crops, houses and public utilities was estimated at Rs. 176.1 million.

Similarly in September, 1988, River Yamuna experienced floods of very high magnitude, flooding many villages and localities like Mukherjee Nagar, Geeta Colony, Shastri Park, Yamuna Bazzar and Red Fort area, affecting approximately 8,000 families (Table 1).

In September, 1995, The Yamuna experienced high magnitude floods following heavy runs in the upper catchment area and release of water from Tajewala water head. Slow release of water from Okhla barrage due to lack of coordination between cross-state agencies further accentuated the problem. Fortunately, the flood did not coincide with heavy rains in Delhi, and could be contained within the embankments. Nonetheless, it badly affected the villages and unplanned settlements situated within the river bed, rendering approximately 15,000 families homeless. These persons had to be evacuated and temporarily housed on roadsides for about 2 months, before they went back to live in the riverbed (Sharma et al. 1996).

Protection from the river by embankments leads to a false sense of safety and development starts taking place in the shadow of these embankments. In the event of failure of these protective works, as has been seen in the form of breaches during past floods, the effect is devastating because the pressure of the entire embanked stretch is released at one point, and According to Ministry of Home Affairs (India)'s disaster management unit, countrywide death toll from floods in various states was 2,404 between June and September 2010. Figure 4 represents area affected by 2010 floods in Delhi. Analysis across various municipal wards around Yamuna river bed shown that in 2010 the flood affected population in Delhi

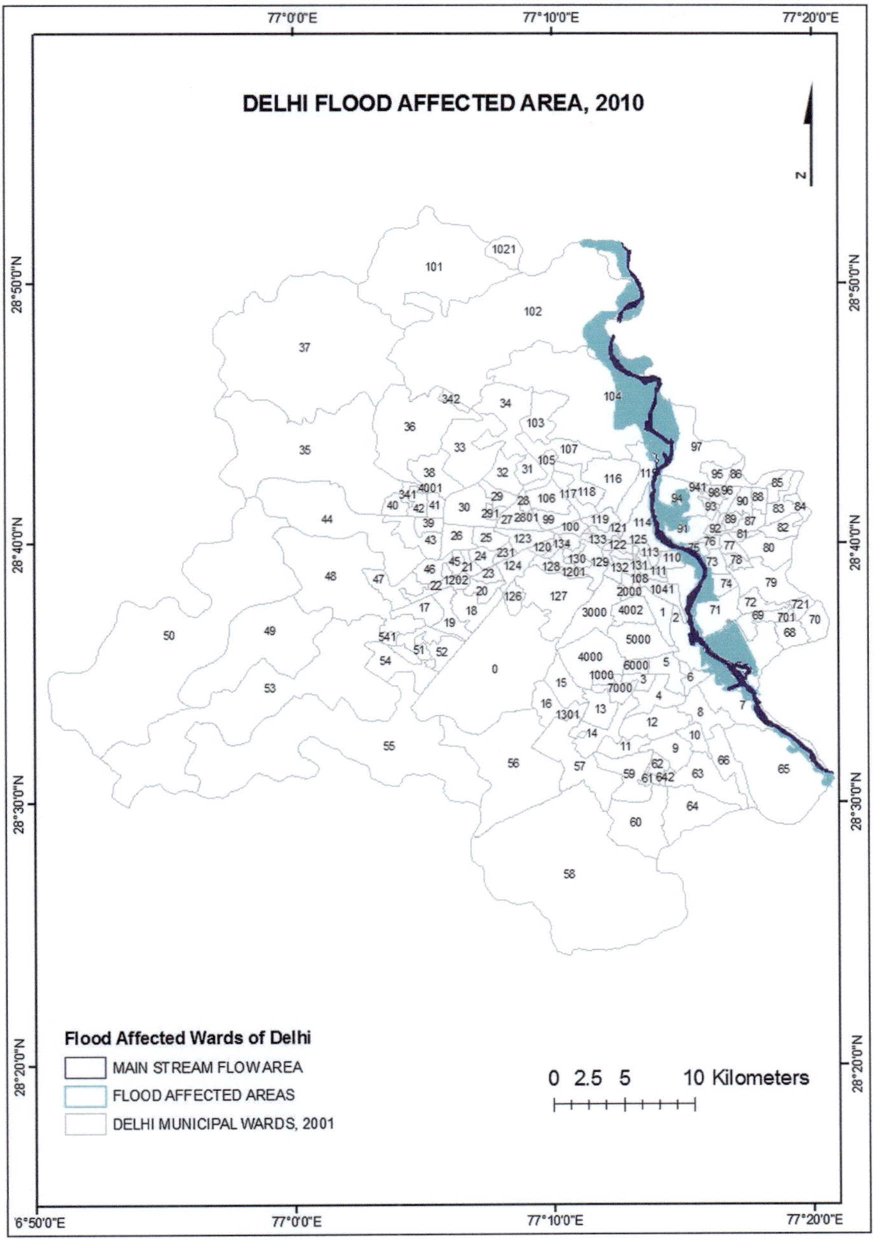

Fig. 4 Delhi flood affected area, 2010. *Source* DSC-RS and GIS, NRSC, Hyderbad

was 173,424 (11.64 %) out of total population 1,490,056. Ward no. 71 was the most affected because of proximity to river bed.

It is the 48.46 % of population of ward 71 living these areas was displaced with the rise in water of River. Around every year, approximately same percent of population is displaced and it takes the people by surprise.

Ward no. 71 is followed by Ward no, 75, 94, 102 and 104 with the flood affected population of 22.21, 15.90, 14.50 and 13.26 % respectively. Ward no. 115 and 65 is the least affected of flood in the year 2010 with only 0.12 and 0.98 % of their total population. Ward no. 74, 2, 91 and 7 were other affected wards with change in water level with a small amount of affected population share 9.09, 6.76, 6.73 and 5.60 % respectively.

The study began with an overview of the data required to prepare estimates of populations at risk of being involved in emergency situations. Since it is impossible to know in advance what events people might confront, the estimates for planning purposes need to be spatially explicit and sufficiently detailed in demographic terms so that they have broad applicability to a number of emergencies. Ideally, population registries would be universally accessible as sources of data at all geographic levels. In reality, censuses of population tend to be the best single source of data because they maximize the geographic coverage of populations and typically have enough detailed characteristics about each person in each household to permit the calculation of estimates of vulnerability. In theory, censuses are also ideal geographically because each household's location had to be known to the statistical agency undertaking the census, so the characteristics of people should be capable of being spatially identified with considerable precision.

In practice, the exact location may not be recorded and so is lost immediately after the data are collected; even if the location is known, it may not be converted to a digital format that can be mapped easily. Therefore, that in much of the world the real issue is not the collection of data per se, but rather what happens to the data after being collected. Census and other data about households and individuals need to be georeferenced (with proper privacy safeguards), linked to accurate maps, and then analyzed by individuals with the appropriate training to undertake tasks.

A major shortcoming of census data (and most population registers as well) is that they are universally collected at places of residence, yet people are often at risk outside of their home. There is no simple answer to this dilemma of estimating the "daytime" populations (assuming that being away from homes is essentially a daytime activity), but modelling based on the results of survey data about out-of-home activities is the most common approach. Most other problems in creating estimates of the population at risk are related to the fact that censuses are not conducted everywhere on a regular basis, and even where they are conducted, the national statistical agency may not have the resources to provide data at a local level, to prepare local-level maps coinciding with the census geography. To work around some of these issues, global population databases such as LandScan were developed to create population 'surfaces' for the globe, but at the moment they lack the breadth of demographic characteristics that would allow users to create estimates of vulnerability beyond population counts and density in a given area.

Conclusion

This study makes use of a derived population distribution dataset to draw inferences about the distribution of local population density. It suggests that applying a population density threshold to this distribution can provide an indicator of population pressure on the land that is traditionally measured with more comparability across regions. In the meantime, 'People and Pixels' (Dobson et al. 2003) approach can take advantage of current remote sensing data, particularly if the data and tools are made widely available and a research community and engages its resources in societal applications. Applicability of LandScan is scale dependent and is cost-effective and easy to use in its raster format. Value of R^2 for states is 0.998 and for districts it drops to 0.664. As resolution increases and thus complexity on ground gets more complex and thus needs more ancillary data to match the reality. There are issues of administrative boundaries, topographical effects and complexities of sealand boundary.

Losses due to natural and man-made disasters will continue to increase because of our continuing population growth and the increase of the concentration of growth in risk-prone areas such as coastal regions, floodplains. On an average more than 1000 people die every year due to floods in India. In 2010 Delhi, along the Yamuna river floodplain about 11 municipal wards were affected. From LandScan datasets it was estimated to about 0.17 million people got affected out of total 1.5 million people residing in these wards. Thus, LandScan estimates are useful enough to locate and estimate the persons under risk of floods. Sea level rise is a great threat to the 30.9 million people of India, who are projected to be environmental refugees if the sea level rises to the level of 20 m above of now. Out of nine coastal states there are five most risk prone, thus about 6 % population might be affected with this change. It is threatening to the basic human right of large number of population. We can easily estimate the population at risk with the LandScan data. Based on above it can be said that LandScan is comparatively accurate and reliable. Allows quick and easy assessment, estimation, and visualization of population at risk and provides high-resolution population distributions. It is a critical component of emergency planning and management, rapid risk assessment, evacuation planning, consequence assessment, mitigation planning and implementation.

References

Allefsen, R. A. (1962). City hinterland relationship in India. *India's*. In R. Turner (Ed.), *Urban future* (pp. 94–116). Berkeley: University of California Press.

Bengtsson, M., Shen, Y., & Oki, T. (2006). SRES-based gridded global population dataset for 1990-2100. *Population and Environment, 28*(2), 113–131.

Bhaduri, B., Bright, E., Cloeman, P., & Urban, M. L. (2007). LandScan USA: A high-resolution geospatial and temporal modelling approach for population distribution and dynamics. *GeoJournal, 69*, 103–117.

Census of India. (2011). Provisional population totals (districts/Su-districts) of India. Retrieved December 24, 2013, from http://www.censusindia.gov.in/2011-prov-results

Clark, J. I., & Rhind, D. W. (1992). Human dimensions of global environmental change. Programme Report 3. International Social Science Council and UNESCO.

Comenetz, J. (2007). Tools and methods for estimating populations at risk from natural disasters and complex humanitarian crises, U.S. Census Bureau, The National Academy of Sciences.

Cutter, S. L., & Emrich, C. T. (2006). Moral hazard, social catastrophe: The changing face of vulnerability along the hurricane coasts. *Annals of the American Academy of Political and Social Science, 604*, 102–112.

Dilley, M., Chen, R. S., Deichmann, U., Lerner-Lam, A. L., Arnold, M., Agwe, … Yetman, G. (2005). *Natural disaster hotspots: a global risk analysis. Disaster risk management series* (Issue No. 5). Washington, D.C.: The World Bank

Dobson, J. E., Bright, E. A., Coleman, P. R., Durfee, R. C., & Worley, B. A. (July, 2000). A global population database for estimating populations at risk. *Photogrammetric Engineering & Remote Sensing, 66*(7), 849–857

Dobson, J. E., Bright, E. A., Coleman, P. R., & Bhaduri, B. L. (2003). LandScan: a global population database for estimating populations at risk. In V. Mesev (Ed.) *Remotely sensed cities* (pp. 267–281). Taylor & Francis.

Emery, K. O., & Aubrey, D. G. (1989). Tide gauges of India. *Journal of Coastal Research, 5*(3), 489–501.

Government of Delhi, Floods. Retrieved March 11, 2013, from http://delhi.gov.in/wps/wcm/connect/DOIT_DM/dm/home/vulnerabilities/hazards/floods

Hoffman, L. A. (1948). India: main population concentrations. *The Geographical Journal, 111*(1/3), 89–100.

Indian Meteorological Department (IMD). UNICEF—Situation Report Bihar Floods 2008 overall Situation Flood Forecast. Retrieved March, 22, 2013, from http://www.static.reliefweb.int/sites/reliefweb.int/files/resources/4D8D801A9B04C621C12574B4004669FB-Full_Report.pdf

Jeffrey, B., & Tschirley. (2005). FAO, United Nations; Mapping global urban and rural population distributions. Retrieved June 4, 2013, from http://www.fao.org/docrep/009/a0310e/A0310E04.html

Linard, C., Alegana, V. A., Noor, A. M., Snow, R. W., & Tatem, A. J. (2010). A high resolution spatial population database of Somalia for disease risk mapping. *International Journal of Health Geographics, 9*(45), 1–13.

Parry, M. L., Canziani, O. F., Palutikof, J. P., van der Linden, P. J., & Hanson, C. E. (2007). Impacts, adaptation, and vulnerability. Contribution of working group ii to the fourth assessment report of the intergovernmental panel on climate change (IPCC). United Kingdom: Cambridge University Press, Cambridge.

Pelling, M., & Uitto, J. (2002). Small island developing states: Natural disaster vulnerability and global change. *Environmental Hazards, 3*, 49–62.

Tobler, W. (1992). Preliminary representation of world population by spherical harmonics. *Proceedings of the National Academy of Sciences, 89*, 6262–6284.

Yeh, A. G. O., & Li, X. (2001). Measurement and monitoring of urban sprawl in a rapidly growing region using entropy. *Photogrammetric Engineering and Remote Sensing, 67*, 83–90.

Vulnerabilities of Relocated Women, A Case of Resettlement in Bawana JJ Colony, Delhi

Vishavpreet Kaur

Abstract 'Cities' which gives the portrait of multi-storied buildings, world class infrastructure, **exploding markets,** pollution, and not only that but long hour traffic jams, crowding of people, unemployment, poverty, growing of slums, crimes, shortage of basic amenities and so on. On one hand we have policy-makers, **city planners**, architectures who call cities as machines of growth which suffice with the **indicator of development,** and on the other hand we have voiceless poor who make city at the cost of **exploitation.** This study was attempted to explore the life of the displaced women who were evicted from **Yamuna Pushta** and were tried to relocate and resettled in Bawana. The question which continually strike during this whole journey was about settling and resettling the life of voiceless. The people who were **evicted,** most were left to fend for themselves with no alternatives and choices. This paper has tried to capture and document the **experiences**, the pain, unheard voices of poor women who had faced this process of exclusion throughout life.

Keywords Cities · Poverty · City planners · Development · Exclusion

V. Kaur (✉)
Centre of Social Medicine and Community Health, School of Social Sciences
JNU, New Delhi, India
e-mail: vishavpreetk@gmail.com

S.S. Acharya et al. (eds.), *Marginalization in Globalizing Delhi: Issues of Land, Livelihoods and Health*, DOI 10.1007/978-81-322-3583-5_13

Introduction

Delhi 'a city for everyone' has continued to attract the rural as well as urban migrants from all over the country. A city which has a place for migrants from rural areas, academicians from all over the world, policy-makers, dhobi, vendors, sky-scrapers, labourers, etc. Cities on one hand gives the picture of glamorous malls, multistoried buildings, exploding markets, congestion, pollution, poverty and unemployment, unauthorized settlements/slums, chronic shortages of basic urban services, lack of community feeling and petty crime. On the other hand, economists and policy makers now acknowledge cities as '**engines of growth**', an indicator of development and a major contributor to the national economy; it is apparent that it is accompanied by growing disparities as well' (Singh and Shukala 2005, p. 1).

As far as Asian countries are concerned, sudden increase in the number of buildings, has acted like a magnet for the workers which finally lead to the proliferation of the informal cities. This invisible urban population caters to the day-to-day services which are required for a planned city. Their presence and requirement in the diversified services marks their importance and significantly contributes to the formal and informal sectors of the cities. The development of the city invites large number of workers without creating any facilities for them which emerge as informal settlements of the workers and service providers. And over a period of time the informal tenement grows in population as new migrants settle wherever they a find an empty space. (Singh and Shukala 2005, p. 1).

Slums: Home and a Hope for Urban Poor

The life of urban poor in slums is characterized by its complete informality. On the one hand the city's growth is fuelled by cheap labour of poor migrants, slum residents, and pavement dwellers, homeless people, etc., on the other hand; there are no provisions to plan for their housing. Due to lack of support the city government, the poor are forced to built their houses in empty public space, but when the authorities decide to the city and make it into a 'world class city', during common wealth games then the house of the same poor, (who has come to city as a driver, domestic maid, street hawker, etc.) are branded as illegal encroachers, criminals, nuisance in the society and they are forcibly evicted and their homes gets demolished.

Journey from Yamuna Pushta to Bawana

Yamuna Pushta—Which Used to Be a Home for 40,000 Families

The Yamuna Pushta (Informal slum settlements) was one of the largest and older slums in Delhi. It was located on the western banks of the river Yamuna Pushta was home to nearly 40,000 families which nurtured more than 1,50,000 people. 'The Yamuna Pushta *jhuggis* (slum settlements) stretch from the old Yamuna Bridge to the Indraprastha Estate Gas Turbine, on both sides of the river. The slums had been developed by the migrant population who had come to the city in search of work. They had been staying there since the last four decades. About 70 % of these families were Muslims. The majority of the people were rickshaw pullers, domestic workers, hand cart pullers, rag pickers, auto drivers, vegetable vendors, beggars, dholakwalas, construction workers ("who had been brought to Delhi by labour contractors during the Asian games in 1982 and had settled in Pushta" (Sen and Bhan 2008, p. 2), etc. These people had migrated to Delhi from Bihar, Bengal, Uttar Pradesh, Orissa, and Jharkhand.

The community ties were very much strong in Pushta. People who shared the same state, same caste, same occupation had been staying together. Pushta had number of slums like Neematala which was dominated by the Bengali population and people from this community were working as rickshaw pullers. Then there were Dhobi ghat, Bihari basti, Moolchand basti, Rajasthani basti, Kisan basti, etc.

Yamuna Pushta had developed well in the last four decades and it had everything from shops to restaurants, from self-help groups to crèches, and various social organizations and all were working with the Pushta residents. Yamuna Pushta was not only occupied by people but it had number of elephants in Hathiwalan basti, horses and goats. In Kisan basti people used to do farming near the banks of river and had been involved in growing vegetables. Pushta was a hub for employment opportunities. A daily wage earner in Pushta used to earn 150–200 rupees daily through his/her labour. So in a way it was home to those people who were engaged in informal sector and have been the vote banks for the politicians but still neglected by the government when it comes to the right to shelter.

Demolition Drive: What Was the Motive Behind in Bulldozing the Yamuna Pushta?

It is actually distressing to note that from last 40–50 years the residents of Pushta had been busy in making their **houses to 'homes'**. From the day one, the poor who had entered the city is struggling hard to survive in the city and working tough in order to make their identity and status in the unorganized sector. The demolition took place under the order of Delhi High Court, which directed the authorities to remove of all the Yamuna encroachments within 2 months of the order. There were mainly two issues on which high court supported their argument for demolition.

- One of the ground for demolition order was that Pushta slum dwellers were, encroachments on the Yamuna river bed.
- And second was the pollution of the Yamuna River caused by the slum dwellers of Pushta.

Logically any encroachment on the river bed means that any construction, any settlement, on the river bed should not be allowed. But what about the Akshardham temple, Delhi Secretariat, Metro rail head quarters, Commonwealth Games Village? And moreover we should not forget that Delhi metro depot uses the river bed ground water to wash trains, and releases their waste water into the river. Bharucha in his book mentions that "A simple example the Metro depot occupies around 52 hectares of land that is river" (Bharucha 2006) Now the question is that why did the government forget about all the above-mentioned illegal structures despite the fact that Pushta slum dwellers had been there for more than last four decades. Did the government wanted to serve only the interest of the wealthier class? This clearly shows that when it comes to the interest of the elite then the rights of the urban poor are sacrificed.

Let us examine the second argument of the court that, Yamuna Pushta slum dwellers **were the main polluters to the river Yamuna**. A study conducted by the Hazard Center in 2004 titled, 'A Report on the pollution of the Yamuna' states that every day around 3,600 million litres of waste water directly goes into the river Yamuna. And out of 3,600 million of water only 0.33 % is accounted by the slum dwellers of Pushta, which is negligible and does not justify the blame on slum dwellers for the pollution of the Yamuna. The clusters do not have the water taps to supply regular water at home. So how come they can be the main culprits in polluting the river?

Vimeldhu Jha from '**We for Yamuna**' mentions that firstly the main source of the pollution of Yamuna happens only at 22 km stretch of this 1370 km long river. And more than 80 % of Yamuna's pollution happens in Delhi in which almost 18 drains of Delhi discharge all their content. Secondly the main source of pollution is industrial waste and municipal pollution and not by those who does not have access to proper water supply. **Jha** further explains that, the slum dwellers were actually cleaning the river because it has been seen that people come in their vehicles (still comes) and stop the vehicles and then throw and dump their garbage. The small children then jump into the black river and collect the bags and reuse the items for their personal use. So in a way these families residing near the river bank are cleaning the river.

Ravi Aggarwal of **Toxics Link** puts a point that that "construction on the river bed is inadvisable as the soil is sandy and has low carrying capacity, a fault line runs through the area on a north-south axis and the area is prone to periodic floods" (Sethi 2005). So it means that if it is a flood prone area then rationally there should be no construction and no buildings on the river bank which means that it is not only the slum dwellers of the Pushta be removed but all the buildings and constructions as well.

Bawana Resettlement JJ Colony

Bawana is one of the resettlement colonies which is situated in the North West of Delhi near the Haryana border. This resettlement colony was developed in 2004, when number of slum dwellers had been relocated from Yamuna Pushta, Pitam Pura, Punjabi Bagh, Vaishali Chowk, etc.

'Unheard Voices': Reflections from the Field Area

> How do you feel when you were asked to demolish your 20 year old home? The home where I came as a bride, given birth to all my six children, brought them up as a good human being. But, everything, everything was shattered, and finished, in just few hours. They came, broke each and everything of my home, and broke my husband investments. I was helpless, everybody was crying, weeping like we all were children. But nobody listened to us. What would a mother do if her 16 years old daughter would be raped? What was her fault? (In **tears**) She went to the field to rest herself but she came and carried herself with all the humiliations, embarrassment, and shame, which she was not able to leave behind. You are asking me that how I am feeling in the Resettlement colony. This is what a resettlement is, where a poor is thrown to the out skirts of the city and losses his/her job, and enjoys in 12.5 km^2 plot… (Sameena, Housewife Bawana Resettlement JJ colony)

It is too early to give a generalized view about the resettlement colonies by reading the above narration, but some where it is providing an insight about a woman who had come to Pushta as a bride, but after moving to a new house she has had not only lost her 20-year-old home but she has lost her dignity, respect which she had maintained from last 20 years. The whole narration also gives an insight about her understanding on resettlement colonies, the way she relates her safety, comfort environment which she felt in Yamuna Pushta. She had tried to relate her husband disease, daughter rape, loss of job and investments to Bawana JJ colony. When her daughter was raped nobody listened to her and she could not raised her **voice** because she is a poor woman and in contrary the powerful people have a right to deliver injustice to the voiceless people without getting and expecting any reactions from the poor.

The field work was done by focusing on some of the important issues which were emerged during the interactions with the respondents. The issues which were revealed by them during the whole research process is given below in the form of pictorial representation (Fig. 1).

But in this paper, the researcher has specifically disused about **the issue of livelihood and issue of health care** (All the issues have been supplemented with the help of narratives of the respondents and their analysis).

Access to Better Work Opportunities

"Employment, or the lack of it, is now universally accepted as the single most important determinant of urban poverty. The employment status and earning power of adults almost invariably determine the well being of the entire family" (Sen and Bhan 2008, p. 57) It should be kept in mind that the only resource that these urban poor have is their own labour. If these people would be thrown out to far flung areas then how, where and to whom they will provide their services in order to survive in metropolitan cities. When families were shifted to Bawana, the High court mentioned that Bawana is a planned industrial area and displaced

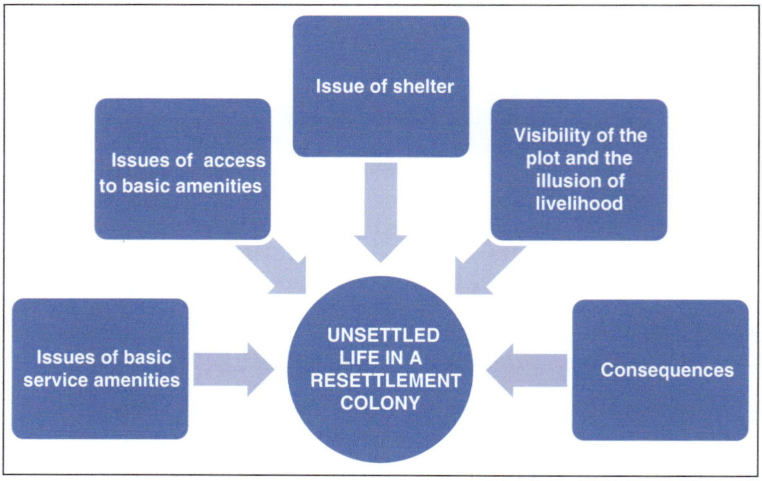

Fig. 1 Unsettled life in a resettlement colony. *Source* (Vishavpreet 2010. *Unheard voices: A study of displaced women from Yamuna Pushta in Bawana*, Delhi, Unpublished M.Phil Thesis, Jawaharlal Nehru University)

families will have an access to better work opportunities as compared to their previous occupation. And it would expand the employment opportunities for the displaced families. **Dunnu Roy** from the hazard center mentioned "When the first resettlement came up after 1977, the area was built around places of livelihood. In fact, the resettlement directive clearly lays down that livelihood is prime for relocation But this is something which was not seen in Bawana resettlement colony.

During the interactions it was frequently revealed that majority of the breadwinner goes to the previous locations, despite of having a plot in Bawana. One of the respondents narrated his story which is given below:

> Who will work for 18 h in these factories, just for 1500 rupees per month? I worked there for 2 months, but instead of giving my salary they told me that, I am really slow in the work so they will not give the salary. I had lost around three thousand rupees for 2 months. In Pushta I used to earn three to four thousand per month. Tell me what is more important for a poor **'a plot on a barren piece of land' or 'good livelihood opportunities'**. This plot costs me around eighteen thousand. But still I am not able to construct the home on this because I don't have that much money. My wife is a TB patient so she can not worked as a domestic helper and also I have seven children to look after, I have five daughters and two sons. My sons go to the school but my all five daughters sit at home and do nothing. We don't have enough money to send everybody to school. It's important for boys to study but it's more important for girls to learn the houses chores work. I have lost all the money that I had saved for the marriage of our children, everything was lost in the demolition. In Pushta we all used to have three meals a day but after coming here we just managed to have only one meal a day. I can't afford to commute daily, so I prefers to stay near railway station and then goes on every Sunday to colony, and gives my family the entire week salary… (Raju, 42 years) (Vishavpreet 2010).

During the interactions with the respondents, they mentioned that the factories in Bawana takes only young girls and don't take older women. Secondly the salary which is given by the factories is not sufficient to run a family. Therefore out of 90 families that have been interviewed, 70 families reported harassment by factory people. Almost all 90 families had already tried their hand in working with various factories. One of the informants stated:-

> My neighbour's daughter was attacked by some factory workers but somehow she managed to escape on that day. But the other day, when she went to the factory with the police, the police blamed the girl for not doing the work properly, then at night she was gang raped by the same factory persons, the girl was not able to bear all this therefore she was sent to her mother's village. Now you tell whose family and which family would like to send their daughters to these factories? Governments have made a joke of our life, because we are poor and voiceless… (Gufrana, 48 years) (Vishavpreet 2010).

The forced relocation has definitely led to the **fall in the income level** of majority of families. But the situation has further worsened because it has directly affected the consumption of food for many families. One of the women during the discussion pointed out that:-

> Here we manage to eat just once a day and that is more than sufficient. In Pushta I used to have three meals a day but after coming here I just managed to eat only once a day. I was not a TB patient but I have got TB in colony because the environment of this colony is not good. (Rafeeta, Unemployed, 30 years).

Another issue which is being pointed by the respondents is about the **loss of community and social ties**. At the time of Pushta the inhabitants of Bawana used to stay within their own caste people and were not bothered about other communities. After moving to Bawana their community life has also been badly affected. Majority of the families complained about the disruptions in social ties. Girls in the community pointed out that they do not feel safe and secure while going out of their home. Rape incidents have also increased after shifting to the resettlement colonies. People complain about bad attitude and behavior of the police and shared that police do not listen to them because they are poor. A lady from the Kanjar community shared her experience. (Kanjar community is from the Rajasthan which makes drums (Dholak). The members from this community are branded as bad people (*gande log*) because of their lifestyle. The women from this community can be seen as having drinks and smoking with their husbands. The inhabitants believed that Kanjar community is also engaged in Black magic. Therefore the families from the other castes and occupation fears in interacting with the Kanjar community).

> We were very good in Puhsta. It is always good to be with our own people. We are traditional drum makers. Be it drying the leather, cutting the wood, everything, was used to be done collectively. But after coming here we have loss everything, our money, our people, because to making a drum is done collectively, if our people are not with us, then how we are going to make the drums? I really miss my people. People say that the condition of Bawana will improve soon. We are hoping for the best (Kanata Rani, 55 years, Drum seller)

Very frequently, respondents mentioned about the assets that they used to have in the Pushta. Majority of the families had TV, refrigerator, cooler, radio, gas cylinder, pedestal fan, etc., and some owned rickshaw also. A few families also had bicycle for commuting. Again and again, respondents wanted me to know that, their condition has really **worsened** after moving to Bawana colony.

The report by UNHCHR (1996) says that "The consequences of forced eviction on families and communities, and particularly for the poor, are severe and traumatic: property is often damaged or destroyed; productive assets are lost or rendered useless; social networks are broken up; livelihood strategies are compromised; access to essential facilities and services is lost; and often violence, including rape, physical assault and murder, are used to force people to comply" It becomes important to understand that slums and slum dwellers are not a problem and threat to cities. They only become a problem when their right to livelihood and right to shelter are not properly addressed. Therefore, we need to integrate the livelihood opportunities with legal housing instead of providing a 'four walled plot on a barren land'.

Issue of Health Care in Bawana JJ Colony

Even though it's more than 8 years to this demolition but still Bawana JJ colony does not have a proper working MCD dispensary. There is no denying the fact that for majority of the poor, the priority for health comes at the end because, livelihood plays the pivotal role in their life, then shelter and finally health. Health care was studied in terms of **availability, accessibility and affordability** (The health care was studied keeping in mind the availability, accessibility and affordability of health services. The views and opinion about the health perception was recorded with the help of unstructured interview and informal discussions with the families focusing on the woman health. Respondents were asked to share their experiences on accessibility towards the health services, to whom they approach for during the child birth, and for day to day illness, And their opinions about the health services in a resettlement colony which is located on the outskirts of the city).

Availability of Health Care in Bawana

Bawana JJ colony is full of local health providers. **Local health provider** means quacks, Bengali doctor, dais and registered medical practioner (RMPs). Majority of the private providers claim that they are RMPs but still no verification has been done by any NGOs working in Bawana. And in every block around 5–10 Bengali doctors are available.

Maharishi Balmiki Hospital is the nearest hospital in Bawana which is located in Puth Kalan and its almost five kms away from the resettlement colony. This is a government hospital. Most of the time, the patients from the colony are not properly attended by the hospital staff. If the case is serious then the patients are referred to the Lokanayak Jai Prakash Narayan hospital (LNJP) which is located at ITO.

There are a number of the NGOs working in Bawana. And every month some NGOs organize the **health camps** in collaboration with various hospitals. But NGOs mention that they are not getting the positive response from these health camps. Even though people do come to the camps but they don't take the medicines regularly. A woman shared her experience of visiting the health camp:-

> "We do go to the health camps. They do a number of health check ups and give number of medicines, so it creates confusion how to and when to eat these medicines. The doctors in these camps give the same medicines to everyone. We are poor people, but it does not mean that we will play with our health by getting the medicines free of cost. Yes doctors in these camps talks to us nicely, but organizing the health camp every month does not solve our purpose" (Noor, 26 years, House wife).

Other Woman Mentioned

> These health camps are organized just for a few hours. The doctors come and do the job and then go away. But I think that these health camps should be organized on a weekly basis. In Bawana colony we do not have any **job opportunities**. So we have to go outside to look for work. We are daily wage earners and cannot afford to miss a single day. So how can we afford to miss our single day just for health camps? But if we would have been in Pushta then it was easy for us to attend these camps. Because in Pushta majority of the population used to work in adjoining areas of Pushta and it was easy for us to attend the camps and then get back to the work. (Rubeena, 45 years, Daily wage earner)

The above two narrations clearly say that organizing the health camps does not solve the purpose. Respondents shared that after coming to Bawana their priorities have changed. In Pushta, they had got some security in their work place because they had been staying for many decades and which lead to the strong ties with the persons for whom they used to work. But after moving to colony, majority of the population had lost their previous jobs which make it difficult for them to ask or to take holiday from their work even if they are ill. Therefore for them health comes at the end after work and food.

Accessibility to Health Care

Accessibility plays a very major role in seeking the health care. All the families interviewed mentioned that they prefer to visit the Bengalis doctors. The health camps and MCD dispensary are not reliable. Importantly, a health camp is not organized on a regular basis. The first and foremost reason given by the residents is that all the local private practioners are easily accessible and secondly sometimes they also check them free of cost when they don't have the money. A woman recalled her time in Pushta and shared:-

> In Pushta everybody was employed. And we had enough savings also. And there was no problem with regard to hunger and food crisis. And whenever we get ill then we go to Kasturba Gandhi That hospital was near from our place and there was no problem like transport. But after coming here we have lost everything. We have become unemployed. The nearest government hospital is the Balmiki hospital and it takes 10 rupees for one side to visit the hospital. What will the poor do? And why we should spend 20 rupees for commuting, if we have Bangalis doctors here. (Ruksana 53 years)

It is clear from the above narration that **Proximity** plays an important role in seeking the health care. Bawana is flooded with local practioners, so whenever the residents fall ill, they first approach the local practioner because they are available to them for 24 h. And if the case is serious they would be referred to Balmiki hospital. Secondly it saves money and time in travelling to other places.

An Older Woman Shared Her Experience

> In Pushta I used to visit the Bangali doctors only. Because I know them from the time I came to Delhi. But after moving to Bawana things were never remain the same. Majority of the families here are facing the problem of discrimination by the hospital staff. The problem of discrimination was completely invisible in Kasturba hospital because the doctors there were aware of the Pushta community. But in Bawana things are completely different. How checkup can be done if the patient is asked to stand near the door? But if a patient comes in a nice dress then he/she would be attended nicely by the doctor. Don't the poor have a right to get a proper treatment from the government hospitals? Then people ask us why we don't visit the Balmiki Hospital? (Rafita Begum, 65 years, house wife)

Affordability of Health Care

During the interview and focused group discussions, various factors were pointed out by the informants for the choice, reasons about health care provider. Majority of the residents preferred to visit the Bengalis doctors or some other local provider. The first and foremost reason given by them is that they can **afford** these doctors. Many of the informants mentioned that even if they don't have money at that time than they will take the money during next visits. Others informed that they don't have that much money to spend on other doctors by commuting. These local private provider are working in the community itself and it was also found that more than 2–3 Bengalis doctors are there in each block.

Community Preferences for Local Health Providers

Majority of the respondents talked about the **Trust factor**. Here by trust, they meant that, they trust the quacks and Bengalis doctors because they have known them from Pushta time. They mentioned that if there is emergency then the local provider himself will refer to the hospital. We know that the Bengali doctors in the community cannot cheat us (Vishavpreet 2010).

One of the Women Shared Her Experience

> Be it small or serious illness I only visit my hakim sahib. My hakim sahib is from the community, therefore he understands us very well. Market medicines do not suit me. The medicines are costly and are not effective. But medicines by the Baba are very effective. My elder son met with an accident and he got permanent scars on his whole body. All the doctors told us that the accident scars will not go. But I did not lose the hope so I asked my son to see the Hakim Baba. Hakim Baba gave him some special medicine. Within 3 months the scars from his body disappeared. If our community has got experienced doctors then what is the need to visit the hospitals. (Rehana, 50 years, house wife)

Second reason they gave was of easy **accessibility**. Respondents mentioned that whenever they fall ill in the Pushta they used to go to Kasturba Gandhi Hospital because it was nearer to their place. And in the case of the emergency also they would take anybody rickshaw and will drop the families to Kasturba Gandhi. But here if the emergency arises then they will not get the any transport at night. And rickshaw puller will take more than 40 min to reach the Hospital. But from Pushta, Kasturba Hospital was only 15 min away from their place.

Third reason they gave with regard to the choice of provider was the **availability of injection and medicines**. The following narration helps in understanding this:-

> Br it is stomach pain or head ache or problem with eye sight, the doctors in balmiki hospital will give the same medicine to everybody. And most of the time the injections and medicine are not available and they tell us to buy from outside. These doctors think that we are not human beings. They are also government servants and they are not our bosses. This was never the case in Machali hospital. There the doctor had formed rapport with us, so they used to treat us seriously. The Bengali doctor gives us the good medicine and injection on the site. The Bengali doctor does not charge the consultation fees for first three visits. (Rajwati, 46 years old)

Fourth reason which motivated the families for the choice of the local health care provider was of **respect that they get from the local private provider**. Informants mentioned that the community doctors treat them with respect, while the doctor at government hospitals tells them not to come closer and stand near the door. Respondents talked about the continuous discrimination they face as “jhuggis wala”. Respondents repeatedly mentioned about the bad behavior of the government doctors. They also feel that the doctor in the community at least talk to them nicely and treats them with respect.

During informal discussion with the women various topics were discussed. But the focus was on birthing. Majority of the woman mentioned that they prefer to give birth at homes by Dais only and only in case of emergency they rush to the hospital. The reasons cited by them are; doctors and nurses don’t behave properly with them in the hospitals and often make rude remarks to them. All women who were interviewed or was the part of the focused group discussion mentioned that they are called as **Jhuggi ki aurtae** by the hospital staff. All of them also stated that, whenever they visit the hospital, they face the same kind of discrimination which actually questions their dignity and identity in the society. These women expressed feelings of their insult, agony and pain when they are treated badly and verbally abused by the hospital staff. Therefore this is also one of the major reasons for the poor utilization of government health services which further motivate them to approach and access the Bengali doctors (Vishavpreet 2010).

Reflecting Back to the Unheard Voices

Yamuna Pushta was a self constructed and self made informal settlement, where as Bawana JJ is a planned resettlement colony. Planned resettlement colony gives an image of a place with better access to basic amenities, better work opportunities, good standard of living and better quality of life apart from planned plots. The above narrations helped us in understanding the better picture of resettlement colonies.

Firstly the experiences of the families' indicate that after moving to Bawana the residents are paying more than they did in the Yamuna Pushta. The problem of poverty had further accelerated because the entire workforce in Pushta was in informal sector but with the security of a livelihood. But after shifting, the urban poor to the outermost periphery of the city their expenses on transportation have gone double and which was negligible in Pushta. Secondly because of non-availability of the proper work opportunities in the colony, majority of the families are going to their previous locations. Thirdly this resettlement has also thrown light on the lives of families after eviction and the consequences of the forced eviction which have directly impacted on the vulnerable groups. The loss of livelihood has crippled the families and issues like education, health have gone out of priorities. The issue of legality and illegality of work has further exacerbated the situation. The unplanned slum of Yamuna Pushta which had been constructed with dreams of many families in a safe and secure environment is now transplanted into an unsafe and unsecure environment in a planned resettlement colony.

Acknowledgment This paper is the outcome of my M.Phil thesis unpublished, submitted to Jawaharlal Nehru University (JNU), titled: A study of displaced women from Yamuna Pushta in Bawana, Delhi and this chapter would have not been possible without the responses and lived experiences of the respondents from the Bawana JJ colony specially women, who took out their time for my queries.

References

Bharucha, R. N. (2006). Yamuna gently weeps: A journey into the Yamuna Pushta slum demolitions, Published by Sainathan Communication.

Government of India. (1996). *Second United Nations Conference on Human settlements: India National Report*. Ministry of Urban Affairs and Employment, New Delhi.

Sethi, Aman. (2005). A site of contestation, Frontline. (Vol. 22, 15) July 16–29.
Sen, K., & Bhan, G. (2008). *Swept off the map: Surviving eviction and resettlement in Delhi.* Yoda Press.
Singh, K., & Shukla, S. (2005). Profiling informal city of Delhi: Policies, norms, institutions & scope of intervention water aid India.
Vishavpreet, K. (2010). *Unheard voices: A study of displaced women from Yamuna Pushta in Bawana*, Delhi, M. Phil Thesis, Jawaharlal Nehru University, Unpublished, pp. 65–82.

Social Vulnerability Mapping for Delhi

Sunita Kumari and Milap Punia

Abstract Marginalization of people in the process of globalization led to increase social vulnerability. This paper addresses peripheralization of social vulnerability in national capital territory. It is based on the analyses of mission convergence data of 1.1 million households across 274 municipal wards of Delhi. In the past, unauthorized colonies have been regularized in Delhi. The total number of *Jhughi Jhopri* (JJ) clusters in 2011 were 687 and number of *Jhuggies* were 0.48 million (Delhi Shelter Board, JJ Cluster list, Govt of Delhi, 2011). (Delhi development report (DDR), 2013), reported reduction in poverty to single-digit figures (9.9 %) in 2011–12, from approximately 13 % in 2004–05. Notwithstanding the wide concern over the present official poverty line, which is indeed an under-estimate of the state of vulnerability. To claim that there has certainly been a decline in absolute poverty levels in Delhi, can be critically looked at from the rest of the papers in this volume, which shows growing marginalization and disparities.

Keywords Marginalisation · Social vulnerability · Mission conversance · Unauthorized colony · NCT of Delhi

S. Kumari (✉) · M. Punia
Centre for the Study of Regional Development, School of Social Sciences, Jawaharlal Nehru University, New Delhi, India
e-mail: choudhary.sunita1@gmail.com

M. Punia
e-mail: milap.punia@gmail.com

S.S. Acharya et al. (eds.), *Marginalization in Globalizing Delhi: Issues of Land, Livelihoods and Health*, DOI 10.1007/978-81-322-3583-5_14

Introduction

Studies on social vulnerabilities in urban localities in India are relatively few and are usually focused on deprivations in terms of infrastructure and services. Studies were mainly by planners and architects focused more explicitly on access of the poor to services and housing infrastructure, and concluded that discrimination was still prevalent on the basis of caste, class, and regional identities. The strength of these studies in connecting poverty to employment and living conditions is that it illustrates the ways in which lack of infrastructure and services, political structure, and hierarchical labor relations influence social and economic mobility (Kundu and Mahadevia 2002). Very few studies have been attempted at disaggregated level of municipal wards (Baud et al. 2008 and Ahmed and Choi 2010). Dupont 2004 analyzed the economic characteristics of the residents by type of settlement at micro-level across resettlement colony, urban villages, unauthorized and regularized colonies, Delhi Development Authority (DDA) flats and slums to study the pattern of social-spatial differentiation and segmentation of the metropolitan area of Delhi.

Delhi is most urbanized state in India with 97.5 % of urban population as per 2011 provisional census results (Census of India 2011). The unplanned areas of the city include Slum and JJ Clusters, resettlement colonies, unauthorized colonies and urban villages. The large-scale land acquisition by DDA, unregulated growth of urban fringes and housing shortage are the genesis of unauthorized colonies in Delhi. In the past, unauthorized colonies have being regularized in Delhi, in 1961 when over 100 colonies were regularized and in 1977 when around 600 colonies where regularized. The total number of *Jhughi Jhopri* (JJ) clusters in 2011 was 687 and number of *Jhuggies* was 0.48 million (Delhi Shelter Board 2011). Delhi government had issued provisional regularisation certificates (PRCs) to over 1,200 unauthorized colonies ahead of assembly polls in 2008 via notification and recently 205 unauthorized colonies were in process of regularization in 2013[1] (Hindu Newspaper 2013). Out of these 205 colonies, 157 colonies came up partly on forest land and while 48 settlement have encroached land belonging to Archeological Survey of India. As per National Sample Survey Organisation (NSSO 2009) sixty-fourth round, about 49 thousand slums were estimated to be existent in urban India in 2008–09, 24 % of them were located along *nallahs* and drains and 12 % along railway lines. In Delhi, 18 notified and 35 non-notified slums were surveyed. Delhi has 6.4 % share of slums in India. Whereas (Bhan 2009) reported about 77 % of total population of Delhi lives in JJ clusters, slums designated areas, unauthorized colonies, JJ-resettlement colonies and urban villages. Delhi has 112 villages, 135 urban villages and 110 census towns form part of the National Capital Territory of Delhi (NCTD). Delhi development report (2013) reported reduction in poverty to single-digit figures (9.9 %) in 2011–12, from approximately 13 % in 2004–05. Notwithstanding the wide concern over the

---

[1]Hindu Newspaper (2013). Notification for Regularization of 895 colonies likely next week. March 2, 2013. http://www.thehindu.com/news/cities/Delhi/notification-for-regularisation-of-895-colonies-likely-next-week/article4468680.ece (Accessed 27.08.2013).

present official poverty line, which is indeed an underestimate of the state of vulnerability, there has certainly been a decline in absolute poverty levels in Delhi. Over a period of time, these transitions have exerted tremendous pressure on available resources, infrastructure and poised a bigger challenge for urban governance.

Henninger and Snel 2002 stressed for the need of graphic representation for spatial information regarding deprivations disaggregated to the lowest level of decentralized planning unit at which decisions on State interventions are made within cities could contribute to improving local governance. Poverty maps are an extremely useful tool for poverty reduction. This is particularly so, if a specific poor area exhibits a lack of public endowments that stifle higher economic growth. Spatial maps pinpoint investment areas that need attention to accelerate economic growth and focus poverty reduction spending. Besides, private expenditure can be heightened in targeted areas for poverty reduction. Gauci (2006) stated that better roads for the poor to have access to markets do not reduce nonpoor use of such facilities. Assessing slums must come from a place-based approach that recognizes place as a shaping force of unique local vulnerabilities. Spatial technologies and techniques are particularly useful in developing a place-based approach to analyzing slum vulnerability. Elbers et al. (2007) simulated and compared the effects on poverty of uniform transfers (whereby all households receive identical transfers) and transfers that are optimally targeted geographically. They show that the use of more highly disaggregated poverty data in targeting cuts the cost of reducing poverty significantly.

Weng (2012) regarded remotely sensed information as important at parcel level for detecting physical features. It provides spatially consistent image information that covers broad areas with both high spatial resolution and high temporal frequency. Therefore, remote sensing is an important tool for providing information on urban land-cover characteristics and their changes over time at various spatial and temporal scales (Herold et al. 2003). The recent land use land cover studies (Gilles and Dalecki 1988) have investigated the causes and consequences of land use land cover change related to human population dynamics (changes in density, composition, and species), and changes in the indices of poverty and well-being. Kundu (2007) examined the differences between periphery and urban center slums in Delhi and found large disparities of local mobilization and political action, which were high in the center compared with the periphery.

This study attempts mapping of social vulnerability across disaggregated level of 272 municipal wards in Delhi. We analyzed a large database of mission convergence survey data 2009 of Delhi Government within geographical information systems to understand the composition and prevalence of peripheralization of social vulnerability in Delhi. This implies that knowledge is needed on the extent, location and concentration of such deprivation in order to be able to make urban governance more effective by targeting interventions where they are needed on priority. This level of poverty analysis is strategic for urban governance because, after the implementation of the 74th Amendment Act to the Constitution, the electoral-ward level is the lowest level of political representation for citizens to local government. Analysis at this level allows us to raise the question of what types of deprivation occur within specific wards and prioritizes the areas of deprivation can be addressed by local governance mechanisms. Second, this gives an opportunity to explore the premise that slums with in municipal wards vary in their nature and the vulnerability of their residents.

Poverty and Social Vulnerability

Poverty is being estimated using various parameters like consumption pattern, expenditure, assessing assets, have or have not of access to resources. But the debate on the proportion (extent) of poverty in India has been a matter of interest to scholars namely for methodological, purpose (targeted/universal), threshold for poverty line, parameters dealing with inclusion and exclusion, rural and urban and ways of how to measure. Broadly, poverty has been discussed under two approaches one is conventional approach where poverty has been described in economic term like people not getting a particular amount within a month is considered as poor or on the basis of consumption level based on certain calorie norms (2400 cal for rural and 2100 cal for urban) and poverty refer to a notional poverty line, other approach of poverty deals with the multidimensional deprivation of life, which has been explained by various scholars with different names like deprivation, vulnerability, social exclusion, etc., including various variables like education, health, political participation, status of employment.

Scholars have used different indicators as per their selected approach (economic or multidimensional). According to (Aggarwal et al. 2007) income is not an adequate indicator for accessing vulnerability; suggested indicators were electricity, drainage, water, toilet, housing condition, education, status of health, credit facility, employment, etc. Assessment of social vulnerability in Turkey (Haki et al. 2004) have explained poverty as social vulnerability with certain variables like employment status, education, household size, ownership of house, age, sex. (Cannon et al. 2003) have used indicators like labor power, education, health, productive resources (land, tools, animal, housing, trees, etc.), kinship network, common property, and source of income. (Cavatassi et al. 2004) in their study on—Estimating Poverty Over Time and Space: Construction of a Time-Variant Poverty Index for Costa Rica have used indicators like no bathroom, no hot water, use coal or wood, dirt floor, dependency ratio, house in bad condition, no washing machine, no electricity, no telephone, unemployed, illiterate, no water, no sewage, occupants per room, and years of education to calculate a poverty index for Costa Rica with using Principle Component Analysis method. A study about the slum and pavement dwellers and squatter in Mumbai by (Karn et al. 2003) suggested indicators like educational attainment of head of household, per capita space in urban poor settlement, water consumption and quality, toilet. (Masika et al. 1997) explained that vulnerability is not synonymous with poverty, but refers to defenselessness, insecurity and exposure to risk, shocks and stress. Vulnerability is reduced by assets, such as: human investment in health and education; productive assets including houses and domestic equipment; access to community infrastructure; stores of money, jewelry and gold; and claims on other households, patrons, the government, and international community for resources at times of need.

There are two main approaches to poverty found in India; first set of approaches limiting poverty to deprivations in area of consumption and income, and second being the set of approaches which recognizes various factors as contributing to poverty (livelihoods approach). Many Indian scholars (Kumar and Aggarwal 2003; Dutta 2008; Chakravarty and Majumdar 2007; Jha 2000; Vashishtha 1993; Dubey and Gangopadhyay 1998a; Dubey and Mahadevia 2002 and Dev 2000) have defined poverty in economic term either consumption or income with conventional poverty lines. But Conventional poverty lines give scant attention to health and social indicators, hence failing to demonstrate the social and health dimensions of poverty. According to (Krishna 2003) the livelihoods approach recognizes a variety of capitals, which make a household capable of producing well-being for its members, or the lack of which prevent them from doing so. (Saith 2005) critiques the first approach because it does not capture adequately what poverty means in the lives of actual households. His main points of disagreement, which also inform stance on poverty issues, are that it does not capture a number of issues influencing poverty in essential ways. First, expenditure lines do not capture the lack of assets which household may have or sell which reduce their vulnerability in the longer term. These include land, homes, larger capital goods which may serve as forms of saving/assets to be sold off only in extreme circumstances. Their loss needs to be counted as part of poverty. Second, health situation of family members can be an assets or liability (where labor is directed to the care economy and ill family members cannot work). Third, approaches, despite the fact that it reduces household's access to state or community-provided resources. Poverty and vulnerability are intimately tied together, yet there has been a recent shift in development discourse to focus on vulnerability as opposed to poverty, with the understanding that poverty is a component of vulnerability (Moser 1998; Beall and Fox 2009). Baud et al. 2008 have adopted livelihood approach in their study about poverty in Delhi, where they have talked about index of multiple deprivations. In which they have selected certain indicators like percentage of literate people, percentage of workers, and percentage of household using banking services, percentage of households having no toilet-electricity, having little space to identify the poor or a deprived person.

In this study, we have considered social characteristics, access to amenities, access to banking services, demographic dynamics, owner ship to house and health all work together to make a household or localities more or less vulnerable. And analysis of all these variables in geographic system gives as an opportunity to interpret the variations between the municipal wards in terms of relative social vulnerability. In other words, municipal wards are likely to be different from place to place even within a city, necessitating an analysis of vulnerability that takes this variation into account. A place-based approach can offer spatially specific insights while maintaining ties to the larger body of vulnerability knowledge. Rashed et al. (2007) boils down urban vulnerability term to one word, 'particularity', emphasizing the complex social, ecological, physical, and spatial dynamics that require vulnerability to be assessed in relation to a specific spatiotemporal context.

Data and Methods

We used survey data 2009 conducted by Mission Convergence, Government of Delhi. The data was collected to identify most vulnerable population in Delhi state. Mission Convergence has been formed with the objective of reaching social services to the economically and socially vulnerable sections of Delhi's population more transparently and more effectively, by a series of reforms including converging and rationalizing all social sector schemes. The basic premise of the methodology for identifying urban vulnerable households and individuals is that it would depend on proxy indicators of income. Social vulnerability and access to public services to further calculate the proxy income and define vulnerability around selected variables. Mission Convergence has collected information on social and occupational characteristics of families through a door to door survey of families only residing in slums, unauthorized colonies and other areas. Survey was done in approximately 1.1 million households or of 5.2 million people residing in notified, non-notified slums, resettlement colonies and unauthorized colonies of the Municipal Corporation of Delhi (MCD).

Remote sensing datasets of Landsat TM of September 22, 2009 of Delhi was used to prepare a land use land cover map. Supervised classification method was used to categorize all pixels in an image into land use/land cover seven classes or themes. The land use land cover classes are high dense built-up, low dense built-up, water bodies, agriculture cropland, dense vegetation (forest), sparse vegetation (including parks), and scrubs and bare soil. Principle component analysis was used to construct an index of social vulnerability. It is a type of factor analysis, based on a statistical technique for reducing data dimensionality by extracting a linear combination, which could best describe these variables and transforming them into one index. Generally, the first principal component captures the greatest variation among the set of variables, can be converted into factor scores, which serve as weights for the creation of the marginality index. Selected variables to construct index were like access to basic services, water, electricity, toilet, bank account, status of employment, house owner ship, status of women, wellbeing in terms of health status or suffering from some kind of disease, and level of literacy.

Results

Land use change in built-up category in 2009 reported an increase of 42 km^2 to already published figure of 522.73 km^2 (Punia et al. 2010) in year 2005. Segregated and low dense built area is more toward periphery and in intermittent areas, between buffer of 5 and 15 km from the central location. Beyond 15 km of buffer, majority land use category was agriculture (refer Fig. 2). Analysis of pattern in Fig. 1, reflects that vulnerabilities are not concentrated at one locality, but

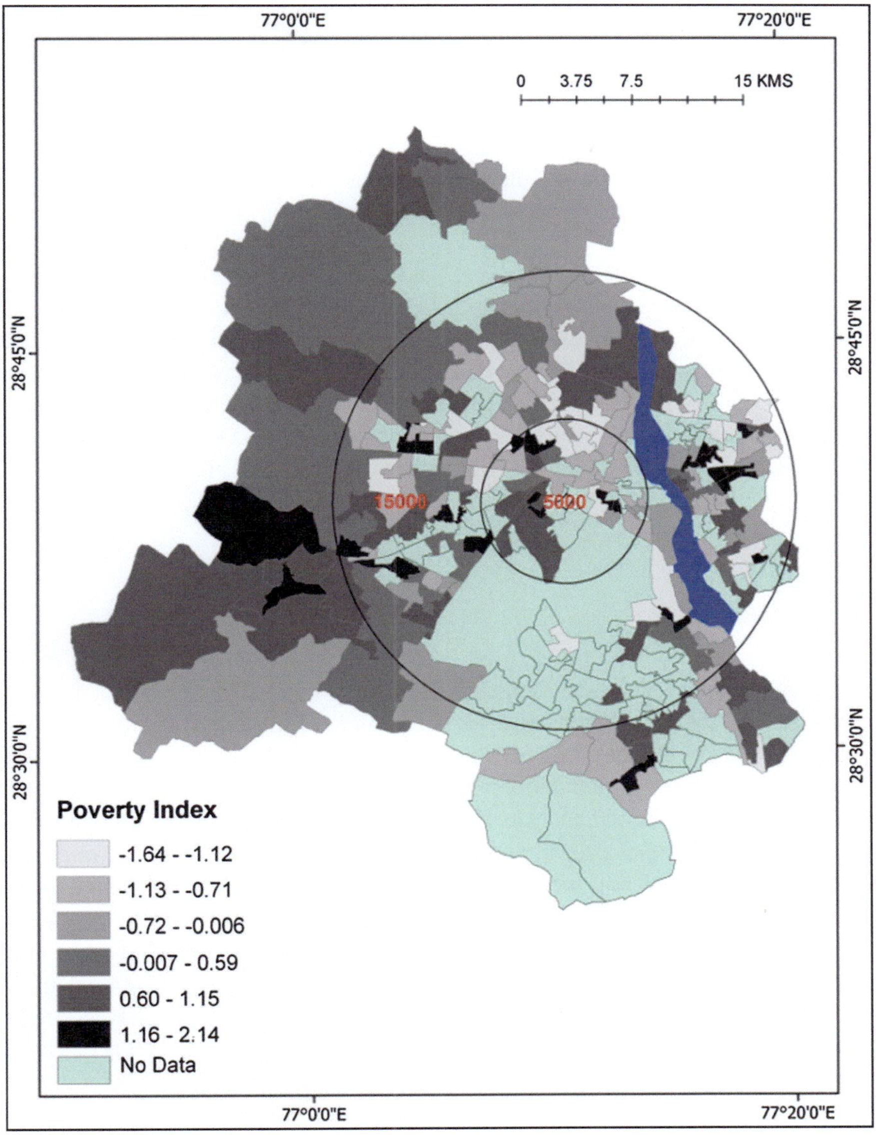

Fig. 1 Proximity analysis and poverty (authors work)

is more pronounced toward the peripheries. However, there are cases of exceptions of occurrence like Wazirpur ward (67), which is located in central part of city. Hereafter, wards numbers will be given in parenthesis after the ward name.

Indicators selected in this study were processed in SPSS statistical software and harmonized in percentage values across municipal wards. Areas of incidence of high levels of social vulnerability are Qasabpura (88), Tagore garden (106), New

Ranjit Nagar (96) and Ram Nagar (87) in central Delhi. Similarly, Hari Nagar (111), Vishnu Nagar (107), Shankurpur (64), West Patel Nagar (94), Mangolpuri West (48), Sultanpuri South (40) and SultanpurMajra (39) in central part of city. Dhirpur (13), Jharoda (8) and Sonia Vihar (272) in north eastern part of the city. Dichaan Kalan (139) and Roshan Pura (137) and Mohan garden (125) in southern-western part. In East Delhi, the municipal wards are like Jhilmil (238), Vishwash Nagar (226), Zaffarabad (250), Welcome Colony (248), Janta Colony(259) and Nand Nagari (243).

Lowest reported index values were in Rohini South (45), second lowest is Model Basti (90) both located in central Delhi and third lowest is in Ashok Nagar (246) which is located in east Delhi. Other areas are Punjabi Bagh (103), Kohat Enclave (63), Ashok Vihar (68), Sawan Park (66), GTB Nagar (12), Model Town (72) and Rana Pratap Bagh, all are located in central part of the city. Some areas of relatively less vulnerability values were located in East Delhi like Ram Nagar (247), Harsh Vihar (264), Mayur Vihar phase 1(209) and Mayur Vihar phase-2 (219).

Peripheralisation

Social vulnerability mapping is useful to display various dimensions of deprivation and its spatial relationships. As the distance from the core increases, the modernity and development related indicators shows a systematic decline, while those linked with social and economic backwardness tend to go up. Same is the case of Delhi, where social and economic indicator reflects the same trend towards peripheries. Municipal wards on peripheries are shelter to poor, who live in degenerated peripheries and find jobs in the industries firms therein or commute to the central city for work.

Dev Nagar, adjoining to Karol Bag (ward No 92) is the identified as central geographic unit in Delhi using geographic information system environment. A buffer of 5 and 15 km from central ward is generated to attempt analysis on the proximity basis. The core is defined as municipal wards within 5 km of buffer from central part of Delhi. The localities beyond 15 km buffer from central ward are categorized as peripheral. Remaining wards between 5 and 15 km are intermittent (refer Table 1). Careful interpretation of land use map generated from Landsat TM dataset reveals that majority of built-up proxy for urban is within 15 km of buffer (refer Fig. 2), so we selected the same distance as a threshold for defining arbitrary peripheral localities for analysis based on distance from the center. As per the selected methodology to attempt analysis on proximity basis, out of total 272 municipal wards, 44 are part of core, 161 part of intermittent localities, and 67 are in category of periphery. Distribution of individual variables is attempted across municipal wards and was differentiated to analyze the prevalence of peripheralisation in Delhi.

Table 1 Spatial distribution of variables across Delhi core (5 kms from *center*), intermittent (between 5 and 15 kms) and periphery (beyond buffer of 15 kms from *center*). (authors work)

Percentage	Core	Intermittent	Periphery
Toilet			
<5	14	58	25
>30	1	7	4
Water			
<5	16	56	17
>30	0	4	3
Electricity			
<5	21	91	38
>30	0	0	0
>10	2	6	2
Literacy			
<5	0	0	0
>30	8	30	8
Banking			
<5	0	1	0
>30	31	107	47
Employment			
<5	9	31	16
>30	18	56	18
House			
<5	30	88	21
>10	1	0	0
Rented			
<5	0	1	0
>30	10	35	16
SC			
<5	0	7	1
>30	18	43	17
>60	6	8	2
ST			
<5	16	74	30
>30	0	2	0
>10	6	14	3

Electricity

Electricity is an essential part of daily life but, however, there are many parts of city where people do not have electricity to light their houses. The central core reported better access to electricity in comparison to intermittent and peripheral wards. There were hardly any wards in the city, where proportion of households devoid of electricity more than 25 %. However, there were eight wards in

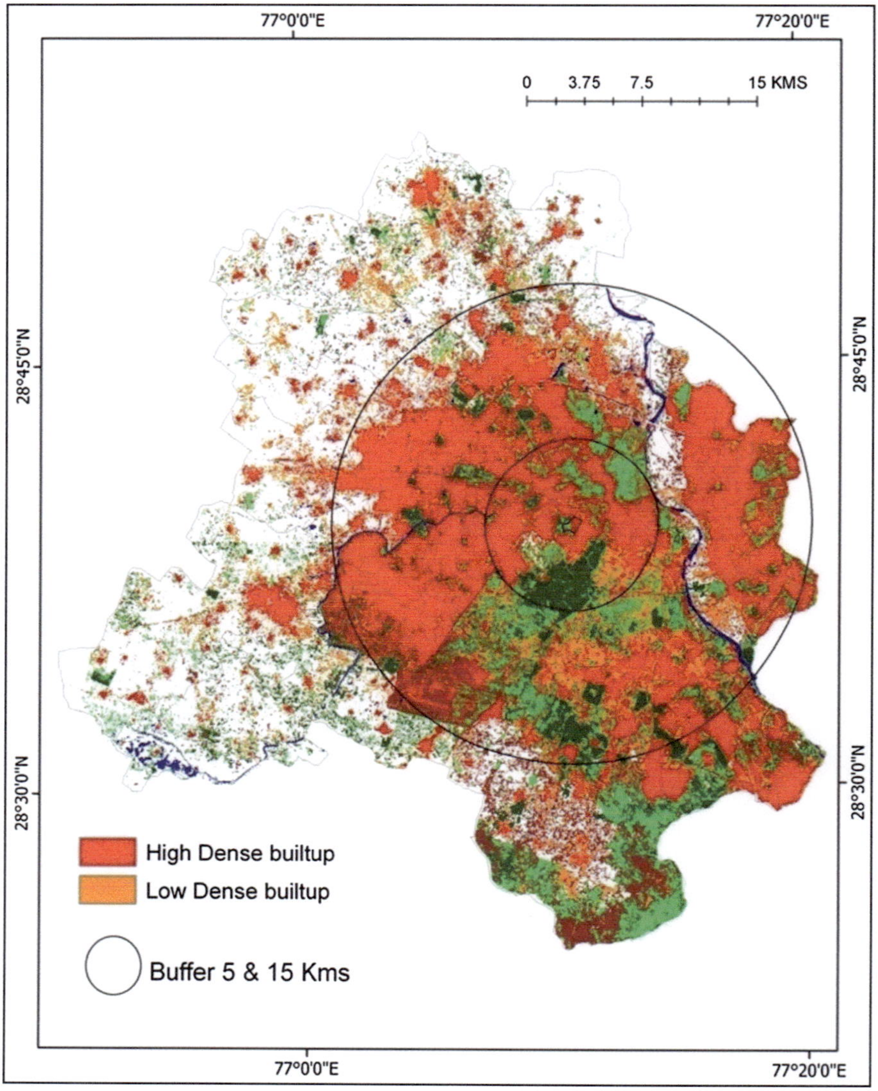

Fig. 2 Land use map for Delhi (authors work using landsat TM of September 22, 2009)

outward areas, where 10 % of households did not have electricity. Wards were like Najafgarh (138), Khera (140) located in southwest periphery of city; Mudka (30), Bawana (28), Sahibabad Daultpur (26), Bhalswa (26) in north. The Census (2011) data reveals that the coverage of access to electricity in the state is nearly universal.

Water

Delhi's core area was better off in terms of access to water; there was hardly any ward where percentage of households was more than 30 %, who did not have access to water in their premises. Peripheral localities like Okhala (206), Kasturba nagar (157) and Sangam vihar (177), reported more than 50 % households did not have access to water. Other wards, where regular supply of water as not maintained were Roshan Pura(137), Dichaan Kalan (139) in south west; and Bankner (2), Bhalswa Jahangir (5), Jharoda (8) in north part of city. In 2011, approximately 81.3 % of Delhi's population received piped drinking water supplied by the Delhi Jal Board, while the residual population accessed water from hand pumps, tubewells, wells, rivers, canals, etc. Disparity in access measured in terms of the distance to the source of drinking water shows a marginal improvement over the same period (Census 2011).

As the global Human Development Report (2006), puts it, "access to water for life is a basic human need and fundamental human right." Lack of safe drinking water can cause death, especially among children. Also, women and children invest considerable effort and time to collect and carry water. Ze´rah (1998) assessed water quality and surveyed about 800 households to conclude that quality of water services in Delhi should be addressed and improved.

Toilets

There were about 11 municipal wards in peripheral areas, where 30 % of households do not have access to latrines. Municipal wards, which represents highest percentage of households without toilet in their premises were Kotala enclave (63) with 97 % in central part of city, Rohini north (45) with 88 % and Lajpat Nagar (155) in south Delhi. Others relatively less worst wards were Mundka (30), Narela (1), Bakhtwarpur (4), Bhalsawa Jahangir (5), Mangolpuri north(48), Pitampura north (54) and Shalimar bagh north (55). As per 2011 latest census, nearly 90 % of the households in Delhi have access to latrines within their living premises. However, 0.24 million households, comprising 7.2 % of the total, use public facilities and 0.11 million households (3.3 %) still use open spaces for defecation. This practice has serious implications not only for health and the environment, but also for the security of women and children, making them more vulnerable to exploitation. Census Slum data (2011), reported close to half the slum households did not have latrine facilities within their premises, which has important implications for the hygiene situation in and around slums. In quantitative terms, out of a total of 0.384 million households residing in the slums in Delhi, which comprise a little more than 10 % of Delhi's total population, nearly 0.192 million households did not have toilets within their premises.

Banking

There were 63 municipal wards out of 189 (those have been surveyed) where majority of households did not have bank accounts. Majority of localities were in peripheries like Khera, Roshanpura, Najafgarh, Dichaan Kalan, Mundka, Nangli, Sakravati, Karala, Begumpur, Bawana, Kakrala, and Mohan Garden. There was exception like where majority had their bank accounts was Shakarpur (223). Samaypur Badli (17) only 2.20 % and Pandav Nagar (224) 18.83 % people did not have account in Bank. Timorpur, MayurVihar Phase-1 and phase-2 were comparatively better off.

Literacy

According to Indian census a person who can read and write with understanding in any language, is considered as a literate. The person may or may not have received any formal education (State of literacy, Census of India 2001).[2] A vast majority (86 %) of the urban poor in Delhi were illiterate compared with 14 % among the urban high income group and urban average of 27 %. The school attendance especially among girls is much lower among the urban poor. The low level of education poses a number of challenges in the adoption of recommended behaviors pertaining to care of mothers and babies (Agarwal et al. 2007).

Spatial distribution of illiteracy across Delhi illustrates decreasing trend from core to periphery. Households in Kasturba Nagar (157) reported illiterate with 57.38 %, second was Ashok Nagar (246) with 48.42 % in east Delhi and third was Model Basti (90) with 48.31 %. Other areas of low literacy were Bawana, Narela on north-western periphery, GTB Nagar, Pusa, Punjabi Bagh, Ashok Vihar, Kahat Enclave, Rohini north and Rohini south in core of city; VivekVihar, KartamPuri, Mustafabad and new Seemapuri in East Delhi; Nizamuddin, Zakirnagar, Minto road and Shakarpur along Yamuna river. Localities with concentration of low illiterates were Bindapur (128) in central Delhi with 6.53 %, Jhilmil (238) in east Delhi with 11.91 % and Meetheypur (202) with 12.16 %.

Employment

Percentage of unemployment was highest among households on Minto Road (81) on western river front of Yamuna River with 80 %, second was Mustafabad (268) in East Delhi with 77.76 % and third was Nehru Vihar (267) with 75.81 %.

---

[2]Census of India (2001). State of literacy (chapter 7), Provisional Totals, Series 1. Office of the Registrar General & Census Commissioner for India, Ministry of Home Affairs, New Delhi.

In east Delhi areas with high percentage of unemployed people were KhajariKhas (269), Shiv Vihar (265), Sabali (263), Harsh Vihar (264), Ramnagar (274), Ashok nagar (246), KartamPuri (258), Dilsad Garden (241), New Seemapuri (242) and Dilshad Colony (240). Percentage of unemployment was reported high in central Delhi and along Yamuna river, including Kamala Nagar (69), KishanGanj (75), Indarlok Colony (74), Rana Pratap Bagh (70), Sawan Park (66), Model town (72), GTB Nagar (12), Majnukatila (78), Ashok vihar(68), Deputy Ganj (274) and Model Basti (90). Along Yamuna are Nizamuddin, Kasturba nagar, Okhala, Pandavnagar, Shakarpur, Geeta colony, Ghandli and Azad nagar.

House

The census of India defines houseless population as the persons who are not living in census house. A census house is referred to a structure with roof. The enumerators are instructed to take note of the possible places where the houseless population is likely to live such as on the roadside, pavements, in hump pipes, under staircases or in the open, temples, mandaps, platforms and the likes (as per Census of India 1991).[3]

Municipal wards, which were located on western periphery, North, and north-western side of city; reported more percentage of people without home than the central, South, south eastern part of city. Wards with homeless population were like Wazirpur (67) with 25.57 % in core, Rani Bagh (59) with 8.85 %, Rohini north (21) with 5.46 %, Baljeet Nagar (93), Pusa (150) and Nangal Raya (110).

Rented

There are several clusters in parts of city like in core Paharganj (89) with 88.55 % of people living in rented houses, Darayaganj (153) with 83.49 % and Rithala (22) with 72.76 %. In South Delhi the areas were like Khanpur (181), Tugalakabad Extension (185), Said-ul-ajab (173), Chhatarpur (174), Kapasahera (143), Bijwasan (141) and Palam (145). In central core Tri Nagar (61), Paschim vihar north(58), Shalimarbagh (55), Model town (72), Kishanganj (75) and Paharganj (89).

Along Yamuna there were wards where number of people living in rented houses was significant like Daryaganj (153), Minto road (81), Nizamuddin (154), New Ashok Nagar (212) and Geeta colony (230).

---

[3]Census of India (1991). Instruction to Enumerators for filling up the Household Schedule and Individual slip. Office of the Registrar General & Census Commissioner for India, Ministry of Home Affairs, New Delhi.

Scheduled Caste (SC)

In case of SC population, there were twenty-three wards where percentage of SC population was more than 55 % like Madipur (104) with 81 %, in core Delhi Model Basti (90) with 80.99 %, Adarsh Nagar (14) with 75.7 %, Sultan Puri east (37) with 76.53 %, Sawan Park (66) with 65.95 %, Kamla Nagar (69) with 63.85 %, Qasabpura (88) with 62.31 % and Pitampura south (53) with 56.41 %. Rohini South (45), Major Bhupinder Singh Nagar (115), HariNagar (111), JanakPuri South (109), Majnuka tilla (78), Pahar Ganj (89); in south east Delhi, Kasturba Nagar (157), Lajpat Nagar (155) and Deoli (178); in east Delhi, Ashok Nagar (246), Ram Nagar (247), Shahdara (237), Dharam Pura (233) and Mayur vihar phase-1 (209); Mahavir Enclave (147) in South west part of Delhi. Out of these only four wards have high level of multiple deprivation, Deoli in south west Delhi, Harinagar and Qasabpura in core Delhi and Shahdara in East Delhi.

Diseases

Nine types of diseases have been included in this survey, namely, tuberculosis, other respiratory diseases, cancer, leprosy, heart disease, mental health, seizure, kidney failure, and paralysis. In case of a pattern of disease, central part of city is better off than localities on the periphery. Pattern of physical disabilities across municipal wards was also interpreted and incidence is toward peripheries, except in Nirmi Colony (65) in central part of city. Similarly, single women households, who could be separated or divorced, were analyzed and found that it constitute a small fraction of total population. Highest percentage of single women households are in Shahdara (237) in east Delhi with 5.85 %, Tagore garden (106) 5.22 %, Ramnagar (87) 4.91 % in central part of city.

There are many urban problems in terms of localities; these are rarely understood as the outcome of emerging process of spatial segmentation into privileged and underprivileged localities. The later are the marginal lands of the city core and peripheral areas bordering inner and outer municipal limits occupied by the poor who are newcomers or are being pushed out from the privileged localities of the city core (Kundu 2000). There are studies from scholars (Dupont 2007, and Bhan 2009), who documented that poor urban slum dwellers are pushed away, year after year, toward peripheral, ill-serviced, and to marginal areas. Baud et al. (2008) used 2001 census data to construct multiple deprivation index and stated that more deprivation do exist in peripheral localities of Delhi. The sites for relocation are found on the periphery or even outside the city, and the residents are dumped in places with no drinking water, no sanitary arrangement, and no roads. High social vulnerabilities levels are synonymous with poor quality of life, deprivation, low literacy and low human resource development. Recently released 2011 census data highlights decease in population growth rate in central district and New Delhi district by 10.48 and 26 % in last one decade 2001–2011. This indicates toward, degree of population being relocated from slum areas to peripheries is far from what has been reported. A major reason for the fall in the decadal growth rate is the wide-ranging removal of slum (*Jhuggi Jhonpri*) clusters from core part of the city since 2001. Major clusters removed during the mid-2000s include the Yamuna Pushta spread along the riverbed in New Delhi District and several clusters within NDMC area.

Conclusion

One of important objective was to quantify the spatiality of social vulnerability index in order to test the idea of existence of peripheralisation in Delhi and that has been proved positive as demonstrated by the results. Wards which have lowest index value of social vulnerability are within 15 kms of buffer, without even an exception. There were 27 municipal wards with low index value, 24 out of these 27 wards reported within 15 kms of buffer area in central part of Delhi corresponding within limits of dense built up area. Individual variables were analyzed from central core part of the city to its periphery. Indicators like illiteracy, no bank account, unemployment and rented house shown concurrence with high level of vulnerability. So intervention programs could focus on improving access/provision of education, skill development programs and appropriate housing. Localities, which reflected concurrence with high level of multiple deprivations, were not concentrated in any particular location. Thus, there is need for further interpretation at micro level for historical and institutional interventions to find out reasons for locational inconsistencies.

The graphic representation as a map not only summarizes a large volume of data concisely, but it also enhances the interpretation of mission convergence data 2009 of Delhi government at decentralized municipal ward level by preserving the spatial relationships among different localities and land use, otherwise was not possible in a tabular data. The socio-economic datasets integrated with land use information exhibited built-up impervious area as proxy for urban and threshold boundary for periphery. One may analyze the extent, spatial distribution, location, and proximity to which geographic relationships and reality could be interpreted. Land use is a factor far more complex than other factors of production and that brings in significant discontinuities in space, thus it has been dealt only to corroborate the geographic setting of Delhi, especially like core being more densely urban and periphery as being more rural and degenerated.

It could be concluded from the finding is that one size does not fit all when it comes to the relationship between municipal wards and vulnerability. The assumption of uniform vulnerability that is so often made across municipal wards/slums is a complex and multifaceted narrative. Since, this data has most of information from slums and unauthorized colonies, aggregated at respective wards. Thus, no two municipal wards are necessarily the same, and this variability should be accounted for.

References

Agarwal, S., Satyavada, A., Kaushik, S., & Kumar, R. (2007a). Urbanization, urban poverty and health of urban poor: Status, challenges and the way forward. *Demography India, 36*(1), 121–134.

Agarwal, S., Srivastava, A., Choudhary, B., & Kaushik, S. (2007b). *State of urban health in Delhi, government of India*. Nirman Bhawan, New Delhi: Ministry of Health & Family Welfare.

Ahmad, S., & Choi, M. J. (2010). Identifying and measuring dimensions of urban deprivation in Delhi: A town level analysis. Infrastructure systems and services: Next generation infrastructure systems for eco-cities (INFRA). In *2010 Third international conference on IEEE Xplore digital library* (pp. 1–5). http://dx.doi.org/, doi:10.1109/INFRA.2010.5679210.

Baud, I. S. A., Pfeffer, K., & Sridharan, N. (2008). Mapping urban poverty for local governance in an Indian mega city: The case of Delhi. *Urban Studies, 45*(7), 1385–1412.

Beall, J., & Fox, S. (2009). *Cities and development*. New York: Routledge.

Bhan, G. (2009). This is no longer the city I once knew. Evictions, the urban poor and the right to the city in millennial Delhi. *Environment and Urbanization, 21*(1), 127–142.

Cannon, T., Twigg, J., & Rowell, J. (2003). *Social Vulnerability, sustainable livelihoods and disasters*. Conflict and Humanitarian Assistance Department and Sustainable Livelihoods Support Office, London: Report to the Department for International development.

Cavatassi, R., Davis & Lipper (2004). Estimating poverty over time and space: Construction of a time-variant poverty index for Costa Rica ESA working paper no. 04–21, Agricultural and development economics division, the food and agriculture organization of the United Nations.

Census of India. (1991). *Instruction to enumerators for filling up the household schedule and individual slip*. Ministry of Home Affairs, New Delhi: Office of the Registrar General & Census Commissioner for India.

Census of India. (2001). *State of literacy (chapter 7), provisional totals, series 1*. Ministry of Home Affairs, New Delhi: Office of the Registrar General & Census Commissioner for India.

Census of India (2011). Provisional population totals (districts/Su-districts) NCT of Delhi. Retrieved December 24, 2013, from http://www.censusindia.gov.in/2011-prov-results/paper2-vol2/data_files/Delhi/Provisional_Rural_Urban.pdf

Census Slum data (2011). Housing stock, amenities & assets in slums—Census 2011. Retrieved October 10, 2013, from http://www.censusindia.gov.in/2011census/hlo/Slum_table/Slum_table.html

Chakravarty, S. R., & Majumdar, A. (2007). Measuring human poverty by population and factor decomposable indices. *Indian Economic Journal, 55*(1), 67–77.

DDR (2013). Delhi Development Report. http://www.delhi.gov.in/wps/wcm/connect/d889268040f180159184bba7591b5f5e/redDHDR2013.pdf?MOD=AJPERES&lmod=-579976292&CACHEID=d889268040f180159184bba7591b5f5e

Delhi Shelter Board (2011). JJ Cluster list, Govt of Delhi. Retrieved December 13, 2013, from http://delhishelterboard.in

Dev, S. M. (2000). Economic reforms, poverty, income distribution and employment. *Economic and Political Weekly, 35*, 823–835.

Dubey, A., & Gangopadhyay, S. (1998). *Counting the poor: where are poor in India* (p. 1). Sarvekshana: Analytical Report, No.

Dubey, A. & Mahadevia, D. (2002). Poverty and Inequality in Indian Metropolises. *Indian Journal of Labour Economics, 44*(2).

Dupont, V. (2004). Socio-spatial differentiation and residential segregation in Delhi: A question of scale? *Geoforum, 35*, 157–175.

Dupont, V. (2007). Conflicting stakes and governance in the peripheries of large Indian metropolises—An introduction. *Cities, 24*(2), 89–94.

Dutta, K. L. (2008). An estimate of poverty reduction between 2004–05 and 2005–06. *Economic and Political Weekly, 33*(47), 61–67.
Elbers, C., Fujii, T., Pete, F. L., Özler, B., & Yin, W. (2007). Poverty alleviation through geographic targeting: How much does disaggregation help? *Journal of Development Economics, 83*(1), 198–213.
Gauci, A. (2006). *Targeting & Mapping Poverty*. Poverty and Social Policy Team, Economic and Social Policy Division: United Nations Economic Commission for Africa.
Gilles, J. L., & Dalecki, M. (1988). Rural well-being and agricultural change in two farming regions. *Rural Sociology, 53*, 40–55.
Haki, Z., Akyurek & Duzgun, S. (2004). *Assessment of social vulnerability using geographic information systems: Pendik, Istanbul case study,* Middle East Technical University, Natural and Applied Sciences, Geodetic and Geographic Information Technologies, Ankara, Turkey.
Henninger, N., & Snel, M. (2002). Where are the poor?: Experiences with the development and use of poverty maps. World Resources Institute.
Herold, M., Goldstein, N. C., & Clarke, K. C. (2003). The Spatiotemporal form of urban growth: Measurement, analysis and modeling. *Remote Sensing of Environment, 86*, 286–302.
Hindu Newspaper (2013). Notification for Regularisation of 895 colonies likely next week. March 2, 2013. Retrieved August 27, 2013, from http://www.thehindu.com/news/cities/Delhi/notification-for-regularisation-of-895-colonies-likely-next-week/article4468680.ece
Human Development Report (2006). Beyond Scarcity, Power, Poverty and the Global Water Crisis. Retrieved May 16, 2013, from http://hdr.undp.org/en/reports/global/hdr2006/
Jha, R. (2000). Growth, inequality and poverty in India: Spatial and temporal characteristics. *Economic and Political Weekly, 35*(11), 921–928.
Karn, S. K., Shikura, S., & Harada, H. (2003). Living environment and health of urban poor: A study in Mumbai. *Economic and Political Weekly, 38*(34), 3575–3586.
Krishna, A. (2003). Falling into poverty: The stages of poverty reduction. *Economic and Political Weekly, 38*(6), 533–542.
Kumar, N., & Aggarwal, S. (2003). Pattern of consumption and poverty in Delhi slums. *Economic and Political Weekly, 37*(50), 5294–5300.
Kundu, A. (2007). Dynamics of growth and process of degenerated peripheralization in Delhi: An analysis of socio-economic segmentation and differentiation in micro-environment. In P. J. Marcotullio & G. McGranaham (Eds.), *Scaling urban environmental challenges: from local to global and back* (pp. 156–178). London: Earthscan.
Kundu, A., & Mahadevia, D. (2002). *Poverty and vulneralibility in globalizing metropolis Ahmadabad*. New Delhi: Manak Publishers.
Kundu, A. (2000). *Urban Development*. MOST Programme, UNESCO: Infrastructure financing and emerging system of governance in India.
Masika, R, Haan, A., & Baden, S. (1997). Urbanization and urban poverty: A gender analysis, Bridge (Development—Gender) Institute of Development Studies University of Sussex, Brighton.
Moser, C. O. N. (1998). The asset vulnerability framework: Reassessing urban poverty reduction strategies. *World Development, 26*(1), 1–19.
NSSO. (2009). *64th round report: Some characteristics of urban slums, 2008–09*. Government of India: Ministry of Statistics and Programme Implementation.
Punia, M., Joshi, P. K., & Porwal, M. C. (2010). Decision tree classification of land use land cover for Delhi, India using IRS-P6 AWiFS data. *Expert Systems with Applications, 38*(5), 5577–5583.
Rashed, T., Weeks, J., Couclelis, H., & Herold, M. (2007). An integrative GIS and remote sensing model for place-based urban vulnerability analysis. In V. Mesev (Ed.), *The integration of RS and GIS* (pp. 199–231). New York: John Wiley and Sons.
Saith, A. (2005). Poverty line versus the poor: Methods versus meaning. *Economic and Political Weekly,* 4601–4610.
Vashishtha, P.S. (1993). Regional variation in urban poverty in India. *Margin,* 483–524.

Weng, Q. (2012). Remote sensing of impervious surfaces in the urban areas: Requirements, methods, and trends. *Remote Sensing of Environment, 117*, 34–49.

Ze´rah, M. H. (1998). How to assess the quality dimension of urban infrastructure. *Cities, 15*(4), 285–290.

Part III
Health and Public Amenities

Disrupted Megacities and Disparities in Health Care

Ranvir Singh

Abstract Space and time are the basic notions which provide basis for all modes of thoughts and beliefs. Spatial dimension of health care encompasses this relationship while addressing the questions of what, where, why, and why there? These concerns became significant especially when the scarcity of resources present a critical situation and access of these resources poses a challenge. In developmental domain, cities have always become challenge with their nature of expansion with shift in demand of different services as well as spatial difference in their demands. Some places in cities become *growth poles* and with enormous pressure on resources, they scramble down and collapse the system. The terms in which the cities are discussed—urban 'explosion,' 'catastrophe'—tend to fit them into a system with lots of problems which are crying out for relief and solutions. Delhi also cannot escape from this enigma and been subjected to increasing socio-economic vulnerability due to increasing poverty, socio-spatial, and political institutional fragmentation and extreme forms of segregation, disparities, and conflicts. In such disrupted environment, it is a challenging task to deliver health care services to the whole city. This paper focuses on spatial expansion of the National Capital Territory of Delhi over recent times and evolution of health care services in the region. Paper further analyzes spatial coverage of health care institutions and their access by the different socioeconomic groups. Geographical information system (GIS) and remote sensing tools and techniques have been used to analyze the phenomenon. Paper concludes that, there are disparities in health care provisioning in Delhi and these health facilities are not equally accessible to all the population. *Distance decay factor* makes people's livelihood cost-effective but it

R. Singh (✉)
JNU, New Delhi, India
e-mail: ranvir.jnu@gmail.com

S.S. Acharya et al. (eds.), *Marginalization in Globalizing Delhi: Issues of Land, Livelihoods and Health*, DOI 10.1007/978-81-322-3583-5_15

affects their accessibility to health care. In such crucial scenario, the evidence-based decision-making needed information which should be very much precise to the real scenario and can explain the phenomena in a simplistic manner. GIS has this strength as its final product appears as an infographic.

Keywords Urban expansion · Urban poor · Disparity in healthcare and access · Space–time relationship

Spatial Dimension of Health

The emphasis on "Spatial" dimension of health care is a model which covers various aspects of Public Health, ranging from disease outbreaks to their epidemiological investigations. This model includes people and communities, and health care service in various environmental setups with their spatial relation with each other. It is clearly evident since ancient times that spatial characteristics of human beings affect their health status. Health indicators are spatial in their nature, which shows occurrence of a disease, some health related event, health status, or some other risk factor. These data elements, when become information, represent a scenario, which need to be very much precise to the real situation. In this context, Pan American Health Organization's (PAHO) analysis group of special program for health analysis mentioned in its epidemiological bulletin that *"The availability of information based on valid, reliable data is a sine qua non condition for the analysis and objective evaluation of the health situation, evidence-based decision-making and programming in health"* (PAHO 2001).

Space and time are among some of the basic notions. They provide a basis for all modes of thought and belief. The importance of space and time is reflected by such expressions as *here* and *there*, *then* and *now*, these references are essential to a conceptual framework of knowledge about the surroundings. In short, occurrence or existence of health indicators relates with space and time. The patterns of disease and human health are intricate, involving a complex interplay of socioeconomic, environmental, and individual factors that vary over both space and time (McKeown et al. 1976). Person, place, and time are the basic elements of outbreak investigations in epidemiology, and maps have been used to track the spread of disease since John Snow mapped the incidence of cholera cases in 1854 for the City of London (Snow 1855).

Eason and Tim (1998), *Gatrell and Loytonen* (1998), *Haining* (1998), *Loytonen* (1998), *Rushton* (1998), *Wilkinson* et al. (1998), *Bohra and Andrianasolo* (2001), *Brabyn and Gower* (2003), *Soret* et al. (2003), *Srivastava* et al. (2003), *Kistemann and Queste* (2004), *Lovett* et al. (2004), *Maheswaran and Haining* (2004), *Malini and Choudhury* (2004) and *Hilton* et al. (2005) used geographical information system (GIS) in their research by emphasizing the spatial component in public health and ranges from health care planning, monitoring as well as evaluation. These authors did intensive research using GIS which helped in analyzing heath care facilities, their accessibility, and distribution; infectious and communicable disease control; information management system; and in broad notion, helped to understand the health disparities.

Access to Health Care

Access to health care can be described along four dimensions: availability, acceptability, financial viability, and geographic/physical accessibility. While availability reflects what resources are available and in what amount, geographic accessibility measures how physically accessible resources are for the population. Combining these measures with acceptance and financial viability, a single index provides a measure of geographic (or spatial) coverage, which is an important measure for assessing the degree of accessibility of a health care network (Ray and Ebener 2008).

Accessibility to a general practitioner is an important health issue that has financial, cultural, and geographical dimensions (Brabyn and Gower 2003). By using GIS, one can estimate minimum both the travel time and distance to closest service provider via a road network, and a least cost path analysis. Assessment of access to health service sites is critical for patients looking to get timely and proper service. Also, access analysis results can be helpful when recruiting health care providers in underserved areas, or when referring patients to nearby practitioners. Assessment of access to Health service sites is a typical spatial analysis, which can be greatly improved by using a GIS (Lu 1998).

A GIS-based study conducted by Bixby (2004) on spatial access to health care in Costa Rica and its equity shows that the mapping of access to health services allowed to identify the geographic inequities, and to pinpoint specific communities in need (Ibid). This study assembled a GIS to relate the 2000 census population with an inventory of health facilities. It assesses the equity in access to health care by Costa Ricans and the impact on it by the ongoing reform of the health sector. It uses traditional measurements of access based on the distance to the closest facility and proposes a more comprehensive index of accessibility that results from the aggregation of all facilities weighted by their size, proximity, and characteristics of both the population and the facility. Half of Costa Ricans reside less than 1 km away from an outpatient care outlet and 5 km away from a hospital. In equity terms, 12–14 % of population is underserved according to indicators such as: having an outpatient outlet within 4 km and a hospital within 25 km.

Distance is a crucial feature of health service use and yet its application and utility to health care planning have not been well explored. A high-resolution map has been developed of population-to-service access in four districts of Kenya by Noor and others (2003). They compared the theoretical physical access (based upon national targets developed as part of the Kenyan health sector reform agenda) with actual health service usage data among 1668 pediatric patients attending 81 sampled government health facilities. Actual and theoretical uses were highly corelated. Patients whom have relatively poor access to government health facilities, traveled greater mean distances as compared to others having better government health facilities. This disparity was varied in rural and urban communities.

To correct inequities in access, policy-level decision-makers should make every effort to optimize the use of scarce resources. One way to do this is focusing interventions in areas identified by these kinds of studies, where impact would be the greatest.

Research Design

Study used mixed methods approach while analyzing the health care facilities, their spatial coverage and their access by different socioeconomic groups. GIS tools and techniques have been used to examine the urban expansion and the spatial coverage of health care facilities in National Capital Territory (NCT) of Delhi. Free satellite images of different years have been used with open source GIS software (i.e., QGIS) to see the urban expansion of the national capital. An innovative approach has been adopted to calculate the built-up area while using the road network and the population density figures. ArcGIS's spatial analyst has been used to analyze the spatial disparity of heath care facilities.

Disparities in utilization of health facilities by higher socioeconomic group and by urban poor from two different zones where health facilities differ in terms of their spatial accessibility have been analyzed within the context of various other socioeconomic factors which enhance or impede the spatial accessibility to health facilities by the mentioned population.

A spatial classification was used to select 200 households from two different socioeconomic groups (50 each from Poor Households and Middle Class Households), in two different locations in Delhi. These locations are different from each other on the basis of their proximity to public hospital. India Kalyan Vihar (Slum Settlement) and Sarita Vihar (DDA Colony) are situated within a distance of 4 km of any public hospital where Goyla Dairy (Slum Settlement) and Ganpati Apartments (Cooperative Society in Dwarka) have no public hospital within a distance of 10 km. A structured interview schedule was used to assess the health care access pattern of the sampled households.

Changing Paradigm of Health Care: Understanding Contours of Delhi

Delhi changed in every aspect since 1912 and the common man experienced this transformation from a vantage point which is strictly and surely out of reach from the outside world. There are thousands of oral histories of the city of Delhi, regarding its evolution. Batra (2010) analyzed that initially old city was acknowledged only for the purpose of creating adequate physical separation between the two cities. The situation of Old Delhi was not improved lately and Hume (1936) wrote that there was a "two-fold problem of congestion, viz, congestion of people in houses and of houses on land…" When Delhi received a deluge of refugee immigrants from then West Pakistan, it grew much larger than its infrastructural capacities. That was the time when DDA took the charge for infrastructural development, but despite the fact that land was available for housing, a constant refrain about the shortage of land for residential purpose shows poor assessment of the DDA for housing the poor. While for the poor only 35 % of the target could be met, for the rich three times more than the planned houses were built (Qadeer 2005). Urban renewal through DDA was set as the approach to planning for redevelopment of the existing city. But the role of DDA in the renewal strategies was biased and benefiting the rich, rather than poor, as envisaged (Maitra 1991; Priya 1993; Hosagrahar 1999; Qadeer 2005).

From the ancient Mughal era till the contemporary global city, Delhi was always at center stage. It functioned like a growth pole and enacted magnificently to attract in-migrants from all over the country. From the beginning of the last century, its population trends got a momentum and in the later half it grew at a remarkable faster pace. In all these years its health care system evolved in different phases, which can be organized as following:

(a) *Indigenous Practices of Health Care* This was the phase of traditional, inherited, indigenous system of medicine in India. Ayurvedic and Unani Tibbia College and Hospital with a consideration of an historical institution in India with special reference to Ayurvedic and Unani medicine, initially started as 'Madarsa Tibbia' in 1889 by *Haziq-Ul-Mulk* Hakim Abdul Majeed Khan Saheb who shares the family history of over 250 years of prominent practice of same medical craft. Institutions' foundation stone was laid down by H.E. Lord Hardinge (the then Viceroy of India) in 1916 and later it was inaugurated by Mahatma Gandhi in 1921 (Khan 2007).
(b) *British Period and the era of Philanthropy in Health Care* British brought allopathic medicine with them and it spread all over the country with British rule. The health care institutions were established with a philanthropic notion and to fortify British Viceregality. Hospitals like Victoria Zanana (now known as Kasturba Gandhi Hospital), Lady Hardinge Medical College for women, Irwin Hospital (now known as Lok Nayak Jai Parkash Hospital), Willingdon Hospital (now known as Dr. Ram Manohar Lohia Hospital), Silver Jubilee Hospital (now known as Rajan Babu TB Hospital) and American Army Base Hospital during World War II (now known as Safdarjung Hospital) were among major contribution of that era.
(c) *Human Resource and the Super-Speciality Care* Bhore Committee report (GOI 1946) reflected acute paucity of trained health personnel and just after independence, it recognized by the Directorate of Ministry of Health. As a result Sardar Vallabhbhai Patel Chest Institute came into existence in 1949.

Nehru's dream of a center of excellence in medical science came true in 1952, when foundation stone of AIIMS was laid with the initiatives under *Colombo Plan*. Later in this phase, institutions like Gobind Ballabh Pant Hospital and Guru Teg Bahadur Hospital were also established to train more health personnel to meet the future need in the public sector. Since 1990 onwards, various public sector hospitals have been established in various parts of Delhi, some of which also cater super-specialty care to the general population.

(d) *Transformation from Charitable Hospitals to Corporate Care During the Times of Privatization* This was (is) the era when the hospitals earlier built with philanthropic motives were transforming into corporate care hospitals. Hospitals like, Mool Chand Khairati Ram, R.B. Seth Jessa Ram and B.L. Kapoor were established after independence by the refugee immigrants who were also having same kind of charitable hospitals on the other side of the border, on the land acquired by the government on concessional lease basis (Qureshi 2001). During the life time of the founders, hospitals were serving well with charity motives but later their family members did not carry the legacy and shifted the main motive from charity to profit making, while converting these hospitals to corporate care hospitals (ibid). In the same realm, Indraprastha Apollo Hospital was built on government land but later failed to serve the urban poor as it promised earlier. Guru Harkishan Hospital was the latest entrapment by private and commercial health care institutions after BL Kapoor Hospital.

Transformation of all these hospitals can be considered as a future challenge in the evolution of healthcare in Delhi. This challenge becomes more serious with the notion that currently all these hospitals are not basically treating the sick but selling the healthcare. In case of Delhi, it is very important to note that, when the health care provisioning is becoming a profit making venture and uses public funds for the same then the whole situation becomes more critical which affects a broad spectrum of ill and sick people, who need immediate attention.

Constantly Changing Cityscape and Urban Poor

In developmental domain, cities have always become challenge through their nature of expansion which comes with shift in demand of different services as well as spatial difference in their demands. Some places in cities become *growth poles* and with enormous pressure on resources, they scramble down and collapse the system. Housing, sanitation, and transportation are some of the major challenges which specifically categorize the cities '*tough to live with*'. In the recent past, especially in the southern hemisphere such terms in which the cities get discussed, tends to fit them into a system with lots of problems which are crying out for relief and solutions. As relief measures and solutions for these problems, cities came up with their zoning and master plans for infrastructural development. But, this infrastructural network in itself is counterfeit social cohesion/collectiveness through *binding of space*. Megacities are origins and motors of multiple problems besides being agents and victims of risks. These cities have often been subjected to increasing socioeconomic vulnerability due to increasing poverty, socio-spatial and political institutional fragmentation and extreme forms of segregation, disparities, and conflicts.

Overcrowding, poor housing, choked drains, high density of insects and rodents, lack of garbage disposal facilities, and poor hygienic conditions are hall marks of urban agglomeration in India. Unplanned and rapid urbanization put a massive pressure on the already dwindling civic amenities. Most of the population which lives in urban areas is lured by massive industrialization, economic and educational opportunities in cities like Delhi, Mumbai, Chennai, and Kolkata, which are already over crowed. Statistics say that about one-fifth of them live in slums (RGI 2001).

New squatter settlements on inhabitable lands on the periphery of the city often came into existence because of *gentrification* or *distance decay factor*. Overcrowded settlements in the city face health problems, many of which are exposed to new types of risks associated with occupational hazards, pollution, road accidents, and poor sanitation conditions. Although urbanization is one of the indicators of development, very fast growth of urbanization in developing countries has created various health care problems.

Delhi was not different in any sense from this entire enigma. Since past 50 years, Delhi expanded from the central part to all its peripheral areas. This expansion in built-up area is increased drastically since 1970s (see Fig. 1). Initially first it started expanding to the periphery and lately the density in the city center and the periphery increased significantly. Currently Delhi is facing many

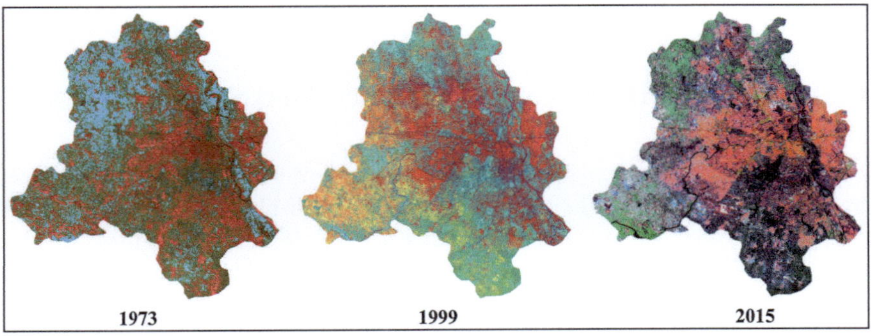

Fig. 1 Urban expansion of Delhi in past 50 years (red hue represents the built-up area) *Note* These images have been generated through LANDSAT Satellite imagery in QGIS. Satellite imageries for year 1973 and 1999 have been downloaded from the Global Land Cover Facility (GLCF) which provides earth science data and products (http://glcf.umiacs.umd.edu/). The recent most Landsat 8 image for 2015 has been downloaded from earth explorer which is a data sharing portal of United States Geological Survey (http://earthexplorer.usgs.gov/)

Table 1 Types of settlements and their share in Delhi's housing

Housing structure	Estimated population in lakh in 2000	% of total estimated population
JJ cluster	20.72	14.8
Slum designated areas	26.64	19.1
Unauthorized colonies	7.4	5.3
JJ resettlement colonies	17.76	12.7
Rural villages	7.4	5.3
Regularized—unauthorized colonies	17.76	12.7
Urban village	8.88	6.4
Planned colonies	33.08	23.7
Total	139.64	100

Source Govt. of NCT of Delhi, 2010a

challenges while distributing the limited resources over its 1483 km^2 area, in such scenario this urban sprawl shows a clear picture that in coming years, civic bodies of Delhi will face a bigger challenge to serve its population. The relationship between demography, health, and health care is rooted in the parallel development of these three concepts (Pol and Thomas 2001). These three concepts are interdependent on each other in terms of their changing nature over a period of time.

While looking deep into this urban expansion—slums, Jhuggi Jhopri clusters and unauthorized colonies represent a larger share of total available housing in Delhi, (see Table 1). From this table, it is clear that over 50 % of Delhi's population lives in some sort of slum area. It seems that growth of such settlements will soon overpower the urban growth by engulfing bigger proportion in the national capital. Delhi needs to be adequately prepared to respond to the enormous health and infrastructure challenges particularly for this marginalized sector of urban population.

Built-up Area of Delhi: Extracting Place from Space

Seventeen million people who live in Delhi represent a complex matrix between physical space and social fabric. Although space and place are sometimes used synonymously the distinction can be made easily while, identifying these inhabitants to their living space. Where space is only a physical location, place represents some attribute with social significance. In the total area of Delhi, there is a vast inhabited region as open scrub, river, and green zones of the city. Only the region of human habitation represents a sagacity of 'place' which deserves equitable distribution of various amenities.

Expanded mode of transportation is one of the basic notions which positively increase the developmental activities and encourage settlements around that network. While considering roads as central measure to see the rather precise version of built-up area (i.e., spatial expansion) of the city, an extensive exercise has been done to map out every single road of NCT of Delhi. In a GIS environment 21,431, roads have been marked with a total length of 60,021 km while using Google map images as base map for all roads.

The size of the settlements (built-up area) beside the roads heavily depends upon the size of population of that respective area. Therefore, to calculate the total built-up area a weightage pattern has been developed on the basis of wards' population density. This exercise calculated the total built-up area of Delhi as 642 km^2 out of its total area of 1483 km^2. 2011 Census' figures for Delhi mention population density of 11,297 persons/km^2. It has been calculated for the entire area (i.e., 1483 km^2) of Delhi. While using the total built-up area of Delhi as 642 km^2, this study calculated the much precise figure of population density of 26,110 persons/km^2. This figure can be projected as more precise than the Census' figures, which also include the 841 km^2 of uninhabited land. For further research this built-up area will be used to look into the spatial distribution of population and health care services.

Disparities in Health Care Facilities in Delhi

Delhi represents a complex structure of health care service providers within its administrative boundaries. Broadly these providers can be classified as—(a) local governing bodies (Municipal Corporation of Delhi, i.e., MCD, New Delhi Municipal Corporation i.e. NDMC and Delhi Cantonment Board, i.e., DCB); (b) State Government; (c) Central Government (Central Government Health Scheme, i.e., CGHS, Directorate General of Health Services, i.e., DGHS, Department of Indian System of Medicine (ISM), Ministry of Ayurveda, Yoga, Unani, Sidhha and Homeopathy, i.e., AYUSH; Employee State Insurance (ESI), Ministry of Labour; and Indian Railways; (d) Autonomous Institutions of State and Center; and (e) Private, Charitable and Voluntary hospitals. All these providers have their own operational boundaries which intermingle with each other's service areas. The lack of operational coordination between these health care service providers creates a situation of overlapping of services in certain areas of the city.

In Delhi, there are 738 hospitals with a total bed capacity of 37,460 beds (see Table 2). Though certain number of health facilities belongs to the other system of medicines but it is important to note that 97.50 % hospital beds are allocated to allopathic system of medicine only. This huge representation also share a diverse representation of many providers where private, charitable, and voluntary hospitals altogether represent the biggest share as 41.23 % of total hospital beds in Delhi.

The difference between public and private hospitals in terms of numbers and their share in total bed strength is inversely related and shows an interesting distribution. Both the sectors (public and private) have a much greater standard deviation than their mean for the total bed strength (see Fig. 2). This extreme variance in bed's distribution represents extreme ends of the curve with much greater

Table 2 Hospitals and bed availability in NCT of Delhi

Name of organization	Hospitals							
	Allopathic		Ayurvedic and Unani		Homeopathic		PHC	
	No.	Beds	No.	Beds	No.	Beds	No.	Beds
-Delhi Govt.	34	7210	2	150	2	150		
-MCD	54*	3951	2	140			5	47
-NDMC	4**	220						
-CGHS	4	101	1	25				
-DGHS	4	3742					3	32
-Dept. of ISM (AYUSH)			3***	116				
-ESI (Ministry of labour)	4	1338						
-Northern railway	2	442						
-DCB/Ministry of defense	3	1832						
-Autonomous (center + state)	4	2786						
-Private hospitals	607#	15175#						
Total	720	36800	8	431	2	150	8	79

* This includes Hospitals, Poly Clinics, IPP VIII and M&CW maternity homes
** This includes Hospitals and M&CW
*** This Includes Hospitals and Yoga Institutes
# From the list of registered nursing homes, charitable and voluntary hospitals in Delhi
Source Govt. of NCT of Delhi (2010b)

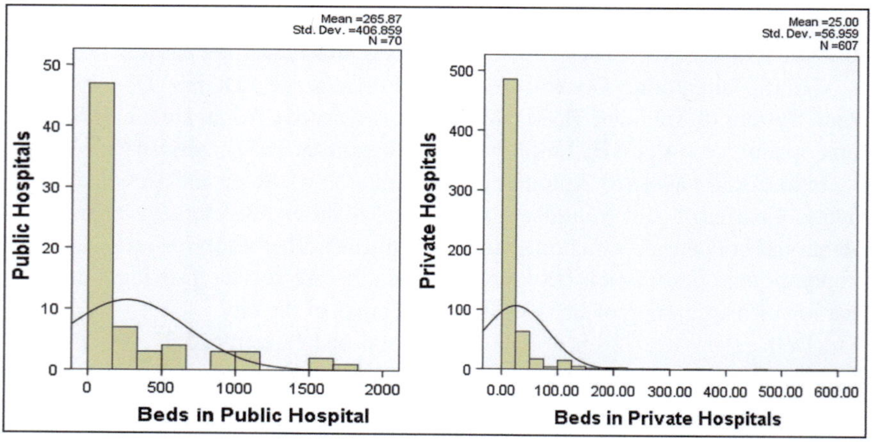

Fig. 2 Dispersed beds strength in public and private hospitals

difference in the magnitude. Where in public sector most of the beds are located in tertiary and super-specialty care institutions, private sectors hospital beds which also represent the enormous strength are distributed evenly. In private sector in total 474 hospitals have up to 20 hospital beds but on contrary in public sector mere 14 hospitals have same kind of bed strength. This extremely skewed bed distribution among primary and tertiary care raise serious concerns over the three-tier public health institutional setup in the city.

Considering this bed distribution, it is relevant to analyze the dispersion till two standard deviations. In private sector where 68 % (one standard deviation) of the hospitals have 0–82 beds, public hospitals represent a much larger range of 0–669 for the same percentage. For 95 % (two standard deviations) private hospitals have hospital beds within a range of 0–139 but public hospitals claim almost eight times high figure in a range of 0–1073. This difference has been analyzed further in an overlay analysis that looks into these beds distribution over the population in nine districts of NCT of Delhi.

Overlay Analysis for Beds Distribution

Study conducted an overlay analysis with all these health facilities and their distribution over nine districts of Delhi. After identifying each hospital with its respective districts' hospital beds distribution has been calculated as per census dataset (see Table 3). Study revealed that Delhi is facing severe spatial disparity in terms of hospital beds' distribution. While having 2.02 beds/1000 population (including Public and Private beds) in total, Central district which is having only 3.45 % of total population got allotted three times higher hospital beds and New Delhi which shares only 0.80 % of population load have more than 13 times bed strength than Delhi as a whole. Northeast and Northwest districts which together share a combined population load of 35 % of total population get much less, 0.98 beds/1000 for their respective populations. In contrast, the Central and New Delhi Districts which share a lesser population load of 4.25 % of total population of NCT of Delhi get a bigger pie of 36.06 beds/1000 population as their share in total bed strength. Per km^2 hospital bed strength also represents almost similar kind of distribution pattern in all these districts.

The spatial disparity in distribution of beds over the total built-up area making it evident that there is no positive relationship between population density and hospital beds distribution over per square kilometer of built-up area. This disparity in total hospital bed strength gets more complicated with private hospitals' role in different districts. While in East district private hospitals provide almost equal bed strength to the population as government hospitals, whereas in Northeast, Northwest, South, and West districts, government hospitals are completely overpowered by private hospitals. This raises a serious question over the disparity among public and private hospitals' beds' distribution.

The disparity in health care provisioning in Delhi has discriminated the access to the population living at the lowest ranking of social, economic, and educational ladder. Distance decay factor makes people's livelihood easy, but it affects their accessibility to health care. Study analyzed this spatial relationship for public and private hospitals' separately and came out with interested findings.

Table 3 Distribution of hospital beds/1000 population in NCT of Delhi

District	Built-up area (km^2)	% age of population*	Hospital beds#		Hospital beds/000 population#			Beds/$km^{2\#}$	Population density/$km^{2\#}$
			Public	Private	Public	Private	Total		
Central	16	3.45	2924	813	5.05	1.40	6.46	233.56	36229
East	54	10.19	2210	1909	1.29	1.12	2.41	76.28	31644
New Delhi	25	0.80	2897	793	21.67	5.93	27.60	147.60	5390
North	37	5.27	2739	1541	3.10	1.74	4.84	115.68	23904
North East	38	13.38	55	326	0.02	0.15	0.17	10.03	58999
North West	142	21.79	1148	1820	0.31	0.50	0.81	20.90	25720
South	118	16.32	2211	4487	0.81	1.64	2.45	56.76	23176
South West	120	13.68	3131	817	1.37	0.36	1.72	32.90	19111
West	92	15.11	1296	2669	0.51	1.05	1.57	43.10	27528
Total	642	100	18611	15175	1.11	0.91	2.02	52.63	26110

* RGI (2011), # Calculated as per built-up area

Spatial Disparities in Health Care Facilities in Delhi

Density of these healthcare institutions has been analyzed in spatial analyst in GIS environment. Figure 3 shows the public and private hospitals' spatial distribution in Delhi. It was revealed that public hospitals and their beds are randomly scattered over NCT of Delhi and not have any clustered patterns. Though the density represented for public hospitals was statistically not significant, it was evident that most of the hospitals are situated only in Central Delhi and New Delhi districts. A&U Tibia College and Hospital, Ayurvedic hospital at Balli Maraan, Hindu Rao Hospital, Kasturba Gandhi Hospital, GLM Hospital, Rajan Babu TB Hospital, MVID Hospital, SPM Chest Clinic, Northern Railways Central and Divisional Hospitals, Ram Manohar Lohia Hospital, Sucheta Kriplani Hospital and Kalawati Sharan Children Hospital, all are situated inside dark blue color band which represent 57 km^2. On contrary, density of private and charitable hospitals makes it very much evident that private sector is flourishing well in West and Northwest districts specifically while having two relatively small clusters in East and South Districts.

When the density test has been done for the distribution of beds in all the hospitals in NCT of Delhi Fig. 4 derived the final result for public and private hospitals, respectively. It was evident that in most of the public sector hospital beds concentrated in and around New Delhi and Central Delhi districts. As it was mentioned earlier that the beds distribution in public sector have a bigger standard deviation from mean, representing some extremes values (hospital beds) and it is because of those extreme values (which certainly represented by some of the bigger health care institutions), most of the available beds in public sector is situated within a very small radius. This dense cluster of government hospital beds falls in the radius of 172 km^2 which covers 39 hospitals with total bed strength of 14292. It is important to note that this cluster represents 26.79 % of total built-up area and has 76.79 % of total public hospitals beds. Private hospital beds are clustered mainly in two regions, Cluster I—On the borders of West and Northwest Districts of Delhi around Tri

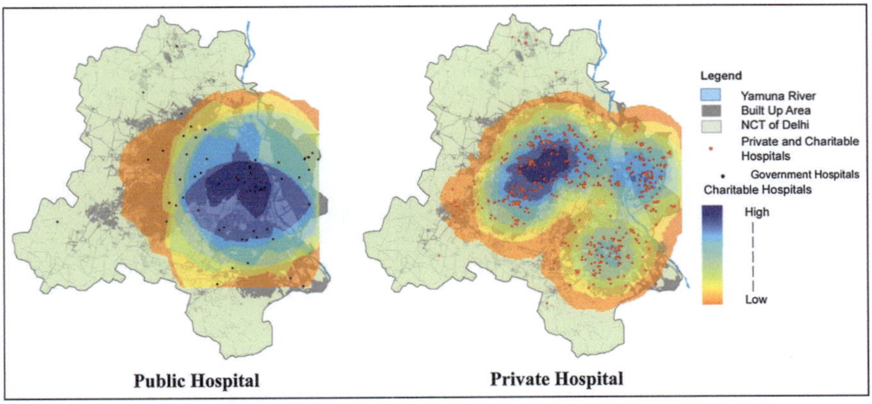

Fig. 3 Density of public and private hospitals

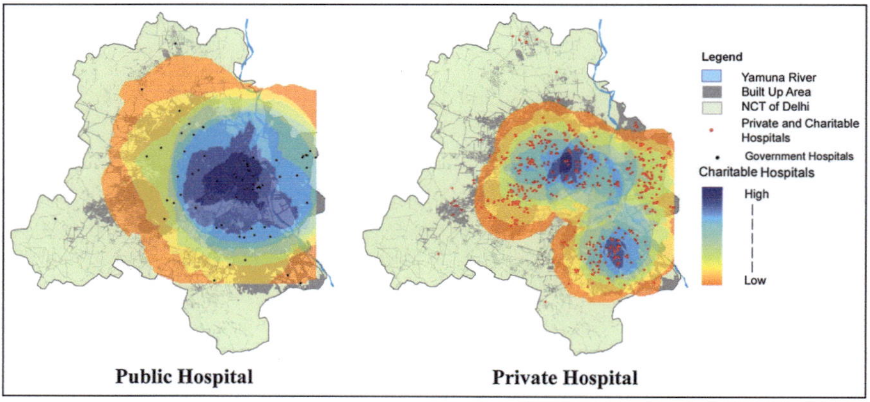

Fig. 4 Density of bed distribution in public, private hospitals

Nagar, Ashok Vihar, Patel Nagar and Punjabi Bagh; Cluster II—In South District of Delhi around Lajpat Nagar, Great Kailash I, II and III. Cluster I represents 65 hospitals with 2370 beds in 42 km^2 area which is 6.54 % of total built-up area and have 15.62 % of total private and charitable hospitals' beds. Cluster II represents 97 hospitals with total bed strength of 4335 in 71 km^2 area represents 11.06 % of total built-up area and claims 28.57 % of total private and charitable hospitals' beds of NCT of Delhi.

In comparison to closely situated public hospitals (most of which were established during British period), private hospitals clustered themselves in three different zones of NCT of Delhi. When, ever expanding city from its core to periphery defined its residential pockets, various service sectors including health care and specifically private health care providers established themselves within a demand supply chain. This change in urban built-up area which basically changes as per the Christaller's Central Place Theory (1933), changed the growth poles of the city and private healthcare providers grew faster and expanded more than the public health care system. The study limits itself for spatial analysis of healthcare facilities, but, the issue of the quality of care and the accessibility with respect to equity are vast domains which needed to be explored further irrespective of public and private health care providers.

Spatial-Temporal Relationship in Access to Health

Space-time relationship of spatial disparities in access to health care facilities among different socioeconomic groups is a complex phenomenon. It was evident that in this relationship mode of transportation is a major decisive factor. Figure 5 explains this relationship where the place of residence, the coverage area (which is the distance of health facility from the place of residence) varies on a time scale where personal vehicles or public transports are the contributing factors which

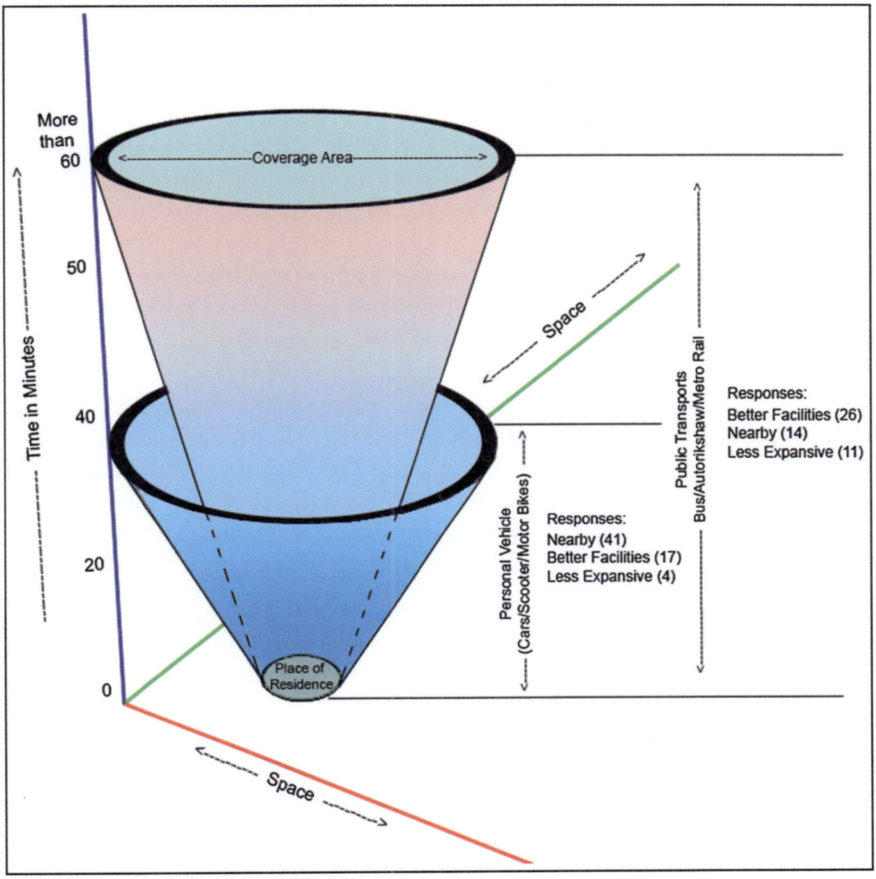

Fig. 5 Space–time relationship between mode of transportation and perceived notions in health care access

are influenced by the perceived notions of proximity and quality. It has also been noted that contributing factors and the notions which influence them, both were heavily dependent on socioeconomic and demographic variables. The comparative notion of good–bad, near–far, and more–less is heavily derived from personal experiences which were distinguished with educational attainment, economic status, place of residence, and the place of migration.

Conclusion

It was evident that in NCT of Delhi, there are spatial disparities in allocation of health care facilities. Where at one end some places have been considered as hotspots for hospitals' beds' congestion, contrarily some places are lacking healthcare facilities to the extreme of being nonexistent in their surroundings. The clustered pattern of health facilities made urban poor more vulnerable especially when they are already situated at the lower end of social ladder.

Polarization of income leads to huge disparity among poor and rich and influence their accessibility to various educational and economic opportunities for them. During the time of need (illness episode), this huge disparity in income influenced the spatial accessibility to health facilities. Whereas the sampled households from lower socioeconomic profile accessed government healthcare facilities after traveling more than 40 min and considering these facilities 'near' in a relative sense, higher socioeconomic sampled households opted nearby private health care facilities with a consideration of perceived good quality of care and less waiting time.

It can also be said that better economic status increased the spatial access but on the other hand it also increased the capacity of affording the nearby private healthcare facilities whenever required. Therefore the urban poor suffer more, have limited access and even when they need these services at the most, the affordability becomes a big challenge/threat for them and puts them at risk.

References

Batra, L. (2010). Out of sight, out of mind: Slum dwellers in 'world-class' Delhi. In B. Chaturvedi (Ed.), *Finding Delhi: Loss and renewal in the megacity*. New Delhi: Penguin.

Bixby, L. R. (2004). Spatial Access to Health Care in Costa Rica and its Equity: A GIS Based Study. *Social Science and Medicine, 58*, 1271–1284.

Bohra, A., & Andrianasolo, H. (2001). Application of GIS in modeling of dengue risk based on socio-cultural data: Case of Jalore, Rajasthan, India, *Dengue Bulletin*, vol. 25.

Brabyn, L., & Gower, P. (2003). Mapping accessibility to general practitioner. In O. Khan (Ed.), *Geographic information systems and health applications*. London: Idea Group Publication.

Christaller, W. (1933). *Central places in southern Germany*, (translated by Baskin, C.W.) Prentice hall: Englewood Cliffs, reprinted 1966.

Eason, A. & U. S. Tim (1998). Using GIS as a management tool for health care assessment and planning. In *Proceedings of the Geographical Information System in Public Health*, Third National Conference held at San Diego, California, August 17–21: 299–310.

Gatrell, A. C., & Loytonen, M. (1998). GIS and health research: An introduction. In A. C. Gatrell & M. Loytonen (Eds.), *GIS in Health*. London: Taylor & Francis.

GOI. (1946). *Report of the health survey and development committee*. Delhi: Ministry of Health, GOI Press.

Govt. of NCT of Delhi (2010a). *Economic survey of Delhi 2008–2009*, Government of Delhi, New Delhi.

Govt. of NCT of Delhi. (2010b). *Delhi statistical hand book—2010*. New Delhi: Directorate of Economic and Statistics.

Haining, R. (1998). Spatial statistics and the analysis of health data. In A. C. Gatrell & M. Loytonen (Eds.), *GIS and Health*. London: Taylor & Francis.

Hilton, B. et al. (2005). Geographic information system in health care services. In James P (Ed.). *Geographic information systems in business*, Idea Group Publishing, pp. 212–235.

Hosagrahar, J. (1999). Fractured plans: Real estate, moral reform and the politics of housing in New Delhi, 1936–1941. *Traditional Dwellings and Settlement Review, 11*(1), 37–47.

Hume, A. P. (1936). Report on the relief of congestion in Delhi. *Vol. I, (Simla: Government of India Press, 1936)*, 20.
Khan, M. A. (2007). *Khandaan–E–Shareefi*, The Generation of Haziq–Ul–Mulk Hakim Abdul Majeed Khan, Hakim Ajmal Khan Memorial Society. Retrieved January 12, 2012, from http://2.imimg.com/data2/YJ/QR/MY-4407593/sharif-manzil.pdf
Kistemann, T., & Queste, A. (2004). GIS and communicable disease control. In R. Maheswaran & M. Craglia (Eds.), *GIS in public health practice*. Florida: CRC Press.
Lovett, A., et al. (2004). Using GIS to assess accessibility to primary healthcare. In R. Maheswaran & M. Craglia (Eds.), *GIS in public health practice*. Florida: CRC Press.
Loytonen, M. (1998). GIS time geography and health. In A. C. Gatrell & M. Loytonen (Eds.), *GIS and health*. London: Taylor & Francis.
Lu, Y. (1998). Health Service Sites Access Analysis using Internet GIS. In *Proceedings of the Geographical Information System in Public Health*, Third National Conference held at San Diego, California, August 17–21.
Maheswaran, R., & Haining, R. P. (2004). Basic Issues in Geographical Analysis. In R. Maheswaran & M. Craglia (Eds.), *GIS in public health practice*. Florida: CRC Press.
Maitra, S. (1991). Housing in Delhi: DDA's controversial role, *Economic and Political Weekly, 26*(7), February 16: 344–346.
Malini, B. H., & Choudhury, P. (2004). Remote sensing applications in the identifications of Malariogenic zones in Visakhapatnam City. In N. Izhar (Ed.), *Geography and health: A study in medical geography*. New Delhi: APH Publishing Corporation.
McKeown, T., et al. (1976). An interpretation of the modern rise of population in Europe. *Population Studies, 26*(3), 345–382.
Noor, A. M., et al. (2003). Defining equity in physical access to clinical services using geographical information systems as part of malaria planning and monitoring in Kenya. *Tropical Medicine & International Health, 8*(10), 917–926.
PAHO. (2001). Health Indicators: Building Blocks for Health Situation Analysis, *Epidemiological Bulletin*, *22*(4): December.
Pol, G., & Richard Thomas, K. (2001). *The demography of health and health care*. New York: Plenum Publishers.
Priya, R. (1993). Town planning, public health and urban poor: Some explorations from Delhi, *Economic and Political Weekly,* April 24, *28*(17), 824–834.
Qadeer, I. (2005). Planning for the health sector: Problems and Limitations of the draft master plan for Delhi 2021. In D. Roy (Ed.), *Blueprint for an Apartheid City*. Hazard Centre: New Delhi.
Qureshi, J. A. S. (2001). *Enquiry report*. Maulana Azad Medical College, New Delhi: High Level Committee for Hospitals in Delhi.
Ray, N., & Steeve, E. (2008). AccessMod 3.0: Computing Geographic Coverage and Accessibility to Health Care Services Using Anisotropic Movement of Patients", *International Journal of Health Geographics*, *7*, 63.
RGI. (2001). *Census of India 2001*. Delhi: Govt. of India.
RGI. (2011). *Provisional census totals of NCT of Delhi*. Delhi: Govt. of NCT of Delhi.
Rushton, G. (1998). Improving the geographic basis of health surveillance using GIS. In Anthony C. G. & Markku L. (Eds.). *GIS and Health*, London Taylor & Francis.
Snow, J. (1855). *Mode of communication: Cholera*. London: John Churchill.
Soret, S., et al. (2003). Understanding health disparities through geographic information system. In O. Khan (Ed.), *Geographic information systems and health applications*. London: Idea Group Publication.
Srivastava, A., et al. (2003). GIS based malaria information management system for urban malaria scheme in India. *Computer Methods and Programmes in Biomedicine, 71*, 63–75.
Wilkinson, P., et al. (1998). GIS in public health. In A. C. Gatrell & M. Loytonen (Eds.), *GIS and health*. London: Taylor & Francis.

Changing Health Care Dynamics: Corporatization and Medical Tourism in National Capital Region

Sunita Reddy

Abstract This paper analyzes the changing landscape of health care in Delhi and National Capital Region (NCR), post independence. How the landscape changed from public service-oriented health care provisioning to privatized and corporatized health care, thanks to liberalization and health sector reforms. The paper further looks at the growth of the corporate sector from critical public health perspective. Based on the secondary sources of literature, health policies and program documents, the paper traces out the growth of private/corporate sector, which has led to marginalization of the poor and dichotomous health care provisioning. Ill equipped, overburdened public hospital services for the poor and state of art, accredited, posh corporate health care sector for the rich, insured and foreign patients, under the captivating term "Medical Tourism."

Keywords Medical tourism · Privatization · Corporate hospitals · Health care · Mega cities

Introduction

Health care since times immemorial is a "service" a Nobel profession, where physicians get a recognition of "Gods who saves lives." Health is also a human right (UN 1948), and in Indian context, it is the responsibility of the welfare

S. Reddy (✉)
Center of Social Medicine and Community Health, School of Social Sciences, Jawaharlal Nehru University, New Delhi, India
e-mail: sunitareddyjnu@gmail.com

S.S. Acharya et al. (eds.), *Marginalization in Globalizing Delhi: Issues of Land, Livelihoods and Health*, DOI 10.1007/978-81-322-3583-5_16

state. Providing comprehensive health services to a Billion plus population in itself is a huge challenge. Since independence, India is struggling to meet its health care needs for its population. Various health policies and programs have been designed to cater to the needs of the population. However, health has evolved from the days of being a mission and now culminated into an industry in the worst sense of the term. This paper analyzes the changing landscape of health care in Delhi and National Capital Region (NCR), post independence. How the landscape changed from public service-oriented health care provisioning to privatized and corporatized health care, thanks to liberalization and health sector reforms. The paper further looks at the growth of the corporate sector from critical public health perspective. Based on the secondary sources of literature, health policies and program documents, the paper traces out the growth of private/corporate[1] sector, which has led to marginalization of the poor and dichotomous health care provisioning. Ill equipped, overburdened public hospital services for the poor and state of art, accredited, posh corporate health care sector for the rich, insured and foreign patients, under the captivating term "Medical Tourism."

Health Care Planning in Post Independence India

India had its share of private care from the beginning. However, Bhore committee (GOI 1946) and Alma Atta declaration[2] of 1978 on Primary Health Care envisaged a holistic comprehensive health care services; preventive, promotive, rehabilitative and curative care, irrespective of their ability to pay. Three-tier health care, primary- secondary- and tertiary services were planned with huge investment in building the infrastructures reaching out to the entire length and breadth of the country. With proper referral system from sub-center (SC) to primary health center (PHC) to community health centers (CHC). The SC serves a population of 5000 in plains and 3000 in hilly and tribal areas. PHC serves for every 30,000 in plain and 20,000 in hilly, tribal and backward areas. CHC serves 1,20,000–80,000 population, these are ideal figures, however, it is not the same for all the regions in the

[1]The paper uses private/corporate sector, which means only the tertiary service private hospitals, which works on corporate management style, where the underlying principle is making profits.

[2]Declaration of Alma-Ata: international conference on primary health care, Alma-Ata, USSR, Sept 6–12, 1978. http://www.euro.who.int/__data/assets/pdf_file/0009/113877/E93944.pdf?ua=1, accessed on 21 Jan. 2016.

country.[3] However, rural and urban distribution of health services is skewed, with 68.1 % all government hospital beds in urban areas and only 31.9 % beds in rural areas.[4]

Private health services both in rural and urban areas, are utmost heterogeneous and of diverse nature; ranging from one doctor clinics to multispecialty and super specialty hospitals. One doctor clinic, with a recognized trained physician, to a non-qualified doctor; a *jhola chaap*, also called Quack, or *Bangali* doctor. They form a very important health care provider irrespective of the negative image they have, are available in emergency, accessible round the clock and affordable. They are the trusted, local man situated in the community, who can be reached any time, especially where the public health services have not reached or nonfunctional especially in rural areas.

From time immemorial, however, there existed traditional and indigenous healing systems existed. Both codified system and non-codified systems existed. Codified systems like: Ayurveda, Unani, Siddha, Homeopathy, Naturopathy, Yoga, existed and continues till today, also exist across the country. The non-codified systems like folk healing, faith healing, herbalists and bonesetters too exist. However, the State always marginalized these indigenous healing systems (Sujatha and Abraham 2009; GOI 1946). In 2005, AYUSH[5] was introduced to integrate the indigenous healing systems into the mainstream, though it is still given secondary treatment and AYUSH doctors are placed in place of Allopathy doctor, in their absence (Rao et al. 2011). Thus, the medical pluralism exists, with its hierarchies in practice (Sujatha and Abraham 2009).

Private care has always been prominent as source of medical care and was encouraged by the state, from the beginning. At the time of establishing the three-tier systems, the private doctors were given incentives to come and serve in the public sector, and was envisaged, that they will be slowly absorbed in the large growing public sector. However, given the low budget for health care, which was around 3 % of GDP in 1960s reducing it to less that 1 % in 1980s and raised to around 1.3 in 1991 and around 2 % with AYUSH, systematically dismantled/ crumbled the public sector. Under the health sector reforms, there were further cuts in budgetary allocation and thus having huge Public Health implications (Qadeer et al. 2001). Public Health Sector, was never strengthened as envisaged at the time of independence, slowly dismantling and purposively disengaging with it, to give rise to parallel, more robust, sprawling private care.

The low resources in Public sector had an adverse affects; lack of essential drugs, old and dilapidated equipment's, lack of ambulance services. As a result,

---

[3]http://mohfw.nic.in/WriteReadData/l892s/rural%20health%20care%20system%20in%20india.pdf.

[4]Central Bureau of Health Intelligence, Ministry of Health and Family Welfare, Government of India. National Health Profile—2007. 2008. Available from: URL: http://cbhidghs.nic.in/index2.asp?slid=987&sublinkid=698.

[5]AYUSH stands for Ayurveda, Yoga, Unani, Siddha and Homeopathy.

the public sector is declared as "inefficient" and nonfunctional, giving an argument and rationale to support the growth of private sector and fill the gaps, which the public sector is creating. However, post 1990s, one can see clear push toward facilitating private sector in all its five year plans from VIIIth plan to XIth plan (Planning Commission 1992–1997; 1997–2002; 2002–2007; 2007–2012). Since 1991, neoliberal government policies supported the private sector and have created conditions for private growth. Various means were suggested, like public private partnerships (PPP) to boost private sector to salvage public sector, with its own caveats to be cautious about. There are ample examples, which show that these PPP models were only beneficial to private sector, where the state remains for provisioning of resources and private sector providing services and makes profits (Qadeer and Reddy 2006; Reddy and Immaculate 2013).

Growth of Corporate Hospitals

Establishing of corporate hospitals can be traced to Dr. Pratap C. Reddy, who came back to India from United States of America and started "Apollo" Hospitals and now chain of hospitals, started as private enterprise (Baru 2003), saw a manifold expansion in terms of its bed capacity and corporate management style. This multi-super-specialty private care was missing from the India's landscape, except for very few well-know and reputed tertiary public hospitals like All India Institute of Medical Sciences (AIIMS). Rich and well-off used to go aboard for treatment. Establishing posh five star health facilities, state of art technology, and well-trained and experienced doctors, with corporate management setup, and national and international accreditation became the highlights and success stories of the corporate hospitals (Baru 2003; Reddy and Qadeer 2006). The returning of an NRI doctor, to establish Apollo, gave a boost to all other doctors to start up their own big corporate hospitals. Well reputed doctors across the nation took up not just doing clinical practice, but establishing super speciality hospitals, which led them the name of doctor- businessmen; be it Dr. Naresh Trehan, Dr. Devi Shetty, and Singh brothers from pharmaceutical industries to set up the chain of hospitals like Medanta, Narayan Hrudayala, Fortis Healthcare Pvt. Ltd., respectively.

The setting up of hospitals, now no more remained as the privilege and ownership for the doctors, once health care became trade and an industry, the health care pie is now being shared by motley of businessmen joining the bandwagon, to set up health care business (Reddy and Qadeer 2010). With the latest being the setting up of tertiary super specialty hospital "Artimis" in Gurgaon, by the Apollo International Tyre company.

Across the four Metropolitan cities in India, Starting from Delhi, Mumbai, Chennai, Calcutta and other big cities like Bangalore, Hyderabad, saw the growth of multi and super-specialty hospitals managed by big companies. Further, these multispecialty hospitals expanded to the two-tier towns, like Pune, Lucknow, Ahmedabad, Kochi, and Trivandrum.

Changing Nature of Health Care in Delhi

Delhi as capital, can boast of best medical care,[6] with some of the reputed names in the public health service sector; All India Institute of Medical Sciences (AIIMS), Safdurjung hospital, Ram Manohar Lohia, Maulana Azad hospital. These hospitals prior to 1990s were the finest institutions, catering not just to Indians, irrespective of their ability to pay, but also for the patients from neighboring countries; Pakistan, Afghanistan, Nepal, Bhutan, Bangladesh. Post 1990s, with the establishment of Indraprastha Apollo hospitals started a chain of private/corporate hospitals in Delhi; Escorts, Sita Ram Bhartia, Rockland, Max Healthcare, Fortis Pvt. Ltd., especially congregated in South Delhi.[7]

This clustering of hospitals in a geographical space gives rise to competition among the corporate hospitals. The latest development is the Medanta a medicity and Artimis in Gurgaon. Some of the big names in the health care industry in Delhi have been established and expanded in the past one and half decade.

There has been shift in the value system of provisioning health care post independence in Delhi. The service-oriented charitable hospitals and philanthropic health care changed its nature to commercial and profit making ventures. Some of the hospitals like Jessa Ram, BL Kapoor, Mool Chand, have changed their nature from trust-based philanthropic to commercial and profitable business ventures. St. Stephen Hospitals, Sir Ganga Ram hospitals, Escorts all started as charitable hospitals but slowly changed to profitable ventures.

These three hospitals, like Mool Chand, Jessa Ram & B L Kapoor hospitals were registered in 1950 post independence after partition, with individually owned charity institutions in Pakistan, were given land in Delhi to set up the hospitals with the help of government subsidies to do charitable health care services. However, Qureshi Committee Report shows that the second and third generation proprietors changed the nature of hospitals from charitable to profitable. Mool Chand which was an Ayurvedic hospital also changed to allopathic hospital (Govt. of NCT Delhi 2001).

Changing nature of health care provisioning also led to sacking of health care personnel's, leading to Public Interest Litigation (PIL) against the hospitals. Delhi government set up Justice A.S. Qureshi committee in 2001 to look into the changing nature of the hospitals (Enquiry Report of High Level Committee for Hospitals in Delhi) and address PIL and whether they were abiding by the lease conditions of the government to look into the subsidies each of these hospitals were given by the government.

The Qureshi Committee sought information from 450 hospitals only 80 responded, 27 hospitals data was presented. Five hospitals (Batra, Ganga Ram,

---

[6]Ranvir's paper in this volume gives the number of hospitals, private and public, number of beds, under different governing bodies and municipalities.

[7]Ranvir's paper gives the concentration and clustering of private hospitals using GIS maps.

G M Modi and Apollo were given land ranging between 11.03 and 17.28 acres. Apollo was given 15 Acres in 1998 by Delhi Government for Rs. 1 per annum with a lease condition to treat 1/3 patients free of cost. Delhi government invested 42 crores in hospitals in 1996, earmarked 140 out of 650 beds for poor. The committee further reported that around 55 hospitals were given land ranging from 10 to 2 acres on throw away prices on lease. St. Stephen and Mool Chand were given 9 acres each. Remaining hospitals received land between 0.88 and 5 acres of land. These hospitals were given tax exemptions for import of technology and also registered as research institutes with tax exemptions.

However, the lease conditions to treat 25 % inpatient (IPD) and 40 % outpatients (OPD) from poor families to treat free of cost, putforth by the land allotting authority; Delhi Development Authority (DDA) were not honored by even single hospitals completely. Out of 27, 13 hospitals provided free OPD care up to 15 % and 12 hospitals gave 40 % OPD care. Majority of hospitals provided less than 10 % of their IPD. Apollo provided only 2 % and Batra and Modi provided 6–10 % IPD care.

Various reasons were given by the hospitals, for not abiding by the lease conditions; lease conditions are not viable, conditions were not clear, how to recognize and identify poor, what kind of services to be given as free were not clear–whether only consultation, or all the services, including medicines and "poor" not defined. Further, it is not possible to provide free treatment due to high cost of drugs. It was reported that serving 40 % free is not viable for the hospitals to run (GOI 1946).

Escort hospital, which started as charitable hospital changed its nature to profitable hospital changing the partnership and Escorts also came with the idea of relieving them from lease conditions by paying 51 crores to DDA. However, the ownership changed and the partnership of Escorts. Dr. Trehan came out of the partnership and started Medanta a medicity in Gurgaon. Escorts then merged with Fortis. The lease conditions continues today, it is a concern that in none of these private hospitals, the beds for patients are full, remain empty as there is no will to admit enough poor patients and treat them. The beds for poor patients often go to the patients from abroad, under medical diplomacy, or to the kith and kin of bureaucrats or politicians as board members referred all patients referred by government to admit (Qadeer and Reddy 2006). Committee described the situation as one who "one buys an expensive cow then hold it by the horn while other milk it" (GOI 1946).

Shifting Priorities: Boost to Medical Tourism

"Medical Tourism" has become a buzzword, for foreign patients to travel to India and other Asian Countries for elective surgeries and treatment. However, the "Tourism" part is often questioned due to the critical conditions in which the

Table 1 The comparative costs between India and other developed countries like US, India, Thailand, and Singapore approximate figures in US Dollars[a]

	US ($)	India ($)	Thailand ($)	Singapore ($)
Heart bypass surgery	130,000	10,000	11,000	18,500
Heart valve replacement	160,000	9,000	10,000	12,500
Angioplasty	57,000	11,000	13,000	13,000
Hip replacement	43,000	9,000	12,000	12,000
Hysterectomy	20,000	3,000	4,500	6,000
Knee replacement	40,000	8,500	10,000	13,000
Spinal fusion	62,000	5,500	7,000	9,000

[a]http://www.nomad4ever.com/2006/12/31/medicaltourism-in-asia-boost-your-healthcare-andreap-the-cost-savings/, accessed on 21 Jan 2016

patient is and the possibilities of sightseeing while they are coming for treatment. Instead a more neutral term "Medical Travel" (Whittaker 2008) and "Medical Exile" (Inhorn and Patrizio 2009) "Medical Refugee" has been used.[8]

It is reported in the media and in business magazines that, India offers world-class medical facilities, comparable with any of the western countries in most of its metropolitan cities. India has state of the art hospitals and the most-qualified doctors in urban areas. Having the best infrastructure, good medical facilities and accompanied with the most competitive prices, the MT is fast growing.[9] The most important factor to promote medical tourism is to showcase the cost differentials, which is around one-tenth in the developing nations to exorbitant prices in developed nations, offering a business and a value proposition. With a caption saying "First World Treatment at Third World Rates" (Table 1).

The web site of department of commerce[10] lists out Medical treatment, wellness and rejuvenation and Ayurvedic and alternate medicine, along with a list of specialty, procedures and locations of all the hospitals across cities in India. Most of these hospitals have accreditation from JCI (Joint Commission of International Accreditation), NABH (National Accreditation Board for Hospitals and Health Care Providers) and NABL National Accreditation Board for Testing and Calibration Laboratories, for maintaining standards. The website also carry success stories and testimonials of the patients from abroad.

[8]For the debate on the terminology of 'Medical Tourism' refer to the article by Ormond Meghann (2011) Medical Tourism, Medical Exile: Responding to the Cross-Border Pursuit of Healthcare in Malaysia. In Minca, C. & Oakes, T. (eds) Real Tourism: Practice, Care & Politics in Contemporary Travel, London Routledge, pp. 143–161.

[9]http://www.medicaltourismindia.com, accessed on 20 Jan. 2016.

[10]www.indiahealthcaretourism.com, accessed on 21 Jan. 2016.

Worldwide MT market is estimated to be worth $55 billion, projected to grow 20 % a year. Annual tally of MT exceeds 11 million people as per patients without borders.[11] Asian countries, Thailand, Singapore, India, and Malaysia are the forerunners in MT.

MT in Major Cities

National Health Policy 2002, (GOI 2002a) clearly supports MT Major hospitals in Chennai, Mumbai, Hyderabad, and New Delhi have recorded a 12 % patient flow from neighboring and South East Asian countries. Patients from the neighboring countries who do not have standard medical services and lack good doctors/facilities in their own countries come to India for treatment. Geo-political reason like the post 9/11, many patients from Middle East and African countries are traveling to India, due to stricter US Visa processes. Patients from US and UK too travel to India, especially NRIs, where the medical care is quite expensive and millions of people uninsured.

Apollo has been a forerunner in health tourism. It has been a choicest destination for patients from Southeast Asia, Africa, and the Middle East. Apollo in Ahmedabad attracts non-resident Gujaratis from the world over. Combination of a Spa and a hospital in Goa, with focus on non-electric surgeries has boosted the medical tourism in Goa. All the hospitals in major cities are listed in the Ministry of Commerce for promoting MT, to name a few, like Apollo, Institute of Cardiovascular Disease, Madras Medical Mission, Institute of Cardiovascular Diseases, Ramchandra Educational and Health Trust, Tamil Nadu Hospital Ltd. The Heart Institute, Vijaya Health Centre, Key Pee Kay Medical Services (p) Ltd., etc. Hyderabad has CDR groups of hospitals, CDR Heart Institute, Medwin Hospitals, Yashoda Hospitals, L.V. Prasad Eye Institute, Apollo Hospital are some of the hospitals treating foreign patients. It has been postulated that the opportunities in the medical tourism market in the country is pegged to a 30 % growth in 2000 and it has been growing at the rate of 15 % for the past five years.

The nature of services in MT is that they do not cater to emergency services. Services provided are largely, knee joint replacement, hip replacement, (largely orthopedic), bone marrow transplant, bypass surgery, breast lump removal, Haemorrhoidectomy, Cataract Surgery, In vitro fertilization (IVF) cycle, cosmetic surgery and cancer treatment, etc. For accompanying kin members, preventive health check is offered. All the patients in India who are elite and those who have health insurance, either private or CGHS (Central Government Health Service) are entitled to treatment in the empaneled private/corporate hospitals in India.

[11]http://asia.nikkei.com/Business/Trends/Asia-leads-industry-worth-55B, accessed on 21 Jan. 2016.

Advertising and Packaging

Medical Tourism is promoted with various catchy advertisements and captions.

> These captions highlights the cost differentials like, "where the cost saved on one MRI could pay for a return ticket, medical tourism is bound to boom",

> "Medical Treatment in USA = A tour to India + Medical Treatment + Savings", "First World Treatment at Third World Prices".

Some captions attracts the nature and beauty of the places, like "Bright sun, blue sea, cosmetic surgery," and "Medical Tourism: Sea, Sun, Sand and…Surgery" forms attractive captions to draw attention.

> One of them is quite open to speak of the business, like, "Your Health is our Wealth".

Interestingly, hitherto the allopathic hospitals only have biomedical procedures, now with the demand for holistic and alternate treatments, the tertiary allopathic hospitals are opening up Holistic centers within the premises, having yoga and meditation, naturopathy, herbal medicine, acupuncture and homeopathy departments. Further, some of them have small space for worship for the relatives to pray, wedding science with religion and place for alternative medicines. The lobbies of the hospitals are plush and waiting rooms for the foreign patients are well maintained. The interiors of the patient's rooms and all the services have standards of three to five star facilities and thus appropriately charged too.

Each of these hospitals and also the agencies, which facilitate MT, carry testimonials on their websites. Quoting some of them, '*Once you reach the hospital, it looks as if you are in any other developed country's hospital*', suggesting that the hospitals did not match with developing country image but the developed ones.

Another interesting testimonial is about the excitement of undergoing cosmetic surgery; "We've had clients who did n't tell their husbands or boyfriends—just said they were going on holiday—and presented a surprise when they came home." "They fly in, recuperate around the pool, and fly out again without anyone noticing they've been under the knife."

MT is promoted through various medical exhibitions and conferences across the globe. Federation of Indian Chambers of Commerce and Industry, FICCI and Confederation of Indian Industry (CII) promotional efforts are reached to the entire medical community through mailers, posters, press conferences, focused presentations. Individual visits to international and domestic medical exhibitions and conferences and also through advertisements and editorial coverage in medical and business magazines. The state too promotes medical tourism under the "medical diplomacy" to strengthen the international relationships and improve relationships with the neighboring countries. Now and then a case or two like Noor Fatima from Pakistan are highlighted in the media, talking of medical diplomacy.

The study by Qadeer and Reddy shows that the satisfaction of the doctors in the public health institutions is the freedom to work without any pressure, freedom to

Table 2 Competition among the hospitals and sales turnover and net profit

Name	Last price	Market cap. (Rs. cr.)	Sales turnover	Net profit	Total assets
Apollo Hospital	**1,381.15**	**19,215.27**	**4,592.79**	**346.59**	**4,677.65**
Fortis Health	174.80	8,095.40	610.64	−33.91	4,276.85
Poly Medicure	325.50	1,435.89	373.69	61.02	250.27
Kovai Medical	641.65	702.11	401.62	38.70	270.82
Indraprastha	70.90	649.96	713.39	32.49	230.16
Opto Circuits	11.60	281.09	140.92	−201.51	2,367.73
Lotus Eye Care	19.65	40.86	29.90	−1.98	50.06

http://www.moneycontrol.com/competition/apollohospitalsenterprises/comparison/AHE#AHE, accessed on 13 Dec. 2015

do research along with the satisfaction of treating the poor. Whereas the doctors in the corporate sector moved from public hospitals, for better pay cheques, high technology care, like robotic surgeries, though are under pressure to perform, ethically or unethically (Qadeer and Reddy 2013). The anecdotal references and social media now and then cover high-rise of cost, exploitation, rude behavior of the staff, over medication and over diagnosis. Next section in this paper will discuss the public health implications of MT and how that leads to inequitable distribution of health care in India in general and Delhi in particular.

Implications of MT

Profit Making

These private/corporate hospitals come with an orientation of profit making, due to its privatized, corporate nature, situated in medical markets. Huge investments go in constructing these super specialty hospitals. The building infrastructure, state of art technology, huge pay scales to the senior physicians, maintenance cost, comes into crores of rupees. The hospitals take few years to break even the cost. Table 2 shows the competition and comparison of the business they are doing, also some of the hospitals showing losses.

The congregation of private and corporate hospitals in a geographical space, as reflected in Ranvir's paper, is concentrated in South Delhi. The plausible reason for competing with each other is to attract patients not just local, but from other countries. The cost of sustaining such huge infrastructure also comes with cost, and also cost cutting in payments to the junior staff. Table 2 shows that huge assets are built in the creation of corporate hospitals and to maintain and sustain they need such turnover. Big hospitals like Fortis show losses of −33.91 crores, whereas the Apollo shows profits of 346.59 crores March 2015.[12] Max Super

[12]http://www.moneycontrol.com/competition/apollohospitalsenterprises/comparison/AHE#AHE, accessed on 13 Dec. 2015.

Specialty hospital showed Rs. 470.71 crores net profit for March 2015.[13] Medanta's net profit for FY 2014 was Rs. 187 crore.[14]

Further, the congregation of these hospitals in posh colonies of major cities, there is a cut throat competition among themselves, trying to attract the patients not just Indians but also the international, under MT. The huge investments, which go in establishing these infrastructures, multifold pay cheques to senior doctors, and running cost, can be sustained only by increasing the cost of care. The implications of such a heavy investments then lead to over diagnosis, over medication, unnecessary surgeries. It comes from a Dr. Shoaib Mohammad confession.[15] These are reported in the media time and again.

Despite the huge profits shown by these hospitals, they have not been abiding by the lease conditions put forth by Delhi Development Authority to serve the poor. There is no mechanism to plough back the profits for general public health care. Further due to lax attitude and no regulation, these hospitals flout rules. There have been media reports and also court cases against these hospitals for profit making and not serving the poor. Four-year litigation, the Income-Tax Appellate Tribunal, said the Devki Devi Foundation (DDF), of which Max Super Specialty Hospital in Saket is a unit, was engaged in "exorbitant" profit making but was not paying taxes in the mask of a charitable institution (Mehta 2015). There were media reports about the patients complaining of exorbitant fees and charging in an accident case in Artimis Hospital.[16]

Studies have proved that this further leads to two-tier system and dichotomous health care, where, poor are left behind seeking health care from the crowded hospitals, lacking emergency services, essential drugs, malfunctioning outdated technology in Public hospitals. On the other hand, the rich, elite and foreign patients can access well equipped private hospitals.

As a result of media highlights of profit making of the hospitals and not abiding by the lease conditions, some hospital's lease deed have been canceled like Escorts.[17] Further DDA changed its policy not to give land on subsidy to hospitals instead auction it on market price in 2001. However, this had far reaching consequences, where charitable hospitals cannot run and only big players can buy. As a result not many takers to buy hospital land from DDA in the recent auction.

---

[13]http://economictimes.indiatimes.com/max-india-ltd/profitandlose/companyid-13435.cms, accessed on 20 Jan. 2016.

[14]http://forbesindia.com/printcontent/38218, accessed on 20 Jan. 2016.

[15]http://www.epw.in/journal/2015/45/commentary/my-market-value.html, accessed on 21 Jan. 2015.

[16]http://www.thaindian.com/newsportal/uncategorized/relatives-create-ruckus-at-gurgaons-artemis-hospital_100613371.html, accessed on 20 Jan. 2016.

[17]http://zeenews.india.com/home/dda-cancels-lease-agreement-with-escorts-hospital_246869.html, accessed on 20 Jan. 2016.

Public Subsidy and Private Sector

The promotion of Medical Tourism in India has larger public health implications, which are not visible to the general public and even to the senior physicians working in Public and Private Hospitals. Very few have the critical understanding of how the public subsidies are going into building of these posh corporate hospitals (Sengupta 2008; Qadeer and Reddy 2013). Majority of them believe that private sector has nothing to do with treating the poor masses and it is the state responsibility. Private Sector is purely for profit business venture and should be treated like one.

The critical public health perspectives on corporate health care show that these hospitals have been established with the support of the State. Given the business proposition and private nature, these hospitals should have been built on their own without state subsidy. But if the subsidy is given, it needs to return back either services or profits to the state. Instead, the state is buying health services from the private sector, after giving all the subsidies, in terms of land lease on throw away prices, tax exemptions on import of technology, and also tax exemption in registering as health research institutes.

Internal Brain Drain

There is a "reverse or internal brain drain[18]" of physicians from public hospitals to private hospitals. The industry gets a pool of medical professional trained in public institutions for fee of Rs. 500 a month, move to work in private hospital leading to indirect subsidy of an estimated Rs. 500 crore per year. These corporate hospitals though give high salaries and perks for the senior doctors, however, the junior doctors and paramedics are exploited, where they are paid less and get more work done (Hazarika 2010). Study by Qadeer and Reddy (2013) also shows that the public hospital doctors felt satisfied serving the poor and also having freedom to work and research.

Conclusion and Discussion

Present government promises to expand health assurance for all. At a time when India is being hailed as a medical destination, it is ironical that patients in government hospitals are suffering due to non-availability of emergency drugs/lifesaving

[18]Hitherto brain drain, where the doctors and engineer left to foreign shores, for better pay opportunities and work culture started returning back calling 'reverse internal brain-drain'. However, with the dismantling of public sector gradually and facilitating the private/ corporate sector, the 'reverse brain drain' is seen, where the public hospitals doctors who have gained expertise, are hired by the corporate hospitals to serve in their hospitals, full time or part time or as consultants drawing huge salaries.

drugs worth a mere Rs. 30–40. Large population is impoverished because of high out of pocket health care expenditure and suffers the adverse consequence of poor quality care. These public hospitals also suffer from gross under-staffing to manage huge patient burden and further there is a long waiting time for surgeries.

More that 40 % of patients admitted to hospital borrow money or sell assets and 25 % of peasant families who needs inpatients care are driven below the poverty line (World Bank 2001).

It is poor who are subsidizing for rich in terms of uses of public health resources in the country, richest quintile consuming three times more services, more public health services as compared to poor. It is believed commonly that the foreign exchange earned will improve general health care. It is also believed that having a monitoring agency in medical field and medical audit is the need of the hour. Which will prove beneficial both to the private and public sector. However, the experience of MT so far is that no such mechanism exists which can plough back mechanism.

Justice Qureshi's report has shown that due to lack of monitoring and regulation, no conditionality's are fulfilled. The expectation of the government that a part of the revenues of private corporate hospitals will revert to the public sector is not materialized; rather the government has subsidized their input prices. Ethical issues have become significant (Borman 2004; Qadeer and Reddy 2013), both in terms of equity and in the more competitive involvement of the market in medical care.

Over the past decade the Indian health system has become ever more dichotomous. Major cities are witnessing this kind of growth of private/corporate health service growth and neglect of public hospitals. Delhi has seen tremendous change in the medical landscape leading to dichotomous service provision. On one hand there is ever growing big plush hospitals for the elite, the insured and the medical travelers from aboard. On the other hand, the overburden, less resourceful and crowded public hospitals are left for the poor, with no emergency medicines in place. There are examples from other countries, which are doing, well in medical tourism; like in Malaysia and Thailand, they too have health care delivery, which is increasingly inequitable. In Thailand there is a huge drain on the public health sector (Connell 2006).

Contrary to the general perception that competition is beneficial to consumers and society at large, it seems to be only partial truth (Godwin 2004). The competition in the health sector can prove detrimental, where the profit is the underlying principle of any trade. Health cannot be treated as any other commodity, placed in the market and arguing that there will be a choice where people can choose the services. Power relations where the doctors either treat, or ill-treat the patient by over diagnosis, over medicalization leads to indebtedness and exploitation. There is an urgent need for framing appropriate policies regarding the regulation of both quality and price of care in the private health sector.

So far there have been misplaced priorities, where the public subsidies have been ploughed into the private/corporate health care, with no benefits to the larger public and especially the poor. Various subsidies and tax benefits to corporate sectors, is unethical leaving the masses at the mercy of limited services. Facilitating the private/corporate sector by the policy shifts have facilitated world best services to the better off, though they these best services are questionable given the cases of overcharging and unnecessary medications being reported.

The draft National Health Policy (2015) by the Government of India has endorsed the goal of providing "universal access to good quality health care services without anyone having to face financial hardship as a consequence." Present government promises to expand health assurance for all. Ironically health ministry officials told Reuters, that more than 60 billion rupees, or $948 million, have been slashed from their budget allocation of around $5 billion for the financial year ending on March 31, 2015.[19] Does that mean mere assurance and no deliverables?

Large population of India is impoverished because of high out of pocket heath care expenditure and suffers the adverse consequences of poor quality care. To bring in the equitable distribution of health care, there is a need for radical restructuring of health care services. India needs to adopt integrated national health care system built around strong public primary care system, with enough financial resources and also with supportive role of private and indigenous systems. Further, there is a need of robust regulations from government and for assuring universal health care (Patel et al. 2015). There is a need to look for strategies and models where masses can be treated. Health care for the masses is an ethical, human rights and human development issue, and needs to be addressed in urgency.

References

Baru, R. V. (1998). *Private health care in India: Social characteristics and trends*. New Delhi: Sage Publications.

Baru, R. V. (2003). Privatisation of health services: A South Asian perspective. *Economic and Political Weekly, 38*(42), 4433–4437.

Borman, E. (2004). Health tourism: Where healthcare, ethics, and the state collide. *BMJ. British Medical Journal, 328*(7431), 60.

Connell, J. (2006). Medical tourism: Sea, sun, sand and… surgery. *Tourism Management, 27*(6), 1093–1100.

Godwin, S.K. (2004). Medical tourism: Subsidizing the rich. *Economic and Political Weekly*, 3981–3983.

Government of India. (1946). *Report of the Health Survey & Development Committee (Bhore Committee) Delhi*. Manager of Publications. Vol. II.

Government of India. (1992). *Eighth Five Year Plan*, 1992–1997. Vol. 2. New Delhi, 1992.

Government of India. 1997. *Ninth Five Year Plan*, 1997–2002. Vol. 2. New Delhi, 1997.

Government of India. (2002a). *National Health Policy II*. Ministry of Health and Family Welfare: New Delhi.

Government of India. (2002b). *Tenth Five Year Plan*, 2002–2007. Vol. 2. New Delhi, 2002.

Government of India. (2007). *Eleventh Five Year Plan, 2007–2012* (Vol. 1). New Delhi: Government of India. 2008.

[19]http://in.reuters.com/article/india-health-budget-idINKBN0K10Y020141223, accessed on 20 Jan. 2016.

Government of NCT Delhi. (2001). *Enquiry Report of High Level Committee for Hospitals in Delhi*. Qureshi: New Delhi. Chairman A.S.
Hazarika, I. (2010). Medical tourism: Its potential impact on the health workforce and health systems in India. *Journal of Health Planning and Policy., 25*(3), 248–251.
Inhorn, M. C., & Patrizio, P. (2009). Rethinking reproductive "tourism" as reproductive "exile". *Fertility and Sterility, 92*(3), 904–906.
Mehta, A. (2015). 'Delhi: Max hospital in tax trouble; found flouting charity clause' Hindustan Times, New Delhi Updated: Apr 05, 2015 08:27 IST.
National Health Policy. (2015). Draft. December, 2014. Retrieved November 28, 2015, from http://www.mohfw.nic.in/showfile.php?lid=3014
Patel, V., Parikh, R., Nandraj, S., Balasubramaniam, P., Narayan, K., Paul, V.K., et al. (2015). Assuring Health Coverage for all In India. *Lancet, 386*: 2422–2435.
Qadeer, I., Sen, K., Nayar, K.R., (eds) (2001). Public Health & the Poverty of Reforms, Sage, New Delhi.
Qadeer, I., & Reddy, S. (2006). Medical care in the shadow of public private partnership. *Social Scientist, 34*(9–10), 4–20.
Qadeer, I., & Reddy, S. (2013). Medical tourism in India: Perceptions of physicians in tertiary care hospitals. *Philosophy, Ethics, and Humanities in Medicine, 8*, 20.
Rao, M., Rao, K. D., Kumar, A. S., Chatterjee, M., & Sundararaman, T. (2011). Human resources for health in India. *The Lancet, 377*(9765), 587–598.
Reddy, S & Mary, I. (2013). RACHI Scheme in AP: A comprehensive analytical view PPP model. *Indian Journal of Public Health, 57*(4), 254–259.
Reddy, S., & Qadeer, I. (2010). Medical tourism in India: Progress or predicament? *Economic and Political Weekly, 45*(20), 69–75.
Sengupta, A. (2008). Medical tourism in India: Winners and losers. *Indian Journal of Medical Ethics, 5*(1).
Sujatha, V., & Abraham, L. (2009). Medicine, state and society. *Economic and Political Weekly*, 35–43.
UN. (1948). Universal Declaration of Human Rights, *United Nations, 1948.*
Whittaker, A. (2008). Pleasure and pain: Medical travel in Asia. *Global Public Health, 3*(3), 271–290.
World Bank. (2001). *'Health nutrition, population sector unit South Asian region, raising the sight, better health systems for Indian poor*. Washington: World Bank.

Heath Care Providers in Delhi Metropolitan Cities

Navin Narayan

Abstract Many studies have been carried out around the issues of health. They cover almost all areas which may offer a potential solution to ensure good health and "health for all". Many perspectives have been used to analyze and understand the issues. Much of the literature which has evolved in public health is contributed by various disciplinary Marxist-perspective-influenced public health researchers to venture into understanding the role of social class in accessibility and utilization in terms of the division between 'have' and 'have-not'; urban and rural; male and female; educated and uneducated; worker and non-worker, among them organized sector and unorganized sector. Principally, there are two actors involved in mission 'Health for all'. One is known as health service seeker and second is health services provider. Most studies have concentrated on only one component—health service seeker, from different angles. Very few have examined the second component of health service provider. The thrust has largely been in understanding the user rather than the provider. This paper is an attempt to understand this second and equally important component responsible for providing health care services from sociological perspective. It comprises three sections. Dealing with 'perspective' pertaining to the fundamental question theoretically; to define the contesting hypothesis around the perspective; and to explain the hypothesis from the data gathered, other issues and concerns in sociological manner. In this attempt, to locate the place of any occupational category in social structure, subjective status perceptions that the category has of itself are of vital importance, in addition to the objective attributes. Therefore, the purpose of the present paper is to analyze the objective attributes of doctors; subjective perception they have of their status mostly in context of the larger society and within the occupational community of

N. Narayan (✉)
JNU, New Delhi, India
e-mail: navinjnu@gmail.com

S.S. Acharya et al. (eds.), *Marginalization in Globalizing Delhi: Issues of Land, Livelihoods and Health*, DOI 10.1007/978-81-322-3583-5_17

health personnel. This study, undertaken in Delhi examines the interpersonal relations between the doctors and their patient in context of social background. To analyze the reciprocal behaviour of the doctors and patients and attributes age, sex, income, rural and urban communities and educational standards and their impact on the interactions and interrelations, in the context of health care providers social backgrounds. Whatever medical services available are good but the availability in the context to provider is not same, because the professionals (as member) is a unit of society which is stratified in account of different level. Hence the available services are still beyond the reach of common man or the quality of service which is provided to them. The concern of this study is that the medical profession comes from the upper status of society and their process of socialization and high-tech education is totally different from the common man, to whom they provide services. The role performance of any professional group partly depends on how far it has been able to change its pre-professional attitudes acquired during the period of primary socialization before entering in the professional training.

Keywords Health care provider · Socialization · Culture of practice · Metropolitan city · Delhi

Introduction

Many studies have been carried out around the issues of health. They cover almost all areas which may offer a potential solution to ensure good health and "health for all". Many perspectives have been used to analyze and understand the issues. Almost all the streams such as Sociology, Economics, Political Science, Psychology, Environment and even History individually or with others have contributed in this regard. Majority of the studies in public health have been conducted from the perspective contributed by these discipline. It ranges from socio, cultural perspective and aspect to the economic. Even environmental angle has been studied. Type of health care institution-public, private—for profit and not for profit are also studied. Marxism as an ideology influenced a lot to the public health researchers. They even ventured into understanding the role of social class in accessibility and utilization from Marxist perspective of division as 'have' and 'have-not'. Further to understand these division axes like urban/rural, male/female, literate/illiterate, worker/non-worker workers in organized and unorganized sector have also been used. Feasibility, accessibility and utilization of health services (India, Morbidity and Utilisation of Medical Services 42nd Round 1989) have also been studied in terms of cost of service, distance of services from health service seeker, culture of health service seeker, etc. Health perception, religion, culture (Sahu, Health Culture of Oraons In the Context of Different Health Institutions 1981), food habit, living condition and employment of health service seeker have also been studied in great amount. Meaning a whole range of factors around the health service seeker have been studied including nutritional status (Chen 1987), urban and rural, poor and rich, utilization and accessibility among male and female and different working condition (Qadeer 1986), social class (Banerji and Singh, Bhopal Gas Tragedy: An Epidemiological and Sociological Study 1985) and even communities–caste base, class base, and sections—workers and non-workers and their classification-organized and unorganized, their conditions—hazardous and nonhazardous and politics of health service for 'have-not' (Zurbrigg 1984).

Principally, there are two actors involved in the mission 'Health for all'. One is known as health service seeker and second is health services provider. Most of these studies address only one component—from different angles—that is health service seekers. Not many studies significantly carried out any serious research on the second component that is health service provider. Perhaps, fundamentally all the study assumes that the problem lies only with one component that is patients (with whole set of other factor) and ignores completely the second, health service provider—their constraints in provisioning of services, for instance. It is reflective from the studies which considers health service provider as a neutral entity with a sacrosanct status enjoining immunity of sorts, and thus nothing is left to understand about this important components. However, medical sociology touched some important area of this second component in early seventies. Ooman (1978), Madan (1972, 1980), Nagla (1988) and few others have done good studies on this second components.

This paper is an attempt to understand this second and equally important component responsible for good and 'health for all' from sociological perspective. It comprises of three sections. Section A deals with 'perspective' pertaining to the fundamental question theoretically, Section B focuses on to define the contesting hypothesis around the perspective. While Section C brings to light to explain the hypothesis from the data gathered, other issues and concerns in sociological manner.

A. Who Are the Health Care Providers?

Health care providers are the main actors in therapeutic process of the health care services. All kinds of diseases whether due to malnutrition or poverty haunt millions of Indians, who go scant or without medical care. It is worthwhile to study systematically the prime agent known as doctors in this therapeutic process of health care service. Always the patient is recognized as more than a disease entity. Sick person is often an anxious person. The anxieties and difficulties as well as the potential for recovery may significantly depend on social ties of the patients' broad situation in family, workplace and in other groups important to him/her. In the same manner, the making of the health care providers must be considered in the light of his/her social and psychological environment. The medical student must not be recognized as a passive receptacle into which new knowledge is being poured.

Sociologists like Kendall and Merton (1958), classified the area of sociological research in medicine into four broad themes (a) social etiology and ecology of disease, (b) social component of therapy and rehabilitation, (c) medicine as social institution and (d) sociology of medical education. Sociological research has been categorized it in two broad categories, 'sociology of medicine' and 'sociology in medicine'. Where the first deals with the organizational structure, role relationship and the functions of medicine as a system of behaviour, thus mainly concerned with the study of medical practice. The second is concerned with collaborative research or teaching and the integration of techniques and concepts. The socialization process of a professional for institutionalized roles is the matter of' sociology of medicine'.

Sociological analysis of medical system and patient care in the Indian context assumes great significance. For an effective application of medical knowledge, it is also important to know the cultural and social pressures, which have a bearing on the response of a doctor to patient. Development of medical and social sciences and recognition of the facts that social environment is significant in etiology of disease and doctor–patient relationship is an important area. The broader perspective developed by the social scientists and their emphasis on interdisciplinary approach helped to understand human behaviour. Identification of the individual with his class or status group influences his social reciprocity. The psychologists consider individual feelings of people to be the basis of class. The subjective identification is the basis of class. A man always has a feeling of belongingness to his class. Persons with similar status and role in different spheres develop certain values attitudes and interests which strengthen 'class consciousness'. An analysis of the correlation of behaviour and various statuses determinants as age, sex rural/ urban residence, religion, caste, education, etc. has proved useful in the study of social phenomena. (Richard 1949 cited in Mathur 1975, p. 36) therefore, it does not appear to be correct to talk about people and their behaviour in general. They should be considered in the context of social categories they belong to.

Above theoretical foundation, health care systems are also applicable. It is clear with the indigenous traditional systems of medicines, where Ayurveda and Unani have identified with Hindu and Muslims religious groups, respectively. This prevents other religious group to enter into this noble profession other than their religion and served their people. Theoretically, the allopathic system being modern and a recent entry into Indian society were open to all religious categories. This suggests that the allopathic system of medicine in India recruits its personnel irrespective of their religious background.

In order to understand the perspective of physicians as a professional group, it is also important to consider the manner in which physicians are selected and trained as medical professionals. Family influence seems to be an important variable in encouraging and reinforcing the ambitions of the future recruitment to the medical profession. Having a parent or close relative who is a physician also seems to be distinct advantage. The decision to study medicine is largely social in character, that is, originates in a social group that is able to generate and nurture the medical ambition (Halls 1948 Cited in Ventkataratnam 1979).

Indeed, the role expectation and performance of the professional group party depends on how far it has been able to change its professional attitude acquired during the period of primary socialization before entering the professional training. All the members of the professional group might not have freed themselves completely from certain pre-professional attitude which may be antithetical to professional values and expectations. From this standpoint, medical students are engaged in learning the professional role of the physician by combing its component knowledge and skills, attitudes and values as a professionally and socially acceptable fashion. Socialization includes more than what is ordinarily described as education and training. Most conspicuous in the process of medicine learning is, of course, the acquisition of a considerable store of knowledge and skills which to some extent occurs even among the least of these students. Beyond this, it is useful to think of the process of role acquisition in two broad classes, direct learning through didactic teaching of one kind or another, indirect learning, in which attitudes, values and behaviour patterns are acquired as by products of contact with instructors and peers, with patients and with members of the health team. It would seem particularly useful to attend systematically to the less conspicuous and more easily neglected processes of indirect learning.

Predominantly, Indian society is a caste-based society and economy is one in which property rights, along with occupations are hereditary, compulsory and endogamous (Thorat 2007). Within this framework, it is necessary to recognize that an unequal and hierarchical assignment of economic rights restricts, obviously, the freedom of occupation and development. In addition of this social and residential separation and isolation due to hierarchical and caste-based society makes the things worse off in choosing the modern occupation/profession even in this politically democratic country. Eventually segregates some—most of the sufferer of caste base society and economy—from the human capability and capacity building processes.

Sociological analysis of professionals is very much needed in country like India which is highly hierarchical. A country like India where social status does decide your career and future prospects. It is also important due to the rampant poverty which forms an *'Identive—social classes'* from some section of society. And further the environment that has provided the member opportunities in the profession of medicine has to be understood so that we can find out whether there are any relation between a particular social environment and the motivation for choosing medicine as a career. This is to understand how different socio-economic group in the community have availed the opportunity provided to them.

B. Contesting Perspective

To explain whether doctor is free from social tie and becomes a mere professional or a product of society only trained in specialized skill of treating ail. As others because before/during/after entering into this professional commitment, he/she who also goes through the entire social process, a part of socialization. In the course of study, two broad contesting perspectives emerges (A) Doctor a Social Product Versus True Professional (B) Doctor a Nobel Person Versus Service Provider.

Doctor: A Social Product Versus a True Professional

Being a social creature, every person goes through a process to learn some basic norms, values, attitudes and form of interaction to others in the prescribed fashion of particular, group or class he/she belongs. There are also some factors like status, wealth, etc. which plays a role as well in constructing the personality. Many sociologists have regarded the family as the cornerstone of society. The external environment and the social structural elements in the community influence the interpersonal relations, the correlation between the status system in the society and the contents and structure of interaction between one units to another units of society. Many studies reveal that 'latent social identities' as to sex, age, residence rural/urban literacy, income groups, etc. influence behaviour. Socialization, one of the foundational concepts in sociology, which points out that when an individual, through socialization, accept the rules and expectations of their society that make up its culture and use them to determine how they should act, means interlined society's cultural rules. (Bilton 1981, p. 10). Thus, socialization enables us to carry out work. Socialization also makes us emotionally sensitive. It binds us with our "environment and neighbours" (cited in Dubey 1989, p. 227).

The role of socialization is very important in the individual's life from two points of view one, individual's 'self' develops through socialization and two, socialization develops his personality and the process of mental interaction. The unification of individual's socio-psychological behaviour reflects in personality. It expresses through the habits, devices and thinking of the individual. Cooley propounded individual's socio-psychological behaviour as means to develop 'Self' which he describes in his 'theory of looking glass self'. Self means 'I' and 'Me'. Self is determined by the individuals thinking about 'Himself'. Cooley believes that the 'idea of self' is a social product. Society, culture and personality are so interdependent that their differentiation poses many problems. The profounder of structural theory explains about the individual's socialization through social facts. In his view, the social fact is a special system of working, thinking and feeling that is beyond and above the individual. Morality, law, religion and the division of labour are social facts. The individual has to behave according to these facts.

Doctor: A Nobel Person Versus a Service Provider

Career is, in fact, a sort of running adjustment between a person and the various facts of life and of his/her professional world. Much is to be learned about career lines, how they are conceived by the students of medicine and how their personal and social backgrounds, school and other training experiences, predispose to turn them in one or another of many directions in which a medical person may go.

We are in a time of great change in the institutions of medicine. Not only is their inner structure changing so that the available positions and careers and the demand made upon those who fill them are in flux as a noble person and a service provider. There are more and more ancillary institutions, more and more connections of medicine with the other concerns and institutions of the world.

The tendency of human behaviour to form characteristics patterns that may be predicated if one knows the social context in which those behaviours appear. It explains those behaviour patterns (or roles) by assuming that persons within a context appear as members of recognized social identities (or positions) and that they and other hold ideas (expectations) about behaviours in that setting (Encyclopaedia Sociology 1992, p. 1681). Role theory is a means for analyzing social system, and roles are conceived as "the dynamic aspects" of society recognized social positions (or statuses). 'Status' according to Linton is a polar position in a reciprocal social interaction. This polar position which he calls 'Status' is a 'collection of rights and duties'. 'Role' according to him is the dynamic aspect of status or giving effect to its right and duties through behavioural enacting (cited in Ventatratnam 1979, p. 96). Roles are viewed as the coping strategies that individuals evolve as they interact with other persons and spoke of the need for understanding others' perspective (role taking) as a requisite for effective social interaction (Encyclopaedia of sociology 1992, p. 1681). Further sophistication was introduced in role analysis. To him, status is a position and role consists of the *activity* the incumbent would engage in were he to act solely in terms of the normative demands upon someone in his position. Role in this normative sense is to be distinguished from role performance or role enactment, which is the actual conduct of a particular individual while on duty in his position (cited in Oomen 1978, p. 15). Moreover, additional insights for role theory were generated by other early authors, particularly Muzafer Sherifs studies of the effects of social norms, Talcott Parson's functionalist theory, which stressed the importance of norms, consensus, sanctioning and socialization, Robert Merton's analysis of role structure and processes, the works of Neal Gross, Robert Kahn and their colleagues, who discussed role conflict and applied role concepts to organizations, Everett Hughis's papers on occupational roles. Theodore Newcomb's text for social psychology, which made extensive use of role concept and the seminal monographs of Michael Banon, Annie—Merrie Rocheblave, and Raghar Rommet as well as Ralf Dahremdorf's essay "Homo sociologicus" (Encyclopaedia of Sociology 1992, p. 1682).

There are contrasting definitions for concepts that are basic role theory. For some authors, the term role refers only to the concept of social position, for others it designates the behaviour characteristic of social position members and for still others it denotes shared expectations held for the behaviours of position members. Role theorists may disagree about substantive issues. For example, some authors use role concepts to describe the social system, whereas others apply it to the conduct of the individuals. Despite these differences, role theorists tend to share a basic vocabulary, interest in the fact that human behaviour is contextually differentiated and is associated with the social position of the actor, and the assumption that behaviour is generated in part by expectations that are held by the actor and others (Encyclopaedia of sociology 1992, p. 1682).

C. Health Care Providers in Delhi Metropolitan City: Area of Study and Data Base

The qualitative and quantitative data[1] used in this section of the paper are collected from southwest district of Delhi popularly known as South Delhi—an area known for posh colony and high-income resident. It is also house of big educational institute like—IIT, AIIMS, JNU and middle and higher middle class/income locality like Huaz Khas, R.K. Puram, Vasant Vihar, and DDA Munirka along with villages like Munirka and Haus Khas. A perfect blend of different income group to study. Locality is mixed as DDA's are occupied by Government employee and business man while villages are occupied by students, strugglers and lower income family. As per DDA's classification, South Delhi comes under 'F' zone due to density of population and availability of infrastructure facility therefore as a result large numbers of private nursing homes come up in this zone.

Nineteen doctors have been interviewed to know about their backgrounds, details and push-pull factor to opt this as a profession. A composite picture has emerged based on the details provided by them. In addition to that, few case studies of patients have also been studied to understand the decisive factor to establish a communication relation between them. The doctors and patients have been contacted at the clinic/service set up identified for the study. One public and 14 private health care centres been studied. Prior appointment has been made, however some have refused as well. The small size of study may be big constraints but findings are eye-openers in many aspects which give an insight to give fresh relook on this 'noble' profession.

Determinants of Doctor's 'Self': A Process to 'Establish Difference'

An important aspect of the development of personality and socialization is the development of 'Self'. Cooley's psycho-social theory of looking glass self focuses on this aspect of individual. For him 'self' means 'I' and 'Me'. Self is determined by the individual's thinking about himself. The infant has no 'self'. It has no interest in 'self'. Its interest in itself awakens only when it becomes conscious of itself. Cooley believes that the idea of 'self' is a social product. So it is also called 'social

[1]Collected for M.Phil dissertation submitted to CSMCH JNU in 2003.

self'. Cooley calls his theory the theory of 'looking-glass self'. The ideas, feelings and tendencies are concerned with 'self'—a process of imagination by which one tries to know what other thinks about them. In the development of 'self', it is important to know not only how people face each other or what they think of each other or what conclusions they arrive at but also to see oneself in the mirror of other's conclusion. Thus, the development of self is the product of society and it is produced by the individual's interaction with other.

A set of the indicators have been put in the interview schedule to understand the doctors' 'self'. It ranges from schooling, parents educational level, father's education and occupation, nativity of respondents and his/her fathers, to the source of the motivation to study medicine and age of decision and future plan after completion of study. Doctors' perception and the factors of consideration about user's health care varies like—educational status, income, occupation, caste, sex or native place and use of technology and cost of cure. It is also to know about the 'social interaction' of doctors as a member of society and exemption if any as a doctor.

Education plays an important role as an agency of socialization. Medium of the instruction in school is also one of the major characteristic to understand the socio-economic background of students in Indian context. Almost all the Government run school imparts education in their respective language. The private school (read expensive) imparts education in English medium. 18 out of 19 have studied in English medium schools.

There is a widely known and very close association between caste and occupation in the traditional social system of India. Thus it is interesting to know the defying traditional association between caste and occupation. Only 15 out of 19 have responded against the question of their caste. Among them, only one belonged to the Schedule Caste and another to backward caste. Data reveals that only one is outside the Brahmin–Vaishya–Kayastha cluster of clean (upper and middle) castes. It is established through examination of surname of respondents except one who mentioned Khandayat as caste from Orissa. Socio-economic development is necessary or prerequisite to enter in any such profession and to map the chances of upward social mobility in hierarchical society of India. Generally, the spread of education is very limited among schedule castes in comparison of upper castes.

An interesting picture has emerged on account of respondents' sex and marital status. Almost equal numbers of practitioners were female (10 out of 19). It should not be considered as equal opportunities available for female folk. It was because of one reason as female practitioners were easily convinced for interview, not a single female doctors who approached have denied. This data was also very interesting because, not a single female doctors from SC been found in the study. A potential explanation of this might be doctors' profession as an expensive education, generally limited family resources of SC, and preference to boy over girl education.

Origin of nativity plays a significant role in deciding the parameter of social mobility. Absolute majority of doctors come from urban (17 out of 19), not only the doctors but their parents were born in urban settings as 15 out of 19 were born in urban settings. Meaning, ambitions of becoming doctors is an urban phenomenon. In fact, modern higher education attracts the urbanites first as they are close to the influence of the institutions of higher learning. The sources by which a 'making of doctor' get influenced are identified as parents, significant relatives and self motivation. The data reveals that by putting parents and significant relatives as in a single category which links with environment stands first as 11 out of 19. Even two respondents have decided to study medicine at tender age of 10 a product of social influence.

Modern system of health service, Allopathy being considered as a neutral system of medicine is also not free from religion biasness. Only one out of 19 respondent is a Muslim. One strong counter argument might be that, majority of the country is of the followers of Hindu religion. However, other religions also have significant presence in Indian population. Therefore, this data is an alarming indicator in many aspect, one underrepresentation of minority religion in higher profession, two even migratory natures of metro cities is still not religion-neutral in terms of opportunity.

The family background plays an important part, to obtain and provide the chances of higher education. The significance of the role of father's education must also be reckoned to be important in this regard. In what ways may education have reinforced or counteracted the particularistic outlook imbibed at home. This is not an easy question to answer, but some clues may be obtained by inquiring the father's education, income and occupation. Not a single respondent's father is below the education of matriculation. Majority of the father—11 were in Government Service followed by business and two each medical professional and other professionals.

'Future plans' is also an interesting and reflecting indictor of concerns of doctors after medical education. More than half—11 respondents decided to establish his/her own clinic/hospitals, while five wished to join government service and two planned to go abroad. This is important to note that more doctors plan to establish unit clinic and fewer want to join government services, but ended in opening a clinic. This reflects the possibility of better returns from the unit than public services but also on the privatization of health sector. It also reflects the diminishing concern to 'return' the expenses incurred on preparing a doctor, considering that many of them became doctor because they wanted to serve people.

A contradictory response received when asked about the factor for performance The term performance here refers to a set of attributes which is considered as a motivational factor to provide service. 'Professional commitment' is articulated as commitment to internalization of a body of generalized knowledge and its conscientious application for community welfare. Commitment is also as a self-imposed professional code of ethics and commitment to work achievement and rewards. But the logical (may be) implication is that commitment to an occupation is to a large extent dependent on the amount of pre-entry investment one makes to acquire the prescribed level of skills. Three doctors consider money as a performance factor while eight out of 19 consider professional ethics as their considering factors.

There is a concern of the study to know the attributes responsible of realization of ideal Vs actual role image of professionals while catering services to the patients. The ideal role image was measured through responses such as sympathetic to the patient, willingness to give more time to a patient if he or she needs it, ability to understand and identify with patients. 12 of 19 consider education status of patients as one of the major considerations for doctors.

Social interaction is the indicator which is used in this study as a process of understanding the desocialization and or expectation of society from the medical professional for the socially accepted norms. Why they are exempted from social obligation. This indicator may be not adequate in sketching the full picture, but it definitely gives some idea. Ten out of 19 respondents said, medical study kept them away from family responsibility, seven said no and only two respondents did not respond to this question. When asked whether they missed any important social event, in the family 14 out of 19 responded positively. But only two out of 19 faced confrontation, for not attending the social events. Most of them 12 out of 19 did not face such confrontation.

Technological development in past 2–3 decades has also an impact on the health care services. A good number of high-tech equipments have come into existence. A new generation of techno-centric doctors is resulted in the increased cost of cure. Doctor's dependence on technology for diagnosis has increased. More than half the respondents think so and, 12 out of 19 believe that technology intervention increase cost of health care. It is quite clear the burden will be more on the marginalized person and doctor's service as business.

Behind the Scene: Social Background of Clientele

Majority of their clientele are from the south Delhi locality of Munirka, and a very small proportion is from other surrounding locality. The wealthy and middle classes form the bulk of their clientele. An attempt was made to enquire about the factors as 'behind the scene' which have any bearing in mind by doctors including education, type of job, residence, look and income level of patients. But the doctors said that they are not interested in that kind of information. They are only concerned with whether the patient could pay for the services used or not. Doctors reveal they are not bothering about the patients' background but 'education and economic status' make difference to establish the relationship with the doctors. During my repeated visits to collect information, I identified following cases for scrutiny to guess the component 'behind the scene' who had come for treatment. Quantifying objectively the base of relation established through this component is difficult. The following interviews with patients could through some light on the issues 'behind the scene'.

Case-I

P is a 40 year old man from the DDA, SFS type residence suffering from minor ailment for the last week. He works in an MNC as an executive and his monthly income is Rs. 35,000. Due to the suffering, he has been consulting this doctor. During the conversation he told that doctor took 5 min for diagnosis in first visit, prescribed medicines and told him to come after a week. This is his second visit, he said. After the initial check up, they exchanged the view on his job-related field and current news and Indian politics over there for 10 min. On the question of patient's background he admits that the economic status and education makes the difference in every sphere of life. He said, they charged more but he could not queue up for the minor ailments like this, in big Government Hospitals.

Case-II

'R' is a 35 year old woman from Munirka village, she is tenant there. Her husband works in a private firm and has monthly income about Rs. 5000. She is suffering from Jaundice and taking treatment for the past 1 month. She almost spent Rs. 3500 on her diagnosis and treatment. She said that doctor does not know about her economic and residential status and never asked her about it and did not suggest anything about the drinking water, she responded. On visiting, he changes some medicine and gives the next date of visit. On question of service, she said that private practitioners provide the best service. And added that it is true they charge more but what we can do. "It is not the grocery shop to change if you do realise, that they are charging more" she quips.

Case-III

'S' was a young man of around 25 years old and visited the clinic while I was having a conversation with one doctor respondent, who was chest specialist and his wife runs a diagnostic centre in same premises. This fellow came with another doctor's prescription to this doctor and asked about necessity and charges of diagnosis prescribed in. This prescription was of his pregnant wife. But doctor neglected the question and in response asked, if it is their first child. He replied, yes and the doctor immediately said that they should go for all the tests and all are necessary and it is not clever to avoid these test. It was important for me to note that doctor did not provide any suitable reason of query. At last doctor also said that you can earn money but not wife. "Come with the patient, I will do something for you" said doctor.

Private Health Care Services: Emergence, Issues, and Concerns

The private sector has been expanding since the past three decades. In India, earlier during the 1950s and 1960s, the presence of private sector institutions was small. But over the years, this sector has been growing and became commercial sectors like others. Nursing home and corporate hospitals is new buzz word in vocabulary of health services. With the increasing penetration of high-tech investigative equipment, investing in medical care has become a profitable proposition and has been an important reason for fuelling the growth of private institutions. The private sector has been largely catering curative services while the public sector has provided both preventive and curative services. Stagnation in public expenditures during the 1970s and the 1980s is also responsible, which has created space for the growth of the private sector. In contrary, government has played a supportive role to the private sector by offering a number of concessions and subsidies from concessional loans, custom duty exemptions to reduction of import duties on high technology medical equipment.

However, there are lots of unaddressed issues and concerned popped up in so-called 'efficient' private service provider.

Introduction of Market Principle: A Flaunt Idea

'More is better' and 'Consumer sovereignty' are the principle which governs the market. 'Consumption' is considered as sole criteria of 'welfare'. Since 'more is better' less consuming is not desirable. 'Consumer sovereignty' means that the consumer knows her/his interest best so whatever she/he wishes to consume should be made available in the market. These principles are contradictory in nature in respect of health service. Corporate service provider's main aim is to maximize the profit by any means. As a result, technology base diagnosis has been increased many fold in corporate setup. Cases of unnecessary diagnosis have been reported many times. As far, the idea of consumer sovereignty is weak in this case. The prime decider is always service provider not consumer himself/herself. Because consumption has link with certain knowledge. Therefore, knowledge holder (doctor) is decider not real consumer (patients). Never, all the information is being shared with patient. Therefore consumer cannot reject any commodity (diagnosis/medicine-even the brand) if he/she wishes so. So the real beneficiary of market principle is service provider not consumer.

Quality of Care: A Myth

A cropped assumption in society is that the private sector provides a better quality services than the public sector. On empirical scrutiny, the assumption 'better quality Service' turns in Myth. It is evident that the private sector attracts and treats persons of 'non-emergency situations' while public sector provides universal access. Therefore, patients load is always higher than the intended capacity. On top of that, general observation is, in the most critical need the private sector refers patient to public sector. Rate of patient turn over, type of patient poverty ridden in public sector while well off in private sector makes comparisons of efficiencies of the public and private sectors difficult. Economic position is one of the prime responsible factors in both acquiring disease and recovering from the disease. Therefore, generalizations between public and private health care services based on 'quality of care' are not possible. Quality of care generally understood in terms of number of patients recovered from disease. Recovery of disease does not solely depend on drug or service but the socio-psychological support patient receives during course of treatment. The second most undeniable argument against the myth is that hospitals are labour intensive organizations which are not only merely dependent on medical expertise but requires the co-ordination of different level of staff to provide quality patient care. It is not enough to have well-qualified specialist alone; it is equally important to have well-trained paramedical and supportive staff for ensuring good quality patient care. Studies on private nursing homes in Bombay (Nandraj 1994) Delhi (Nanda and Baru 1993) and Hyderabad (Baru 1998) have shown that paramedical and supportive staff often work for very low wages and are not qualified for the work that they do.

Culture of Practice: Non-transparency

Unlike the other profession, a doctor receives most trust and faith from his clients in the society. The reason lies in the history, where doctor is a person who helps the patient in recovering from the pain and also helps back to work. It is due to his or her acquired knowledge and special skill and also a non-selfish action. Now-a-days, desire to earn more money takes them to unethical practice or a culture of practice based on non-transparency. Over-medicalization, increasing use of technology and unethical practice are a few manifestation of this non-transparent culture of practice. Dependency of sufferer on doctors and historical image of the profession helps professionals to hide behind them and form the open critical scrutiny of their conduct. The doctors prior to technological revolution were independent healers. They examined, diagnosed, investigated and treated the patients under one roof. They could be compared to the artisans of medieval times. The increasing technological use in diagnosis and the treatment has, therefore changed the practice of medicine from 'caring' to mere 'curing'. Thus, the changes in the organizational set up of individual medical practice are not limited to the change in the doctor–doctor relationship and doctor–patient relationship but the very social position of the doctor as a health care provider has changed. The doctor has indeed become an essential part of the market strategy of the health care industry.

Introduction of Health Insurance: New Big Boss

The health care insurance is also introduced in Indian market. Medical insurance is heavily promoted by Government as a means of providing and covering the cost of health care service. But this premium-based service sector is also facing problems and very India-specific constraints (Vyasulu September 27, 2008). Insurance is a market-based service but not necessary that everyone, who is willing to pay premium, can buy the service for example; senior citizen above the age of 80 and diabetic sufferer (often excluded of diabetic-related ailment). Generally, who needed the most of such services denied the same to them. In addition to this, the policy documents—printed in unreadable font of the premium hides many important points. The 'small prints' become a big issue. Often dental problems and buying spectacle do not come under the policy. On top of that, this new big boss does have two-pronged effect. One side, it helps in the increasing usage of hi-tech high-cost medical care in the private sector. Once they know that a patient is covered under the insurance, they may charge high rates, or includes item that have not been provided. This is a common complaint in India. Other side of coin is role of private bureaucracy hired by insurance company to manage the business (profit making at any cost) and to deny as maximum amount they can, generally in the name of "following rules". Often the work of such supervisor is judged by savings they make for the company.

Health Care in 'Consumerist Society': Consumer Concerns and Empowerment

In this era of consumerism, free market economy and information explosion, how one can empower the consumer to utilize health care services more effectively without endangering doctor–patient relationship which is based on trust? The consumer rights and consumer responsibility gain equal importance. An irresponsible use of the rights may lead to a distorted and expensive health care delivery as seen in USA today. The current Indian scenario, despite great technological advances and specialization in medicine, health care still depends greatly on trust, care and compassion. Unfortunately, in the blind present of scientific knowledge, the human side of doctor–patient relationship is often forgotten and the doctors should find time to listen to their patients and allay their anxieties. This would humanize medicine. The piece meal and dehumanized health care that is available today causes a lot of consumer dissatisfaction and arelargely responsible for the litigations in consumer protection councils.

On the one hand, they demand the status of an industry for financial support including the grant of status of infrastructure, providing a level field for health care, giving nursing homes the status of small-scale industry, loans and further reduction of import duties on medical equipment; and on the other hand, they want to retain the privileges of a welfare institution. They defend unfair market and trade practices under the garb of professional independence. They have interpreted the new economic policy as being one which promotes the market forces without enforcing any regulations and allows private providers to practice without obligations to ethics or patients/users.

Conclusion

In this attempt to locate the place of any occupational category in social structure, subjective status perceptions that the category has on itself are of vital importance, in addition to the objective attributes. Therefore, the purpose to analyze is not only the objective attributes of doctors but also subjective perception they have of their status mostly in two contexts; one is the wider society and within the occupational community of health personnel. This study, undertaken in South of the Delhi Metro, which comprised the posh colony as well as middle class colony, with the urbanized village, describes the interpersonal relations between the doctors and their patient in context of social background. To analyze the reciprocal behaviour of the doctors and patients, and attributes such as age, sex, income, rural and urban communities and educational standards and their impact on the interactions and interrelations, in the context of health care providers social backgrounds are studied. Whatever medical services are available is good but the availability in the context to provider is not same, because the professionals (as member) are a unit of society which is stratified in account of different level. Hence the available services are still beyond the reach of common man or the quality of service which is provided to them. The concern of this study is that the medical professional comes from the upper status of society and their process of socialization and high-tech education is totally different from the common man, to whom they provide service. The role performance of any professional group partly depends on how far it has been able to change its pre-professional attitudes acquired during the period of primary socialization before entering in the professional training.

The main findings of this study is that most of the physicians were of high caste and class background, English medium-educated, urban born and/or brought up, at least second generation children, higher status of father, educated mother, small family size, luxury lifestyle, most of the clinics were in shopping mall and some were in residential locality. The findings of this study about social background of physicians and their socialization process were very close to the findings of other scholars and studies conducted by other academic and institutions discussed earlier. It is a pity that the scenario has not changed even after the 'Globalised economy' and after half the century of democratic political system. Still the health profession, physicians have been moulded and trained as a separate entity in society. Due to their high-class background, hi-tech training, and society bestows respect to them makes them a person "for society" and not "with society". Therefore, the urgent need is to understand the profession in its holistic way with large sample size. It may give impetus to relook the policy to ensure the diversity-social, religious, and linguistic and nativity—in profession. Thereafter, the mission health for all could be realized progressively.

References

Abidi, N. F. (1993). *Women physician: Role and role conflict*. New Delhi: Manak Publication.

Anita, N. H. (1990). Medical education: in need of cure. *EPW,* 1571–1573.

Banerji, D. (1974). *Anatomy of the medical profession of India*. New Delhi-: Mimeographed CSMCH/SSS/JNU.

Banerji, D. (1985). *Health and family planning services in India: An epidemiological socio-cultural and political perspective.* New Delhi: Lok Prakashan.

Banerji, D. (1990). Medical profession and social orientation of health services in India. *Seminar.*

Banerji, D. (1981). *Poverty, class and health culture in Indian,* (Vol. II). New Delhi: Parachi Prakashan, 1981.

Banerji, D. (1973). "Social Orientation of Medical Education in India." *EPW.*, 3rd March 1973.

Banerji, D., & Lakhan, S. (1985). Bhopal gas tragedy: An epidemiological and sociological study. *JNU News*, 1985: 15–19.

Baru, R. V. (1994). The Rise of Business in Medical Care. *Health for Millions*, *2*(1).

Baru, R. V. (1998). *Private health care in India-social characteristics and trends*. New Delhi: Sage Publication, New Delhi.

Baru, R. V. (2000). Privatisation and corporatisation. *Seminar*, May 2000, 489.

Bhat, R. (1999). Regulations of private health sector in India. In *Private Health Sector Growth in Asia-Issues and Implications*, by William N. B. Ahmadabad: IIMA.

Bilton, et al. (1981). *Introductory sociology.* New York: McMillan Press Ltd.

Bloom, S. W., & Wilson, R. N. (1972). Doctor-patient relationship in hospital. In H. E. Freeman et al. (Eds.), *Hand book of medical Sociology*, (pp. 315–339). New Jersey: Practice Hall Inc.

Centres, R. (1949). *The psychology of social class—A study of class*. USA: Princeton University Press.

Chandani, A. (1985). *The medical profession—A sociological exploration*. New Delhi: Jainsons Publication.

Chen, L. C. (1987). Malnutrition and Mortality. In C. Gopalan (Ed.), *Combating malnutrition: Basic issues and practical approaches*, pp. 47–57. New Delhi: Nutrition Foundation of India.

Coe, R. M. (1978). *Sociology of medicine*. New York: Me Grawhill.

Cokerhem, W. C. (Ed.). (1989). *Medical sociology*. Printince Hall: New Jersey, USA.

Committee, ICMR/ ICSSR. (1981). *Health for all—An alternative strategy.* Pune: Indian Institute of Education.

Dak, T. M. (1991). *Sociology of the health, Jaipur*. India: Rawat Publication.

Dent, M. (1993). Professionalism, educated labour and the state hospital medicine and the new managerialism. *The Sociological Review*, *41*(2), 244–273.

Dingwell, R., & Lewis, P. (Eds.). (1983). *Sociology of the profession-lawyer, doctors*. McMillan: Hong Kong.

Dubey, S. M. (1987). Profession of medicine in India. In S. K. Chandani and A. Lal (Eds.), *Readings in Medical Sociology,* pp. 100–110. New Delhi: Jain Sons Publication.

Dubey, S. M. (1975). *Social mobility among the profession-study of the profession in a transitional Indian city.* Bombay: Popular Publication.

Eckland, B. K. (1972). Social Biology. In H. E. Freeman (Ed.), *Handbook of Medical Sociology*, p. 108. Englewood, New Jersey: Prentice Hall, Inc.

Elliott, P. (1999). Sociology of the profession. In *Encyclopaedia of Sociology* (Vol. 4, London: McMillan).

Enos, D. D., et al. (1976). *The sociology of health care-social, economic and political perspective*. Newyork: Praeger Publication.

Frankenberg, R. (1981). Allopathic medicine, profession and capitalist ideology in India. *Social Science and Medicine* (pp. 115–125).

Friedson, E. (1975). *Profession of medicine.* New York.

Giddens, A. (1973). *The class structure of the advanced societies*. London: Hutchinson.

Gore, M. S. (1978). *Social sciences in professional education*. New Delhi: Committee Report.

Government of India. (1989). *Morbidity and utilisation of medical services 42nd round.* National sample survey type 364, New Delhi: Central Statistical Organisation.
Government of India. (1995). *Report of the group on medical education and support.* Health service and medical education—A programme for immediate planning, New Delhi: Ministry of Health & Family Welfare.
Harlambos, M. (1988). *Sociology-themes and perspectives.* New Delhi: Oxford University Press.
Illich, I. (1976). *Medical nemesis—The exploration of health.* London: Marion Boyans Publication.
Jackson, J. A. (Ed.). (1970). *Profession and professionalisation.* London: C.V. Publication.
Jacob, J. M. (1988). *Doctors and rule—A sociology of professional value.* London: Routledge Publication.
Jaffery, R. (1978). Allopathic medicine in India—a case of deprofessionalisation. *EPW.*
Jeffery, R. (1988). *The politics of health in India.* London: University of California Press.
Jesani, A., & Anantharam, S. (1989). *Private sector and privatisation in the health care services: A review paper for ICSSR-ICMR.* Bombay: FRCH.
Jones, L. (1994). *The social context of health and health work.* New York: McMillan.
Lentin, B. (1994). *Doctors and patient—Life under consumer protection act.* New Delhi: TOI.
Madan. (1972). Doctors in a north indian city-recruitment, role perception, and role performance. In S. Suberwal (Ed.), *Beyond the village-sociological exploration*, pp. 77–110. IIAS.
Madan, T. N. (1980). *Doctors and society.* New Delhi: Vikas Publishing House.
Madan, T. N. (1972). Doctors in a north Indian city-recruitment, role perception, and role performance. In S. Seberwal (Ed.), *Beyond the village-sociological exploration*, pp. 77–110. IIAS.
Mathur, I. (1975). *Social and organisational structure of hospital.* Jaipur: Rawat Publication.
Merton, K. (1958). Medical Education as a social process. In *Patient. Physician and Illness*, pp. 321–322. New York: The Free Press of Glencoe.
Merton, R. K. (1957). Some preliminaries to a study of medical education. In R. K. Merton (Ed.), *The Student Physician*, pp. 6–7. USA: Cambridge Mass, Harvard University Press.
Morris, D. (1965). Health profession its challenges and perspective. In Freeman (Ed.), *Medical Sociology.* New Jersey: Prentice Hall.
Nady, A., & Visvanathan, S. (1990). *Modern medicine and its non-modern critics—A study in discourage in dominating knowledge.* London: Clarendon Press, Oxford.
Nagla, M. (1988). *Medical sociology.* Delhi: Printwell Publication.
Nanda, P., & Baru, R. (1993). *Private nursing homes and their utilization—A case study of Delhi.* New Delhi: VHAI.
Nayar, P. K. (Ed.). (1982). *Sociology in India—retrospect and prospect.* BRPC: New Delhi.
Ogburn, W. F., & Nimkoff, M. F. (Eds.). (1972). *A handbook of sociology.* New Delhi: Eurasia Publication House Ltd.
Oomen, T. K. (1978). *Doctors and nurses-A study in occupational role structures.* Delhi: McMillan.
Park, C. (1985). *Doctors and medicine in early renaissance.* New Jersey: Princeton.
Phillips, M. (1985). *Doctor dilemma—Medical ethics and contemporary science.* John Dawon: Harvester Press.
Qadeer, I. (1986). *The XI world sociological conference.* New Delhi.
Qadeer, I. (2011). *Public health in India.* New Delhi: Daanish Books.
Ramamurthi, B. (1992). Medical college, doctors and health care. Delhi: The Hindu.
Sahu, S. K. (1991). *Health culture in transition—A case study of Oraon tribe in rural industrial city.* New Delhi: Khama Publication.
Sahu, S. K. (1981). Health culture of Oraons. In *The Context of Different Helath Instituions. Ph.D Thesis Submitted to CSMCH, JNU.*
Shorie, H. D. (1994). Doctors and patient—A sacred tie. New Delhi: Hindustan Times.
Solidarity, W. (2000). Critical condition—A report on workers in Delhi's private hospitals. New Delhi.
Taylor, K. (1976). *Doctors for the villages.* London: Asia Publication.

Thorpe, G., et al. (1971). *The affluent worker in the class structure*. Great Britain: Cambridge University Press.

(TOI), Editorial. (1994). What Ails Medicine? *TOI.* New Delhi, 31st June 1994.

Ventataratnam, R. (1979). *Medical sociology in an Indian settings*. Madras: McMillan.

White, L. P., & Wooten, K. C. (1986). *Professional ethics and practice in organisational development—A system analysis of issues, alternatives and approach*. NewYork: Praeger Publication.

Young, Kimball. (1969). *Sociology—study of society and culture*. New York: American Book Company.

Zurbrigg, S. (1984). *Rakku 's story—structure of ill health and source of change*. Banglore: For Centre for Social Action.

Access to Maternal and Child Health Care: Understanding Discrimination in Selected Slum in Delhi

Sanghmitra S. Acharya and Golak B. Patra

Abstract Discrimination in the name of 'caste', 'class' and 'gender' is very much prevailing in Indian scenario. But the gender-based discrimination can be called as multiple discrimination, as a same person comes under the deprived caste (*dalit*) as well as the deprived gender (women). In case of the access to the health care services by the women it has been experienced the everywhere in India and in the cases of *dalit* women it can be found the extreme. Delhi is the capital of India representing the people from almost all Indian States. The slums in Delhi are bearing the similar population distribution as well. Being the lowest income quintal living in slums, people are experiencing the poor access to the health care services in general. In case of the Maternal and Child Health (MCH) it has been deterioration of the services. There are multiple factors responsible for the poor health care services and success to it by the people. Economic factor can be one of the major factors but in the cases of Kusumpur Pahari we cannot strike out the system of discrimination based on the caste in particular. This study has been undertaken to probe into the intermediate factors that responsible in discriminating access the MCH care as well as the general health care by the women in the study area. The study slum has represents mixed culture of population representing rural Indian as well as the modern; as it is situated in the National Capital Region (NCR) of Delhi. Hence, this study has been trying to understand the pattern of discrimination in accessing health care by the people in general and by the women in particular.

S.S. Acharya (✉) · G.B. Patra
Centre of Social Medicine and Community Health, School of Social Sciences, Jawaharlal Nehru University, New Delhi, India
e-mail: sanghmitra.acharya@gmail.com

S.S. Acharya
Indian Institute of Dalit Studies, New Delhi, India

S.S. Acharya et al. (eds.), *Marginalization in Globalizing Delhi: Issues of Land, Livelihoods and Health*, DOI 10.1007/978-81-322-3583-5_18

Keywords Health · Maternal and child health · Discrimination · Urban slum · Dalit · NCR

Introduction

Social exclusion is concerned with the causes of poverty, specific nature of essential needs in different societies, access to the services and opportunities which enable meeting the needs, and civil and political rights of the individuals. Poverty is an important determinant of access to health care services (Zurbrigg 1984); and most poor are *dalits* as well as most *dalits* are poor.[1] Poverty evolves a different health culture and affects perception of illness and utilization of care. A rather national picture was generated regarding the utilization of the health care services by the scheduled communities after the National Health and Family Surveys (NHFS) (IIPS 1995; IIPS and ORC Macro Internaltional 2000; IIPS and Macro Internaltional 2007) were conducted and spurt of research papers emerged. It was evident that the level of utilization is much lower among the *dalits* as compares to the non-*dalits*. (Ram et al. 1998; Acharya 2002; Kulkarni and Baraik 2003). Social exclusion is a way of examining how and why individuals and groups fail to have access to or benefit from the possibilities offered by societies and economies. It is multidimensional and encompasses lack of access to goods and services; and also exclusion from security, justice, representation and citizenship. It is related with inequality in economic, social, political and cultural spheres. It is important to identify those who include and exclude, and to understand how and why they do so. These agencies can be social groups, state, business enterprise, military, local authorities, religious bodies, or local elite. Those excluded have a role in promoting their inclusion. Social exclusion can be understood at different levels—national, regional, institutional, social groups or individual. Social discrimination is, therefore, related to lack of access to services and goods offered by societies. Social and religious groups appear to accentuate social discrimination by denying certain opportunities pertaining to social and religious practices and access to services to some and not to others. Caste-based discrimination is permanent in nature and differs from exclusion that is created and recreated by the operations of social and economic forces. It focuses directly on the nature of the lives people live and disadvantages they experience (Thorat et al. 2006). It is a part of basic institutional framework and institutional arrangement within a nation and refers to institutions and rules that enable and constraint human interaction.

Caste-based social exclusion in access and utilization of health care can be understood as complete exclusion of certain social groups such as *Dalits* in access and utilization of health care. There is denial of certain services. There can also be

[1]More than one-fourth (27 % among rural and 24 % among urban population), are *Dalits* in the population below poverty line. Among *dalits*, 36 % are below poverty line as compared to dominant castes. (NSSO), 55th Round, 1999–2000, as quoted in Shah et al. (eds.) Untouchability in Rural India, Sage Publications New Delhi.

selective inclusion or partial denial services to the discriminated groups reflected in access to some and not to the other services. There can be unequal care access in terms of time spend with; tone and use of derogatory words for; dispensing of the medicine via a medium to; and not touching the discriminated groups by the provider. Unfavourable or forced inclusion in providing certain services such as health camps; and exclusion from certain service provisioning such as health camps, health education programmes, water supply, electricity and infrastructure too can be understood as caste-based social exclusion. As an attribute of individuals, caste-based social exclusion focuses directly on the health status of *Dalits* and disadvantages they experience. They are isolated, lack social ties to local community, voluntary associations, trade unions or even nations. They are disadvantaged in their ability to use their legal rights and constitutional provisions effectively. They are unable to overcome both consumption and work related disadvantage. Public goods and services which should be available to all are limited to a select few based on the caste hierarchy. They are isolated, lack social ties to local community, voluntary associations, trade unions or even nations. They are disadvantaged in their ability to use their legal rights and constitutional provisions effectively. They are unable to overcome both consumption and work related disadvantage. Forced inclusion or exclusion, partial or complete, amounts to discrimination (Thorat 2002). Social exclusion can be distinguished as an attribute of individuals; and as a property of societies. As an attribute of individuals social exclusion focuses directly on the nature of the lives people live and disadvantages they experience. As a property of society, exclusion could be an outcome of group identity and affiliation.

Conceptual Framework

There are ample evidences of the practices of discrimination against the *dalits* in different spheres and varied forms. Access to civic amenities and social facilities has always been a concern in the context of the *Dalits*. Although the constitutional provisions have been in place for penalizing those practising discrimination, yet it continues to thrive. Discrimination against *dalits* has metamorphosed over time from overt, open and accepted norm to subtle, invisible, hidden and 'unaccepted' behaviour. In the present context the divide is between those who had the benefits in the past and were oppressing the *dalits* in the worst possible way as their right; and those who have now been given certain privileges as part of the positive discrimination policy of the state. In the past the former had internalized oppressing the oppressed as their right and the latter had internalized being oppressed as their normal lives. This continues even today, though with a difference. What used to be obvious and overt earlier has become subtle, covert and surreptitious. Resentment of non-*dalits* towards the *dalits* is present and gets reflected in various forms, in sporadic incidences across the country.

Discrimination is likely to be present in the health care access in the forms of refusal to observe certain norms which are mandatory in care giving, but are often violated while rendering care to the *dalit* care seekers. These may be manifested in the form of refusal to touch, enter into the house, and share the seating place, sharing the food and water, and transportation. The spheres in which discrimination is likely to be visible are care delivery 'spaces' which could be the care centre or the users' house.

What are these factors which continue to reign over and above constitutional provisions? What is it that makes the religion which claims to be 'all embracing' and touted as 'a way of life' has failed to accept some its own people? It becomes imperative, therefore, to understand the factors which still fuel the element of discrimination experienced by the *dalits* at various levels and in different forms and spheres.

Identity is important in understanding social interaction. It is socially located because it is through this concept that the personal and the social are connected. Identity provides links between the personal and the social, self and society and is relational. It is constructed through relations of difference, such as 'us' and 'them'. Identity also has to accommodate and manage differences. Formation and establishment of identity involves locating and transgressing boundaries. The *dalit* identity places the individual in certain social realm which superseded other attributed acquired and innate. Recognition of self in relation to others often leads to two starkly opposite responses—docile, on one extreme and volatile on the other. Consequently, there are evidences of prevalent discriminatory behaviour such as not placing the medicine on hands of a *dalit*; and the helpless acceptance of such care; not sitting on the designated places in fear of being rebuked and insulted. On the other end of the social identity scale, assertive recognition of self is likely to reflect anger and discontent; and may also lead to lesser discrimination due to the fear of the notoriety of anger. There is also a possibility of genuine positive response from the others to the assertion (Box 1).

Box 1: Sensing Identity…

A sense of identity can be a source not merely of pride and joy but also of strength and confidence. It is not surprising that idea of identity receives such widespread admiration from popular advocacy or loving your neighbour to high theories of social capital and of communitarian self-definition

… and yet identity can also kill- and kill with abandon. A strong and exclusive sense of belonging to one group can in many cases carry with it the perception of distance and divergence from other groups. Within group similarity can help to feed between group discord

Defining the Concept of Discrimination in Health Care Access

On the basis of the foregoing understanding, discrimination in accessing health care can be understood as complete exclusion of *Dalits* from accessing health care. There is denial of certain services and selective inclusion or partial denial of services to reflect access to some and not to the others. There can be unequal care access in terms of time spend with; tone and use of derogatory words for; dispensing of the medicine via a medium to; and not touching the discriminated groups by the provider. Unfavourable or forced inclusion in providing certain services such as health camps; and exclusion from certain service provisioning such as health camps, health education programmes, water supply, electricity and infrastructure too can be understood as caste-based social exclusion. As an attribute of individuals, caste-based discrimination focuses directly on the health status of *dalits* and disadvantages they experience. Discrimination in access to health care service can thus, be understood through three basic forms:

- Complete exclusion or complete denial of health care services
- Partial denial or selected exclusion of health care services
- Unfavourable inclusion or forced inclusion for certain services.

The state health care system entails to provide services to all without any discrimination. However, if a group of people are completely excluded from availing some services for whatever reasons, it may be termed as *complete exclusion*. Many a times some people have access to some services and not to other. Also they may be discriminated by the services providers and co-users at the place of services delivery in terms of priority and proximity. They may have access to some services and not to others. This is *partial denial or selected exclusion*. This can be visualized in two ways—differential treatment by the health providers; and differential treatment by the co-users of the care. There can be differential treatment by the health providers. There are different types of care provider, public sector, private sector, nonprofit/NGO sector. The providers are from different streams of care—allopathic, homeopathic, indigenous/traditional. The treatment can be differential in terms of providing no, less, or wrong information; providing discriminatory treatment at the place of delivery of care; involuntary inclusion or exclusion in some schemes; discriminatory treatment during emergency and home visits; and behaviour and attitude of the provider.

The co-users of the care can discriminate in use of space for waiting. Their behaviour and attitude can be derogatory, dominating and suppressing. They may be surpassing rules to use the services when it is actually due to the people from the discriminated groups (pushing them back in the queue). In access to water and electricity too, there are evidence of such discrimination. There can also be differential treatment for certain services. There can be forceful inclusion in certain services for some specific groups. There could be some forceful inclusion to participate in health camps; sanitation and cleaning of the village; local self-governing bodies like Panchayats, in case of mothers. There are also chances that some people are forced to avail some services in spite of their unwillingness. This may be considered as *unfavourable or forced inclusion*.

Discrimination in access to health care is mostly observed in the disparity in care provisioning at the health care centre by the providers—doctor and the supporting staff; and at home during the visit by the health worker. Discrimination in access and utilization of health at the health centre is likely to be practised during diagnosis and counselling, dispensing of the medicine, laboratory tests; while waiting in the health centre, and in paying the user fee. Discrimination during diagnosis may be measured in terms of time spend in asking about the problem, and touching the user during diagnosis. Discrimination during dispensing the medicine can be measured in terms of the way medicine is given to the user—kept on the palm, kept on the window sill/floor, someone else is asked to give. Discrimination in the laboratory can be measured in terms of direct touching of the user for the tests and x-ray. Discrimination while waiting and payment of user fee can be measured in terms of duration of waiting, space for waiting, waiting till the other dominant castes have been provided care, attitude of the paramedics towards them while they wait. Discrimination during payment of user fee, if any, can be measured in terms of actual amount being paid, time spend for waiting to pay and space for waiting and a separate queue for payment.

Discrimination at home during the visit by the health worker may occur while entering the house, touching the user, sitting, drinking/eating in the user's house and while giving medicine and information regarding health camps/programmes to them. Selective dissemination of information regarding health camps and programmes; and exclusion of *Dalits* in accessing certain type of services where touch is involved (such as vaccination) also reflect on the traditional notion of polluted and pure and the consequent discrimination.

Thus, discrimination can be practised by different providers across spheres and forms. Present policies and programmes for health care and against discrimination; awareness regarding them and ability to use them culminate in the experience of discrimination, expressed as complete or partial exclusion; and forced inclusion in access to health care services.

The forms include duration of interaction; touch; speaking gently; use of derogatory words or phrase; and long waiting time. The personnel include doctor; lab technician; pharmacist; and grassroots level health workers such as Auxiliary Nurse Midwife (ANM)/Village Health Worker (VHW)/Lady Health Visitor (LHV); and Anganwadi Worker (AWW).

On the basis of this typology, study is designed to collect information on some forms of discrimination in different spheres and practised by different providers; and probable consequences of such practise.

Purpose of the Study

With this background, therefore, the present paper aims to understand the nature and patterns of caste-based discrimination (henceforth referred as discrimination) in access to health care practised in different forms; and the consequences of such practices. This is one of the initial studies to explore caste-based discrimination in health sector. There are problems in defining the very concept of discrimination in health. Typology to understand it; and empirical methodology to measure it are still evolving and yet to fully develop. Thus, the specific objectives are to:

1. Identify forms of social discrimination experienced in accessing health services.
2. Study the consequences of discrimination; and identify the best practices that improve access to health care.

Study Design

The Study was conducted in Kusumpur Pahari, a notified slum, located behind the Central Bureau of Investigation (CBI) colony in Vasant Vihar. It is inhabited by more than two lakh migrants. Social composition of the population suggests that about one-fourth belong to Other Backward Castes (OBC); more than half are high caste; about 17 % belong to scheduled castes and about 8 % are scheduled tribes.

The methodology adopted in the present study deals with database and sample design. The second part is on methods of measurements which includes selection of indicators; ranking of indicators; construction of a composite index; and content analysis of the narratives obtained from the Consultative Meetings and discussions held during the fieldwork.

The methods used included both qualitative and quantitative techniques. Tools and techniques used for the primary data include individual interviews, in-depth interviews, group discussions, consultative meetings, exit interviews and observation through structured household schedule and semi-structured questionnaires, check lists and field notes. Some of the GIS (Geographic Information System) based images of the selected villages were also used for mapping purposes. In addition to these, photography has also been used to illustrate some observations.

The field work was done in selected Blocks with the women aged 18–45 years age; health care providers, government officials, NGO personnel, activists, community leaders and policy makers were identified for the conduct of the field work. Houselisting was done to identify households with mothers and children.

Profile of the Study Area

Kusumpur Pahari is a notified slum, located behind the CBI colony in Vasant Vihar, New Delhi is inhabited by more than two lakh migrants. They mainly comprise of daily wage earners like domestic workers, labourers, painters and construction workers. Situated alongside the remnants of the endangered Delhi Ridge Area around Vasant Kunj, Kusumpur Pahari is a slum cluster more in the form of an urban village. The area is divided into five blocks A, B, C, D and E. Approximately there are around 20,000 households in the area. The inhabitants of the area includes migrants mostly from Uttar Pradesh, Rajasthan and Haryana; followed by the migrants from Tamil Nadu, Bihar, Jharkhand, West Bengal and a few also from Nepal.

Demographic Characteristics

As regards the age sex composition of the study participants, there were 462 of which 50 % each were men and women. It is important to note that the sex ratio is lowest in the age group 25–39 which is economically most active and thus reflects on the process of male selected migration prevalent among young adults in search of livelihoods to the urban areas (Table 1). Concentration on younger ages, 0–4 and 5–14 highlights the need for child health care services. Unsurprisingly, the female population is highest in the age group 15–39 (103) because of the likelihood of marriage migration which would have required them to join the spouse in the due course. These women are active both economically and reproductively. Therefore, there is evident need of the maternal health care services for them in addition to child health. What is conventionally labelled as young population 15–24, has the highest sex ratio (1864) in the study area. Unlike the macro scenario, in this case the high level of sex ratio may not be speaking of empowerment of women. Evidences, as discussed later, show that many of the girls have accompanied their families so as to facilitate the services which can be accessed by their male siblings. For instance, in the age group 5–14 there are fewer boys than girls. They appear to be taking over odd jobs, both at home and outside to release the boys from the drudgery and engage in activities such as schooling; and sometimes work as a vendor or part time worker too.

Majority of the residents are engaged in unorganized sector and it includes construction workers, domestic maids, rickshaw puller/auto drivers, car painters and rag pickers. There are people engaged in lower rank of the government services but their numbers are very few. Few people are also working in private sectors as guards, peons, gardener, etc., and some of them are also self-employed in their own business. But overall the household income is mostly dependent on unorganized sector.

Table 1 Age group and sex ratio

Age group	Male	Female	Total	Sex ratio
0–4	54	55	109	1019
5–14	48	58	106	1208
15–24	22	41	63	1864
25–39	89	62	151	697
40–59	14	13	27	929
60 and above	4	2	6	500
Total	231	231	462	1000

Source Prepared from the primary data collected from the study site (authors own source)

Educational Status

About one-third of the study participants are Illiterate. Less than one-fourth is educated up to primary (22 %) and middle (21 %) level. About 7 % have completed 10 years of schooling and done matriculation or secondary school. While all educational attainment is lopsided in favour of boys, it is encouraging to note that equal number of boys and girls each reported to have done some technical or professional degree like medical, engineering, or law. There are eight boys to one girl who have graduate degree (Fig. 1). This corroborates the possibility that the girls aged 5–14 years are engaged in activities other than education and are in reality facilitating their siblings to be educated.

The girls do not show an interest to get educated and subsequently, employed. They are not allowed to study beyond matriculation because of the economic reasons. According to some parents of the study area:

> If girls are sent out for studies they will run away with some boy. They are not allowed to work according to their desire. Parents give more money to boys. All this is because we go to a different house after marriage and they also have to spend for our marriage. (Focus Group Discussion/FGD, Block C)

Girls are not even allowed to walk alone in the slum for fear of security and "integrity". Few persons involved with NGOs come to teach sometimes but since the girls are not allowed to move out and usually have to move in a group, these teachers are unable to cover as many girls as they may have wanted.

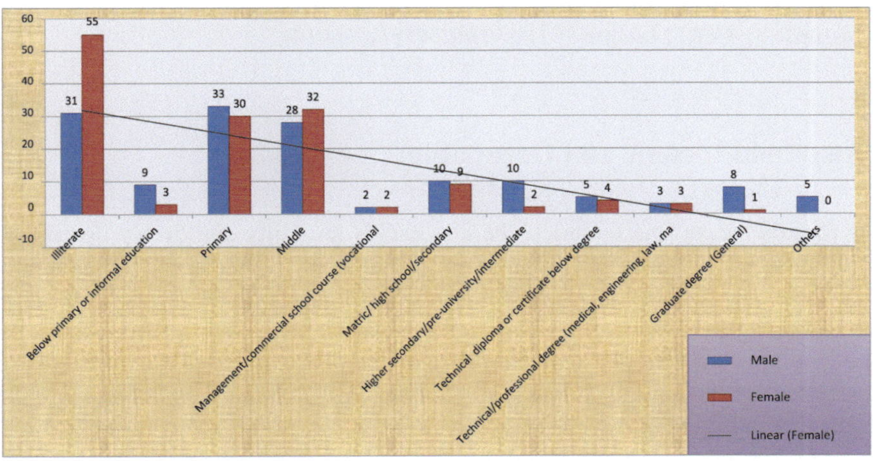

Fig. 1 Educational status of 7 years and above. *Source* prepared from the primary data collected from the study site (authors own source)

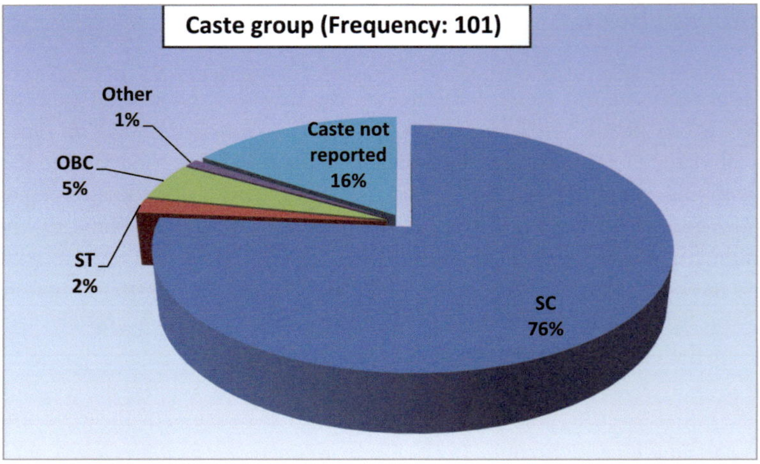

Fig. 2 Social structure in kusumpud pahari. *Source* prepared from the primary data collected from the study site (authors own source)

Social Groups

Most of the families belong to the scheduled castes (76 %) is evident from Fig. 2. The households belonging to Scheduled Tribes, Other Backward Castes and others comprise only 6 % of the total study participants. About 16 families did not report caste on account of their following religion other than Hinduism. However, the follow-up visits, discussions and observations suggested that they were *Dalit* Muslims (3), OBC Muslims (9) and *Dalit* Christians (4).

Household Income and Occupation

As regards the income quintiles, the households are fairly and evenly distributed with about 17 % falling in each quintile (Table 2). It is only in the third quintile that there are 18.2 % households. About 13 % households reported no income. These were the households which were established separately to claim rights on the land and the dwelling unit. For all practical purposes they were attached to their 'parents' household. It was also reported that many of them were using the housing unit for the purpose of sleeping only. Thus, labelling them as families was more appropriate than households.

The main occupation of the household respondent is regular employment in private sector (9.1 %) followed by casual labour in nonagricultural other than public work (4.5 %). Closely following is the regular employment in public sector and traditional service occupations such as shoe making/mending, washing and

Table 2 Income quintile and their distribution

Income quintile	Households/families	%
1	80	17.3
2	80	17.3
3	84	18.2
4	77	16.7
5	82	17.7
Total	403	87.2
No reported income	59	12.8
Total	462	100.0

Source prepared from the primary data collected from the study site (authors own source)

Table 3 Main occupation of the household

Main occupation	Engaged	%
Self-employed in agriculture/fishery/orchard	2	0.4
Self-employed in nonagriculture	14	3.0
Regular salaried/wage employee in government	17	3.7
Regular salaried/wage employee in private sector	42	9.1
Casual wage labour in public works	4	0.9
Casual labour in agriculture/horticulture	2	0.4
Casual labour in nonagriculture other than public works	21	4.5
Domestic work but also engaged in free collection of goods	2	0.4
Traditional service occupation (cobbler, dhobi, barber)	18	3.9
Total	122	26.4

Source prepared from the primary data collected from the study site (authors own source)

ironing clothes, and hair cutting/styling; which is offering work to less than 4 %. Other works like self-employment, domestic work engages very small share of the households' members of the study (Table 3).

Occupational Opportunities Among Young Migrants

In case of both the sites there is a marked mental strain among the youth girls and boys as to their employment possibilities. The girls pointed out that they should be given some training in tailoring, embroidery or even knitting so that they can earn some money from home itself (FGD3, Block E). In case of socio-economic programmes for the vulnerable groups the emphasis has been largely on skills passed on and vital aspects such as availability of credit and linkages for marketing are often ignored. Quite often the organizations are unable to continue training on a regular basis and this causes slow progress in the training process. The paucity of

Table 4 Duration of stay in slum by household

Duration in years	Frequency	%
2–5	8	7.9
6–10	13	12.9
10+	53	52.5
For generations	25	24.8
Total	99	98.0
Could not recall	2	2.0
Total	101	100

Source prepared from the primary data collected from the study site (authors own source)

resources, nonavailability or nonrenewal of the grants in time and also the lack of specialist trainers or an exclusively training department in the organization are some of the reasons for this. However sporadic functioning, apart from slowing down the momentum and pace of work also results in loss of credibility and image in the eyes of the community. Furthermore, the vocational schemes are being taken up without a pre-assessment of felt needs of the communities and also the market feasibility of the schemes. With reference to women, the programmes being offered provide them meagre incomes, which are insufficient for their economic independence.

The process of peopling in the slum directs toward the in-migrating populations which accommodate in the slums in the urban areas. In case of Kusumpur Pahari too, more than half of the residents have been living there for more than 10 years and a quarter of them claim to be living there 'for generations' (Table 4).

Accessibility of Basic Services in Kusumpur Pahari

Kusumpud Pahari a recognized slum can be demolished any time. Residents of the area have not had adequate access to basic facilities for the last 4–5 decades. The main source of water is the water tanker that comes in the slum from Delhi Jal Board (DJB). It supplies water 88 % study participants. Due to presence of pucca motorable road passing within the slum, the tanker can come inside. Each household has a fixed quota of water and it is generally not sufficient for them. Moreover fetching the water from the main road to the respective household is also very difficult given the uneven terrain of the area. There are borewells present in the slum but the quality of water is not good so, they use the water from borewell mostly for cleaning. There is a hand pump at the extreme end of the slum, in the Block B which supplies water to about 7 % study participants (Fig. 3). Residents use water from this hand pump for drinking purpose as the tanker cannot reach them.

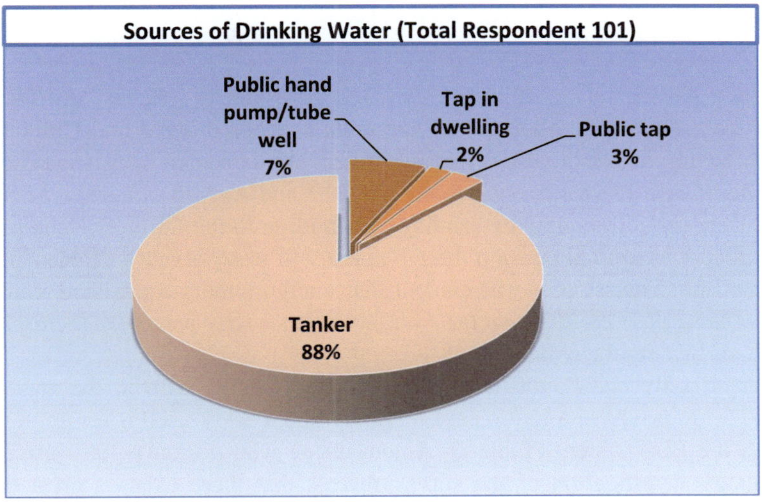

Fig. 3 Main source of drinking water in the slum. *Source* prepared from the primary data collected from the study site (authors own source)

Most houses are semi-pucca, about 60 %, followed by pucca (15.8 %). There are 11 % of households who are living in *khaprail* houses. Most of the study participants lived in own houses (68.3 %) which are *pucca* and have electricity (97 %). Open drainage mark the study slum. None of the families have their own private toilet. Very few families have constructed their own private toilets. There exist three public toilets, one is not in working condition other two although in better condition but nobody goes there. Resident confine to nearby forest area. More than 87 % use this area for defecation and only 8 % use the public latrine (Table 5). There is one garbage disposal unit in the slum, where garbage is collected and taken away by the municipality department. But it hardly functions as garbage is not collected regularly by the municipality department.

Table 5 Type of housing in the study area

Type of housing	No. of households	%
Pucca	16	15.8
Semi-pucca	61	60.4
Khaprail	11	10.9
Kuchcha	13	12.9
Total	101	100
Own house	69	68.3
Houses having electricity	98	97

Source prepared from the primary data collected from the study site (authors own source)

Government Schemes and Programme

The study participants were aware of some government schemes and had benefitted from them too. About 41 % knew about Reproductive and Child Health related (RCH); and about 34 % had benefitted. While nearly 54 % were aware of Integrated Child Development Scheme (ICDS) and *Anganwadi*, only 17 % benefitted from the programme by sending the children to the Centres. None of them had availed widowhood pension though about 7 % knew about it (Table 6). In the course of the discussion, it was evident that many mothers considered it undesirable to *'make their children eat the AWC food'* since they perceived themselves as capable of feeding the children.

There is only one Public Distribution System (PDS) shop in the area. More than 56 % do not have a ration card and only about 30 % used it for getting food through the PDS system (Table 7). Among those who do, only 30 % use it. The preliminary investigation of the survey reveals that there exists a great deal of irregularity in supply coupled with malpractices as people are not getting their required share. There are around twelve ICDS centres present in the slum. But it has not been very effective as people are mostly resorting to nearby private schools for their children. Moreover people are not enthusiastic about the ICDS services as they feel it has not been able to deliver and there is a general sense of discontent with the service.

Table 6 Awareness of government schemes/programme and their use

Name of scheme/programme	% Families	
	Awareness	Used/benefited
Reproductive and Child Health (RCH) services	40.6	33.7
Janani Suraksha Yojna (JSY)	13.9	3.0
ICDS/Anganwadi	53.5	16.8
Mid-Day-Meal (MDM) Scheme	27.7	6.9
Scholarship for Child	9.9	4.0
Old Age Pension	8.9	3.0
Widow Pension	6.9	–

Source prepared from the primary data collected from the study site (authors own source)

Table 7 Distribution of household with ration card and its use

Response regarding PDS	With ration card		Use ration card/PDS	
	Families	%	Families	%
No	57	56.4	26	25.7
Yes	36	35.6	30	29.7
Total	93	92.1	56	55.4
Do not know	8	7.9	45	44.6
Total	101	100	101	100

Source prepared from the primary data collected from the study site (authors own source)

Many of them in the lower income quintile, as compared to higher quintile, do not have the ration card. The ones who have the ration cards in the lower income quintile use it more than those in the higher quintiles.

> 'I earn about Rs 100 per day by selling the 'raddi' and 'kabaad' that I collect through the day, to the 'kabadiwala' in Block C… I had got the form filled for getting the ration card almost a year ago. I am still struggling to get the ration card even after paying Rs 200 to Raji Saheb- the local facilitator' (In-depth Interview, women aged 32, Block D).

Krishna ji (named changed) is employed with an NGO and earns around Rs. 12,000 per month has got the ration card which she mostly uses as a document for identity.

Health Care Services in Kusumpur Pahari

There is no denying the fact that for majority of the poor priority for health comes at the end because livelihood plays the pivotal role in their life, then shelter and finally, health. (Kapadia-Kundu and Kanitkar 2002; Kumar et al. 2003; Sharma and Sita 2000; Sundar and Sharma 2002). Health services inside the slum are a mix of voluntary sector and private sector. The nearest government health facility is located at the distance of 1 km. It is the Safdarjung hospital which is about 10 km away. There are two health centres run by the voluntary sectors. These centres are mostly focused on immunization of children, antenatal care of the mother and child care. There is a weekly mobile homeopathic clinic that comes to slum every Monday.

Reported Illness Among Household Members

Poor water and sanitary conditions lead to adverse health outcomes in the households living in the slums (Duggal and Sucheta 1989; Nandraj et al. 1998; Karn et al. 2003). Morbidity of any kind was reported by 53 families. From among them, most of the family members reported to have suffered from common fever (56 %) followed by cough and cold (22 %). Other ailments like diarrhoea and pneumonia was reported by about 6 % each. Conjunctivitis (2 %) and fracture of limb (2 %) was also reported (Fig. 4).

Private facilities as well as informal health services are also present in the slum. Private facilities are present in the form small clinics. Kusumpur Pahari also has numerous chemist shops and informal/local health providers. The informal health providers are also called "Bengali doctor" and sometimes just 'doctor', who are in demand mostly for providing health services at a very low rate. We tried to study the health seeking behaviour keeping in mind the issue of availability, accessibility and affordability. The residents of the slum approach the local health provider/informal health providers because of the following reasons

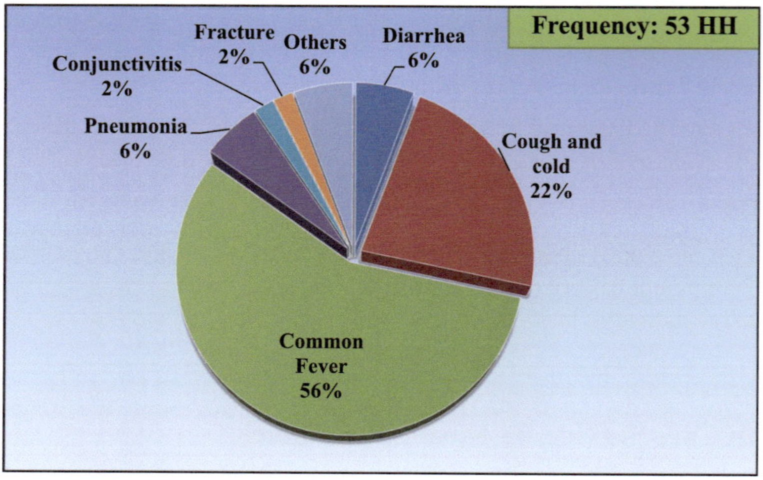

Fig. 4 Different types of diseases. *Source* prepared from the primary data collected from the study site (authors own source)

- The people trust the local health provider,
- The proximity is playing an important role,
- They do not take money during the initial visits,
- They talk nicely to patients and give them respect,
- Use of injection plays an important role for the residents.

Maternal and Child Health

Prevalence of illness was higher in the slums than in the resettlement areas (Sundar and Sharma 2002). Studied maternal and child health in urban Maharashtra by surveying 8,575 women, living in slums, council towns and municipal corporations, who had delivered within 12 months or less of the survey. In the slums, only 34 % women reported a birth interval of more than three years, while in the nonslum areas it was 51 %. With regard to women's health, a study was conducted by Institute of Medical Health, Pune in 1998 in 27 slums in Pune. The study revealed that 44 % of women did not take treatment for Reproductive Tract Infections. People resort to diverse source of health care for antenatal care, delivery and postnatal care. Although this slum is located at the heart of the city the deplorable condition of mother and child health can be witnessed here as people still practise home delivery with the help of traditional birth attendants (*dais*) with minimal/no antenatal care or no vaccination of the children under age of five.

Reliance on government facility for delivery is prominent in the area as going to private facility will mean high expenditure. Nonetheless people do go to private

Table 8 Income quintile and medical assistance during birth

Income quintile	No		Yes		Total	
	No.	%	No.	%	No.	%
1	24	82.8	5	17.2	29	100
2	19	59.4	13	40.6	32	100
3	19	61.3	12	38.7	31	100
4	14	60.9	9	39.1	23	100
5	9	33.3	18	66.7	27	100
Total	85	59.9	57	40.1	142	100

Source prepared from the primary data collected from the study site (authors own source)

hospitals for delivery as they are not satisfied with the functioning of government services. Women felt that the time spent waiting is very high in Safdarjung hospital. Moreover, they are not happy with the kind of service they get. One of the women narrated her experience as follows:

> These doctors get money from the government. They treat us as if we are 'coming from the streets'. They give the same medicine for cold, cough, fever etc. I really wonder that how can they write the medicine for us without checking us properly. It's all about the game of money and power. If we will look nice they will talk to us nicely. (In-depth Interview, women aged 23, Block A)

Health seeking behaviour for maternal and child health to a large extent was determined by the income and the disparity also followed the same line. But certain cultural norms also influenced the utilization of MCH services and it was evident in case of immunization of children, use of ICDS services and assistance during time of delivery.

About 60 % women of the study households did not use any assistance during birth. The share of those who used, however, increases with each income quintile. About 67 % of those who used are from the fifth income quintile (Table 8).

It is evident from the study that different sources are used for accessing care. As regards place of delivery, of the total 141 reported during the study period, about 69 % were at home, followed by 25 % at the Primary Health Centre (PHC) or the dispensary (Table 9). Most home (79 %) and PHC/Dispensary (28 %) deliveries were in the income quintile three. Only one delivery was reported to have occurred in private hospital in income quintile one.

Social Constraints in Nutrition and Breastfeeding

Gender discrimination becomes quite evident not only in terms of education but also nutrition. Girls eat after all the men and boys have eaten. Even when no one is at home, the socialization process has been such that the consciousness towards one's own health is absent. The girls reported in the focus group discussion (FGD)

Table 9 Place of delivery and income quintile

Income quintile	Home		PHC/state dispensary		Government hospital		Private hospital		Total	
	No.	%	No.	%	No.	%	No.	%	No.	%
1	23	76.7	5	16.7	1	3.3	1	3.3	30	100
2	20	62.5	9	28.1	3	9.4	0	0	32	100
3	23	79.3	5	17.2	1	3.4	0	0	29	100
4	16	69.6	5	21.7	2	8.7	0	0	23	100
5	15	55.6	11	40.7	1	3.7	0	0	27	100
Total	97	68.8	35	24.8	8	5.7	1	0.7	141	100

Source prepared from the primary data collected from the study site (authors own source)

that often they do not cook if alone and eat whatever is left over. Certain cultural practices prevalent in their native rural continue in the city of their choice too. This increases their vulnerability. The women of the *Paasi* community (Scheduled Caste) stated-

> … after delivery the mother can breast feed only when the Pandit (local priest) allows and he usually says after two days. Then the breast is cleaned with warm water and the feeding begins. (In-depth Interview, Women aged 36, Block B

This effectively means that the infant is missing out on the immunity producing colostrums. In some communities, the practice is to clean the breasts with the paste of the leaves plucked from the trees and then the colostrums is squeezed out near the tree close to the place of worship.

Issues and Concerns

The foregoing analysis needs to be placed within the socio-economic and cultural framework so as to identify the various strands of social, cultural, economic and other constraints of the vulnerable groups in access and equity of health services. Even though the RCH programme emphasizes the need to speak about women in the context of development, much of the efforts revolve around finding medical solutions to women, and children's health problems. There is a need to visualize health in the context of overall development, which involves effectively addressing the issues of literacy, nutrition, gender inequalities and social discrimination.

Generally the very poor go to the government hospital and those who are a relatively well-off go to the private practitioners. The Traditional Birth Attendant (TBA) and the private doctor ask for Rs. 500 each time they deliver a baby. Often people ask them to reduce the charges, but believed that:

> …everybody becomes poor when it comes to giving money for deliveries.

Quite often the women go for check-ups only after four months of pregnancy when there is stomach ache or vomiting; and their work starts getting affected-

> …Doctor told me I was in my fifth month …I was thinking it was just the beginning of the fourth month.

Although they seem to be fairly conscious about immunization of the children, they do not appear to be very regular in taking medicines, weight and blood pressure for themselves as expectant mother. So, most of them are contacting the health care service providers or visiting the facilities almost half way through the pregnancy. The economic factor is essentially impacting the health behaviour of the vulnerable population (FGD, 4 Block A).

Utilization of Services

Utilization of care and counselling services depended on the availability of providers. In the study area, availability was poor. Some of those available were used while others were not for reasons as varied as distance, time, availability of the provider and awareness regarding the availability of the service(s). The youth in Kusumpur Pahari considered the services at the nearby hospital as satisfactory. However, they did point out the shortage of medicines and the *out-dated equipment like tubes and syringes being used.* In contrast to this some young people preferred private doctors since they were nearer to their residence as compared to the district hospital (FGD, 2 Block D). They also pointed out that the doctors do not come to the center regularly and punctually. A young adult said,

> … after coming so far to the Centre, when the doctor is not there then, we have no other option but to go to the private doctor. (In-depth Interview, a Man aged 20, Block C)

Experience of Caste Discrimination in Accessing Health Services

Respondents in the study area have reported accounts of caste discrimination prevalent in the ICDS centers. One of the respondents said that children from the *Dalit* community are seated separately from those belonging to other castes for mid-day meal programme. The ANMs and other health workers visit the *Dalit* households less frequently. Like their native villages, they live in the outskirts of the slums too. Most of the part inhabited by them is poorer in already poor infrastructure. The drains are mostly open and often overflowing, with water supply and electricity often missing. There are evidences of street brawl due to caste identity related reasons at the time of filling water from the tanker which is a major source of water.

Spheres and Forms of Discrimination

In the spheres of discrimination such as dispensing of medicine, counselling, waiting, conduct of pathological tests; no evident experiences was reported. However, subtle references such as *'tumko toh sab kuch muft mein milta hai...'*[2] was reported by one of the users in reference to the caste status and affirmative action for education and job (in-depth Interview, women aged 37, Block A). Dispensing of medicine was perceived as the most discriminating sphere by most users. Consulting the care providers for referral was least discriminating in terms of perception as well as experience. As regards the forms of discrimination, physical immediate expressions of interaction—touch (tough roughly/do not touch) and conversation (speak gently) appear to be the areas perceived as most discriminating. The providers of health care services are perceived as most discriminating by most users (FGD1, Block D). The users suggest that public sector providers are more discriminating.

Discussion

The concept of health as a right and therefore the need to demand services as a right is all-together absent for the youth. In fact, the study interviews reflect the viewpoint that the health system is being perceived by the communities as a bureaucratic government operation which must be availed of services only when absolute necessary and that too rather guardedly.

Regular house-to-house contact by health workers essentially needs to be taken up to reach the majority of the vulnerable populations. The objective of the household contact is to inform the communities about the health facilities available and to inform them about the general as well as reproductive health issues; facilities available for treatment and ways and means to prevent any form of infections.

Camps can be organized separately for men and women target groups. This would need active collaboration between the PHCs/Urban Health Post, voluntary organizations/NGOs, private practitioners, community opinion leaders, youth groups, women *sangathans/mahila mangal dals*/Self Help Groups, literacy groups and other such civil/volunteer groups. Each camp needs to be attended by male and female health workers separately and assisted by community volunteers/peer educators. The health workers need to discuss the problems of the target group in reference to cases, symptoms and complications. They also need to disseminate information on transmission and its prevention and control of diseases which

[2]When translated, literally means that the one being spoken to gets everything free of cost. The reference is being made to the perception of high caste of the reservation policy which enables the vulnerable population to access certain resources and services. This was evident from one of the in-depth interviews.

are seasonal and can be prevented by little care. Health care workers would be required to keep a record for those who are referred for treatment so that they can make follow-up visits to ensure complete cure of the patients.

References

Acharya, S. (2002). Health care utilisation in rural north India—A case of Nirpura, District Meerut. Study undertaken as part of the MHSP, CSMCH-EU Project. Unpublished Report. Centre of Social Medicine and Community health, School of Social Sciences. Jawaharlal Nehru University. New Delhi.

Duggal, R., & Sucheta, A. (1989). *Cost of health care: A household survey in an indian district*. Bombay: Foundation for Research in Community Health/ICMR Sponsored.

IIPS. (1995). *National Family Health Survey (MCH and Family Planning), India 1992–93*. Bombay: International Institute for Population Sciences (IIPS).

IIPS and ORC Macro International. (2000). *National Family Health Survey (NFHS-2), 1998–99*: India . Mumbai: International Institute for Population Sciences (IIPS).

IIPS and Macro International. (2007). *National Family Health Survey (NFHS-3), 2005–06*: India: Volume I Mumbai: Institute for Population sciences (IPS).

Kapadia-Kundu, N., & Kanitkar, T. (2002). Primary healthcare in urban slums. *Economic and Political Weekly*, December 21.

Karn, S. K., Shikura, S., & Harada, H. (2003). Living environment and health of urban poor. *Economic & Political Weekly, XXXVIII*(34) (August 23, 2003), 3575–3586.

Kulkarni, P. M., & Baraik. (2003). Utilisation of health care services by scheduled castes in India. Working Paper IIDS. New Delhi.

Kumar, S., Shigeo, K., & Harada, H. (2003). Living environment and health of urban poor: A study in Mumbai. *Economic and Political Weekly*, August 23.

Nandraj, S., Madhiwalla, N., Sinha, R., et al. (1998). *Women and health care in mumbai: A study of morbidity, utilisation and expenditure on health care in the households of the metropolis*. Mumbai: Centre for Enquiry into health and Allied Themes.

Ram, F., Pathak, K. B., & Annamma, K. I. (1998). *Utilisation of health care services by the underprivileged section of population in India—Results from NFHS*.

RGI. (2002). *Rajasthan data highlights: The scheduled castes, census of India 2001*. http://www.censusindia.net/scstmain/dh_sc_rajasthan.pdf

Sharma, R. N., & Sita, K. K. (2000). *Cities*. Economic and Political Weekly, October: Slums and Government. 14.

Sundar, R., & Sharma, A. (2002). Morbidity and utilisation of healthcare services: A survey of urban poor in Delhi and Chennai. *Economic and Political Weekly*, November 23.

Thorat, S. (2002). Oppression and denial: Dalit discrimination in the 1990s. *Economic and Political Weekly, 37*(6) (Feb 9–15).

Thorat, S., Mahamalik, M., & Panth, A. S. (2006). Caste, occupation and labour market discrimination—A study of forms, nature and consequences in Rural India. Indian Institute of Dalit Studies. Study Sponsored by ILO, New Delhi.

Zurbrigg, S. (1984). *Rakku's story: Structures of ill health and the source of change*. Bangalore: Centre of Social Action.

Life on Streets: Health and Living Conditions of Children in Delhi

G. Dilip Diwakar

Abstract 'Street-living Children' is the most vulnerable category among the street children as they are living alone without any adult protection. The study was conducted to fill the gaps in the available literature on understanding the life at street and their experience in seeking care from public health institutions. The study also attempted to examine how various factors interplay in determining the life of the street children. Information on health problems and pattern of health seeking behaviour was also sought from the health providers. The study was conducted in two locations of New Delhi that is Hanuman Temple and New Delhi railway station. In-depth interviews and focus group discussions with children were used for understanding their health condition and experience of public institutions. Doctors, paramedics, NGOs workers, shopkeepers, police personnel and other key personnel were also interviewed to get a comprehensive understanding on the problems of street children. The study showed that they ran away from home at a very early age to escape from the coercive environment. However, the life at street makes them more vulnerable to physical and sexual abuse, harassment by police and lack of access to basic amenities. The constant threat and coercion enforced made them to act coercively towards others and get addicted to drugs to cope with the harsh realities. Some of them do involve in crime and other delinquent behaviours. The poor living condition and harassing environment predispose them to high level of morbidity in the form of accidents, injuries and infectious disease. The negative experience with public health institutions leads to delayed health seeking which in turn aggravates their health problems. Most of the time they seek treatment in emergency care unit. Based on the findings this paper proposes some suggestions and recommendation to address the problem of the street children in Delhi.

G. Dilip Diwakar (✉)
Department of Social Work, Central University of Kerala, Kerala, India
e-mail: dilipjnu@gmail.com

S.S. Acharya et al. (eds.), *Marginalization in Globalizing Delhi: Issues of Land, Livelihoods and Health*, DOI 10.1007/978-81-322-3583-5_19

Keywords Street children · Health condition · Exclusion · Coercion · Health-seeking behaviour

Introduction

Migration of adults is mainly the effect of both push and pull factors. However, the reason for children landing up in the city varies from that of the adult. Though majority of the adults were attracted and pulled towards the cities for better opportunities but in case of children it was mostly the push factors which forced them to land up in the nearby cities and towns. Some of the reasons were (1) To escape from family problems including rejection, (2) To escape from work demands in the home, (3) To earn money for themselves and support their families, (4) To find shelter (WHO n.d).

The street children problem gained political, academic and international concern recently in late 1980s and early1990s. Because of the magnitude and increasing number of street children in Latin America and other developing countries, street children are called by different names in different countries. In the developed country they are labelled as 'homeless youth', 'runaways' or even 'throwaways'. In developing countries street children are named after their main survival activities. In India they are called mainly as rag pickers (WHO 1993). There is no recent official data on the number of street children, the UNICEF survey indicated, there are about 100 million street children in the world and in India there are about 11 million street children (Kant 2004; Benitez 2011). As per the recent survey of Save the Children in association with Institute for Human Development, in Delhi there are about 51,000 street children (Nayar 2011).

UNICEF categorized Street children into three categories based on their relationship with families—(1) street-living children, (2) street-working children, and (3) children from street families. Street-living children are who ran away from their families and live alone on the streets. Street-working children are who spend most of their time on the streets fending for themselves, but return home on a regular basis. Children from street families are who live on the streets with their families. According to UNODC (http://www.unodc.org) there are four categories of street children they are (1) child on the street, (2) child of the street, (3) child a part of a street family, (4) child in institutionalized care.

Of these categories 'street-living children' are the most vulnerable as they are living alone without any adult protection. They have been physically, sexually and psychologically harassed by the police, government authorities, elderly peers, employers and other miscreant elements. Public authorities and police have the opinion that street children are juvenile delinquents and they involve in all illegal activities. However, a sociological understanding informs that they live in a coercive environment both with the family later on the street which forces them to involve in delinquent behaviour.

Street children are excluded from the main society and deprived of food, education, shelter, and even live without the basic necessities such as sufficient potable water, sanitation, and health services. After they reach the city/town they mostly stay in railway station, bus stops and terminal, under bridge, pavement, etc. They were denied of all the basic rights including their childhood. This study was conducted with an aim to understand the poor living condition and harassing environment which predispose them to high level of morbidity in the form of accidents, injuries and infectious disease. The negative experience with public health institutions further leads to delayed health seeking which in turn aggravates their health problems. Most of the time they seek treatment in emergency care unit. This paper will propose some suggestions and recommendation to address the problem of the street children in Delhi.

Theories on Child Delinquency and Crime

The biological and psychological theories exist long back to understand delinquent behaviour of human being. However, the relatively newer stream, the sociological theories on delinquency gave much comprehensive understanding on the delinquent behaviour. As human being is a social animal and the social surrounding plays a dominant role in changing his behaviour and it is an intrinsic characteristics. There are many social theories which tried to explain crime and delinquency of the juveniles some of them were

(1) Stain theory by Robert K. Merton,
(2) Differential Association Theory by Edwin H. Sutherland's
(3) Social learning theory by Arnold Akers
(4) Social control theory, by Travis Hirschi and self-control by Gottfredson and Hirschi
(5) Differential Coercion Theory by Colvin

Though there are many other theories in Criminology to understand the crime and delinquency, the theories which could be of some help to understand the nature and behaviour of runaway children were taken for discussion in this paper the other theories were not discussed.

The Stain theory mentions that nonconforming behaviour arises out of social circumstances in which individuals or groups experience normative confusion or disruption. Confronted with a new, traumatic, or frustrating social situation (social strain), some people respond in a deviant and perhaps criminal manner. Merton had identified five possible behavioural patterns for individuals while they respond to culturally approved goals and institutionalized means for achieving those idealized goals. There are (a) Conformity, (b) Innovation, (c) Ritualism, (d) Retreatism and (e) Rebellion. Of these typology the retreatism is rejecting both the culturally approved goals and institutionalized means. As it seems to them unachievable so they get frustrated and retreat from social system and culture. The runaway children could be part of this category as they move out of family and also indulge in drug, alcohol and delinquent activities without having any goal in life. However, this theory does not explain the factors contributing for the children to make this decision. Their living condition, the struggle they encounter in the family due to poverty or other structural problem are not discussed. Moreover, it was not explained where they learn this behaviour from nor the role of family and friends (Thompson and Bynum 2013).

The differential association theory mentions that criminal behaviour is learned through interactions with other people. Through the interaction and communication with the people involved in criminal activities they learn their values, attitudes, techniques and motives. The greater the frequency, duration and intensity in those environment they are more likely to become deviant. It does not focus on why they become criminal or the structural factors into account. The primary group, family and friends, in the early childhood provide the learning of both conforming and nonconforming activity. In the adolescence along with family the school, leisure, recreational and peer groups form the primary group. The secondary and reference groups can also indirectly provide the context for learning if an individual differentially associates themself with the behaviour, norms, values, attitudes and beliefs. The priority, duration and intensity of the association have influence on the behaviour. However, Aker when talks about the Social learning theory he sees differential association as only one part of the learning and he mentions that other factors which influence a person's behaviour are the definition, differential reinforcement and imitation (Aker and Jenning 2009). Though this theory partially addresses where the children learn the nonconformity behaviour. However, the learning of nonconformity behaviour alone cannot explain fully why the children run away from the family, as there are many children with nonconforming behaviour continues to stay at home. Secondly, it does not explain why some children are pushed to an environment where they learn nonconforming behaviour, whereas, other children escape from those environment even they also live in the similar circumstances.

Social Control asserts that ties to family, school and other aspects of society serve to diminish one's propensity for deviant behaviour, when these links become weak or are not well established. Unlike the social learning theory which tries to explain why people engage in deviant behaviour it tries to explain why people refrain from criminal behaviour. The attachment to those within and outside family, commitment to activities in which an individual has invested time and energy, involvement and the belief in wider social values thought to interact and affect individual behaviour. The Self-control theory forms the general theory borrowing notions from routine activities theory, ration choice theory and other psychological theories on crime. It illustrates the process of occurance of crime as follows (1) an impulsive personality to (2) lack of self-control to, (3) the withering of social bonds to, (4) opportunities to commit crime and delinquency and (5) deviant behaviour. Though it explains the minor offending, however, these theories does not help us to understand the behaviour of runaway children. As children are mostly forced or coerced to move out of the family and not because of impulsive personality (Ministry of Children and Youth Services n.d).

Colvin (2000) defines coercion as a force that compels one to act because of the fear or anxiety that it creates. Coercion is experienced in interpersonal and impersonal contexts, the interpersonal contexts of coercion are the control relationships that one encounters in various settings, including the family, school and governmental agencies. Impersonal contexts of coercion include the economy or any other structural situation beyond one's control. Finally, Colvin argues that individuals are not passive receivers of coercion. Through their responses to coercive control, they elicit more coercive control leading to a continuous "vicious cycle" of coercion. The coercion may cause social-psychological deficits that may increase the propensity to nonconforming activity. Repeated exposure to coercion may lead to weak social bond to the authority figure. Further, an individual's confidence to create positive outcomes or prevail against outside forces is diminished, lowering their self-efficacy, self-control and creating a feeling of powerlessness (Colvin 2000; as cited by Gaspar 2013).

Coercion also takes away an individual's ability to act for his or herself, creating an external locus of control. Colvin theorizes four possible relationships. These are: (1) type I, consistent, non-coercive; (2) type II, erratic, non-coercive; (3) type III, consistent, coercive; and (4) type IV, erratic, coercive. Each relationship varies on the schedule of coercion it delivers, the various social-psychological deficits it creates, and the criminal involvement it fosters. The type IV erratic, coercive control is characterized by inconsistent punitive reactions to non-compliance and weak to non-consistent social support. The inconsistent monitoring of behaviour aids in the development of low self-control, allowing the individual to get away with behaviour at times, giving them some sense of autonomy (ibid).

Erratic coercive discipline in the home will foster coercive behaviour in a child. It develops social-psychological deficits in the child including anger, low self-control, control imbalances, and coercive behaviour modelling. Children who display social-psychological deficits in school are more likely to be placed under tight control structures. So, the children were not allowed to involve in pro-social activities which makes the children frustrate. This theory helps to understand the situation of the children who take drastic decision like to run away from home to escape from the coercive environment both in family, school and locality. However, it does not explain where they get the information/learning on living an independent life in the cities and towns street (ibid).

Second, to understand the health status of a population we need to understand the interaction between host, environment and agents, health is very complex subject. To identify the determinants, we need to understand the dynamics of the interaction between the host, environment and the agent. The biological factors, social, economic, political, demographic and cultural factors and factors in the form of active intervention are specifically designed to change the epidemiological behaviour of the health problems (Banerji 1973). The application of medical technology also plays a role in determining the health problems.

The health condition of the street children can be understood by studying their physical environment, social environment and the agents. Socio-economic and cultural factors helps to understand the host. The living condition and access to basic amenities, demography helps to understand the environment. In case of street children the disease causing agent though has a role to play, however, mainly the physical and social environment and their living condition acts indirectly as agent and causes disease to the children. The runaway children do not seek treatment immediately after any illness because of the coercive environment in which they live and because of lack of support system like family.

Conceptual Framework

Impersonal context of coercion faced by the children because of poverty and unemployment in the rural villages affects the poor families. Some cope with the help of friends, relatives and caste networks, however, others have very difficult times to manage the families. The financial constraint in the family to meet the everyday needs force the children to move out of school and take work at a very early age. The children not readily accept to take up work at that young age when other children in the villages go to school and play with friends and siblings.

The structural factors do affect the interpersonal relationship in the family. The parents get busy with work to manage the daily subsistence. Not able to give much care and love for the children, their monitoring on the activities of the children become irregular and weak. They use coercive method when they find out they are not going to school regularly, not showing interest in studies or not willing to participate in work to support them financially. In some cases the alcoholic, step father/mother and siblings, physically abuse them when they are not conforming to their expectation. The erratic coercion used by parents/sibling might create frustration and anger in the children. This may also create social-psychological deficits among the children. This further pushes them in coercive environment in the school and peers. Even in the schools they face problems due to the social-psychological deficits. As suggested by the Merton it forces the children to retreat from the culturally approved goals and the institutional means. When they encounter people who have also rejected culturally approved goals and the institutional means and having nonconformity attitude they get along with them well. Also learn their values, norms, attitudes, belief and behaviour. The propensity and the duration with them change their values and norms and intensify their belief. This instigates the children to move out of the family in search of an autonomy and freedom.

The hostile situation in the street and struggle to get the food, shelter and basic services further intensifies their problem. The coercion from the police, government authority, employer and peers make them believe in coercive ideation. Start using coercion to make their ends meet. They get addicted to drugs to survive the hostile situation in the street. Also get involve in delinquent activities to get food and drugs. As their survival in the street become difficult they are not bothered to meet their health needs even when they fall sick. As the doctors do not approve their nonconformity attitude and expect them to take medicine regularly and stop drugs. They avoid taking treatment as long it becomes life threatening.

Research Design and Methodology

This study was done at two levels by reviewing the literature at the first level and second used the qualitative information collected in the primary study to bridge the gap. Institute for Human Development (IHD) with the support of 'Save the Children'[1] have carried out a census study on street children in Delhi in 2011. The

[1]An nongovernmental organization working for the rights of the children.

report will be used to understand the situation of street children. To understand the existing gap in the report the qualitative information from the primary study conducted will be used. Especially the health problems and the health seeking behaviour of the children were not captured in the IHD report, the finding from the primary study will substantiate those information. Additionally, the literature from government documents, document available online, books, NGOs publications and articles were studied. Literature on status and living condition, deviant behaviours, health problems, and health seeking behaviour are reviewed.

The IHD census study was carried out during July–August 2010. This study will provide information on their geographical location, nature, demographic profile and details about night shelter. The qualitative data was collected during September–January 2005 in two commercial hubs, namely New Delhi Railway Station and Hanuman Temple (Cannought place) in New Delhi. About 20 street children were selected, 10 from each area for the in-depth interview. Apart from them eight key informant interviews (NGO's, police, shop owners and public) were conducted. To understand the health seeking behaviour and health problem of street children 9 doctors and 3 paramedics were interviewed. Four focused group discussions were conducted among the children, 2 from each area.

During the fieldwork, the first one month was spent to build rapport with the children. It was felt gaining confidence of the children and getting acquainted with the area before the actual data collection was important. This one month time period helped a lot to build a good working relationship with the children. Latter in the month of January, the data collection was started it took 3 months to complete the data collection in both the area and with other key informant.

The study used mixed methods of data collection, quantitative informations were taken from IHDS survey and qualitative information were collected from the field. In-depth interviews were conducted with the children, health personnel and other official coming in contact with the children. Other techniques used include quasi-participant observation and focused group discussion. A semi structured interview schedule was adopted to understand the life of these children.

Key Findings

i) Children's Profile

The census study carried out by Institute for Human Development (hereafter IHD) identified about 50,923 children below the age of 18 living and working in the streets. Of these children about 36 % are children from street families, 29 % street-working children and 28 % street-living children and 7 % no response. There are about only 20 % girls found on the street including all categories. Majority 61 % of the children are above 6 years and below 15 years (Table 1).

The qualitative study was undertaken among 20 street children in Hanuman Temple (Connaught Place) and New Delhi Railway Station also reflected majority 16 children were above 6 and below 15 years (Fig. 1).

Table 1 Distribution of types of street children

Type of children	Population	Percentage
Children on road/street	14,214	27.9
Children on road/street working	14,793	29.0
Children on road/street people	18,350	36.0
No response	3566	7.0
Total	50,923	100

Source Institute for Human Development & Save the Children 2011

Fig. 1 Distribution of the social group. *Source* Institute for Human Development 2011

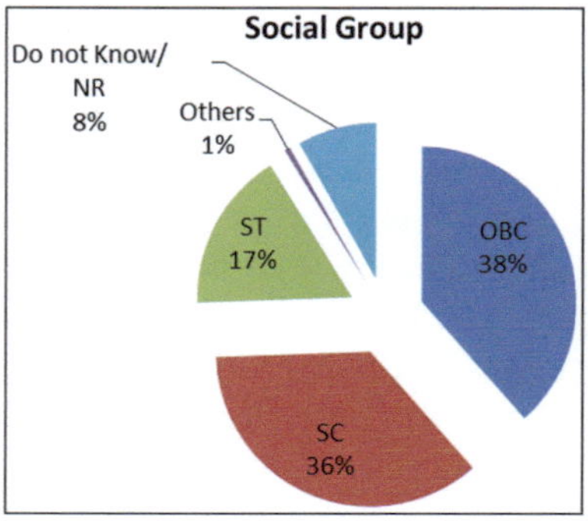

Data on Social group shows about 36 % belong to Scheduled Caste, 38 % from Other Backward Caste, 17 % from Scheduled Tribe and less than 1 % belonged to ‘Others’ category. This clearly shows more number of SC and ST children are in the street in proportion to their population. However, in case of others it is very less; it implies the poverty and vulnerability faced by the children in the lower caste are more. The religion wise classification shows about 75 % belong to Hindus, 17 % Muslim, 1 % Christians and the remaining did not answer (Table 2).

While looking at the education status of the children the data shows about 50.5 % of the street children were not literate. Only 23 % had received some form of informal education and another 20 % had received some kind of education (13 % pre-primary; 4 % up to primary; and 2.4 % up to middle school).

Table 2 Education status of the children

Education level	Total	Percentage
Illiterate	25,716	50.5
Informal	11,829	23.2
Below Primary	6682	13.1
Primary	2054	4.0
Middle	1222	2.4
Secondary and above	102	0.2
NR	3318	6.5
Total	50,923	100

Source Institute for Human Development & Save the Children 2011

Table 3 Type of occupation

S. No	Type of occupation	Total	Percentage
1	Begging	7479	14.7
2	Rag picking	10,354	20.3
3	Sell flower, newspaper, fruits and other item on the road	7728	15.2
4	Cleaning cars and two wheelers	3838	7.5
5	Working in roadside stall or repair shop	6188	12.2
6	Working in small hotel or tea stall	2085	4.1
7	Whatever available	4629	9.1
8	Working in manufacturing units	621	1.2
9	Others	2701	5.3
10	NR	5300	10.4
	Total	50,923	100.0

Source Institute for Human Development & Save the Children 2011

Even the qualitative in-depth interview with the children in Hanuman Temple and New Delhi Railway station also informed that majority of the children are illiterate or studied below primary (Table 3).

While looking at the occupation pattern of the children, the data shows about 20 % of the children engaged in rag picking and the second majorly about 16.3 % engage in road side stall (including hotel and tea stall), third about 15.2 % engaged in street vending (sell flower, newspaper, fruits and other items on the road), fourth about 14.7 % engaged in begging and the remaining engage in other jobs which are available readily for them.

Even in the Hanuman Temple and New Delhi railway station all most everyone in New Delhi Railway station and few in Hanuman temple are engaged in rag picking, and some of the children in Hanuman temple work in the food and flower stall during Tuesday and Friday. Some of them engage as server in the party and carry light on the head during marriage season.

NDC3 a resident of New Delhi Railway while explaining his work pattern, he said

> …we collect water bottle and food mostly from Rajdhani and Shatabdi train.[2] Even we check trains, which terminate at New Delhi Railway Station. Because in these trains we get lot of bottles so we prefer these trains. We can earn up to Rs 50-60 in a train. If we check in more trains we can earn more than 150. It mainly depends upon how many people are competing in a train. I collects bottle alone but some children collect bottles in groups and share the money after they sell the mall (heap of bottles).

HTC8, while sharing about his nature of work he described that:

> *"In Hanuman Temple I go for catering work they paid Rs. 110 per day for 24 h work. It is very strenuous and it is only a seasonal job".*

[2]They are special trains, which provides food for all the passenger packed in aluminium foil.

Table 4 Reason for landing up in street

S. No.	Reason for landing up in street	Frequency	Percentage
1	Ran away from home	2783	5.5
2	Parent sent me away	6409	12.6
3	In search of jobs/income	9001	17.7
4	Came with family members	9903	19.4
5	Lost family while travelling/ visit	723	1.4
6	Lost family during calamity	309	0.6
7	Kidnapped	256	0.5
8	There was abuse	210	0.4
9	Poverty/hunger	17,323	34.0
10	Just landed here	191	0.4
11	Others	202	0.4
12	NR	3613	7.1
Total		50,923	100.0

Source Institute for Human Development & Save the Children 2011

HTC6 is from U.P, shared about his work nature:

During the marriage season we go for carrying light. They pay Rs 60-70 per night. Most of the time we have to carry the light for a long distance along with the marriage procession. It creates body and backaches. Sometime even I also get pain in the chest. Even then without missing the opportunity I try to go for two marriages since it is seasonal job, I tried to capitalize the opportunity.

Reason for Landing in Street

The study of IHD shows majority 34 % landed up in street due to poverty and hunger, 37.1 % came with family/in search of jobs and income, about 12.6 % reported parents sent me away and 5.5 % reported they ran away from home (Table 4).

Coercion at Home

The qualitative information from Hanuman temple and New Delhi railway station on why the children ran away from home indicated that inter play of many factors pushed the children to streets out of home. Impersonal context and interpersonal context of coercion by poverty and interpersonal context of coercion in the family, school and peers played a major role in pushing them out. In some cases to support the family financially, they were discontinued from their studies. Many reported that they have to do both household chores and help in agriculture work if they deny or went out to play with other children they were beaten up.

HTC2, while he describe the reason for runaway, he said

Father passed away stayed so I stayed with his brother and sister-in-law. Though I do all the household work but my sister-in-laws complains to my brother, he beats me thinking that I have not done any work and went out to play. This frustrates me a lot.

Work at home leads to poor performance and later they dropped out of school. The heavy workload combined with lack of care and affection affected the children psyche negatively. They felt alienated from other children and did not find much time to mingle with other children and enjoy their childhood. The dejection by their parents and loneliness made them feel that there is no one to understand them and help them. Moreover, in schools they get severe punishment for not doing homework and poor performance.

HTC3, while he describe the reason for runaway, he said

> *Father passed away so I stayed at uncle home with my family. The poverty of family had infused in his mind that unproductive childhood are wasteful.*

The parents are illiterate could not help them in studies and they fail to motivate them. It creates anger and frustration among the children as they have to struggle both at home and outside (school/workplace). Even there are some cases that the children got used to smoke and use "gutka" (intoxicating tobacco/beetle nut) at their work place and their parents came to know and beaten them badly. In some case, the alcoholic father/sibling beat them for not going work and earning money.

Most of children come from outside reported that they have come in contact with someone who informed him about Delhi and that they can go there and have an independent life with more fun. Even the children ran away from home also learnt about the street life from some elders or known person. The hard life and recurring punishment instigated the children to move out of their home.

Coercion at Street—At the Work Place and while Accessing Basic Amenities

At Job Though they thought the life at street would be of fewer struggles. But, they were forced to work for more than 12 h in a day for low wage. Most of the hotel owners exploited them and they did not provide them food properly and were forced to sleep outside or sleep in a small room without proper ventilation. Even in many cases they were not paid their salary when asked they were physically abused. Most of them reported that they were verbally and physically abused by the employer for not concentrating on work and for not doing hard work. Sometime they were asked to work till late night if they refuse they were beaten up by the employer. If they ask for more food they were beaten, anything they ask to the employer they either physically or verbally abuse them, this has become part of their life.

NDC5, while describing about his job, he said

> *He worked in a hotel in New Delhi Railway Station for 2 months but when he asked for the salary, the owner refused to pay and had beaten him black and blue. The owner was a very awful person he not even gave him good food to eat. He left the job and moved to New Delhi Railway station with his street friends. Then he started collecting water bottles from the train.*

In the New Delhi railway station, they were not allowed to enter the station to collect the bottle. The police beat them whenever they see them in the station. The children said they were treated very badly just like a dog.

As the jobs are very limited there is always fight between the kids on who will get that work. On Tuesday and Friday the need 2–3 children to clean outside the temple and they get paid Rs.50. Usually the elder kids take the job if any new person attempts to do that job they will be beaten up by the elder kids. Similarly, in the railway station there will be fight who will first board the Shatabdi and Rajdhani train as they can get more bottles and aluminium foil in this train.

Sleep The roads are busy so till mid night they cannot sleep because of vehicle noise. The dust and smoke inhaled by children creates respiratory tract infection among these children. Tuesdays and Fridays are auspicious for Hanuman Temple so the place will be very busy all the shops will be open till 12 a.m. They have to sleep after all the shops are closed or after the city becomes calm and they have to get up early in the morning before the shop owner reaches there or the city wakes up. So, the children have to go to bed after that. In the railway station as the trains comes even during the night time they hardly get sleep. Along with that, when the railway police come for the visit in the morning they drive and chase them away. They hardly sleep 5–6 h in a day that too they get a very disturbed sleep.

NDC10 a respondent from New Delhi Railway Station describes the availability of place:

> *"Earlier we slept beneath the big peepal tree, but after the place got cleaned the police started drive us away from that place. So it is difficult to find a place to sleep".*

HTC5, while sharing about place to sleep, he described that:

> *"Usually they beat them while they were in deep sleep and they will not let them to sleep and they simply drove them away".*

During winters and rainy season they have more problems. In the winter for almost 3 months the weather is very harsh and sleeping in the street is very difficult. In the rainy season most of the places are wet so finding a shade and a dry place is very difficult. Mostly in those day they did not get sleep many days. The less sleep and constant threat creates psychological disturbance among children and makes them restless, moreover it also hampers the next day's work.

Peer Pressure and Coercion

The peers are the most influential part in the life of runaway children. As they do not have any support in the street they mainly depend upon each other for help. However, the relationship between them are not always smooth, most of the children reported that fights are very common among them. Fight happens even for small things and ends up in stabbing and severe injury. Whenever, a runaway child come to location, the elder peers living in the street try to dominate them and create lots of problem; beat them and tell them to move away from that place. Because the livelihood opportunities are very limited, it may invite more trouble to them. If they are submissive and listen to the demands of elder peers then they allow them to stay.

HTC8, while sharing about his nature of work he described that:

> *"Fight among them is very common, fails to pay money, steal money while asleep, garbing ones 'mall' (collected waste material) or his solution. They tease each other and it ends with fight with breaking head or stabbing with blade. Then after some days they will join together, because 'aak ungle se thali bachtha nahi'(in one hand we cannot clap)".*

Most of the children take some kind of drugs and become very aggressive even a casual talk end up in fight. The fight for them is showing of dominance, supremacy and power. So, whenever they felt threatened they will fight with the other to prove their dominance. Use of violence and force, as a principle ('coercion ideation'), to get things done, forms very strongly in the minds of the runaway children.

Having mark in the face is very common among the street children. Whenever, they have fight they put mark in the other person face to show everyone that he is weaker than him and has to listen to what he says. In each locality there are one or two children whom all the children are scared off. Some children keep the surgery blade in the mouth, they can drink water and eat while having blade in their mouth, nobody can identify that they are having blade in their mouth, if they have fight they use to offend the opponent.

HTC2, while he describe described about his mark on his face, he said

> *"Previously he was good looking and fair now he got a mark in his face, thinks he looks like criminal so he wants to stay away from family. Some days back in Phar Gang some kids snatched 400 and put a mark in his face with blade when he resisted giving money. This makes him as if looks like a 'gunda'(goons)".*

Drugs and Delinquent Behaviour

Most of the children are often in the clutches of drugs; the main reasons behind these are peer influence, to dominate other children, responding 'better' to outsider who are arrogant and rough, other children and authority, family problem, escaping reality, loneliness, to make themselves part of some group, to escape from the shivering cold, etc. They get addicted at their early age, some of them even at the age of eight. Mostly the street children are addicted to glues, nail polish, cigarette lighter refills, hair spray, paint thinner, gasoline, correction fluid, injections, alcohol, charas/ganja, and other pharmaceutical drugs. In the study area, the children mainly take solution correction fluid/whitener used for erasing (which has toluene, an intoxication substance), ganja (marijuana), bhang (an intoxicating substance made from the seeds of a fruit tree), *bidi (smoke made of tobacco rolled in dry leaves)*, *gutha*, smack (brown sugar) and cigarette.

They involve in petty crime during lean season and when they need money for the drugs. Mostly they involve in petty crimes to fulfil their basic needs in the street. None of the respondent has reported that they involve in big crime. Primarily they are very thin, weak so they do not involve in big crimes. When they have withdrawal syndrome from the drugs, they need money to have drugs (solution) it forces them to involve in illegal activities starting from stealing the money from other street children while sleeping, taking their collected bottles and stealing footwear from the temple to sell. They reported that some elder peers are involved in pickpocketing and robbery. Police beat the pickpockets and the thieves very brutally so they try to stay away from these big crimes.

HTC2, while describing his involvement in delinquent activities, he said

> *"If we have tootan (a physical state when they don't get drugs) during late night they will take stone or any object to threaten people to grab money. If they refused to give money*

they even break their head and steal the money from the passer-by. Even they will snatch mobile phone, pick pocket and steal during that time to get the drugs".

Shelter Home

Most of the children have been put in the shelter home, some stayed for months and few stayed for years. The children said the shelter home provides food, clothes, education, recreation and health facilities. Many of the children reported that they like to stay in the shelter home, however, most of them ran away from the homes because of their addiction to drugs, influenced by elder peers to escape and visit many places, beaten by the elder peers.

"He got shelter after few days of his arrival in PRAYAS, a NGO working for street children. Food, clothes, education, recreation and health facilities were provided in the shelter home. He liked the shelter, he stayed in the shelter for 1 ½ years then along with his friends he escaped from the shelter as he wanted to go visit many places in Delhi". (HTC5)

"He stayed in Salam Balak Trust (SBT) shelter home for last three years his seniors in the shelter home used to beat him whenever he tried to come out of the shelter for socializing with his old friends. He could not complain to the authority, which would irk the seniors again resulting into further beating so he ran away from shelter". (HTC7)

Some of the elder street children reported the children home has jail. There are lots of restrictions, the newly runaway child may like the home but the children stayed in the street for long time and got addicted to substances and enjoyed a free life will not like it and sees it as 'jail'.

"He was caught by police and put in Children Home, which he refers as 'jail'. He was there for 5 ½ months, then his father came and took him back home. He stayed in home for two months and again he ran away". (HTC10)

Most of the children reported that when they fall sick or met with an accident they approach the social worker and persuade them to stay at home. Once they recover they immediately run away from there and come back to street.

Aspiration

Most of the children did not believe in the culturally set goals and the institutional means to achieve it. This is also one of the reasons which made them to run away from home. The situation in which they lived was not conducive enough to have dreams and aspirations on their future live. So, they want to escape from that situation so they ran away from home in the aspiration for better life. However, life at street is much more difficult so it does not provide an opportunity to have aspirations and dreams. They said living each day is a struggle in the street, so they live life for that day.

They have very small aspiration like same money to go for films or visit different places. Some save money to visit home during festivals and not many of them had any aspirations. Second, the aspirations come from the social milieu and from the people surrounded by them, here, in the case of street children their surrounding the shop keepers, police authorities, government officials and general public sees them as delinquent, illegal resident and criminals. The people surround (other street children) them also live in the same condition, so they were not motivated and does not have any dreams or aspirations.

Health Problems of Street Children

The street children both in New Delhi Railway Station and Hanuman Temple do have access to potable drinking water, water for bathing, food to eat, place to sleep, and no sanitation facilities. All this makes the children prone to common illnesses along with this the drug use among children creates lots of respiratory disease. Interview with a recall period of 6 months for common illness and last 5 years for chronic illness revealed that they have fever, cough and cold, skin disease, cuts and wound, chest pain, stomach pain, dysentery, kidney problems, dog bites and rat bites, eye sight, mouth ulcer, respiratory problems, chicken pox, accidents, epilepsies, back pain, throat pain and blood vomit. The study accepts the presence of other diseases but these were seldom reported by the children.

The social worker who was one of the key informants, informed about Sexually Transmitted Infection (STI) among street children in Hanuman Temple. Even, researcher came across a child who had some problems in genital area so he took him to Kalawati Hospital there the doctor diagnosed the problem as STI. Later on, the child accepted that he had sexual intercourse with other street child and it was common among them. Even the social worker later conformed few other children in Hanuman Temple also face similar problem. The researcher came to know about this issue at the end of his field work, this made the researcher to realize that the children did not disclose all the information even after having good rapport and trust.

Except the chronic ailments like chest pain, kidney problem, respiratory problem, accidents, chicken pox and dog bite; rest of the ailments were faced by the children in the recall period of last 6 months. There were about 9 of them had cuts and wound due to accidents and fight; 8 of them had abdominal pain, fever this winter and respiratory problem; 7 had cold and cough in this winter; 5 of them had chicken pox and chest pain and 4 of them have skin problem. Moreover, they also face the rest of the above-mentioned problems. Many of them face more than one health problems. Here one thing to be noted is that the self-reported morbidity is very less among these children. Consequently, the number of health problems may go up if we do clinical examination.

Mostly the respiratory, kidney problems are related to sniffing of correction fluid (which has Toluene) by the street children. It is a clear, colourless liquid with a distinctive smell. It is used in making paints, paint thinners, fingernail polish, lacquers, adhesives, and rubber and in some printing and leather tanning processes. Low to moderate levels can cause tiredness, confusion, weakness, drunken-type actions, memory loss, nausea, loss of appetite, and hearing, colour vision loss and affect the nervous system. These symptoms usually disappear when exposure is stopped. Inhaling High levels of toluene in a short time can make one feel light-headed, dizzy, or sleepy. It can also cause unconsciousness, and even death. High levels of toluene may affect one's kidneys (http://www.atsdr.cdc.gov).

Utilization of Health Services

Children in Hanuman Temple and New Delhi Railway Station can avail services from the government hospital such as Kalawati Hospital, Lok Nayak Hospital, Lady Hardinge, Ram Manohar Lohia and NDMC Hospital. Apart from these hospitals, they can avail service also from mobile clinics and community-based health intervention by NGOs and shelter home. Children in New Delhi Railway Station have more options than the Hanuman Temple children. Many NGOs are working in New Delhi Railway Station which offers health services. Some bring general medicines during their visit to the locality, it helps the children to take medicine if they face any health problem. In case of serious illness the children prefer to go to Kalawati and Lok Nayak Hospital.

If they have major health problems or met with accidents, which hampers them from doing work then they go to the shelter home run by NGOs. They stay there till they recover and later they move out of the shelter.

NDC1, a resident of New Delhi Railway Station explained what he does if he falls sick:

> *"Very often I have fever; bhaiya (male social worker) took me to the hospital. Even this winter I had fever 3-4 times; I took medicine from didi (female social worker from Salaam Balak Trust) for cold and coughs. This winter I visited hospital 3 times to take treatment for chest pain, which I have stopped few months back, as the pain increased I visited hospital now. I have never visited hospital alone, they pose lot of quires and they will not treat me properly. So I always go with 'bhaiya', so that they will treat me well. 'Bhaiya' force the doctor to provide good treatment".*

Mostly the children go to hospital with the social worker, police, and with some well-wishers as they feel insecure going alone to the hospital. Even the youth above 18 years will not go to hospital alone. If children met with accidents, the information will be given to police. The case then becomes a Medio-Legal Case (MLC). Some times on seeing their pathetic condition or if they fall unconscious, some persons feel pity on them and take them to hospital.

Problems in Accessing Services

Though very few children accessed government health services, many of them availed services from the NGOs, pharmacist, etc. In both the areas, the 'Butterflies'[3] mobile clinic comes weekly. Many children prefer pharmacist as they were not satisfied with the treatment from the mobile treatment.

NDC2 explained why he does not prefer the mobile clinic:

> *"I had fever so I took medicine from the mobile clinic even after two days it did not recover. Latter I went to the pharmacist and I took medicine for Rs.2 and slept in the hot sun for some time, the fever immediately went off".*

Many children shared in the mobile clinic the tablets given were not effective and they do not recover quickly, however, they behave with them very well. Some go to the shelter home for treatment. The only problem is that they have to stay

[3]NGO working on health care provision for street children.

there so they prefer it only when they have major ailments. Regarding government hospitals, the following observation is relevant:

NDC5 a resident or New Delhi Railway Station shared his experience,

> *"Once I visited Kalawati Hospital, for a cut in my hand they did dressing and gave medicine. The hospital was very crowded so I was hesitant and scared to go to hospital. Moreover, I had to spend one half a day this treatment and also have to travel far to reach the hospital".*

Problems in Using Public Health Services

The children face lot of hindrances in accessing public health services as:

a. OPD will take at least 2–3 h and they have to wait in long queue. Moreover, they need some address to get the OPD card. So, they will not go to the OPD. Emergency care is only for accident cases, sudden acute pain, vomiting, respiratory problem, etc. If they go for minor illness they will send them back and refer them to OPD. So, only for the major ailments they go the hospital.
b. Hospitals will not provide all the medicines. Sometimes doctors prescribe medicine outside and they have to purchase medicine paying from their own pocket. So, they feel anyway we are purchasing the medicine from outside then why take pain to go to hospital.
c. Some children feel they have not received good treatment from public hospital. As, even after medication they do not get well soon.
d. Mostly they do not complete the full course of treatment, as they have to purchase medicines from outside medical shop. It scares them to meet the doctor again, if they have recurring problem.

They are very scared to move out of their locality as it may invite them lot of problem. Moreover, they were very scared to meet the doctor and other government officials. Most of the children felt that doctors wanted to avoid them; so they were asking them to shuttle unnecessarily from one place to another. Moreover, they were scared to explain their problem to the doctors.

Doctors' Perspective

The children experience gives the one sided view of the problem, to verify the facts, as well as to get an comprehensive understanding on their health problems the researcher approached the doctors and paramedics in the two nearby government hospital, Kalawati Saran Children's Hospital (here after it will be mentioned as H1) and Lok Nayak Hospital (here after it will be mentioned as H2). The children during the interview reported majority of them have visited these two institutions in case of emergency. So, these two institutions were selected for this purpose. Interviews with doctors in emergency care (causality ward), general physician and specialities like ENT, eye and orthopaedics were interviewed. Mainly the issues related health seeking behaviour, major health problems and the hurdles they face in accessing and utilization of health services from the institution were explored.

Utilization of Services by Street Children:

Three medical doctors from both the hospital were interviewed from the Casualty ward. They have conform that the street children come often but they never came alone, either they came with social worker, well-wisher or with police. They usually came across medico legal case with the street children. Three doctors from specialties like ENT and Eye were interviewed from H1; they told that they hardly came across street children. If at all they come they will not come alone they will come with some adults. An orthopaedic and a surgery doctor were interviewed in H2. They told that they mainly came across accident cases and the unknown cases came with police. They mainly come under MLC. H1SN told that "*We will treat them and refer them to some NGOs and rest they will take care*". Even the T.B health officer of H1 shares the same perception. He felt were very scared to approach the hospital to avail treatment.

Nature of Illness and Usage of Services

Almost all the doctors from both the hospitals said that street children come mainly for accidents, high fever, chest pain, wound, etc. H1SN said that they usually approached the hospital in death bed. H1D5 said that they never come to hospital for common illness. The orthopaedic, surgery doctor and the H1D5 of the emergency care said that mainly street children approach hospital for accident case that too police bring them to the hospital. Only H1D1 of general OPD said she come across children with all sort of ailments.

Majority of the doctors have a general opinion that the street children come for treatment which is irregular and liable to stop at any time. H1D1 said, *"they take treatment until they recover partially; after that they will not come. Even if they were hospitalized they stay in hospital without any caretaker. A street child was hospitalized stayed for 3 days after a partial recovery, he immediately ran off from the hospital. This is the same case with other hospitalized street children. They do not come regularly"*. H1D5 worked in psychiatry and drug de-addiction before he came to casualty ward. He said that there were many street children in the shelter home not having access to drugs. Somehow, they did not stay there for long time. They go out and steal things and start taking drugs. Initially they take drug out of curiosity and later they get addicted. They take drugs for reducing pain, sweating, lethargy, etc.

Most of the doctors reported that they do know that these children cannot afford to purchase the medicine outside, so they provide all the medicines which they could provide from the hospital. *"H1D1 said that in very rare case he prescribes medicines to purchase from outside shop"*. *"H1SN said that it is a lame reason that we are not providing medicine which stops them from taking treatment from the hospital"*. Most of the doctor also said that if they come with NGOs, they will get the medicines for the children. "*H2D2 said that he discharge street children with lots of drugs after their recovery*". We provide treatment without any discrimination whether they are rich or poor.

Suggestion and Recommendations

The poverty and coercion at home by the parents and sibling leave the children without love and affection. The family and society fail to build trust and hope in the life of the children. This leaves the children with anger and frustration. The children lose beliefs in the existing cultural goals and institutional means of achieving it, forces the children to lose belief in the existing institutions and structure. The excessive pressure, frustration, anger and coercion creates social-psychological deficits among the children. Even at the school and in the surrounding environment the children start facing similar problems. This forces the children to run away from home to escape from all problems. This is accentuated when people in similar situation provide a hope to have better life in the city. They run away from home and land up in street, however, the streets are worse than their home. But, they manage to eke out a living in that difficult situation. The condition of the children is further worsened when they get into the clutches of the addictive substances. When there is no or limited availability of children home to rescue then immediately they reach the street the situation worsens.

A proper prevention method is the most needed at this point of time to stop the children run away from home. The family should be oriented on not to use coercive methods on children. For the children in the street they need protection, rehabilitation and repatriation, that too at a very early stage. The children should be identified immediately after they land up in the street before they get addicted to the drugs. Otherwise the rehabilitation and repatriation becomes very difficult.

Proper counselling should be given to the parents and children before repatriation, so as to understand the problems better and avoid using coercive method and provide proper care and affection. This will help to address the problem so that the children will not be forced to run away from home again. The parents should be taught better parenting practices and not to use coercion so as to make the children's home a happier place to live in. The children also should be given proper counselling and bring hope and belief in the cultural goals and institutional means. Both family and the government should build necessary supportive system for the poor children to strengthen their hope and belief.

Street children face lot of minor and major health problems as the health institution is not much responsive they do not prefer to take treatment at the early stage, which worsens their condition further. So, the health system should be more responsive and approachable. Moreover, the environment in which they live has direct impact on their health condition, so as long as they stay in street there will not be any improvement in their health status.

For children in need of care and protection, currently, there are 60 registered home catering services to boys, girls and special children; it includes observation homes (Delhi Police Juvenile Justice Unit). However, the children home in Delhi are not child friendly, it lacks basic facilities, and they were treated harshly like delinquent children. They did not receive any sort of love, care and affection in the home. So the children does not prefer to stay at government, even they are scared because of ill-treatment. So, instead of staying at children home they prefer to stay in street at hostile weather. So, it is time for the government to make all its children home a "child friendly home". Proper education and vocational training should be given to the children to become economically self-sufficient and to contribute to the development of the nation.

Acknowledgments I take this opportunity to thank my guide Dr. Sanghmitra S. Acharya and Dr. Rajib Dasgupta for their support and valuable comments to bring in this work more meaning full. I would like to thank Dr. Sachidananda Sinha for giving very useful comments to make the paper more specific. I would also like to thank Varun and Asghar and other team members of Aman Biradari, organization working for street children in Delhi, and all the respondents for their support and cooperation to complete my M.Phil field work timely and meaning full manner. Usual disclaimers apply.

References

Aker, R., & Jenning, W. (2009). Social Learning Theory. in J. Miller (Eds), *21st Century Criminology: A Reference Hand Book.* (pp. 3223–332), Retrieved from Thousand Oaks: Sage Publication, Inc. doi:10.4135/9781412971997.n37

Banerji, D. (1973). *A Long Term Study in 19 Indian Villages.* Un published. Centre of Social Medicine and Community Health, Jawaharlal Nehru University. New Delhi: JNU.

Baron, S. W. (2009). Differential Coercion, Street Youth, and Violent Crime. *Criminology, 47*(1), 239–268.

Benitez, S.T. de (2011). *State of World's Street Children: Research.* Consortium for Street Children. Street Children Series 2. London.

Bhaskaran, R., & Balwant, M. (2011). *Surviving the Streets.* Institute for Human Development and Save the Children. New Delhi: Institute for Human Development. Retrieved from http://resourcecentre.savethechildren.se/sites/default/files/documents/5332.pdf

Colvin, M. (2000). *Crime and Coercion: An Integrated Theory of Chronic Criminality.* New York: St. Martin's Press.

Delhi Police Juvenile Justice Unit. Special police unit for women and children. Retrieved from http://www.dpjju.com/

Gaspar, C. R. (2013). *Differential Coercion and Homelessness: A Criminological Approach to Homeless Street Youth in Mexico (Unpublished master's thesis).* Canada: Department of Sociology. Queen's University.

Information Change India (n.d). *On the street where they live.* Retrieved July 17, 2006, from http://www.infochangeindia.org/Childrenlstory.jsp?recordno=228&storyofchangev=

Institute of Human Development & Save the children. (2011). Surviving the Street: A census of street children in Delhi by the Institute for Human Development and Save the Children http://resourcecentre.savethechildren.se/sites/default/files/documents/5332.pdf

Kanth, A.K., Prayas Juvenile Aid Centre Society, Harris, B., & Casa, A. (2004). Street children and Homelessness. *CYC—Online.* (68) September. Retrieved from http://www.cyc-net.org/cyc-online/cycol-0904-Homelessness.html

Ministry of Children & Youth Services(n.d). Review of the Roots of Youth Violence: Literature Reviews (Vol 5, Chap. 12). *Social Control and Self-Control Theories.* Retrieved from www.children.gov.on.ca

Nayar, L. (2011). A Tough School. *The Outlook.* Retrieved from http://www.outlookindia.com/article/A-Tough-School/271591

Thompson, W. E., & Jack, B. (2013). *Juvenile Delinquency* (9th ed.). United Kingdom: Pearson.

World Health Organisation (n.d). A Profile of Street Children: A Training Package on Substance Use, Sexual and Reproductive Health including HIV/AIDS and STDs (Module 1). Retrieved from http://www.unodc.org/pdf/youthnet/who_street_children_module1.PDF

World Health Organization. (1993). Programme on Substance Abuse. (WHO/PSA/93.7). Retrieved from http://pangaea.org/street_children/world/who3.htm

Socio-Economic Disparities Among Youth in Delhi: Issues and Challenges

Chandrani Dutta and Kanhaiya Kumar

Abstract Around 21 % of Indian population is youth. Youth is considered as the demographic dividend of the country. The paper shows even in a developed region like Delhi disparity across gender and social groups exist. Women from lower economic background face multiple disadvantages. Further this paper raises the concerns about marginalization of youth in Delhi, where one fifth of its main workforce is constituted by youth. They highlighted the disparity in their health status, gender-based discrimination in sex ratios and also unemployment of different social groups from different classes, in Delhi. Policies of the Government like National Youth Policy and Rashtriya Kishore Suraksha Yojana are positive directions but need to be nurtured in full force so as to reduce the existing gaps and ensure the prospects for each and every young individual in the country.

Keywords Social and mental health · Youth · Gender disparities

Context

Around 21 % of the India's population is youth. Young age is a very crucial period in an individual's entire life span. It encapsulates the earlier years when a person is supposed to spend in school, the middle years in higher education and in the latter

C. Dutta (✉)
Indian Institute of Dalit Studies, New Delhi, India
e-mail: chandrani@dalitstudies.org.in

K. Kumar
Centre for Social Medicine and Community Health, School of Social Sciences, Jawaharlal Nehru University, New Delhi 110067, India
e-mail: adikanha.jnu@gmail.com

S.S. Acharya et al. (eds.), *Marginalization in Globalizing Delhi: Issues of Land, Livelihoods and Health*, DOI 10.1007/978-81-322-3583-5_20

years, one is mostly in various forms of employment. Therefore, youth comprise both the adolescent period and the early years of adulthood. The entire span of years during the youth period therefore is very important from two different levels, first, one must take into account the individual level needs (social and mental health) of the young population, which if not catered to lead to disruption in the normal growth of the individual. On the other hand, this kind of disruption further leads to frustration, anger, sudden outbursts and also even more harmful aggressive behaviour which has a detrimental impact on the community and at large the society. All around the world, antisocial behaviour has got manifested from the youth population who has been denied the expectations they have had from the society. In most circumstances, lack of educational opportunities at the school-going age and lack of suitable employment opportunities in the early adult years lead to tensions which have serious implications on the young individual itself and the society. Youth is considered the demographic dividend[1] of the country. The increase in the working age group with the rise in the youth population signifies growing investment and less spending on the dependent population.

Across different cultures, the youth cohort is found to experience certain changes ranging from biological changes (onset of puberty), cognitive changes (emergence of more advanced cognitive abilities), emotional changes (self image, intimacy, relation with adults and peer groups) to social changes (transition into new roles in the society) (Acharya 2015). It is this period when social interactions increase with friends of same or opposite sex. These interactions get manifested in many forms like entering into relationships, marriage, pregnancy and childbearing. Therefore the immediate social environment, the family, school, neighbourhood through the agents like parents, siblings, relatives, teachers, school mates, peers and neighbours are responsible in shaping the behaviour of the individuals from this cohort. Therefore in all the forms of interactions, youth associating with the positive agents have a positive and constructive influence on their lives and the contrary happens in case of negative agents leading to deviant behaviour. In most cases, such deviant manifestations take place in behavioural disorders and use of harmful substance like smoking and consumption of alcohol and even drugs. The social and economic development of the youth is to a considerable extent a consequence of family background, opportunities available and fair access to these opportunities, and the policy environment in the country which is instrumental in reducing the gaps in demand and supply of resources to each and every

[1]'The Demographic dividend is the accelerated economic growth that may result from a rapid decline in a country's fertility and the subsequent change in the population age structure. With fewer births each year, a country's working-age population grows larger in relation to the young dependent population. With more people in the labour force and fewer young people to support, a country has a window of opportunity for rapid economic growth if the right social and economic investments and policies are made in health, education, governance and the economy. Investments in today's youth population can position a country to achieve a demographic dividend, but the gains are neither automatic nor guaranteed. (Source: 'The Potential of Youth for a Demographic Dividend: Investing in Health, Education, and Job Creation' at the International Conference on Family Planning, Addis Ababa, Ethiopia, November 12–15, 2013).

individual (Acharya 2015). The 'Social Learning Theory' according to Comerci (1990) provides explanation regarding the likelihood of an individual especially someone young, indulging in troublesome behaviour (Comerci 1990 cited by Acharya 2015). The development of the individual depends upon the opportunities available to him and her and exposure to the kind of society, the positive influences inculcated by him or her. Absence of a positive growing environment leads to disorder, conflict in the mindset, frustration which many times lead to depression, behavioural disorders which might lead to offence. Therefore, education in the early years and proper employment opportunities in the later years of youth are crucial in the development of the personality of the young individuals.

Youth has got associated with negative stereotypes for instance, delinquency, drug abuse and violence for a long time. It is one age cohort which not only needs importance from the family level but from the society and hence, policy makers need to see this cohort from these multi-dimensional perspectives. Young people need to realize their rights to education, health, to live free from discriminatory practices and violence. Lack of opportunities on these lines creates disillusionment among the young vibrant minds. Student unrest got widespread during the 1960s in Europe which made international agencies take the agenda on youth. Policies on youth needed to identify the strength hiding in youth which if rightfully channelized would help in development, peace and democracy (Acharya 2015). In Asia, 1978 was a turning point for the youth when UNESCO convened a meeting on 'Youth Mobilisation for Development'. The UN recognized 1985 as the 'International Year of the Youth'. Ministry of Youth Affairs and Sports (2014). Policy makers therefore need to channelize investments on the development of youth keeping in mind that informality is prevalent along with youth unemployment and there lie problems with job quality.[2] In addition to this, one must keep in mind, that youth is not a singular entity. It embodies, gender, social and economic status of the individual and also the region from where they belong. Youth as the demographic dividend highly depend on "good policies" and in the absence of quality in the government institutions formulating such policies, the potential of the youth remain unexplored (Chandrashekhar et al. 2006).

The central purpose of this study is to examine the status of youth in Delhi in terms of socio-demographic indicators of development and the disparities existing in the young population across social groups in Delhi. Data from the secondary sources, like Census of India, National Family Health Survey and other documentary sources, have been utilized in constructing the paper. The paper is structured in such a manner as to examine the status of youth in general from the point of view that a healthy young population in a country is also the potential human resource of the country where the outcome should be the equitable development of the entire youth population irrespective of their region where they belong, gender, and their social and economic status.

---

[2]http://blogs.worldbank.org/developmenttalk/youth-bulge-a-demographic-dividend-or-a-demographic-bomb-in-developing-countries accessed on 9 November 2015.

Youth in India

Office of the Registrar General of India (2011). According to the 2011 Census, an estimated 358 million people belong to the age group 10–24 years, which comprised 31 % of the country's population. By 2020, India is estimated to become the world's youngest country with 64 % of its population in the working age group. This rise in young population is supposed to take place mostly in urban areas. While it is true that this spurt in working age population have positive implications on demographic dividend, disparity both at the social as well as at the spatial level exists, creating imbalances in the positive outcome of such dividend. Against this backdrop, Indian policy makers have to strengthen the existing policies in such a manner so that critical issues concerning the youth especially with reference to health, sexuality, access to basic facilities and skill development can be streamlined in meeting the demands. So far there is limited proportion of youth with formal skills, the largest share is found in the state of Kerala followed by Maharashtra, Tamil Nadu, Himachal Pradesh and Gujarat. The state of Maharashtra had the highest share and Bihar the lowest among those who were undergoing training in various kinds of skill development programmes (Acharya 2015).

Physiological, social and emotional changes taking place during this age group bear considerable importance on the interactions and social behaviour of this cohort. While skill development and formal education help in boosting the potential to become economically empowered, nutrition, sexual and reproductive health, mental health, preventing injuries and violence (including gender based violence), substance use, non-communicable diseases also need to be addressed. Demographic dividend borne out of the youth population stands on the pillar of good physical, social and mental health.

Status of Youth in India with Special Reference to Health

The physical, mental and social well-being of the young population is a country's resource. It is important from that point of view to appraise both the quotient of well-being as well as illness the youth in India are subject to. A young individual needs to be free from any diseases, sickness, should have the freedom to pursue education of his or her choice, and also work in place of choice. In addition to that, an informed young population is a necessary advantage. Young people should be aware of their basic rights as well as responsibilities. The National Family Health Survey III (2005–2006) (Parasuraman et al. 2009) on Youth revealed certain crucial points which highlight the status of India's youth. It listed out certain key characteristics of the youth population in India. It revealed that a considerable portion of India's youth lacked education and many remained illiterate. Out of them, most were found to be employed. Early marriage and childbearing and rearing is found to be a huge burden carried by the youth in the country. International Institute for Population Studies (IIPS) and Population Council (2010). Most of the young have very low nutritional status and had a risky lifestyle, with very low prevalence of family planning practices, and young men indulging in substance use, which have severe health implications.[3] These findings point out the significance of access to reproductive health information and services among adolescents and youth, to avoid unplanned pregnancies and to prevent STDs including HIV/AIDS (Parasuraman et al. 2009). For young individuals adequate access to family planning information and services would help in delaying their first pregnancy till the point they are physically, psychologically and socially equipped for childbearing. Health programmes are important to prevent the adverse effect of lifestyle risks among youth and adolescence who indulge in substance use like drugs, alcohol and also consumption of junk food which is leading to obesity along with sedentary lifestyles.[4] Therefore the need for increased investments on child survival, reproductive health needs of both married and unmarried youth, improve quality of schools, enact and legally enforce prevention of early marriage and promote participation of youth in every fruitful exercises.[5] (authors' emphasis).

Delhi is a state with very high per capita income, and the life of the young population undergoes a lot of challenges posed by a highly urban, modern economy. Delhi as a state with the National Capital offers multitudes of advantages for the growing population both in terms of good educational opportunities and variety of employment opportunities. The state of Delhi along with Maharashtra and Karnataka are the main destinations for education purposes while Bihar, Uttar Pradesh, Kerala, West Bengal and Rajasthan are the source states for migrants. On

[3]'Most youth are exposed to some form of media. Female youth are more likely than male youth to belong to the lowest wealth quintile and less likely to be in the higher wealth quintiles. Majority of the unmarried youth live in nuclear households, whereas the majority of the married youth live in non-nuclear households. Many youth are economically active. Many youth are married and many youth are heading households. Most youth lack basic knowledge of women's menstrual cycle. Messages about family planning are not reaching all youth. Many youth have not heard of available modern contraceptive spacing methods. A majority of youth lack comprehensive knowledge of HIV/AIDS. Most youth desire a small family, most young men have a positive attitude toward contraception, but some are misinformed about it. Youth attitudes towards gender roles are, in general, no more egalitarian than the attitude of the older cohort age 25–49. Early childbearing defines India's fertility pattern. Both traditional and modern methods of contraception are popular among youth. The pattern of contraceptive use by youth reveals son preference. Youth have a large unmet need for family planning. Early marriage leads to early initiation of sexual activity among young women. There is evidence of higher risk sex among male youth unprotected by condom use. Tobacco use and alcohol consumption by youth are matters of concern. Sexually transmitted infections (STI) and STI symptoms are not uncommon among youth, particularly sexually active unmarried male youth. Prevalence of lifestyle diseases such as diabetes among youth is a matter of concern. Under-nutrition is very common among youth. The high prevalence of spousal violence is a continuing hurdle to the achievement of health goals and gender equality.' (Compiled from National Family Health Survey, 2005–2006).

[4]'The Potential of Youth for a Demographic Dividend: Investing in Health, Education, and Job Creation' at the International Conference on Family Planning, Addis Ababa, Ethiopia, 12–15 November 2013.

[5]http://www.prb.org/Publications/Articles/2012/demographic-dividend-factsheet.aspx, accessed on 9 November 2015.

the other hand, NSS 2007–2008 data had revealed that the states of Delhi, Gujarat, Maharashtra and Karnataka receive 64.1 % of the migrants from other states in the country who belong to the age group 15–32 years, who come to these states looking for employment opportunities (Chandrashekhar and Sharma (2012); Chandrashekhar and Sharma 2014).

The region serves as the melting pot for young across the country from diverse social, religious groups with varying economic conditions. Delhi, being mostly urban and having a considerable growth in manufacturing and retail sector under the neo-liberal regime, is the favoured destination for many young individuals looking for work. Better lifestyles in the state attract others from surrounding and far flung regions which create additional pressure on the service providers. Policy makers need to take into account this factor of exceeding demand on public services like basic amenities, health and education. Delhi offering better lifestyles attract youth who become potential contributors to the demographic dividend. The youth in Delhi therefore get exposed to both the hardships of poverty as well as the dazzle of posh lifestyles. Considering the age, neither they are too young nor are they old enough to take important decisions and get very easily swayed by the peer groups which have both positive as well as negative influences as is evident from the reckless lifestyles many young ones come face to face with.

As found from the National Family Health Survey, youth in Delhi reflect relatively better lifestyles and access to certain crucial health services like institutional deliveries among women, antenatal care and also contraceptive prevalence (Fig. 1). However, from the same dataset on the Youth certain aspects have come out which could thwart the development of this cohort. For instance, Figs. 2, 3, 4 and 5 reveal that even if the youth in Delhi are more exposed to mass media, therefore more well informed than the national level aggregates, and have better health situations (Figs. 4 and 5), there exists considerable gender gap, especially

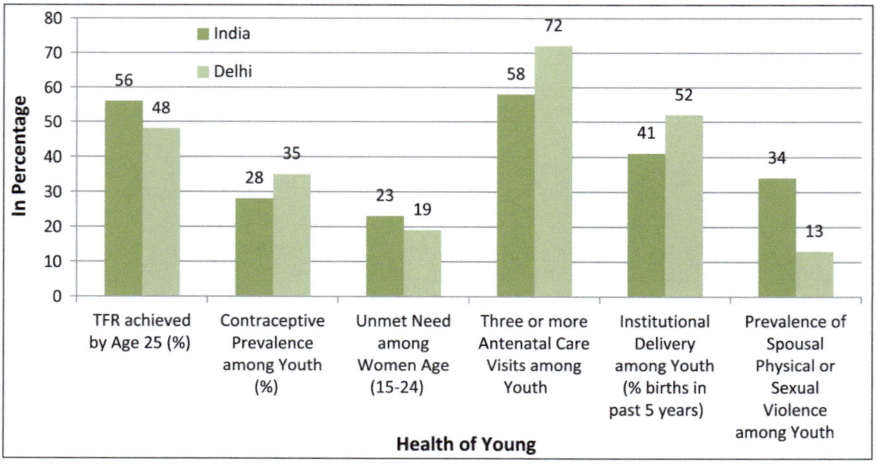

Fig. 1 Situation of youths in India and Delhi, 2005–2006. *Source* Prepared from National Family Health Survey III, 2005–2006 (Profile of Youth)

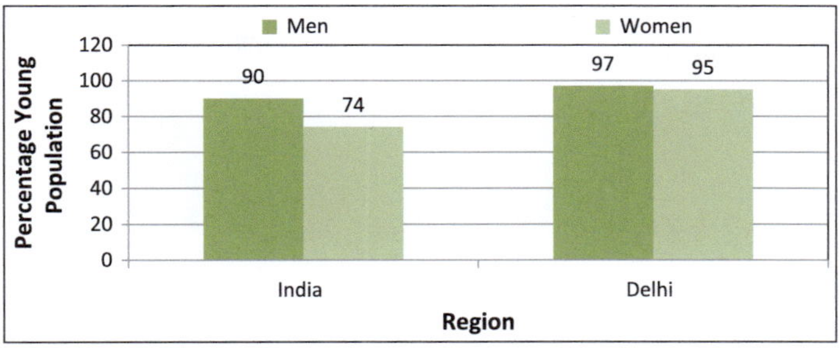

Fig. 2 Exposure to mass media among youths in India and Delhi 2005–2006. *Source* Prepared from National Family Health Survey III, 2005–2006 (Profile of Youth)

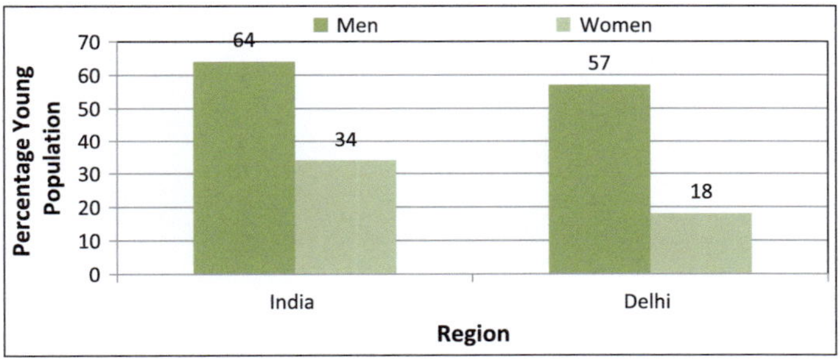

Fig. 3 Employment of youths in India and Delhi, 2005–2006. *Source* Prepared from National Family Health Survey III, 2005–2006 (Profile of Youth)

young women are found suffering from anaemia relatively more and have been found to be abnormally thin than men in India and also in Delhi which indicate the low nutritional status of women in the country. Young women are found less in employment than men (Fig. 3) and the gender gap in case of Delhi is quite high.

These findings therefore need to be taken into consideration strongly in the discourse of youth as demographic dividend. These findings pose as concerns as the true potential of demographic dividend could be exploited only with a healthy and balanced development of the youth where there is no disparity across various population subgroups. On that note, the next section would reflect the status of youth with respect to their demographic, social and economic status taking help from the 2011 Census data.

Demographic Profile of Youth in India and Delhi: A Special Reference to the SCs Vis-à-Vis Non SC Youth Across Districts in Delhi

About one fifth of the population of Delhi is youth. It ranges from 22.2 % adolescent and 22.1 % youth in North East Delhi to 18.2 % adolescents in Central

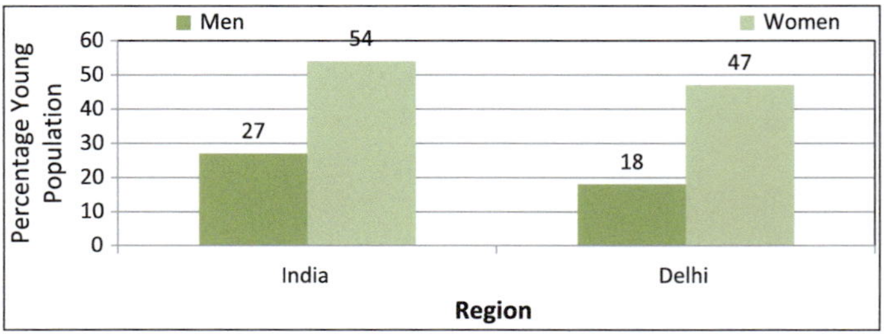

Fig. 4 Anaemia among youth in India and Delhi, 2005–2006. *Source* Prepared from National Family Health Survey III, 2005–2006 (Profile of Youth)

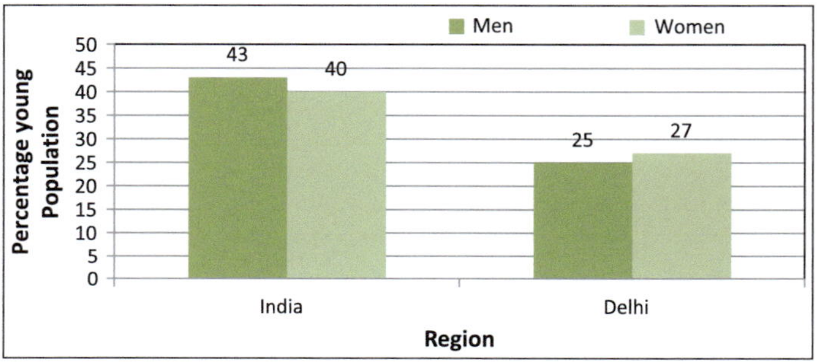

Fig. 5 Youths who are abnormally thin in India and Delhi, 2005–2006. *Source* Prepared from National Family Health Survey III, 2005–2006 (Profile of Youth)

and 19.5 % youth in West Delhi. As regards, the sex ratio, among the adolescents, rural south Delhi (704) and urban South West Delhi (794) has the lowest sex ratio. Among the youth, lowest sex ratio is in the North West Delhi (802) for rural population and South West Delhi (794) for urban population (Table 1).

On the basis of social groups, New Delhi has the highest proportion of adolescent SC population (26.22 %), while over all youth population is highest in Central Delhi (25.81 %). Rural adolescent sex ratio is highest in East Delhi (1000) and 878 in urban areas of East Delhi. On the other hand, over all youth SC sex ratio was highest in rural areas of East Delhi and in urban areas of Central Delhi had the highest SC sex ratio (924). Sex ratio of the SCs has been relatively better compared to the Non SCs in Delhi (868 for SC and 820 for Non SCs). Except in North East Delhi, all the other districts have revealed higher sex ratios among the SCs compared to the Non SCs.[6]

[6]SC connotes Scheduled Caste population and the Non SCs constitute that population subtracting the Scheduled Caste population from the total population.

Table 1 Demographic profile of young population of Delhi, 2011

S. No.	Area	% of young population		Sex ratio of adolescent pop.		Sex ratio of youth pop.	
		% of total adolescent (10–19) pop.	% of total youth (15–24) pop.	Rural	Urban	Rural	Urban
1	India	20.9	19.2	901	892	907	910
2	NCT of Delhi	19.7	20.4	791	822	822	829
3	North West	20.5	20.7	802	806	804	816
4	North	19.7	20.4	777	838	880	845
5	North East	22.2	22.1	796	858	802	876
6	East	18.6	19.6	820	826	917	844
7	New Delhi	18.6	21.7	000	829	000	764
8	Central	18.2	20.2	000	854	000	853
9	West	18.6	19.5	794	809	971	815
10	South West	18.6	19.9	782	794	853	794
11	South	19.9	20.5	704	830	683	829

Source Computed from Census of India 2011

Socio-Economic Status of Delhi Youth

Delhi has revealed better results in terms of literacy across both male and female population compared to the aggregate national estimates. However, there lies district level, rural/urban and gender wise differences. Among the adolescents, New Delhi has the highest literacy rate (96.16 %). male literacy rates are relatively higher than female literacy; however, the differences are less. The district of New Delhi has recorded the highest male literacy rate (96.32 %). Highest female literacy is found in the district of East Delhi (96 %). Among the youth, literacy is highest in the district of New Delhi, with male literacy highest in the South West and highest female youth literacy is found in the district of New Delhi (Table 3). SC youth literacy is highest in the district of New Delhi; male literacy also highest in New Delhi, while SC female literacy is found to be highest in Central Delhi.

In case of adolescent SC, literacy is highest in North East, while male literacy is highest in New Delhi (96.13 %) and female literacy is highest in Central Delhi (Table 4). In terms of literacy, Non SCs have relatively better literacy levels than the SCs. While the pattern remain the same in case of gender differences, when Non SCs and SCs male literacy levels are generally higher than SC and Non SC females, but it should be noted that across majority of the districts, SC females have relatively lesser literacy levels than the Non SC females. Another point which is evident is compared to the Non SCs and SCs, both male and female literacy rates are better in the Eastern, Central parts of the state compared to the other districts.

Table 2 Demographic profile of young population by social group of Delhi, 2011

S. No.	Area	% of SC young population		Sex ratio of SC adolescent pop.		Sex ratio of SC youth pop.	
		% of total SC adolescent (10–19) pop.	% of total SC youth (15–24) pop.	Rural	Urban	Rural	Urban
1	India	17.52	17.13	890	913	893	931
2	NCT of Delhi	18.61	18.65	845	865	861	868
3	North West	21.18	21.29	851	852	845	849
4	North	20.10	20.60	782	890	776	889
5	North East	16.90	17.50	765	868	829	873
6	East	19.25	19.08	1000	878	2000	889
7	New Delhi	26.22	25.12	000	853	000	852
8	Central	25.56	25.81	000	893	000	924
9	West	17.21	17.01	822	865	1009	859
10	South West	15.94	15.57	845	843	914	840
11	South	17.36	17.34	839	875	726	882

% of Total SC Adolescent (10–19) Pop = SC adolescent pop/total adolescent pop*100
Source Computed from Census of India 2011

Table 3 Proportion of Total Literates of Young Population by Gender of Delhi, 2011

S. No.	Area	Total literacy rate of young population					
		Adolescent			Youth		
		Total	Male	Female	Total	Male	Female
1	India	90.05	91.74	88.17	86.14	90.04	81.85
2	NCT of Delhi	94.99	95.23	94.70	93.17	94.19	91.93
3	North West	94.51	94.80	94.15	92.27	93.57	90.68
4	North	95.90	95.82	96.00	94.26	94.70	93.75
5	North East	94.17	94.25	94.07	91.83	92.86	90.66
6	East	96.13	96.24	96.00	94.71	95.34	93.96
7	New Delhi	96.16	96.32	95.97	94.95	95.27	94.53
8	Central	94.32	93.37	95.43	92.30	91.36	93.40
9	West	94.33	94.70	93.88	92.56	93.52	91.39
10	South West	95.90	96.26	95.45	94.76	95.94	93.29
11	South	95.40	95.89	94.80	93.59	95.01	91.88

Table 4 Percentage of total literacy rate of Young Population by Social Group and gender of Delhi
Source Computed from Census of India 2011

Profile of Work Participation Among the Youth

The economic profile of the youth population in Delhi reveals that 21.65 % of the young population are main workers, out of that male main workers constitute 34 % and female 6.68 %. Central Delhi has the highest main worker population

Table 4 Proportion of total literates of young population by gender and by social group, Delhi, 2011

S. No.	Area	Total literacy rate of young population by social group					
		Adolescent			Youth		
		Total	Male	Female	Total	Male	Female
1	India	88.80	90.63	86.76	83.32	88.07	78.05
2	NCT of Delhi	93.95	94.38	93.46	91.46	93.11	89.56
3	North West	93.17	93.71	92.54	90.18	92.12	87.89
4	North	94.31	94.54	94.05	91.90	92.96	90.70
5	North East	95.39	95.49	95.27	93.19	94.36	91.85
6	East	94.96	95.10	94.80	92.63	94.01	91.09
7	New Delhi	95.32	96.13	94.37	94.06	95.86	91.96
8	Central	95.16	94.65	95.73	93.34	93.36	93.32
9	West	92.49	93.00	91.91	89.69	91.42	87.68
10	South West	93.78	94.43	93.01	91.58	93.59	89.21
11	South	94.14	94.95	93.21	91.75	93.95	89.26

Source Computed from Census of India 2011

among the youth, which is also in case of males (40.02 %). On the other hand, female main worker population was highest in New Delhi (9.99 %). The pattern is similar for overall male main workers among the adolescents. On the basis of rural/urban distribution, both among youth and adolescents, highest proportion of main working population is found in the urban areas of Central Delhi. On the basis of social groups, highest proportion of SC young main workers is found in West Delhi (25.13 % total, 40.81 % male, 6.87 % female). Among adolescents, similar pattern is observed.

Analyzing the data on the basis of SC versus Non SC population subgroups, it is found that out of all the main workers, workers from the age group 15–24, the young workers, are relatively higher among the Scheduled Castes compared to the Non Scheduled Castes across most of the districts of Delhi. It is similar among young marginal workers in North, East, Central, West, South West and South Delhi. On the basis of gender, it is found that male main and marginal workers are higher than female among the youth.

On the basis of category of work,[7] among the main workers, it is found that among youth, SCs are in higher proportion than Non SCs working in Other Work category. Female main workers in the Other Workers category are relatively less than the male workers and even lesser among the SC population in the state of Delhi.

[7]Other workers have been considered as proportion of cultivators, agricultural labourers, household industry, who have been found to be in very less proportions.

Discussion and Concluding Remarks

The above findings show that youth in Delhi are relatively better off than the national level estimates. The earlier discussion on the advantages of Delhi being the state having the National Capital could be considered for such improved conditions. However, this study has attempted to shed light on a very important issue, which is balanced development. It has tried to bring out the problem of disparity in social and economic outcome among today's youth in the country and especially Delhi. The study has shown that even in a developed region, like Delhi, disparities exist. It exists across gender and it exists across social groups, SCs and the Non SCs in particular. The study has also pointed out the multiple disadvantages faced by women from lower social background. There is relatively less literacy among SC women than the Non SC women. Even work participation shows similar patterns. Therefore, in the discourse of demographic dividend, which Delhi definitely scores very high, gaps across gender and social groups create worrisome situations. Sex ratio which is a crucial indicator of human development also reveals that youth in Delhi is highly imbalanced. It needs to be mentioned that sex ratio among the Non SCs are much lower compared to the SCs. The analysis has depicted certain findings than SCs are more in employment than Non SCs. On the other hand, the SC has lesser literacy rates compared to Non SCs among the Youth. This implies the kind of work mostly availed by the SCs are in the unskilled and semi-skilled labour. Women remain within the households to do domestic chores, while men go out to work thereby showing male preference in employment opportunities. Women and especially women from the lower social groups have been socially and economically deprived. It is important to consider that women who are educated are more likely to work outside home and add to the economic development of the family and also the society. Development of a region depends on the contributions from each and every individual, especially the youth where education, health and employment are crucial pillars. In all the analysis it has been found out that women have remained far behind, especially women from lower social groups like the SCs. However, regions where a section continuously remains lagging, potential of exploiting the demographic dividend remain unutilized. It is imperative for governments to realize that a healthy transition from youth to adulthood is important, through availability of proper education and job opportunities.[8] Policies of the Government like National Youth Policy and Rashtriya Kishore Suraksha Yojana are positive directions but need to be nurtured in full force so as to reduce the existing gaps and ensure the prospects for each and every young individual in the country. Therefore, it needs to be reiterated again and again, of the importance of three strategies, strengthening health programmes, expanding educational opportunities for all and creating good quality jobs. All these together would help in achieving accelerated economic growth arising out of a demographic dividend.

[8]http://www.prb.org/Publications/Articles/2012/demographic-dividend-factsheet.aspx, accessed on 9th November 2015.

[*The authors owe immense gratitude to Professor Sanghmitra S. Acharya, Director, Indian Institute of Dalit Studies, for her guidance and crucial suggestions*]

Appendix

See Tables 1, 2, 3, 4, 5, 6, 7, 8, 9, 10, 11, 12 and 13.

Table 5 Proportion of total main worker of young population by gender of Delhi

S. No.	Area	Total main worker of young population					
		Adolescent			Youth		
		Total	Male	Female	Total	Male	Female
1	India	8.27	11.06	5.17	24.30	34.30	13.29
2	NCT of Delhi	5.62	8.78	1.77	21.65	34.05	6.68
3	North West	5.83	9.13	1.75	21.74	34.59	5.98
4	North	6.24	9.60	2.21	21.35	34.08	6.30
5	North East	5.92	9.77	1.42	20.72	35.23	4.13
6	East	4.97	7.71	1.66	20.67	31.91	7.35
7	New Delhi	5.60	8.72	1.83	23.97	34.65	9.99
8	Central	7.58	12.60	1.71	24.60	40.02	6.52
9	West	6.26	9.50	2.26	23.54	35.76	8.55
10	South West	4.91	7.54	1.59	21.66	32.94	7.51
11	South	4.83	7.39	1.75	20.60	31.68	7.22

Source Computed from Census of India 2011

Table 6 Proportion of total main worker of young population by space, Delhi, 2011

S. No.	Area	Total main worker of young population					
		Adolescent			Youth		
		Total	Rural	Urban	Total	Rural	Urban
1	India	8.27	8.70	7.20	24.30	25.51	21.74
2	NCT of Delhi	5.62	5.27	5.63	21.65	20.39	21.68
3	North West	5.83	6.04	5.82	21.74	22.06	21.72
4	North	6.24	5.61	6.25	21.35	18.30	21.42
5	North East	5.92	6.70	5.91	20.72	21.97	20.70
6	East	4.97	3.65	4.98	20.67	21.32	20.67
7	New Delhi	5.60	0	5.60	23.97	0	23.97
8	Central	7.58	0	7.58	24.60	0	24.60
9	West	6.26	3.67	6.27	23.54	16.45	23.56
10	South West	4.91	3.44	5.02	21.66	17.36	21.95
11	South	4.83	8.94	4.81	20.60	26.60	20.58

Source Computed from Census of India 2011

Table 7 Percentage of total main worker of young population by social group and gender, Delhi, 2011

S. No.	Area	Total main worker of SC young population					
		Adolescent			Youth		
		Total	Male	Female	Total	Male	Female
1	India	8.91	11.95	5.51	25.33	35.36	14.21
2	NCT of Delhi	6.31	10.04	2.01	21.43	35.46	5.25
3	North West	6.78	10.73	2.13	22.46	37.27	5.00
4	North	7.36	11.72	2.46	22.66	37.77	5.66
5	North East	5.58	9.17	1.45	19.10	32.48	3.76
6	East	5.31	8.50	1.68	19.45	32.50	4.78
7	New Delhi	5.33	8.73	1.35	20.56	32.55	6.49
8	Central	6.47	10.59	1.85	22.37	37.47	6.04
9	West	8.11	12.57	2.96	25.13	40.81	6.87
10	South West	5.87	9.24	1.86	20.96	33.86	5.70
11	South	5.25	8.33	1.73	19.51	32.26	5.04

Source Computed from Census of India 2011

Table 8 Percentage of Total Main Worker of Young Population by Space, Delhi, 2011

S. No.	Area	Total main worker of young population					
		Adolescent			Youth		
		Total	Rural	Urban	Total	Rural	Urban
1	India	8.91	9.22	7.86	25.33	26.38	22.25
2	NCT of Delhi	6.31	6.03	6.32	21.43	20.67	21.45
3	North West	6.78	6.56	6.79	22.46	21.87	22.51
4	North	7.36	5.34	7.38	22.66	21.43	22.67
5	North East	5.58	5.72	5.58	19.10	18.85	19.10
6	East	5.31	0.00	5.31	19.45	11.11	19.45
7	New Delhi	5.33	0	5.33	20.56	0	20.56
8	Central	6.47	0	6.47	22.37	0	22.37
9	West	8.11	5.12	8.12	25.13	17.78	25.15
10	South West	5.87	4.00	6.02	20.96	16.68	21.30
11	South	5.25	16.89	5.19	19.51	39.65	19.42

Source Computed from Census of India 2011

Table 9 Proportion of young population among SCs and Non SCs, Delhi, 2011

Area	Non SCs			Scheduled caste		
	Persons	Males	Females	Persons	Males	Females
INDIA	19.0	19.4	18.7	19.7	20.2	19.3
State—NCT OF DELHI	20.0	20.5	19.4	22.8	23.0	22.5
District—North West	20.2	20.8	19.4	23.1	23.5	22.7
District—North	19.9	20.2	19.6	22.6	22.7	22.4
District—North East	21.9	22.0	21.8	23.2	23.5	22.9
District—East	19.0	19.5	18.5	22.8	22.9	22.6
District—New Delhi	21.2	22.1	20.1	23.3	23.3	23.2
District—Central	19.9	20.4	19.3	21.2	21.4	21.0
District—West	19.0	19.7	18.2	22.4	22.7	22.1
District—South West	19.5	20.0	18.9	22.3	22.6	22.0
District—South	20.0	20.5	19.5	23.0	23.1	22.8

Source Computed from Census of India 2011

Table 10 Sex ratio of the young population among SCs and Non SCs, Delhi, 2011

Area	Sex ratio	
	Non SCs	Scheduled caste
INDIA	909	902
State—NCT OF DELHI	820	868
District—North West	806	849
District—North	835	889
District—North East	876	872
District—East	834	889
District—New Delhi	737	852
District—Central	829	924
District—West	806	859
District—South West	790	845
District—South	817	881

Source Computed from Census of India 2011

Table 11 Proportion of literates among SC and non SC population in Delhi, 2011

Area	Non SCs			Scheduled caste		
	Persons	Males	Females	Persons	Males	Females
INDIA	86.7	90.5	82.6	83.3	88.1	78.0
State—NCT OF DELHI	93.6	94.4	92.5	91.5	93.1	89.6
District—North West	92.8	94.0	91.5	90.2	92.1	87.9
District—North	94.9	95.1	94.6	91.9	93.0	90.7
District—North East	91.5	92.5	90.4	93.2	94.4	91.9
District—East	95.2	95.6	94.7	92.6	94.0	91.1
District—New Delhi	95.2	95.1	95.5	94.1	95.9	92.0
District—Central	91.9	90.7	93.4	93.3	93.4	93.3
District—West	93.1	93.9	92.2	89.7	91.4	87.7
District—South West	95.3	96.4	94.1	91.6	93.6	89.2
District—South	94.0	95.2	92.4	91.8	93.9	89.3

Source Computed from Census of India 2011

Table 12 Proportion of young main and marginal workers among the SCs and the Non SCs in Delhi, 2011

Area	Non SCs			Scheduled caste		
	Persons	Males	Females	Persons	Males	Females
Proportion of young main workers						
INDIA	15.2	14.9	16.3	17.3	17.5	16.8
State—NCT OF DELHI	13.5	13.4	14.2	16.4	17.0	12.7
District—North West	13.9	13.9	13.7	17.5	18.3	12.4
District—North	13.1	12.7	15.5	16.4	17.0	12.9
District—North East	16.6	16.4	18.0	16.2	16.6	12.9
District—East	12.0	11.8	13.6	15.1	15.9	11.1
District—New Delhi	12.8	13.1	11.8	14.0	14.9	10.3
District—Central	14.7	14.8	13.9	14.9	15.3	12.7
District—West	13.2	13.0	14.5	17.9	18.5	14.7
District—South West	12.8	12.7	13.5	15.7	16.2	12.7
District—South	12.9	12.7	13.9	15.5	16.0	12.3
Proportion of young marginal workers						
INDIA	24.7	27.3	22.2	24.2	26.9	21.2
State—NCT OF DELHI	27.0	28.1	24.5	27.3	29.1	22.7
District—North West	28.4	29.9	24.4	27.7	29.9	21.3
District—North	27.3	28.6	24.5	28.8	31.0	23.2
District—North East	30.4	30.7	29.4	26.8	27.9	23.5
District—East	26.5	28.0	23.2	28.4	30.4	22.5
District—New Delhi	28.7	30.1	26.2	27.3	29.6	21.2
District—Central	26.0	26.5	24.8	26.1	27.1	24.0
District—West	27.8	29.2	24.5	28.2	30.0	23.6
District—South West	25.5	26.3	23.9	27.0	28.7	22.7
District—South	24.5	25.5	22.1	26.3	27.5	22.8

Source Computed from Census of India 2011

Table 13 Proportion of other workers (main) among the youth SC and Non SC population, Delhi, 2011

Area	Non SCs			Scheduled caste		
	Persons	Males	Females	Persons	Males	Females
INDIA	45.85	50.53	32.46	40.16	44.28	28.32
State—NCT OF DELHI	95.25	95.19	95.59	96.29	96.70	93.06
District—North West	95.25	95.16	95.87	96.33	96.74	92.72
District—North	94.4	94.37	94.63	96.24	96.68	92.97
District—North East	92.5	92.94	88.26	96.64	97.04	92.64
District—East	95.31	95.14	96.09	96.83	97.1	94.8
District—New Delhi	98.2	98.31	97.73	97.17	97.5	95.24
District—Central	93.69	93.71	93.51	93.7	94.53	88.07
District—West	95.96	95.79	96.83	96.17	96.75	92.12
District—South West	96.24	96.24	96.24	96.10	96.45	93.60
District—South	96.53	96.38	97.29	96.72	96.92	95.20

Source Computed from Census of India 2011

References

Acharya, S. S. (2015). *Youth in Development discourse and demographic dividend: Connecting the axes of social inclusion. Demographic challenges in India*. New Delhi: Bookwell Publishers.

Chandrasekhar, S., & Sharma, A. (2012). Internal Migration for Education and Employment among Youth in India, Chapter 6 in State of the Urban Youth, India 2012: Employment, Livelihoods, Skills. Report Commissioned by UN-HABITAT's Global Urban Youth Research Network and Published by IRIS-KF. http://www.igidr.ac.in/pdf/publication/WP-2014-004.pdf.

Chandrashekhar, C.P., Ghosh, J., & Roychowdhury, A. (2006). *The 'Demographic Dividend' and Young India's Economic Future*. Economic and Political Weekly. December 9, 2006, pp. 5056–5064.

Chandrashekhar, S. & Sharma, A. (2014). International Migration for Education and Employment among Youth in India. Indira Gandhi Institute of Development Research

International Institute for Population Studies (IIPS) and Population Council. (2010). *Youth in India: Situation and Needs 2006–2007*. Mumbai: IIPS.

Ministry of Youth Affairs and Sports. (2014). *National Youth Policy*. Government of India. 87 pp.

Office of the Registrar General of India (2011). *Special Tabulation on Adolescent and Youth Population classified by various parameters for India, States and Union Territories*. Census of India 2011.

Parasuraman, S., Kishor, S., Singh, S.K., & Vaidehi, Y. (2009). *A Profile of Youth in India*. National Family Health Survey (NFHS-3), India, 2005–2006. Mumbai: International Institute for Population Services; Calverton, Maryland, USA: ICF Macro.

Condition of the Aged in National Capital Territory of Delhi

Bhaswati Das

Abstract A population is called ageing when the proportion of aged 60 or 65 years is increasing in total population. This is a dynamics of decline in fertility and mortality which may be modified by migration of young population in a specific geographical region. To understand the condition of the aged, the study relied on different official secondary data sources. National Capital Territory of Delhi is the capital of India and while coping with globalization, the city has experienced large amount of growth in creation of economic opportunities which has attracted a large number of young male migrants. It has provided the region a relatively young age structure with lesser proportion of aged population than the country's average. Elderly sex ratio also, which otherwise favours females is favouring males in this region. Commensurating with previous studies it is observed that even in the capital city, women headship is low when they are in the union and they get headship of the household with increase in age and mostly when they are not in the union. Living arrangement is distressing where nearly 2 % of the households are exclusively all-aged households irrespective of the number of persons in the household. Little less than half (46 %) of the male elderly in 60–69 age group are working as main worker, which is extremely high. This has reduced the number of economically dependents in Delhi. However, it is important to mention that proportion of pensioner is also quite higher in Delhi than country as a whole. High work participation may be linked with the lesser morbidity of the Delhi's elderly where both the incidence and rate of hospitalization are substantially low. However, surveys have observed that crime against the elderly is much higher in Delhi than it is in many other urban centres in India. Delhi Government has shown its concern in

B. Das (✉)
Centre for the Study of Regional Development, School of Social Sciences
in Jawaharlal Nehru University, New Delhi, India
e-mail: bhaswati@mail.jnu.ac.in

S.S. Acharya et al. (eds.), *Marginalization in Globalizing Delhi: Issues of Land, Livelihoods and Health*, DOI 10.1007/978-81-322-3583-5_21

this and taken initiative to address the same. However, a comprehensive database focusing on elderly is required for Delhi as it is experiencing fast change.

Keywords Elderly in Delhi · Ageing process · Living arrangement · Health condition · Working elderly

Introduction

Technically any population whose average age is rising can be said to be ageing, but usually the term is more specifically used with reference to an increase in the proportion of persons aged over 60 or 65 (Kurek 2007). The age structure is an indication of the dynamics played by the most important factors for demographic change, i.e., fertility and mortality. Transition from high fertility to low fertility instals the supply of young in the population in one hand and increase in the span of life retains large population for long. This initiates the process of ageing which is primarily determined by fertility trends and secondarily by mortality trends (Mirkin and Weinberger 2001; Golini 2003; Supan and Jurges 2008). Ageing as a challenge was first recognized in 1940s, shortly after the inception of the United Nations. Government of Argentina first submitted a draft declaration on old-age rights to be considered in General Assembly in 1948. Population ageing again drew attention in 1969 with government of Malta submitted the topic to the General Assembly. It was only on 1978 the General Assembly decided to convene the first world assembly on ageing. As a result of that First World Assembly on Ageing was held in Vienna in 1982. The Vienna International Plan of Action on Ageing is the first international instrument on ageing, and provides the basis for the formulation of policies and programmes on ageing. It again took 20 long years to reflect a global consensus on the social dimensions of ageing that has evolved during preceding decades through multilateral activity and work conducted at the United Nations which took a shape through the Madrid International Plan of Action on Ageing and the Political Declaration (UN 2002). Madrid recognized the rising median age and increase in life expectancy. The Second World Assembly on Ageing in 2002 gave a clarion call for "building a society for all ages". It focuses on three priority areas: older persons and development; advancing health and well-being into old age; and ensuring enabling and supportive environments (WHO 2002). The population ageing has had far-reaching effects on economy. The first of these effects is on the economy's potential growth rate. Decline of working age population has reduced labour supply and thus has pushed down economic growth in Japan. Globalization has made the life of the aged more challenging, especially in the developing countries. Here, as part of globalization all age group population including children, youth, women and the old are undergoing a change in terms of their lifestyle, world outlook and the relationships in the society. While others can adopt with the changes, old are in an anomic mind which push the aged in periphery, making them marginal (Nair 2014). Also globalization has reduced capacities of developing countries by influencing policies in regards to healthcare, economic security and education; as a result, these nations face an uphill task in providing basic social protective services for their ageing population (Mukherjee 2008).

Madrid declaration thus, identified three major sets of research areas which include (i) socio-psychological support; (ii) economics of support and (iii) bio-medical aspect of health.

A large part of the condition of the aged depends on the support they receive from the family, especially in India, as the state funded benefits for elderly population are meagre. The status of elderly is high in agricultural economy than any 'exploitative economy' which is mostly non-agricultural (Kuntz and Lee 1987).

A general trend seems to be that the elderly and their families are becoming more responsible for their own economic security, health care and well-being. Intergenerational support systems are diminishing as a result of the new cultural paradigm that emphasizes the individual over the family. Moreover quick demographic changes such as reductions in family size, increasing migration of the young and economic crises leading to the problem of breaking of intergenerational support system (Ham et al. 2009). Participation, which is one pillar of 'active ageing', includes participation in socio-economic activities. However, it is important to note that continuing with work after retirement age may be out of compulsion or by choice. The tenet that work-ability may improve with improvement in mortality has been examined by the scholars (Feldman 1983) but conclusions varied. However, it is said that the reciprocity of support within family relations contributes to the well-being of elderly parents rather than unidirectional provision of support to the children and the absence of support exchange has a detrimental effect (Dowd 1975; Kim and Kim 2003). In the current cohort of aged, people at least have taken birth during 1950s. The socio-economic condition was widely varying by gender as there was low level of educational and economic participation among women during that time. Women's economic participation was restricted leading to their subordination which restricted their decision-making (Alam and Yadav 2013). Thus, headship in a household[1] which is mostly determined by the decision-making power, remains inordinately ambitious for a woman in the presence of their father/husband. It has been seen that women in India acquire headship mostly with age through the loss of their spouse (Das and Vemuri 2009). Thus, these complexities in the life course get imprinted in the condition of the aged. Living arrangement, support system these are increasingly becoming concern to describe the condition of the aged. The condition of the aged cannot be discussed without considering their gender as their role in society is always remained segregated.

Condition of the aged in NCT of Delhi is very typically could be understand with the above mentioned three broad aspects. However, data on those very

[1]The Census of India 2001 has defined 'Head of the household' as one who was recognized to be so by the household. In such a person vests the chief responsibility of managing affairs of the household as also the decision making on behalf of the household. Thus, the title implies for its holder a status in the society and supremacy in the household.

aspects of the elderly are lacking especially for Delhi. For that matter, Delhi elderly issues could not attract much attention of the researcher, probably because of the very young nature of its population. Present paper is an effort to understand the condition of the aged of Delhi with respect of the overall situation of the country. It also will attempt to analyze Delhi's demographic situation in terms of the ageing process in India. Discussion thus will be divided into broad two sections: (i) ageing process in Delhi and (ii) socio-economic profile of the aged. While discussing about socio-economic condition of the elderly, the economic activity, headship by marital status and the health status will be highlighted.

Data and Method

The present study is based mostly on secondary data. Since age data is the most basic demographic data, thus Indian census since its inception collects information on population characteristics by age. Census of India provides a major data source for any ageing study. For the present study, mostly Census of India 2001 and 2011 has been used. Migration information has been limited up to 2001 as 2011 census data is not yet been available. Other than that data as it is available from different Sample Registration System reports are used to understand natural increase in Delhi. National Sample Survey of 60th Round which has emphasized on morbidity and health care, 2004 has been the only source to understand aspects of health in recent most time. Health condition is analyzed using that data.

Lack of any micro-data restricts the analysis of the condition of the aged in NCT of Delhi. However, for the current purpose, mostly descriptive statistics are used which are often put into the perspective of space and time. Wherever relevant, data is presented by gender. Different cartographic methods are used to represent the facts suitably.

Ageing Process in India and in Delhi

Like many other Southeast Asian countries, India is also experiencing rapid fertility decline, increase in life expectancy and a rapid change in age structure since Independence. During 1950s, 1960s and 1970s, the variation in median age was less than 1 year whereas between 1980–1990, it was 1.3 years and adding 2.5 years more between 2000 and 2010. It is seen that in some developing countries demographic transition was much faster than the developed countries. Even in India regional variation is so wide that one can see the context of both developed and developing block demography. Thus a considerable regional variation in age structure is observed in this vast country. It has been observed that in past 40 years, the decline in death rate for the country as whole is sharper than what Delhi has observed for the same time period. But level of mortality remained consistently higher for the country as a whole than it is observed for Delhi. Almost same is true for the birth rate also where country is showing a steady decline during the past 40 years but maintaining a higher level always. Delhi, on the other hand had shown a decline but with large amount of fluctuations. However, the decline in birth rate is almost same for the country as well as for Delhi (Fig. 1).

In demographic studies on ageing, scholars have shown that while through ageing process, workforce experiences a shrinkage, by mitigating international

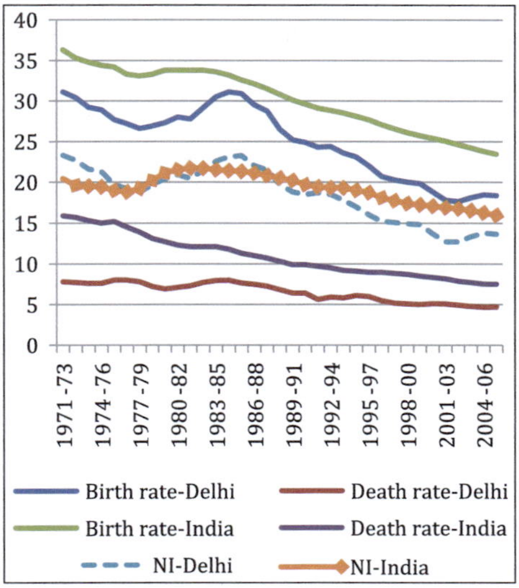

Fig. 1 Natural Increase (NI) in India and in Delhi: 1971–2006. *Source* Sample Registration System data of respective years

migration that is checked by several countries (Supan and Jurges 2008; Bloom et al. 2008). Though at the national level migration has little role to play in determining age structure, at the local level it could be an important factor, depending upon the volume of migrants. Despite being a region of low fertility and low mortality for a longer duration of time, proportion of elderly remained low in Delhi because of net inflow of young age population in the territory.

Population projection for Delhi (ORGI 2006) estimated that in 2026 Delhi will have 10 % of its population as elderly when India will have 12.4 %. It also has estimated that old-age dependency will show an increase of 73 points between 2001 and 2026 (from 119 to 192) for India and an increase of 67 points (from 81 to 148) for Delhi during the same time period. The life expectancy has been projected to be 73.5 for the males and 77.4 for females in Delhi during 2021–2025. Life expectancy for India, however, will be lower at 69.8 years for the males and 72.3 years for the females. Thus it appears that in the next decade also age composition of the state of Delhi will largely be determined by young age migration flow.

India is a country where every citizen enjoys the right to move freely throughout the territory of India (Article 19 (1/d)). Delhi experienced a heavy inflow of migrants and over the past 4 decades more than one-third of its population was comprised by the migrant population and expected to remain so in 2011 also (Fig. 2). 2001 census had shown that net migration flow in Delhi was 1.7 million during preceding decade (ORGI 2001). Thus the proportion of 60+ population is only 6.8 % compared to 8.6 % in the country as a whole in population census 2011 (Fig. 3). Migration, which is age and sex selective, has a strong impact in the population characteristics of Delhi. Contrary to the declining sex ratio of the country over the decades, sex ratio among the elderly favours the females in India (Das and Vemuri 2009). However, since migration is sex selective, sex ratio among

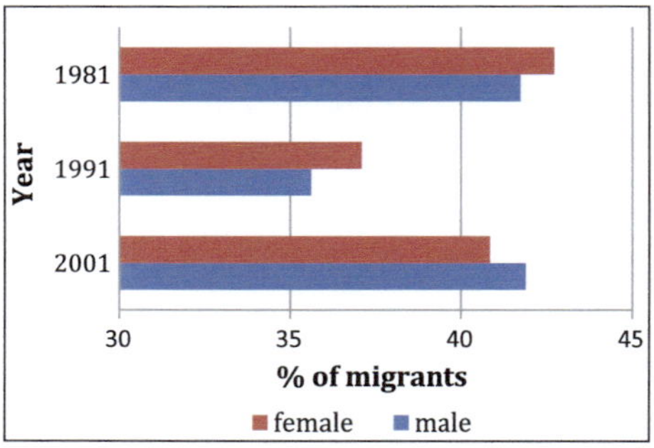

Fig. 2 Percentage of migrants to total population in Delhi by sex. *Source* Based on Census of India of respective years

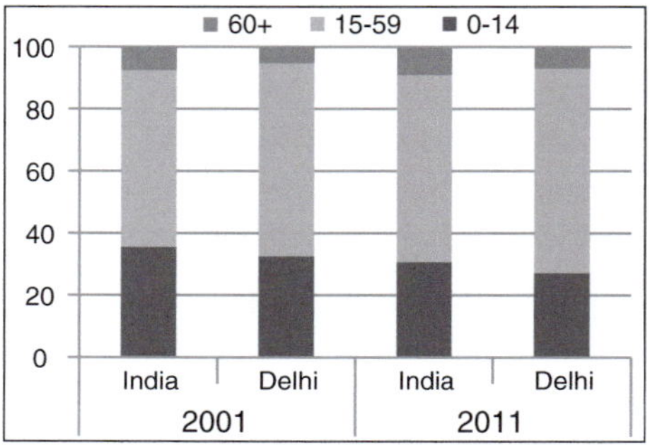

Fig. 3 Age structure in India and Delhi. *Source* Based on Census 2011

Table 1 Sex ratio among the aged in India and in Delhi

Sex ratio	India	Delhi
1991	930	855
2001	1029	964
2011	1033	989

Source Census of India, 2011

the 60+ population in Delhi favours the males (Table 1). Nonetheless the growth rate among the elderly women for Delhi is much higher than it is observed for the country as a whole. Overall Delhi is a young state and is expected to remain so in the next decade.

Socio-Economic Condition of the Aged

Among the various socio-economic factors which may describe the condition of the aged, only few of the factors will be discussed, considering their importance in an urban setup. Within this family headship by marital status, living arrangements are of special consideration to see the social status whereas, economic participation and dependence is considered to understand economic situation of the elderly. In a way these factors are linked to describe the condition of the aged specially the women as women's economic dependence on their husband links their fortune to those of their husbands. Because wives are typically 5–10 years younger than their husbands, the probability of being widowed is also high for a woman (Cain 1986).

Marital Status and Household Headship

Marriage is near universal in India. Many literatures reveal that married persons are better in all economic and social aspects than those who are single and the worst condition is observed among those who are widow. Among the elderly there is hardly any variations observed between the country average and Delhi (Table 2). Overall pattern shows that currently married men are much higher than currently married women, whereas among the women proportion of widow is much higher than male. The high incidence of widowhood is an important factor in the low status of many elderly South Asian females (Martin 1990). Widows have more health problem because they tend to live with children and their families, and sometimes family problems can lead to mistreatment (Badithe and Ali 2003). Srivastava (2010) has observed that widowhood is predominant among the elderly women due to the substantial age difference between marriage partners, due to the differential life expectancy between male and females. Further she also added by saying that the rate of remarriage among males is much higher than among the females so the number of widows is higher than the widower in India. Gulati and Ranjan (1999) in this context, noted that (a) the incidence of widowhood steeply increased with the advancing of age among both men and women in India and (b) the incidence of widowhood, among women of 70 years and above, is very high in India, particularly relative to that of men in the same age group. Marital status of the elderly women is also indicative of their social status as widowhood imposes various restrictions on women. These social restrictions also deter them to venture out the labour market which probably they have not thought in the presence of their spouse. Or in many other situations they were restricted to do so. However, some of them force to take up work in the absence of their spouse, for their own maintenance and for the maintenance of their family.

The prevalence of patriarchal family system in India allows male member of the family, more often the eldest male member, to be the head of the household. A female member becomes the head only when she is living alone or when there are only female members in the family (Sivamurthy and Wadakannavar 2001). Rajan and Kumar (2003) also found that the highest proportion of female headed households was found among widowed and divorced women. Over the age women headship never crosses 50 % marks when they are within the union (Fig. 4). The present distribution is contrary to the findings of Sivamurthy and Wadakannavar (2001), where both currently married and never married reported fewer headships

Table 2 Marital status of the elderly by gender

	India		Delhi	
	Male	Female	Male	Female
Never married	2.89	2.04	2.8	2.0
Currently married	82.12	49.57	81.5	52.7
Widowed	14.61	47.80	15.5	44.9
Separated	0.44	0.30	0.1	0.2
Divorced	0.08	0.15	0.1	0.1

Source Census of India, 2011

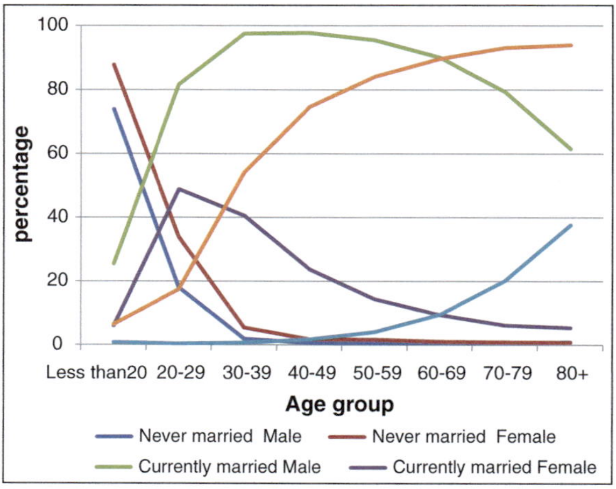

Fig. 4 Headship by marital status and age in NCT of Delhi, 2011. *Source* Based on Census 2011

with growing age. Burden of headship comes to women when she is widow, thus mentally and physically fragile and the most vulnerable.

Living arrangement of the elderly: Families are observed as the centre for providing support and care to its members. Living arrangement of the aged actually observes the household structure, i.e. with whom the aged are staying. Traditional families where co-residence of the older parents along with their adult children was predominant started declining in the developed countries over last century (Kramarow 1995). Population ageing in the developing countries is coinciding with rapid socio-economic and demographic changes. Thus changing family composition provides an indication of the human support available for the aged. The general pattern of living arrangement for the elderly in this rural society seems to be with spouse closely followed by with married children and unmarried children (Audinarayana et al. 1999). The household size is an indication of the degree of jointness among the generations. If more and more people are living together, the elderly are likely to get better attention including care during sickness (Rajan and Kumar 2003). A study on quality of life and living arrangement among the Chinese Canadian elders observed that elders will have higher well-being if they are the heads of household, rather than their children. It also has observed that living arrangements have no effect on the quality of life of married elders whereas living alone negatively affects well-being/social isolation of the widows (Gee 2000). The filial piety at societal level provides well-being and life satisfaction.

Delhi, which is mostly urban in nature, shows only 0.8 % one-member household (Census 2011) where aged person is the only family member. Though the percentage figure is low, the number of household hidden behind it is 28,192 (Table 3). There are another 38,000 two-member households where both the members are aged and 1085 three-member households where all three members are aged. Together they form 2 % of the total households. Within one-member households, it is important to note that proportion of households with only one female

Table 3 All-elderly households by number of members in the household

	DELHI (NUMBER)	
	Male	Female
One-member HH	11,414	16,778
Two-member HH	38,331	38,017
Three-member HH	1398	1857

Source Census of India, 2011

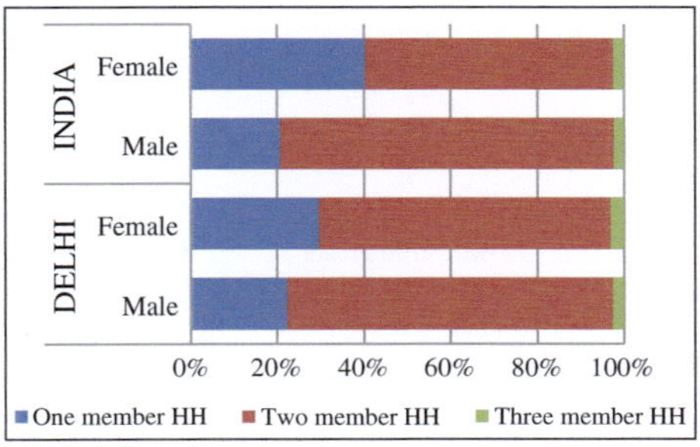

Fig. 5 Distribution of all elderly households by gender, 2011. *Source* Based on Census 2011

aged member is high for India as well as for Delhi. Among two-member households, gap in the proportion of male–female is less in Delhi. It is assumed that they are mostly the elderly couple who are living alone (Fig. 5).

Economic Characteristics of the Elderly Population of Delhi

With increase in the number of the aged in the society, policy has started to orient itself to use this experienced group of population for the development activity. While defining active ageing, World Health Organisation (WHO 2002) spelt out that it is the process of optimizing opportunities for health, participation and security. The participation referred to continuing participation in social, economic, cultural, spiritual and civic affairs. For the developed countries with longer life spans, if people work longer, they can keep their consumption level high and need only to save at the same rate as before for old age (Bloom and Canning 2008). Thus they can maintain a healthy economic life. For Delhi, it has been observed that overall 38 % of the males and 5 % of the females are main workers (Census of India 2011) and there is an increase in this share since 2001 (Table 4). Percentage of elderly who still work has been analyzed by major old-age group. According to 2011 census, there is an increased percentage of population in 60–69 years age group is main workers among both males and females.

On the contrary, percentage of marginal workers among the elderly is extremely low among both males and females and across all the old-age groups. A study in Punjab has revealed that workforce participation among the elderly is predominantly influenced by economic compulsions (Alam and Yadav 2013). In preindustrial societies, the flow of transfers was from the middle aged and old to the young which is a phenomenon of the developing countries (Lee 2000). The compulsion of work is pronounced from high percentage of main worker even in the 80+ age group in Delhi. However, one cannot ignore the fact that life expectancy is positively related with

Table 4 Main worker among the aged by sex: Delhi and India

	2001		2011	
	Male main worker (%)	Female main worker (%)	Male main worker (%)	Female main worker (%)
60–69	43.28	5.87	46.47	6.49
70–79	25.74	3.07	22.94	2.84
80+	17.32	2.19	19.24	2.94
60+	35.79	4.76	37.99	5.20

Source Census of India, 2011

Table 5 Marginal worker among the aged by sex: Delhi and India

Age group	2001		2011	
	Male marginal worker (%)	Female marginal worker (%)	Male marginal worker (%)	Female marginal worker (%)
60–69	1.91	0.91	2.34	0.9
70–79	1.31	0.5	1.33	0.57
80+	0.84	0.36	1.21	0.52
60+	1.63	0.75	1.98	0.78

Source Based on Census 2011

income. Thus, people of high income areas are expected to live longer (Preston 1975). NCT of Delhi, being a high income area, expected to observe better health condition among the aged which allows them to continue in gainful employment for longer period of time. Thus their participation as marginal worker which means less than 6 months of work in a year is negligible both among males and females (Table 5).

Dependency is an indicator of vulnerability of the aged (Alam and Yadav 2013). Occupation of the non-workers asked in population census, reveals the major kind of engagement of the aged. It has observed that pensioners (28 %) and rentiers (1.5 %) are substantially more in Delhi as compared to India as a whole which has resulted into a low dependency status among the elderly. No other major states have more than 1 % rentiers among the aged except Delhi.

Gender dimension in dependency needs special attention to understand the vulnerability of the aged population. It has been observed that a small proportion of the aged women are pension receivers because they had low work participation rate than the males at all working age group, making them economically marginalized and non-eligible for pension (Das and Vemuri 2009). While trying to place Delhi with respect to pension, it appeared that no major state has as high proportion of male pension receiver as Delhi (Fig. 6). For the females, however, situation is slightly different where states like Himachal Pradesh, Uttarakhand, Haryana, Odisha, Chattisgarh and Andhra Pradesh have higher percentage of pension receivers. But most interestingly, hardly few of the states which have faired than Delhi in terms percentage of pension receivers have not positioned them better in terms of dependents (Table 6).

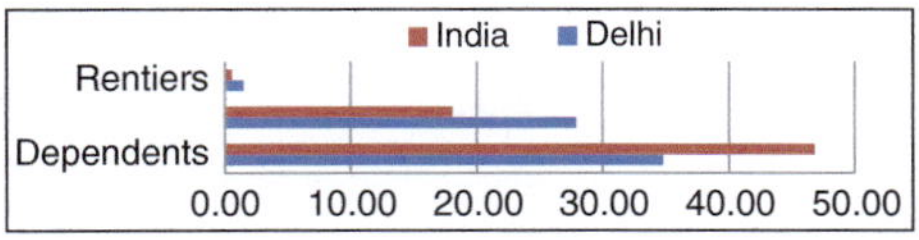

Fig. 6 Non-worker by main activity, 2011. *Source* Based on Census 2011

Census dose not collect information with respect to the amount of pension they receive. Thus, higher proportion of dependent in spite of higher proportion of pension receivers in some states is an indication towards low amount of income from pension. At the same time all the occupational categories are non-overlapping in nature. Thus it is difficult to conclude whether the pensioners are also dependent or not. To elucidate this further, main non-economic activity of the marginal workers, as available from census, is analyzed. It has been observed that only 1 % of the marginal workers among the females are also pension receivers. Delhi rank second among the major states (Punjab 9 %). All other major states have recorded high percentage of pension holder work as marginal worker mostly because pension is not sufficient enough for their survival.

Health Condition

While considering the well-being of the aged, health occupies the core position. It is mentioned that by 2030, 45 % of Indians' health burdens will be borne by the older population with a high burden of non-communicable diseases (Arokiasamy et al. 2010). However, there is hardly any data source than NSSO, which has provided information on the health status of the elderly. In the current paper only prevalence of ailment, hospitalization and major chronic illness is processed.

NSSO collects information on incidence of ailment between 1 day and 15 days prior to the survey. For the current study only longer duration of ailment is considered. With respect to the prevalence Delhi appeared quite healthy as only 126 per 1000 of the population in the state have reported any ailment 15 days prior to the survey. This figure is substantially lower than the national average where 310 persons per 1000 have reported any ailment in the same reference period of time. Different studies have shown that ailment and disability is more among the aged women than among men (Alam and Yadav 2013; Arokiasamy et al. 2010; Das and Vemuri 2009; Rajan 2001).

Ailment is a subjective response where respondents' perception influences the status. However, since the reference period is only of 15 days chances of recall error is less, but it has the probability of getting affected by the seasonality of disease with relation to the data collection period. Thus a question on episode of hospitalization was asked with a reference period of past 365 days. The cases of hospitalization are less affected by self perception on health and also expected to be less affected by recall error. In this case it has been observed that Kerala (26.2 %), Karnataka (13.3 %), Tamil Nadu (17.5 %), Gujarat (15.3 %), Haryana (16.7 %) and Rajasthan (12.3 %) reported more hospitalization among the aged than it has been observed in Delhi (10.4 %). Thus, the aged population in Delhi is considered to be less morbid (Table 7).

Delhi may be better than some of the states in terms of ailment prevalence rate for short duration but the situation is not very healthy in case of long duration or

Table 6 Positioning Delhi for the pensioners and dependents among the aged population by sex: 2011

More pensioners among males	More pensioners among females	Less dependents among males	Less dependents among females
Chandigarh (67.6), Puducherry (63.8), Andaman and Nicobar Islands (63.9)	H.P (19.6), U.K (17.3), Chandigarh (18.0); Haryana (29.2); Tripura (18.7); Odisha (19.6); Chattisgarh (23.2); Andhra Pradesh (25.7); Puducherry (40.2), Andaman and Nicobar Islands (22.4)	HP(31.6); Chandigarh (17.0); U.K (29.2); Haryana (31.4); Nagaland (25.8); Lakshadweep (17.5); Puducherry (24.8)	Punjab (29.4); Chandigarh (22.6); Haryana (28.8); Goa (32.2); Lakshadweep (24.1) Puducherry (30.3), Andaman and Nicobar Islands (28.6)
52.0	**12.4**	**34.1**	**35.2**

Figures in bold are with respect to Delhi in relevant indicator, 2011

Table 7 Distribution of the aged by type of disease they suffered, 2004

Disease type	Delhi	India
Waterborne communicable	9.0	9.5
Heart disease	16.0	9.4
Hypertension	9.5	4.5
Respiratory including asthma	6.0	9.1
Kidney disorder	6.40	5.8
Diabetes	2.70	3.7
Psychiatric disorder	1.90	0.5
Cancer	4.9	2.2
Accident	5.30	7.4
Fever of unknown origin	12.80	4.1
Cataract	8.20	11.2
Others	17.30 %	32.6

Source NSS 60th Round

persistent health problem. A larger proportion of aged in Delhi are suffering from some of the life style diseases like heart disease, hypertension, kidney disorder, cancer than the average observed at the national level. Psychiatric disorder is also quite high among the elderly population in Delhi. Along with the life style disease, Delhi has recorded a very high percentage of population who suffered from fever (12.8) of unknown origin and this proportion is more than three times higher than what is observed for the country as a whole.

Conclusion

Delhi, the capital of India attracts population from across all over India. Its characteristic feature is that a vast majority of the population are migrant from different parts of the country. Thus the state carries a cosmopolitan character. Its economic vibrancy attracts a large number of youth which keeps the state young inspite of low natural growth rate (Das and Bhusan 2014). However, sociologists on the other hand, have expressed the belief that alienation increases when people move from a small, intimate community to an urbanized, industrialized, and complex society (Parker 1978). Thus, it is prudent to believe that the aged in Delhi are worst affected by this alienation because of their restrictive mobility, physical fragility and powerlessness. They are vulnerable to different crime against them. Help Age India (2011) has done a study in twelve major cities of India and reported different kinds of elder abuse. They also have observed that NCT of Delhi tops the list in terms of crime against elderly.

Commensurating with the challenges, several steps have been taken by the Delhi government to improve the lives of the aged. Delhi Development Authority (DDA) has drafted a proposal to create the biggest housing project for the elderly built with government participation in the country. The plan is to construct around

4,500 one-room flats for the elderly on rental basis with common kitchens, canteens, medical and recreational facilities (ToI 5 July 2014). Government also has taken initiative to open recreational centres in different DDA localities where aged population can come and interact and play indoor games. Delhi police has initiated Senior Citizen Security Cell. The officers from this cell make personal visit to the registered houses where elderly is living alone. Registration with the Delhi Police is encouraged to ensure safety and security of the aged.

Finally, it is important to mention that because of its young population characteristics, Delhi's elderly received less attention from researchers. It also lacks in-depth and robust data to do further research. Delhi as a capital, experiences the wave of changes specially resulted from globalization, most severely. While Delhi is planning to be the smart city, more data base and research on marginal section of the population including the elderly is urgent need of the hour.

References

Alam, M., Yadav, P. (2013). Building Knowledge Base on Population Ageing in India: Status of Elderly in Punjab, 2011 (India: UNFPA), December 2013.

Arokiasamy, P. et.al. (2010). Longitudinal Ageing Study in India: An investigation of the health, social and economic well-being of India's growing elderly population. IIPS, Harvard School of Public Health, RAND Corporation

Ashok, B. T., & Ali, Rashid. (2003). Aging research in India. *Experimental Gerontology, 38*(6), 597–603.

Audinaryana, N., Sheela, J., & Kavitha, N. (1999). Living arrangements of the elderly women in a rural setting of South India: Patterns, differentials and determinants. *International review of modern sociology, 29*(2), 37–48.

Bloom, D.E. & Canning, D. (2008). Global Demographic Change: Dimensions and Economic Significance. In A. Prskawetz, D.E. Bloom & W. Lutz (Eds.), *Population Ageing, Human Capital Accumulation, and Productivity Growth, Population Development Review, Supplement* (Vol. 34)

Cain, Mead. (1986). The consequences of reproductive failure: dependence, mobility, and mortality among the elderly of rural South Asia. *Population Studies, 40*(3), 375–388.

Das, D.N. & Vemuri , M.D (2009). Gender Differences among Older persons: A Study Based on the 2001 Population Census of India. In *Gender Issues in Develoment-Concerns for the 21st Century*, eds. Bhaswati Das and Vimal Khawas. Jaipur: Rawat Publication

Das, D.N., Sweta, B. (2014). Magnatism in India's Metros-A Study on migrants choice of destination. *Social Change, 44* (4), 519–540.

Dowd, J.J. (1975). Aging as exchange: A preface to Theory. *Journal of Gerontology*, 584–594.

Elder Abuse & Crime in India. (2011). Help Age India. New Delhi.

Feldman, J.J. (1983). Work Ability of the Aged under Conditions of Improving Mortality. *The Milbank Memorial Fund Quarterly. Health and Society*, Special Issue: Aging: Demographic, Health, and Social Prospects(pp. 430–444).

Gee, E. M. (2000). Living arrangements and quality of life among Chinese Canadian elders. *Social Indicators Research, 51*(3), 309–329.

Golini, Antonio. (2003). Current demographic setting and the future of aging. The experience of some European countries. *Genus, 59*(1), 15–49.

Gulati, L., & Irudaya, R.S. (1999). The added years: Elderly in India and Kerala. *Economic and political weekly*, 34(44), 46–51.

Ham-Chande, R., Palloni, A., & Wong, R. (2009). *Aging in developing countries: building bridges for integrated research agendas*. IUSSP, Policy and Research Papers.

Helpage India. A Report on Elder Abuse and Crime in India. (2011). India (https://www.helpageindia.org/images/pdf/ElderAbuseCrimeIndia11.pdf)
Kim, I.K., & Kim, C. S. (2003). Patterns of family support and the quality of life of the elderly. *Social Indicators Research, 62*(1–3), 437–454.
Kramarow, E.A. (1995). The elderly who live alone in the United States: Historical perspectives on household change. *Demography, 32*(3), 335–352.
Kuntz, M.I., Garry, R.L. (1987). Status of the Elderly: An Extension of the Theory. *Journal of Marriage and Family, 49*(2), 413–420.
Kurek, S. (2014). Population ageing research from a geographical perspective-methodological approach. *Bulletin of Geography. Socio-economic Series* 8 (2007):2949. PedagogicalUniversityoCracow, http://www.bulletinofgeography.umk.pl/8_2007/S_Kurek.pdf (4 December 2014).
Lee, R.D. (2000) Intergenerational Transfers and the economic Life Cycle: A Cross Cultural perspective. In A. Mason and G. Tapinos (Eds.) *Sharing the wealth: Demographic Change and Economic Transfers between Generations.* Oxford University Press.
Martin, L.G. (1990). The status of South Asia's growing elderly population. *Journal of Cross-Cultural Gerontology, 5*(2), 93–117.
Mirkin, B., & Weinberger, M.B. (2001). The demography of aging population Population Bulletin of the United Nations, *Living Arrangements of Older Persons.* Special Issues No. 42/43, (2001): pp 37–53.
Mukherjee, D.(2008). Globalization without social protection: Challenges to aging societies across developing nations. *The Global Studies Journal, 1*(1), 225–241.
Nair, L. V. (2014). Ageing in India-A conceptual clarification in the background of globalization. *European Scientific Journal, 10*(2), 379–392.
ORGI. (2001).http://censusindia.gov.in/Data_Products/Data_Highlights/Data_Highlights_link/data_ highlights_D1D2D3.pdf (downloaded on 5 December 2014).
ORGI. (2006). Population projections for India and states 2001–2026—Report of the technical group on population projections constituted by the national commission on population. Government of India.
ORGI. (2011). http://www.censusindia.gov.in/2011census/hlo/HLO_Tables.html. Accessed on 5 December 2014.
ORGI. (2011). http://www.censusindia.gov.in/DigitalLibrary/TablesSeries2001.aspx. Accessed on 5 December 2014.
Parker, J.H. (1978). The Urbanism-Alienation Hypothesis: A Critique. *International Review of Modern Sociology, 8*(2), 239–244.
Preston, S. H. (1975). The changing relation between mortality and level of economic development. *Population studies, 29*(2), 231–248.
Rajan, S. Irudaya, U.S.M., & Sarma, P.S. (2001). Health concerns among India's elderly. *The International Journal of Aging and Human Development, 53*(3), 181–194.
Rajan, S. Irudaya, & Sanjay, K. (2003). Living arrangements among Indian elderly: New evidence from national family health survey. *Economic and Political Weekly, 38*(1), 75–80.
Sivamurthy, M., Wadakannavar, A.R. (2001). Care and support for the elderly population in India: Results of a survey rural North Karnataka. 2001. Available: http://www.iussp.org/Brazil2001/s50/S55_P04_Sivamurthy.pdf.
Srivastava, V. (2010). *Women Aging.* New Delhi: Rawat Publications.
Supan-Axel Börsch & H. Jurges (2008). Changes in Health Status and Work Disability. In A. Börsch-Supan et al. (Eds.) *Health, Ageing and Retirement in Europe (2004–2007)—Starting the Longitudinal Dimension* (pp. 230–238). Mannheim: MEA.
Times of India. (2014). Delhi Development Authority plans to build 4,500 flats for the elderly, *Times of India*, November 5, 2014.
United Nations. (2002). Political Declaration and Madrid International Plan of Action on Ageing, Second World Assembly on Ageing, Madrid, Spain.
World Health Organisation. (2002). *Active ageing: A Policy Framework.* Geneva: UN.

Water and Sanitation and Public Health Issues in Delhi

Ajit Kumar Lenka and Golak B. Patra

Abstract India has more than one billion people who live in different ecological, social and cultural regions. Providing safe water and improved sanitation to such a large and diverse population is a challenge. Socio-economic development, education, poverty, awareness, and practice of rituals add to the complexity of providing water and sanitation; and consequent to good health of people. Around 5 million people die due to waterborne diseases annually. More than 1.5 million children are estimated to die of diarrhoea alone each year in India. In developing countries, some 2.6 billion people invest a significant proportion of their household time or money in securing drinking water or a private space to defecate. Over 9 % of the global disease burden could be prevented by better management of water, that is, supply, conservation and sanitation. Water is fundamental to addressing diarrhoea, cholera, malaria control, Guinea worm eradication; and non-communicable conditions such as fluorosis, arsenicosis, hydration-related effects and exposure to modern pollutants. Public health perspective in water management provides opportunities to improve population health and reduce costs. Accessing drinking water continues to be a problem for more than 32 % households even today in India. Despite an estimated total of Rs. 1,105 billion spent on providing safe drinking water since the First Five Year Plan was launched in 1951, lack of safe and secure drinking water continues to be a major economic burden. In 2000 water quality monitoring was accorded a high priority. The Government of India launched the National Rural Drinking Water Quality Monitoring and Surveillance

A.K. Lenka (✉) · G.B. Patra
Centre of Social Medicine and Community Health, School of Social Sciences,
Jawaharlal Nehru University, New Delhi, India
e-mail: ajitlenka.lenka@gmail.com

G.B. Patra
e-mail: gulu.jnu@gmail.com

S.S. Acharya et al. (eds.), *Marginalization in Globalizing Delhi: Issues of Land, Livelihoods and Health*, DOI 10.1007/978-81-322-3583-5_22

Programme (NRWQMSP) in February 2006. This paper endeavours to examine the status of water supply to the vulnerable populations in the slums of Delhi and the challenges involved between different stakeholders on water management. It includes the quality of water supplied and events of illnesses with probable association to water quality.

Keywords Water and sanitation · Health · Waterborne disease · Slums · Delhi

Introduction

India has more than one billion people who live in different ecological, social and cultural regions. Providing safe water and improved sanitation to such a large and diverse population is an enormous challenge. Differential level of awareness, socio-economic development, education, poverty, practices and rituals add to the complexity of providing water and sanitation; and consequent good health to people. Around 38 million Indians are affected and around five million people die due to waterborne diseases annually. More than 1.5 million children are estimated to die of diarrhoea alone each year. The economic burden thus faced is estimated at $600 million a year. In developing countries, some 2.6 billion people invest a significant proportion of their household time or money in securing drinking water or a private space to defecate. Over 9 % of the global disease burden could be prevented by better management of water, that is, supply, conservation and sanitation. Water is fundamental to addressing diarrhoea, cholera, malaria control, Guinea worm eradication; and non-communicable conditions such as fluorosis, arsenicosis, hydration-related effects and exposure to modern pollutants. Public health perspective in water management provides opportunities to improve population health and reduce costs.

The provision of clean drinking water has been given priority in the Constitution of India, with Article 47 conferring the duty of providing clean drinking water and improving public health standards to the State. The government has undertaken various programmes since independence to provide safe drinking water and sanitation. Despite an estimated total of Rs. 1,105 billion spent on providing safe drinking water since the First Five Year Plan was launched in 1951, lack of safe and secure drinking water continues to be a major economic burden. Accessing drinking water continues to be a problem for more than 32 % households even today. In 2000 water quality monitoring was accorded a high priority. The Government of India launched the National Rural Drinking Water Quality Monitoring and Surveillance Programme (NRWQMSP) in February 2006.

Study Methodology

The current paper attempts to examine the challenges of water supply to the vulnerable populations in the slums of Delhi. The quality of water supplied and events of illnesses with probable association to water quality has been analyzed through this study. The present study is mainly undertaken using the secondary sources of data. Major sources are the Survey Reports, like National Family Health Survey (NFHS), District Level Household & Facility Survey (DLHS), National Sample Survey organization (NSSO), and Census Reports. Some of the micro studies have been used for the study as well.

People Living in Slums

In India, the number of people living in towns and cities is growing rapidly both as a result of natural urban growth and migration into towns and cities from rural areas. This adds significantly to the number of people living without safe drinking water or adequate sanitation in urban areas. It also causes more unemployment and poverty, widening the gap between the urban rich and the urban poor who lack access to a whole range of basic services in addition to the clean water and sanitation, including health care, education, transportation, housing, security, information and justice. Due to the rapid urbanization[1] and population explosion, the management of water and sanitation is a major problem in urban areas. Most people in the urban slums[2] are vulnerable to access resources for their life and livelihoods. State is often not in a position to address the needs due to reasons varying from invisibility of such population to lack of funds. Invisibility due to inappropriate and incomplete identity documents deprives them of many services including the ones as basic as water and sanitation. It therefore becomes imperative to examine the condition of such people, especially when efforts such as Jawaharlal Nehru National Urban Mission (JnNURM)[3] have been put in place.

The economic growth depends on the quality and availability of infrastructure services like: roads, transportation, electricity, water supply, sanitation and solid waste management facilities in any urban area. As per the 2011 census, 31.2 % population lives in urban areas in India and the rate of growth of urban population has been increasing. About 65 % of the gross domestic product (GDP) is contributed by urban areas. Due to the growth of urbanization, there is a problem in providing basic services to the population residing in urban area.

As per the Census Report 2011, 17.4 %, of the population in urban areas were living in slums. It amounted to million people consisting 137.49 lakhs households who were living in slums in 2543 reported towns spread over 26 states and Union Territories. In India, 21 % of urban population are living in poor condition and

[1]Urbanization is a process people are living in a particular environment and majority of the population are engaged in less agricultural activities.

[2]A Slum, for the purpose of Census, has been defined as residential areas where dwellings are unfit for human habitation by reasons of dilapidation, overcrowding, faulty arrangements and design of such buildings, narrowness or faulty arrangement of street, lack of ventilation, light, or sanitation facilities or any combination of these factors which are detrimental to the safety and health (Census 2011).

[3]JnNRUM-Jawaharlal Nehru National Urban Renewal Mission, The aim is to encourage reforms and fast track planned development of identified cities. Focus is to be on efficiency in urban infrastructure and service delivery mechanisms, community participation, and accountability of ULBs/ Parastatal agencies towards citizens (MUD 2011).

Table 1 Population living in Delhi Slums

Sl. No	Year	Slum population (Lakh)	Total population (Lakh)	Share of Delhi population living in slums (%)
1	1951	0.6	14.4	4.4
2	1973	4.9	40.1	12.3
3	1983	5.7	61.7	9.2
4	1990	13.0	81.1	16.0
5	1997	30.0	108.1	27.6
6	2001	21.5	127.4	16.9
7	2010	21.6	153.1	14.1
8	2011	NA	NA	17.4

Source Slum Department, Municipal Corporation of Delhi (MCD) from 1951–2001, Census, 2011
NA Not Available

they do not get access to basic facilities in urban areas. Eighty percentage of urban population have access to safe drinking water but the quality and quantity vary; 36 % household had waterborne toilets that are connected by public sewerage system while 46 % household have waterborne toilets. In urban areas, there is high amount solid base generated every day and the west management becomes difficult (GOI 2009; RGI 2011). Table 1 shows the slum population in Delhi.

Challenges of Water Supply and Sanitation of the Urban Poor in Delhi
At present, more than 65 million people are living in slums in Delhi (The Hindu 2014). Delhi, the metropolis and the National Capital Territory of India, has the forth largest number of urban households (14.6 %) living in slum areas followed by Chennai (28.5 %), Kolkata (29.6 %) and Greater Mumbai (41 %), (Census 2011). As per the NSS 69th[4] Round, 53.4 % households, living in slum areas, have access to improved sources of drinking water in Delhi. At the same time 99.3 % households living in non-slum areas have improved source of drinking water. Only 24 % households living in slum areas used improved source of toilet facilities and members of one out of six households defecate in open areas (NFHS-3 2005–06). It is one of the cities in India where highest municipality waste (9,500 tonnes) is generated every day which becomes difficult to manage. Only one thousand tonnes municipality waste are treated every day whereas 5,700 tonnes waste are dumped at landfill sites (The Indian Express 2014a, b, c and d). In slums, the condition of water supply and sanitation is very poor due to various challenges like, economic, political, sociocultural, environmental, infrastructural barrier, administrative barrier, technological barrier and educational barriers. It leads to the poor condition of the people living in slums in Delhi. These barriers are discussed below.

[4]As per the National Sample Survey (NSS) 69th Report based on Key Indicators of Drinking Water, Sanitation, Hygiene and Housing Condition in India (NSSO 2013). http://mospi.nic.in/mospi_new/upload/kye_indi_of_water_Sanitation69rou_24dec13.pdf.

Economic Challenges:
The access to water supply and sanitation is a fundamental need. All human beings should be able to access it as a right. Safe drinking water and proper sanitation are important conditions for poverty reduction. But in the developing and under-developed countries, the condition of water supply and sanitation is very poor. It is due to the poor economic condition. According to World Health Organization (WHO), 884 million people do not have access to safe drinking water and 2.6 billion people do not have access to sanitation facilities (WHO-UNICEF 2002). In developing countries, the water supply and sanitation condition are very poor due to the high access cost. People have poor health condition due to lack of proper water and sanitation. The poor access to water supply and sanitation has a barrier to improve the health of the people. The lack of access to water supply and poor sanitation condition are major factors for the high mortality rate in developing countries. Every year, 1.8 million people die of diarrhoea and 90 % children under five die due to the inadequate water supply and sanitation condition (Haller et al. 2007).

Minh and Hung (2011) study shows that in developing countries, people's economic growth and health condition depend on improved sanitation condition. Poor sanitation results in a number of diseases worldwide and 10 % of total global burden of disease is due to the poor sanitation and unsafe water supply. Due to the poor sanitation, various diseases are increasing like diarrheal, acute respiratory infection, undernutrition and other tropical disease.

Water is important for life. Without water existence is in danger. Water and disease are closely related, contaminated water is the cause of waterborne diseases and diarrhoea is the one of them. Rapid urbanization is the major cause that creates pressure on infrastructure like water supply and sanitation. The stress on water supply affects it quality, particularly, of those belonging to lower economic households living in slum areas with inadequate infrastructure. The low economic status households mainly experience waterborne diseases and the diarrhoea is a major one of them, caused by polluted water (Dasgupta 2004).

The policy makers and general public have not fully realized the importance of improvement in sanitation as a solution to reduce various diseases. The government also failed to interpret that improved sanitation is an important part of economic growth. India is a country, where inadequate sanitation condition is the primary drive of economic deprivation. A line could be drawn that, every state has been rendered more significant for the water and sanitation and must invest more for access of adequate sanitation. Achieving Millennium Development Goal (MDG) of sanitation will help in stimulating economic growth in developing countries like India.

Poverty is another important reason for poor sanitation infrastructure in India. (Bhan and Jena 2004), on their paper, discussed about the poor households who pay more than their larger part of monthly income for accessing basic services. People living in slum areas are facing more health-related problems because of the poor hygienic condition. When rich people are disproportionately contaminating the environment, only poor people are suffering. In India, particular castes are involved in cleaning the wastes, but they are treated as unclean untouchables due to the presence of caste system in various forms and shapes in society. India will not be clean unless and until the existing caste system is not eradicated from its roots (Teltumbde 2014).

Every year, millions of children under 5 years die due to diarrhoea which is the result of poor water supply and sanitation condition. The survey also demonstrates importance of oral rehydration therapy because of the high burden of diarrhoea among children below 5 years of age all over the nation. Cost-effective solutions to improve water supply and sanitation do exist. These 'software related' interventions include providing education, social marketing of good hygiene practice and regulation of drinking water supply and monitoring of water quality for positive impact on health and reduced diarrhoea among children under 5 years. The use cost-effective intervention has been used due to giving importance role of water supply and sanitation in health sector. But we always perceive that water and sanitation generally involves only physical infrastructure, water supply sanitation is only a programme and always misunderstand the role of water supply and sanitation in health sector (Varely et al. 1998).

Bajpai and Bhandari (2001) stated that in India, millions of people were facing problems related to water supply to fulfil their daily requirements. In India, people mainly living in urban areas are primarily dependent on supply water for day-to-day life, but in many cities and towns in India, people cannot access tap water provided by municipalities. In many cities and towns in India, access of water supply to those who are economically poor is difficult. The household economic condition is an important determinant to access water supply, so both the policy makers and academics need to pay more attention to water supply and invest in water supply based on economic capabilities of the households.

The issue of inequality, quality, affordability and accessibility to the water supply among the poor slum dwellers of Chennai, Tamil Nadu was highlighted by Anand (2007), The access to water supply is very important in a poor household, those are poor, do not have access to water supply services and many private tanker supply drinking water which is quite costly. The study conducted in Chennai showed that, the quality of water varied based on household income, those with high-income households, had access to good quality of water and poor have substandard quality of drinking water.

The present government has started *Swachh Bharat Abhiyan* (SBA) on 2 October 2014 for cleaning India and building toilets for making India open defecation free. Two lakh crore rupees will be spent on SBA over the next 5 year as per the consideration of both rural and urban development ministries. The central government is also planning to give responsibility to corporate sector for fulfilling this mission. The mission also focuses on eradication manual scavenging and solid waste management and converting waste into wealth (The Hindu 2014).

Majority of the slums in Delhi do not have safe drinking water, improved toilet (even no toilets), and separate space for cooking, proper ventilation and electricity facilities in their housing units or in public. The Data shows that in Delhi 60 percent Households who have been settled in slum areas they don't have window facilities in their house and only 24% household used improved toilet facilities (NFHS-3 2005–06).

Political Challenges

In India, millions of people migrated from rural to urban in search of better life and livelihood. But due to the poor economic condition they live in slums. They are unable to access basic amenities. Provisioning of services and facilities in slums is influenced by different factors, political contact is one of them. Political factor has an important role in accessing basic amenities. The political accessibility is crucial for the survival of the slum dweller to get basic amenities in urban areas India. During election period, the political leaders make many promises about providing facilities slum areas but after winning they have many boundaries to enter the slum.

Slums are marked with unplanned settlements with limited access to all facilities specially water supply and sanitation services. The unhygienic living condition often causes illness. There are livelihood issues and often human dignity is at stake due to poor security and safety, especially of women and girls. Thus barriers in access include social position, political links and cost of accessing water services and location and distance from the source of water (Bouselly et al. 2006).

In 2011, studying the access to water inequality in Delhi through feminist political ecology framework, Truelove found that in urban areas accessibility to water clearly highlights the existing inequalities for women, which they had to face in everyday life due to social and gender differences. He also found that the distribution of water supply in Delhi is broadly based on the power and inequality. Those who are affluent and powerful would get access to clean water easily, while those who are poor and powerless, mainly living in slums, would have to be on the mercy of concerned authorities. Due to scarce water supply, these poor people, especially poor women and girls, are forced to fetch the water from the tankers to meet their basic need. The growth of slums is a major problem in India. Various programmes are implemented by the government, NGOs, donor agencies to solve the problem. But disparities existing in slum areas act as disabling factors in solving the problems. Most of the programmes, opportunities and resources are accessed by some section of the population who are financially better off than the others (Agarwal and Taneja 2005).

Figure 1 shows that as per the NSS 69th[5] Round, in Delhi 53.4 % households are living in slums have access to improved source of drinking water. Whereas 99.3 % of the household living in non-slums have access to improved source of drinking water (NSSO 2013).

With the announcement of the *Swachh Bharat Yojona (SBA)*, the country, the ministers, the bureaucrats, and the armed forces personnel joined in SBA to 'clean' different parts of India, particularly Delhi. The Health Minister of Delhi, in his address during the cleanliness drive as a part of SBA in Nirman Bhawan categorically stated that '*Swachh Bharat* is linked with *Swastha Bharat*'. The Environment Minister reflected his participation in SBA by 'banning' the use of plastic

---

[5]As per the National Sample Survey (NSS) 69th Report based on Key Indicators of Drinking Water, Sanitation, Hygiene and Housing Condition in India (NSSO 2013). http://mospi.nic.in/mospi_new/upload/kye_indi_of_water_Sanitation69rou_24dec13.pdf.

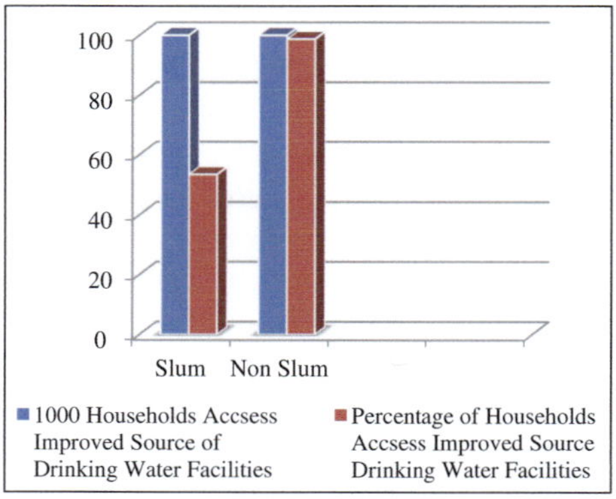

Fig. 1 Improved source of drinking water supply facilities per thousand households living in slum and Non-slum areas 2013. *Source* NSSO 69th Round 2012

bottles—*'no more plastic bottle... in environment ministry'*. State Minister also promised to build one lakh toilets in school. All the politicians, government officials are campaigning for SBA but nobody seems to be saying anything about those cleaning the city every day, and for whom nothing is changing in their lives. In Delhi, a safai karmachari[6] said that *''our salaries still low, most of us working contract basis and we rarely get our money on time but never get pay slip. Delhi might become clean but we will remain poor and untouched'*. Another safai karmachari mentioned that *'It does not make any differences, we haven't get salary on time so we can't celebrate any way'* Another safai karmachari said that *'I fell sick and could not able to work for a month, later I had stop working. But my bills still with the Delhi municipal department and I haven't seen a single paisa' The Indian Express* 2014a, b, c *and* d.

The current government and other party members have also taken initiatives for fulfilling the aim of SBA. In Delhi residential areas, the Aam Admi Party (AAP)[7] members have taken initiatives for cleaning garbage through the support of residents using WhatsApp and helpline number. The party proposed to lodges complaint to the local Municipal Corporation for garbage collection. The ruling party has also taken initiative by sending messages to general people of Delhi by submitting the photographs of garbage stock anywhere in Delhi to inform local civic authorities and what action will be taken for those complaints will also be updated every day. Both the ruling party and other parties are taking responsibility for the BSA but the outcome will be seen only in the future (The India Express 2014a, b, c and d).

Sociocultural Challenges

The caste system in India is the mother of all challenges in accessing the water and sanitation facilities by all the slum dwellers. Not only in Delhi but in all parts

[6]As per the concern of Department of Law, Justice and Legislative Affairs "Safai Karamchari" means a person engaged in, or employed for, assisting in disposal of human excreta, or any sanitation work (DLJ&LA 2006).

[7]Aam Aadmi Party (AAP) is a national political party of India.

of the country it is considered that fetching water is the sole duty of the women and girls. It has seen even more rigid when the education level of the household or the community is low. Those are mainly staying in slums in urban areas.

Superstitions and cultural practices are yet another set of barriers to the access of water supply and sanitation facilities. Many disabled people are not accessing safe drinking water supply and sanitation facilities, both in rural and urban areas. In Bangladesh people believe that, disability is a disease transmitted by infections due to karmic punishment. Therefore, disabled persons are banned from using public facilities like latrines. According to the Statement of the Committee for the Right to Sanitation (45th session, E/C.12/2010/1) of the United Nations Committee on Social, Economic and Cultural Right, *'States must ensure that everyone, without discrimination, has physical and affordable access to sanitation, in all spheres of life, which is safe, hygienic, secure, socially and culturally acceptable, provides privacy and ensures dignity'*. Access to safe water supply and sanitation is positively impacting on health and growth of the economic condition of the society (Noga and Wolbring 2012).

(Jha and Nitish 2010) Access to water supply and sanitation is governed mainly by the economic, technological, institutional as well as social factors. In the urban areas those living in slum, due to the poor economic condition cannot get piped water connectivity because the government worker takes extra charges. The leakage in piped water is another reason for lowering the pressure of water which is a major problem for slum population to collect water from tap. The social and religious views of purity act as barriers in accepting indoor latrines because of perceptions associated with rituals. Large sections of population are facing difficulties to access health care resources because of social discrimination. This defeats the very purpose of universal health care which is based on the principle of universal coverage for all members of the society. Caste system is very complex and intricate and it plays a major role in accessing the basic services like water sanitation and health care is difficult to establish (Acharya 2013).

The government of India started the *'Swachh Bharat Abhiyan (SBA)'*[8] initiative for clean India and changing daily practices of millions people who practice open defecation. Building toilets alone is not going to address the problem of open defecation unless there is a change in peoples' behaviour and mindset. Because even who have a toilet repeatedly prefer for open defecate. Due to the practices of open defecation hundred thousands of babies are dying in India. Majority of the people have more knowledge regarding smoking, having tobacco and drinking alcohol are negative or harmful impact on health but very less people have knowledge on the bad impact of open defecation. Lack of information, education and communication even after 15 years *Total Sanitation Campaign* leads to lower level of knowledge on sanitation. So it is important to make awareness along with the construction of the infrastructure for the better sanitation. Government must take

[8]The government of India implemented a scheme for total sanitation programme both urban and rural areas.

priority for constructed toilets and in same time also must take priority for its own dedicated staff to change people's behaviour for open defecation free (ODF), (Gupta and Hathi 2014).

Environmental Challenges

The growth of urban population, particularly slums is an important reason for environmental problems in the cities in India. The situation in the megacities is devastation. The government is unable to fulfil basic needs like water supply, sanitation and infrastructural facilities. Every year millions of people migrated to the urban India and live illegally and forcefully in the government acquired land. The factors responsible for environmental problem include colonial laws characterized by inequitable access to sanitation services, lack of funding for urban slum dwellers by the governments, failure to manage urban growth and increase slums. In the post-colonial period, the state has been dominated by the group of people interest in public funds to provide private goods for the sanitation development. The government provided sanitation services for urban poor but due to the lack of political pressure, government failed to implement the policies for improving their living condition (Chaplin 2011). In addition, poor management administrative status is also responsible for the reducing the water supply (Bownder and Chattri 1984).

In India, accessing clean drinking water for the entire population is a fundamental right as per the consideration of Supreme Court on December 2000 under the Article 21. In India, the drinking water is collected mainly from various sources such as ground water and rivers. Mainly groundwater and rivers are now polluted because of untreated industrial effluent and untreated sewerage. In general, if the ground waters are polluted due to the industrial effluent and untreated sewerage then it takes time up to hundreds of years for normal condition. A study conducted by Central Pollution Control Board, New Delhi mentioned that 12 major rivers are polluted and the quality of water was very terrible and does not fulfil the parameters those are required. Here in Delhi, Yamuna River is polluted due to the contamination of untreated sewerage (Ramachandraiah 2001).

Growth of chemical factories and breakdown of the sewerage system facilities in cities are important factors for the pollution of river and source of drinking water in urban areas. In micro level, those living in slum areas basically are urban poor they are living in unhygienic condition, the lack of sewerage, water supply and sanitation facilities, create major environmental problems and its severely effects people health (Kundu 1991). In 2012, Sabat conducted a study on the underlying causes of environmental degradation and its impact on Bhubaneswar city of Odisha. Due to the environmental degradation, various problems emerge like, excessive heat in summer, scarcity of drinking water supply in summer, air pollution and water pollution. The main cause of environmental degradation is mainly the uncontrolled growth of population, poor drainage system, poor sanitation system, deforestation and improper management solid waste. Vijaya et al. (2010) define the ground water plays the most important role of natural resources especially in the coastal urban areas in Puri town in Odisha, where people are dependent on ground water for drinking purpose but the quality of water is deteriorating due to the lack of proper sewerage system.

Administrative Challenges

Panda and Agrwala (2003) on their study show that the inadequate provisioning such as lack of infrastructure, human recourses, poor quality mechanism for water supply and sanitation are the main reasons for poor condition water supply sanitation in Delhi slum areas. Those funds sanctioned by the government were not properly utilized in the slum areas. As per the 11th five year plan, the government had sanctioned 73 crores for providing drinking water supply and sanitation in slum areas. The money has been sanctioned through two scheme plans such as Grant in Aid Augmentation of water supply and Water supply for Resettlement colonies but twenty crores are not utilized. In twelfth year plan also only 4.8 crores have been sanctioned to Delhi Jal Board (DJB)[9] for providing drinking water supply in slum areas. In Delhi where, 1,058 Notified Slums[10] and 2,075 Non-Notified slums[11] has not possible for providing proper drinking water supply in limited resources. So, due to limited funds it has not been possible to cover proper water supply and sanitation facilities in all slum areas. Even the sanctioned money was not also utilized properly for water supply and sanitation.

Infrastructural Challenges

It is very much evident that most of the urban slums are congested and pushed to the unhealthy locations in any part of a city. In case of Delhi, the similarities are found. Slums are scattered through the city but there are minimal infrastructures for the dwellers. Some of the slums are situated in illegal and government-owned lands. And as a result they provided no public health facilities or the facilities are provided poorly. Slums situated in Yamuna banks are facing extreme odds during the monsoon.

The urban growth increases informal settlements in urban areas. The facilities can be provided for formal units. Therefore, residents of informal settlements like slums are unable to access public health services especially water supply and sanitation. (Solo et al. 1993) A study was conducted in Mumbai where the slum sanitation programmes within the adequate sanitation programme in informal settlement in slum areas. The slum sanitation programme is offered as a solution to the

---

[9]Delhi Jal Board is responsible for production of water in Delhi and its distribution in the area under the control of Municipal Corporation of Delhi. The Board also supplies water in bulk to N.D.M.C. and Delhi Cantonment. Besides, the Board is responsible for collection, treatment and disposal of sewage in Delhi http://delhi.gov.in/wps/wcm/connect/d38fb2804ff1fee7bf28bfd9d1b46642/Water+Supply+WU89.pdf?MOD=AJPERES&lmod=-336682211&CACHEID=d38fb2804ff1fee7bf28bfd9d1b46642 Accessed on 13/9/2014.

[10]As per the 2011 census "All notified areas in a town or city notified as 'Slum' by State, UT Administration or Local Government under any Act including a 'Slum Act' (Census 2011) https://www.google.co.in/?gfe_rd=cr&ei=34GRVOSDNY_V8geT04CQBg#q=definition+of+slum+as+per+census+2011".

[11]As per the 2011 census Identified Slum is a "A compact area of at least 300 population or about 60–70 households of poorly built congested tenements, in unhygienic environment usually with inadequate infrastructure and lacking in proper sanitary and drinking water facilitie (Census 2011) https://www.google.co.in/?gfe_rd=cr&ei=34GRVOSDNY_V8geT04CQBg#q=definition+of+slum+as+per+census+2011".

solve sanitation problems of the slum areas is mainly based on partnership, participation and cost recovery. The programme suggested that user fees to be charged for the sanitation facilities offered. It also argued that the programme is a flexible approach in urban sanitation intervention for policy infrastructure, technical infrastructure and cost recovery.

Diseases related to the water and sanitation in the Slums:
The inadequate water supply and sanitation condition is the cause of diarrhoeal disease and mortality among children under 5 years in developing countries, especially in slum areas. Every year, 15 % of children die due to the unsafe water supply, poor sanitation and unhygienic condition in low- and middle-income countries. In a study in Bangladesh, the effect of improved sanitation in urban areas was studied through the changes in weight and height of 153 children who used latrine. It was evident that children using latrines reported fewer incidences of diarrhoea. Use of latrines also created safe and hygienic environment (Buttenheim 2008). Another study shows that poor water supply, sanitation and unhygienic condition are related to undernutrition. In India, 53 % of the population goes for open defecation and 48 % below 5 years are stunted. There are evidences that if proper water supply and sanitation can be ensured, hygienic condition are likely to prevail, and problem under nutrition controlled in India (Champers and Mendoza 2013).

Esery et al. (1991) study shows that, poor water supply and sanitation cause of the various diseases like, Ascariasis, Diarrhoea, Dracunuculiasis, hookworm infection, Schistosomiasis and Trachoma. The improved sanitation and water supply can protect people from the diseases and 144 studies analyses in the study. The study concludes that the personal water supply and domestic hygienic conditions are important to reduce the rates of these diseases and sanitation facilities reduced the diarrhoea mortality. A study conducted among the urban poor in Mumbai city, showed that there is high prevalence of diseases due to the poor water supply, sanitation and unhygienic condition. The data shows that annually 61,468 cases of diarrhoea, typhoid and malaria are reported. The high prevalence of diseases in the slums is due to the various reasons like, the slums being situated near polluted waterways, the lack of sewerage and sanitation facilities in the communities, personal hygienic condition is very poor due to the less availability of water supply, poverty and lack of environmental education. The poor environmental conditions are the cause of people suffering in the slum and the data collected from 1,070 household in four slums. The paper concluded that the safe adequate water supply and sanitation facilities reduce diseases and decrease mortality rates (Karan and Harada 2002).

Knudsen and Sloofen (1992) in their study 'Vector Borne Diseases Problems in Rapid Urbanization', show that the growth of urbanization process results in high population growth, unhygienic condition, increasing urban poor and the degrading environment condition. In slum areas due to inadequate water supply, garbage collection services and surface water drainage system create serious vector bone diseases such as malaria, lymphatic filariasis and dengue as major public health problem because of the growth of urbanization. The Municipal Corporation is taking important part in using community resources and spraying pesticide to control

Table 2 Water-related diseases

Waterborne Diseases: caused by the ingestion of water contaminated by human or animal faeces or urine containing pathogenic bacteria or viruses; include Cholera, Typhoid, Amoebic and bacillary dysentery and other diarrheal diseases
Water-washed Diseases: caused by poor personal hygiene and skin or eye contact with contaminated water; include scabies, trachoma and flea, lice and tick-borne diseases
Water-based diseases: caused by parasite found in intermediate organism living in contaminated water; include Dracunculiasis, Schistosomiasis, and other Helminths
Water-related Diseases: caused by insect vectors, especially mosquitoes, that breed in water include Dengue, Filariasis, Malaria, Onchocerciasis, Trypansomiasis and Yellow fever

Sources Dirty Water: Estimated Deaths from Water-Related Diseases 2000–2020, Pacific Institute Research Report, Peter H. Gleick, August 15, 2002, Online access

of waterborne diseases. Bhunia et al. (2006) in their study shows that inadequate water supply and poor sanitation is the reason for cholera in West Bengal. Two hundred and ninety cases are reported on diarrhoea from various health care facilities and the attack rate is highest among the children in a certain period of time. Following Table 2 is showing some of the water-related diseases.

Discussion

The growth of urbanization is a worldwide phenomenon. In India, 31.16 % of total population are living in urban area as per the 2011 census. The growth of urbanization took place mainly due to migration of people from rural to urban areas in the misery of poor economic condition. In Delhi, 14.6 % urban households are living in slum areas as per the census 2011. Various challenges have emerged in urban areas due to rapid population growth. These problems are: growth of slums, housing, and lack of good transportation, crime, environmental, water supply and sanitation. But the public health service to the urban poor is one of the sensitive issues to be addressed by the urban local body.

The government has various schemes for the water supply and sanitation. But now it is the time to implement those programmes in the effective way to address the problem. In the slum areas those have better economic condition had more drinking water and toilets facilities than the others who are poorer in the same slum. A particular section of society engaging in sanitary work and the government provides very less facilities and payments for their work. Technology needs to be developed specifically for sanitation works in such a way that it can be used. The government has provided community or individual toilets facilities for urban poor in slum areas, without water supply which affects proper functioning of the toilets. The government needs to be more focused on availability of water connection in the toilets. In the slum areas majority of the people have toilets but they still continue to defecate in open. This needs more focus on awareness to change peoples' behaviour on open defecation. Monitoring of water business is much needed. Many international and national companies are promoting bottled water business. Poor people are further getting marginalized from accessing water as they are unable to afford it. Funds for developing water supply and sanitation in slum areas remain often unutilized while the problem continues. So it is important ensure proper use of the funds allocated for the purpose which they are meant. This can be a way to address the present need.

References

Acharya, S.S. (2013). Universal health care: pathways from access to utilization among valunerable population. *Indian Journal of Public Health 57*, (4).

Agarwal, S., & Taneja, S. (2005). All slums are not equal: Child health condition among urban poor. *Indian Pedriatrics, 44*, 233–244.

Anand, P.B (2007). Semantics of success or pragmatic of progress: an assessment of India's progress with drinking water supply. *The Journal of Environment Development*, 32–57.

Bajpai, P., & Bhandari, L. (2001). Ensuring access to water in urban households. *Economic and Political Weekly*, 3774–3778.

Bhan, G., & Jana, A. (2013). Of slums or poverty: Notes of Caution from Census 2011. *Economic and Political Weekly, xlviiI*(18), 13–16.

Bhunia, R., Ramchandran, R., Yvan, H., & Mohan, G. D. (2006). Cholera outbreak secondary to contaminated pipe water in urban area, West Bengal. *India. Median J Gostroenterol, 28*(2), 62–64.

Bouselly, L., Shreekant, G., & Debjani, G. (2006). Water and Urban poo. *NIUA WP*, 1–27.

Bownder, B., & Chattri, R. (1984). Urban Water Supply in India: Environmental issues. *Urban Ecology 8*, 295–311 (Elseiver Science Publisher).

Champers, R., & Von-Mendoza, G. (2013). Sanitation and stunting in India under nutrition's blind spot. *Economic Political Weekly xlviii, 25*, 1–4.

Chaplin, S. E. (2011). Indian cities, sanitation and the state: the politics of the failure to provide. *Environment and Urbanization, 23*(1), 57–70.

Dasgupta, P. (2004). Valuing health damages from water pollution in Uraban Delhi, India: A health valuing health production function approach. *Environment and Development Economics, 1*, 83–106.

Esery, S. A., Potash, J. B., Roberts, L., & Shiff, C. (1991). Effects of improve water supply and sanitation on Ascariasis, Diarrhoea, Dracunculisis, Hookworm, infectious, Schistosmiasis and Trachoma. *Bulletin of the World Health Organization, 5*, 609–621.

Gupta, A, & Hati, P.(2014). A Sanitation Sena for India. http://indianexpress.com/article/opinion/columns/a-sanitation-sena-for-india/. Accessed 15 March 2014.

Haller, L., Guy, H., & Bartram, J. (2007). Estimating the cost and health benifits of water and sanitation improvement at global level. *Journal of Water and Health, 05*(4), 1–14.

Jha, & Nitish (2010). Access of the poor water supply and sanitation in india: salient concept, issues and cases. *International Policy Center for Inclusive Growth 62*.

Karan, S. K., & Harada, H. (2002). Field survey on water supply, sanitation and associated health impacts in urban poor communities: A case from Mumbai city India. *Water Science and Technology (IWA), 45*(11–12), 269–275.

Knudsen, A. B., & Sloofen, R. (1992). Vector borne diseases problems in rapid urbanization: new aproches to vector control. *Bulletin the World Health Organization, 70*(1), 1–6.

Kundu, A. (1991). Micro environment in urban planning: access of poor to water supply and sanitation. *Economic Political Weekly, 26*(37), 2167–2171.

M-Buttenheim, A. (2008). The sanitation enviornment in urban slum: implication for child health. *Population Enviornment 30*, 26–47 (Published Online).
Minh, H. V., & Nguyen, V. H. (2011). Economic aspects of sanitation in developing countries. *Environmental Health Insight, 5*, 63–70.
National Family Health Survey (NFHS-3).(2006). Health and Living Conditions in Eight Indian Cities, 5–118. http://pdf.usaid.gov/pdf_docs/PNADQ634.pdf
National Sample Survey, 69th Round. (2013). Key Indicators of Drinking Water, Sanitation, Hygine and Housing Condition in India, 3–48.
Noga, J., & Wolbring, G. (2012). The economic and social benefits and the barriers of providing people with disabilities accessible clean water and sanitation. *Sustainability, 4*(11), 3023-3041.
Panda, G. R., & Agarwala, T. (2003). Punlic provisioning in water and sanitation study of urban slum in Delhi. *Economic & Political Weekly XLVIII, 5*, 24–28.
Peter, H.G. (2002). Dirty Water: Estimated Deaths from Water-Related Diseases 2000–2020, Pacific Institute Research Report, August 15, 2002. http://www.pacinst.org/wp-content/uploads/sites/21/2013/02/water_related_deaths_report3.pdf
Ramachandraiah, C. (2001). Drinking water as a fundamental right. *Economic Political Weekly, 36*(8), 619–621.
Solo, T.M., Eduardo, P., & Steven, J. (1993). Constraing in providing water and sanitation services to the urban poor. In *Water and Sanitation Health Projects, Bureau for Research and Development Agency for International Development Under WASH* Task No.338, 1–48.
The Hindu. (2014). 65 Million People Live in Slums in India, says Census Data. New Delhi: http://www.thehindu.com/todays-paper/tp-national/tp-newdelhi/65-million-people-live-in-slums-in-india-says-census-data/article5188234.ece. Accessed on 1/9/2014.
Teltumbde, A. (2014). An Ambedkar for our times. http://www.thehindu.com/opinion/lead/an-ambedkar-for-our-times/article5859610.ece/. Accessed 21 June 2015.
The Indian Express. (2014a). Aam Aadmi Party Opens Helpline to Report Grabge in Each Locality, New Delhi. http://indianexpress.com/article/cities/delhi/aap-opens-helpline-to-report-garbage-in-each-locality/. Accessed on 5/9/2014.
The Indian Express. (2014b). BJP Leaders Told to Report Daily Cleanliness Drive. New Delhi. http://indianexpress.com/article/cities/delhi/bjp-leaders-told-to-report-daily-on-cleanliness-drive/. Accessed on 5/9/2014.
The Indian Express. (2014c). Delhi's Waste Size. New Delhi. http://epaper.indianexpress.com/354904/Indian-Express/12-October-2014#page/12/1. Access on 12/9/2014.
The Indian Express. (2014d). Ministers Give Own Tuch to Cleanliness Drive New Delhi. http://indianexpress.com/article/india/india-others/ministers-give-own-touch-to-cleanliness-drive/. Accessed on 3/9/2014.
Varely, R.C., Travid, J., & Chao, D.N. (1998) A reassessment of the cost-effectiveness of water and sanitation interventions in programmes for controlling childhood diarrhoea. *Bull World Hhealth Organ, 76*(6), 617-631
Vijay, R., Abhinav, S., Ramya, S.S., & Apurba, G. (2010). Fluctuation of Ground Water in an Urban Coastal City of India: A Gis- Based Approch. *Wiley Online Library 25*, 1479–148.
Vijay, R., Khobragade, P., & Mohapatra PK. (2010). Assessment of groundwater quality in Puri city, India: an impact of anthropogenic activities. *Environmental Monitoring and Assessment, 117*, 409-418.

Solid Waste Management and Health of Workers

Jagdev C. Sharma

Abstract At the policy level state has made a transition from Laissez Faire to Regulator to Facilitator mode globally and so is the case in India. Since the adoption of New Economic policies it has got momentum in every arena and similar is the case vis-a-vis waste management. In contemporary times urbanization is a global phenomenon, but its ramifications are more pronounced in developing countries. Natural growth of population, reclassifications of habitation and migration trends are important in urban population in India. Global experience shows that when a country's urban population reaches almost 25 % of the overall population (as in the case of India), the pace of urbanization accelerates. Due to rapid urbanization and uncontrolled growth rate of population, Solid Waste Management (SWM) has become an important issue in India. Municipal bodies and other organizations in India render SWM services. Though it is an essential service, it is not given due attention which it deserves and also the services are poor. Presently, the SWM systems are assuming importance due to population increase in municipal areas, scope for legal intervention, emergence of newer technologies and rising public awareness towards cleanliness. Human activities create waste. The way these wastes are handled, stored, collected and disposed, they can pose a risk to the environment and to the public health. Where intense human activities concentrate, such as in urban centres, appropriate and safe SWM are of utmost importance to allow healthy living conditions for the population. In India municipal corporations are primarily responsible for solid waste management and with growing urban population are facing financial crunch. The scarce revenues earmarked for the municipalities make them ill-equipped to provide for high cost involved

J.C. Sharma (✉)
Government College, Sarahan, Sirmaur, Himachal Pradesh, India
e-mail: jagdevjnu@gmail.com

S.S. Acharya et al. (eds.), *Marginalization in Globalizing Delhi: Issues of Land, Livelihoods and Health*, DOI 10.1007/978-81-322-3583-5_23

in the collection, storage, treatment and proper disposal of waste. They collect waste from municipal bins and depots. A substantial part of the municipal solid waste generated remains unattended and grows in the heaps at the collection centres. Open dumping of garbage facilitates breeding of disease vectors such as flies, mosquitoes, cockroaches, rats and other pests. The present paper endeavours to understand the load of Municipal solid waste collection and the situation of those engaged in the process.

Keywords Solid waste management · Waste management workers · Health · Municipal bodies

Introduction

Society is a complex reality which cannot be understood in totality from a single perspective. Society as MacIver and Page would define is the "web of social relationships" which means different actors and institutions engaged in a meaningful way with each other. Max Weber has tried to understand this meaningful engagement or interaction of the different 'actors' through the concept of 'Social Action' wherein he defines sociology as an interpretative understanding of social action through their causal explanation.

Different thinkers have tried to understand the phenomena of development through different disciplinary boundaries from time to time. Emile Durkheim would analyse it as an evolution from simple form to complex form of evolution. The simple society is characterized by 'mechanical solidarity' where population was relatively scarce and more or less homogeneous with almost identical necessities and complex society is characterized by 'organic solidarity' with heterogeneous population and with varied necessities. The word 'Organic' Durkheim has borrowed from Herbert Spencer's 'Organic Analogy' where he has tried to compare 'Society' with an 'Organism' and postulates that like an organism survives as a result of proper and coordinated functioning of its different parts which are functionally related to each other in a similar way society is a result of interaction between different parts and institutions which are functionally interrelated to each other. Therefore it is very important to understand the interconnections or the interconnectedness between different aspects of social life.

With the passage of time the society has evolved from the primitive communism stage to the simple agrarian society to the modern complex industrial society. On the passage of transformation from one stage to the other the human beings have engaged themselves in the process of production and consumption at varied levels and in the process of production–consumption, they started generating waste which is voluminous and needs equal attention. The process of waste management involves the waste management workers who are at the last echelon within the waste management system, but their contribution is not lesser in any sense than anyone else within the waste management system.

Solid Waste Management

Solid waste management includes all activities that seek to minimize the health, environmental and aesthetic impacts of solid wastes. Solid waste is the discarded or the unwanted material in the form of garbage or refuse resulting from household or domestic sectors (food waste, plastic, paper, glass), industrial, commercial, healthcare sectors, mining and agricultural (leaves, vegetables) operations, from community activities and accumulates in streets and public places which sometime contains biomedical waste, discarded electronic items as well. This solid waste is categorized as municipal solid waste, construction and demolition waste, hazardous waste, abandoned vehicles, etc. Municipal solid waste generation is at ever-increasing rate with the increase in economic prosperity and urban population. Solid waste management is a worldwide phenomenon. Improper management of solid waste causes hazards to inhabitants. It is a big challenge all over the world for human beings.

Solid Waste Management (SWM) has become an important issue in India. Municipal bodies and other organizations in India render SWM services. Though, it is an essential service, it is not given due attention which it deserves and also the services are poor. Municipal Solid Waste Management is a part of public health and sanitation, which is enshrined in Seventh Schedule[1] (State List—List II) and solid waste management in Twelfth Schedule (Entry 6) of the Indian constitution under Article 243 W[2] and is entrusted to the municipal government for execution. Presently, the SWM systems are assuming importance due to population increase in municipal areas, scope for legal intervention, emergence of newer technologies and rising public awareness towards cleanliness. Human activities create waste. The way these wastes are handled, stored, collected and disposed, they can pose a risk to the environment and to the public health.[3] Where intense human activities concentrate, such as in urban centres, appropriate and safe SWM are of utmost importance to allow healthy living conditions for the population. This fact has been acknowledged by most governments. However, many municipalities are making efforts to provide even the most basic services. In our country municipal corporations are primarily responsible for solid waste management. But with the growing population and urbanization municipal bodies are facing financial crunch and can no longer cope with the demands. The limited revenues earmarked for the municipalities make them ill-equipped to provide for high cost involved in the

[1]Seventh Schedule contains three lists: List I—Union list, List II—State list, List III—Concurrent list, List II contains the subjects which comes under the state's discretion.

[2]Article 243 W deals with the powers, authority and responsibilities of municipalities, etc. Entry 6 in Twelfth Schedule empowers municipalities for public health, sanitation conservancy and solid waste management.

[3]Public Health here includes both the health of the public in general and the health of the waste management workers who are handling and dealing with the waste every day.

collection, storage, treatment and proper disposal of waste. Municipalities are able to provide secondary collection of waste. They collect waste from municipal bins and depots. A substantial part of the municipal solid waste generated remains unattended and grows in the heaps at the collection centres. Open dumping of garbage facilitates breeding of disease vectors such as flies, mosquitoes, cockroaches, rats and other pests. The services provided by the municipal authority are, often inefficient. It is estimated that as much as 30 % of the municipal wastes are left uncollected in urban centres (Venkateswaran 1994). The problem of SWM in Delhi is being looked at in the present study, to find out the problems and prospects of solid waste management. A detailed investigation was made regarding the methods of practices associated with sources, quantity generated, collection, transportation, storage, treatment and disposal of solid waste in Delhi. The present paper endeavours to understand the load of municipal solid waste collection and the situation of those engaged in the process.

Problem of Waste Management and the Scenario in India

The problem of waste seems to have arisen because of its very nomenclature. One really need to ask oneself **is it really a waste or a resource? Why has the situation become so critical in India today?** According to a survey conducted by the Ministry of Urban Development in India 1.6 lakh metric tonnes which is equivalent to 16 crore kilograms of waste is generated every day and municipal corporations are supposed to take care of it. The total waste quantity generated by the year 2047 is estimated to be about 260 million tonnes per year. It is estimated that if the waste is not disposed off in a more systematic manner, more than 1,400 km^2 of land, which is equivalent to the size of city of Delhi, would be required in the country by the year 2047 for its disposal (EBTC 2011). The per capita waste generation in cities varies from place to place and size of the population along with economic prosperity of the region, but one thing is common in all the cities of India that the waste is generated, stored and collected in mixed form, which contains both biodegradable (wet waste) and non-biodegradable (dry waste) in mixed form which also contain injections, needles, batteries, etc.

In some of the places even if the efforts are made to collect separate waste at household levels through door-to-door collection schemes again the waste is mixed at collection centres, for want of proper disposal mechanisms. The generated waste is dumped in dumping sites or dumping grounds mostly untreated resulting in creation of 80–100 ft high mountains of waste spreading on acres of land. This untreated waste emanates poisonous gases contaminating the nearby environment and simultaneously the rotten mixed waste generates the leachate which gets mixed with ground water which is again dangerous.

Solid Waste Management and Health of the Waste Workers

Health as defined by the World Health Organization is a state of complete physical, mental and social well-being and not merely the absence of disease or infirmity. Looking from this perspective the health issues of safai karamcharis and the waste management workers are very critical. In municipal waste management one needs to ask: What are the risks in various alternatives for resource recovery? Who or what is threatened? What is saved or protected? Decisions about environmental risks are made in the face of uncertainties beyond common experience, particularly for new technologies. While many concerns have been raised about the potential harm from MSW management to the environment, general public, and wildlife, the risks and consequent costs of occupational hazard in waste management activities have received relatively little attention in the rush to adopt or adapt new technologies. The attitudes of many concerned with various hazards of MSW management appear to be rather blasé regarding worker health and safety.

This lack of attention appears to stem from the presumption that, however MSW is handled, workers will either be protected by or that liability will be reduced by appropriate management by the responsible contractor/agency. Further the skill/education level for MSW workers as to other manufacturing and production areas, the general absence of workers' and professional operators' organizations, the tardiness of state in creating certification and training standards for operators, and the public's inclination to ignore the full costs of waste management also contribute to this issue. In the name of contractualization of waste management services citing the reason of lack of financing and infrastructural resources, municipal bodies want to do away with its responsibilities, but that puts the double burden on contractual workers one lesser payment for the work done and secondly not the proper supply of equipment to do the job which one would be having entitlement to as a government employee. Worst of all is the condition of rag pickers who to eke out their living would be toiling in mixed dumped garbage which may be having broken glass, blades, batteries, etc. risking their lives and above all listening all ill names from the general public and the contractors who have got the right over the waste.

The Waste Generation and Management in Delhi

Delhi, which is the largest municipal solid waste producer in the country, generates around 8,500 tonnes of solid waste daily. The figure has come out in the Economic Survey presented by the then Chief Minister in Delhi Assembly in March 2012. The report said 500–600 MGD (Million Gallon Daily) sewage is also generated in the city each day. It said the city also produces around 10 metric tonnes of biomedical waste daily while a total of 583 metric tonnes of plastic waste is generated every year. The economic survey identified vehicular exhaust as main source of air pollution and said number of vehicles registered in Delhi has increased from 24.32 lakh rupees in 1994–95 to more than 74 lakh rupees in March 2012. (http://www.moneycontrol.com/news/wire-news/8500-tonnessolid-waste-generated-dailydelhi_840537.html)

The urban local bodies such as Municipal Corporation of Delhi (MCD), New Delhi Municipal Council (NDMC), and Delhi Cantonment Board (DCB) are responsible for solid waste management in Delhi. MCD alone manages almost 95 % of the total area of the city. The above authorities are supported by a number of other agencies. The Delhi Development Authority (DDA) is responsible for siting and allotment of land to MCD for sanitary land filling. Delhi Energy Development Agency (DEDA) under Delhi Administration (DA) is responsible for solid waste utilization projects aiming at biogas or energy generation in consultation with the Department of Non-Conventional Energy Sources (DNES), and Ministry of Environment and Forests (MoEF), Government of India. The Department of Flood Control of Delhi Administration looks after the supply of soil to be used as cover for sanitary landfills by the MCD. Sewage management is taken care by Delhi Jal Board (DJB) which works under Delhi Government. Similarly other bodies such as Ministry of Urban Development (Central Government), non-governmental organizations, resident welfare associations and societies, private operators and waste pickers the most significant informal sector, etc. also contribute in solid waste management in different capacities at different levels.

Authorities in Delhi proclaim that waste management is in a state of crisis-waste is commonly dumped in the open illegally and the existing landfills are over capacity. For example, Delhi's Chief Minister, claimed, "The Municipal Corporation of Delhi (MCD) was inefficient and corrupt as was proved by the accumulation of garbage across the city" (The Hindu 2012). This narrative portrays the failure of management rather than a public health and urban planning issue. But from a public health perspective it needs to be analysed in a holistic and comprehensive way and the solutions need to be derived accordingly. (Seth et al. 2012) in their paper Delhi's Waste Conflict analyses the policy shift in twenty-first century in Delhi in three phases viz. The first phase began in 2005 when Delhi municipalities floated tenders for private firms to collect, segregate and transport municipal solid waste. The terms of these contracts distort integrated waste management with the logic of "more waste, more money" because companies are compensated for the amount (in tonnage) of waste they transport to landfills (regardless of whether it is recycled). The second phase is a plan to divert waste from Delhi's three landfills, viz. Okhla, Gazipur and Bhalswa to waste-to-energy plants to process waste into refuse-derived fuel (RDF) that is incinerated to generate electricity in the process. The third phase which has just began, extends the reach of private firms to household by granting them the right to door-to-door collection, transfer and transportation of municipal solid waste for the development of an integrated municipal solid waste processing facility (including a waste-to-energy plant) and an engineered sanitary landfill.

Owing to the nature and composition of solid waste in India is largely organic, and the heavily techno-centric approach alone does not seem to be successful.

Solid waste is often disposed without the expectation of compensation for its inherent value. However, it is increasingly being recognized that some of the value of refuse could and should be recovered. In economically less developed countries, poverty is the major reason why thousands of people are involved in the (informal collection), sorting and processing of solid waste. A number of recyclable materials, for example, glass, rubber, plastic, etc. in the MSW are suitable for recovery and reuse. It has been estimated that the recyclable content varies from 13 to 20 % and in Delhi 15 % of MSW is recyclable. A survey conducted by Central Pollution Control Board revealed that waste pickers play a key role in SWM by eking their livelihood from it. In India 40–80 % plastic is recycled. In Delhi, there are more than 100,000 rag pickers and the average quantity of solid waste materials collected by one rag picker is 10–15 kg/day. About 17 % of Delhi waste handling is done by rag pickers, who collect, sort and transport waste for free of cost, as of the informal trade in scrap, saving the government Rs 600,000/- daily (Sharholy et al. 2008). Second, owing to the organic nature of solid waste particularly household waste and vegetable, fruit market, etc. or commercial places like hotels, dhabas etc. the waste can be collected separately instead of allowing it to get mix with rest of the solid waste and can be fed to the stray animals by keeping them at one place and the fresh cow dung can be used for bio-methanation which would give us the fuel for cooking and the remnant can be vermin composted which is also known as black gold and can be used as manure in agriculture which indeed has a value/cost. This entire process will need less than 72 h or else decomposing of this biodegradable vegetable leaves, etc. would take nearly 40–45 days to decompose and will emanate a foul smell in the process. Third the traffic jams/accidents because of stray animals in search of searching food in garbage bins/community bins would also be taken care of. The segregated plastic can be recycled and can be used in tarring of roads which have a durability compared to the present tarring mechanism of roads. This entire sequence of reusing and recycling of waste at every stage is reducing waste at every level and leaving very less to go to the landfill sites. Instead of seeking to capitalize on the effectiveness of the informal sector and institutionalizing its participation in waste management, the MCD sought to radically transform solid waste by resorting to such policy shifts as mentioned earlier. The formal and informal sectors are intricately linked as waste passes through very distinct stages in both the formal and informal systems as it is processed and ultimately either disposed of in a landfill or recycled.

Urban Local Bodies often cite the reason of lack of Resources such as Financing, Infrastructure—Land and manpower. At present the municipal solid waste management system comprises of only four activities, i.e. waste generation, collection, transportation and disposal, But the Municipal Solid Waste Management system involves activities associated with generation, storage, transfer and transport, processing, recovery and recycling and disposal of solid wastes. A thorough check and management need to be taken care of at every stage of waste management system. The same can be shown in Tables 1and 2.

Table 1 Waste management

Present system of waste management waste generation,	How waste management should be taken care of Generation,
Collection,	Storage, (separate for both biodegradable and Non-biodegradable)
Transportation, and	Transfer and transport, (separately)
Disposal	Processing and treatment,
	Cost recovery and recycle, and
	Disposal of solid wastes

Table 2 Roles and responsibilities for solid waste management

Sr. No	Functional element of SWM	Responsible agency/organization	Monitoring authority
1	Collection	D-T-D/MC/waste pickers	CPCB/SPCB
2	Transfer and transport	MC	SPCB
3	Processing and treatment	PPP	MC/SPCB
4	Cost Recovery and recycling	PPP	MC/SPCB
5	Disposal	PPP	MC/SPCB

Policy Recommendations and Suggestions

In order to make the SWM system participatory in true sense, there is a stringent need for adoption of ***integrated comprehensive approach***, an approach that is people-centric and which represent the people in every aspect at different levels. All the agencies whether private or public need to work in coordination with each other to attain sustainability.

The primary requisite for introducing this paradigm shift, we need to ensure responsible governance from the public authorities. While the provision for proper sanitation and clean living conditions is the prerogative of the citizens, a shift of responsibility can be suggested. In the waste management system, citizens become responsible for their waste, while the government concentrates on larger welfare aspects of the people. The role of the government in this context is to provide the right kind of environment, social infrastructure, institutional capacities, and legal framework for the public to take up and implement the waste management schemes. New capacities, infrastructure and training facilities need to be adopted for composting, recycling, and recovery. The capacities of formal system can be enhanced by increasing the role of informal sector. The legal framework of waste management in the country also needs to be reviewed. The relevant laws should focus on a resource conservation and recovery approach and clearly spell out guidelines for waste management. The newer instruments of waste management such as Extended Producer Responsibility (EPR), take-back policies, and packaging laws need to be included in the relevant rules and laws. The tax payer's money should not go to buy 'obsolete' or 'dumped' technology, but should go towards investment in an infrastructure that clearly aims at recovery of resources as well as financial returns. Apart from this there in inevitably the need for creating mass awareness about the proper handling of garbage with responsibility, this could be done through direct interaction programmes and grass-roots level campaigns. These local actions should be based upon a global vision and should incorporate the global changes in paradigms of material use and management.

On the basis of literature review, the following suggestions can be made for dealing with the problem of garbage disposal in India in general and specifically in Delhi:

- The informal policy of encouraging the public to separate municipal solid waste and market it directly to the informal network appears to be a better option.
- Public awareness should be created among masses to inculcate the health hazards of waste.
- To recognize and realize the potential of benefits of 4R's, i.e. Refuse, Reuse, Reduce, and Recycle.
- Door-to-door collection on regular pre-informed timing should be practised either by municipal corporation Safai karamcharis or by incorporating informal sector or voluntary organizations/NGOs and also by encouraging the public participation in the collection of garbage.
- Currently, at the level of waste generation and collection, there is no source segregation of compostable waste from the other non-biodegradable and recyclable waste. Proper segregation would lead to better options and opportunities for scientific disposal of waste.
- The separate collection bins must be appropriately designed with features like metallic containers with lids which do not allow rain to pour in and prevent the access of monkeys and other wandering animals to the waste inside the bins.
- To adopt the suitable means of collection of waste generated by traders dealing with the trade in fruits, vegetables and fast food corners, etc.
- Slaughter house waste should be properly regulated and the solid waste they produce should be prevented from mixing with community waste.
- Hospital and other infectious waste should not be allowed to be dumped in community bins. Biomedical wastes should be disposed off in consonance with the standards and guidelines laid down under the biomedical rules.

Conclusion

"Alma Ata" declaration way back in 1978 had envisioned "Health for All by 2000" irrespective of their paying capacity. The Alma Ata declaration views Health as a means for development and not as the end result of development. Therefore, every individual has the fundamental right to seek a healthy environment to live in. Associated with fundamental rights are fundamental duties, so every individual has the fundamental duty to keep the environment safe and free from pollution. Creating environmental awareness among general masses is equally important. There is a need to sensitize masses towards the environment and related problems by inculcating environmental ethics and creating civic sense. Since the benefits of ***4R's, i.e. Refuse, Reuse, Reduce, and Recycle***, have not been formally recognized till now in SWM system, so there is an inevitable need to adopt three 4R's principle at each level.

Cleaner cities attract people and investment. Cleanliness is an indicator of good urban governance and management. Poor solid waste management practices affect the health and amenity of cities in multiple ways—by transmitting disease to residents and waste workers, by clogging drains and sewers, through contaminated leaching, and through visual and smell impacts.

Successful improvement in SWM in Delhi requires in both upstream and downstream activities. Upstream improvements in collection efficiency will inevitably lead to greater quantities of waste deliveries downstream. Downstream changes in reduction and disposal may act as a key to spread change upstream. This can be achieved by an optimum synthesis of hardware and software approaches. Hardware refers to the appropriate technology and software refers to the agencies which have deeper links and rooted connectedness in the community by involving the informal sector for effective solid waste management.

References

Durkhiem, E. (1900). Sociology and its scientific domain, translation of an Italian Text entitled " La sociologia e il suo dominio scientific" http://en.wikipedia.org/wiki/%C3%89mile_Durkheim

European Business and Technology Centre. (2011). *Waste Management in India—Snapshot*. EBTC New Delhi. www.ebtc.eu

PTI. (2012, March 19). 8,500 tonnes of solid waste generated daily in Delhi. http://www.moneycontrol.com/news/wire-news/8500-tonnessolid-waste-generated-dailydelhi_840537.html?utm_source=ref_article

Ramachandran, R. (2001*). Urbanisation and Urban Systems in India*. New York: OUP.

Rao, M. S. A. (Ed.). (1991). *A reader in urban sociology*. New Delhi: Orient Longman.

Registrar General of India, Census of India. (1991). *District census handbook.*

Registrar General of India, Census of India. (2001). *Primary census abstract, compact disk, digital data*

Ross, E. (1994). The origin of public health: concepts and contradictions. In D. Peter (Ed.), *Health through public policy—The greening of public health*. London: Green Print.

Sarkar, P. (2003). *Solid waste management in Delhi—A social Vulnerability study*. New Delhi, India: Toxic Link.

Seth, S. et al. (2012). *Delhi's Waste Conflict, Economic and Political Weekly*, Vol XLVII No. 42, pp. 18–21.

Shah, G. (1997). *Public health and urban development—the plague in surat*. New Delhi: Sage Publications.

Sharholy, M. et al. (2008). *Municipal solid waste management in Indian Cities—A review, waste management 28*, pp. 459–467. www.sciencedirect.com

Sharma, J. C. (2007). *Solid waste management initiatives—An exploratory study of solan town* (Himachal Pradesh), M. Phil Dissertation (Unpublished). New Delhi: Centre of Social Medicine and Community Health, School of Social Sciences, JNU

Sheel, S. (1994). *Social area analysis of Delhi metropolitan city*, Ph. D. Thesis, New Delhi: Centre for the Study of Regional Development, School of Social Sciences, JNU

The Hindu. (2012, March 5). *MCD trifurcation will benefit Delhi.*

Venkateswaran, S. (1994). Managing waste: Ecological. *Economic and Social Dimensions in Economic and Political Weekly, XX, 19*, 2907–2911.

Weber, M. (1961). *The Urban community in theories of society (vol. 1).* New York: The Free Press of Glencoe.

Wirth, L. (1938). "Urbanism as a way of life". In R. Sennett (Ed.), *Classic essays on the culture of cities*. New York: Appleton-Century-Crofts.

Living in Blight in the Globalized Metro: A Study on Housing and Housing Conditions in Slums of Delhi

Dipendra Nath Das and Sweta Bhusan

Abstract Studies on contemporary urbanization have put a lot of emphasis on the conditions of the slums which presently are almost universal phenomenon in the developed and the developing countries alike. But the magnitude and the nature of the problems suffered by these spatial units vary regionally depending on the skewed behaviour of the combination of socio-economic and demographic variables. Slums, often referred to as the urban blight, suffer from insufficiency of infrastructures and civic amenities, filth and dingy ambience and the health hazards of the residents are directly related to such stressful environment and living conditions. The living conditions on the other hand is greatly reflected in the type of the dwelling unit, the density of the occupance, the availability of proper ventilations to name a few and the socio-economic status of the occupant on the other. However, it is also true that the conditions in the slums cannot be straight-jacketed as studies have revealed a great deal of variations in the so called homogenous urban space. Therefore, the present study attempts to assess the housing and housing conditions in the slums of Delhi and would proceed to measure whether the choice of such dwelling units has any causal relationship with the various socio-economic and the demographic variables. Furthermore, attempt has also been made to congregate the findings on the basis of the regional variations the conditions of living of the slum dwellers. For the purpose of the study 13 slums well distributed geographically had been selected in Delhi.

Keywords Urbanization · Slum · Housing · Living conditions · Level of poverty

D.N. Das (✉)
Faculty in the Centre for the Study of Regional Development (CSRD),
Jawaharlal Nehru University, New Delhi, India
e-mail: dipendra02@gmail.com

S. Bhusan
CARE India Head Office, New Delhi, India
e-mail: swetajnu@gmail.com

S.S. Acharya et al. (eds.), *Marginalization in Globalizing Delhi: Issues of Land, Livelihoods and Health*, DOI 10.1007/978-81-322-3583-5_24

Introduction

The slums are a manifestation of urbanization in the third world post-industrial cities. They are associated with filth, squalor, wasted human and natural resource and fallacy on part of both the authorities as well as the common people in augmenting the inclusive growth structure on the part of the larger society. For a sustainable and assimilated urban growth trajectory, however, there should be a thorough understanding of the workings of slum as well as non-slum demographics, their resource potential, limitations and obstacles. Post-industrial urbanism, which had impacted the United States of America's urban growth in the mid-twentieth century, had its effect felt in the third world about three decades later. But the reflection of the post-industrial phenomenon shares a common thread in the developed and the developing nations in a sense that one of the most distinct features of the urban space was the presence of '*tenement city*' or the city of unskilled work (Knox 1995, 1996). These spatial units serve as home for the ones engaged in irregular employment, limited job security and therefore enjoy little benefit of making headway for good. However, the relief comes from the fact that the conditions in the slums cannot be straight-jacketed as studies have revealed a great deal of variations in the so called homogenous urban space and the living conditions are directly dependent upon the interactions between the innumerable socio-economic and demographic parameters. The crux of the problem lies in the fact that the occupants of these tenement settlements are not an unnecessary appendage to the urban system or the urban way of living. They serve the city dwellers in many ways providing them with variety of services quintessential for the smooth running of the day-to-day livelihood. Therefore, it is not at all a good idea to disown their existence in the urban space, rather an all round development of urban space would be there ones these toiling masses are incorporated in the mainstream urbanism through policy implementation and betterment of their living conditions.

Cities are a reflection of the cohesion of the urban planning, development and the interventions on a city are mainly in response of proper planning, management, governance and schemes of development. The call of the day is to build smart cities that are the *cities of tomorrow, characterized by smarter options for the consumers of urban network, rapid actions for individuals and to the extreme powered by automated decision making tools which in turn would make nations smarter* (Vinod Kumar 2014). Delhi, the capital of India, with a population of 16.3 million in the 2011 census, has emerged in a big way in the last quarter of the twentieth century. It is the topmost competitor in the race of the global cities from India and in many ways has the credentials to turn out to be a smart city (if not the smartest) of the nation, thereby emerging prominent in the list of the globalized metros of the world. The matter of awe lies in the fact that close to 12.00 % of the total households in Delhi thrives in the slums adding up more than 3 lakh in terms of absolute numbers (Census 2011). This fact surely raises a great alarm looking at Delhi from the perspective of a contending city of *smart growth* or *a globalized metro*.

Since independence, India has formulated several programmes related to provision of basic amenities in the slums. The Five-Year plans of the country with

Table 1 Population distribution in the four major metros between 1901 and 2011, India

Year	Population in million			
	Delhi	Mumbai	Chennai	Kolkata
1901	0.2	0.8	0.5	1.5
1911	0.2	1.0	0.6	1.7
1921	0.3	1.3	0.6	1.8
1931	0.4	1.3	0.7	2.1
1941	0.7	1.7	0.9	3.6
1951	1.4	3.2	1.5	4.7
1961	2.4	4.5	1.9	5.7
1971	3.6	6.6	3.1	7.4
1981	5.8	9.4	4.2	9.2
1991	8.5	12.6	5.3	11.0
2001	12.9	16.4	6.6	13.2
2011	16.3	18.4	8.6	14.1

Source Computed from the Census of India, 2001 and 2011

their explicit objective to remove poverty have also considered policy measures to improve the living conditions among the urban poor. In the fifth Five-Year Plan, the first formal attempt was made to eradicate poverty by inducting "Slum Clearance and Slum Development Scheme" under the "Minimum Needs Program" which encompasses basic needs in a broader perspective. In the successive plans a greater weightage was given to the provision of reasonable level of living and basic amenities of the poor. In the beginning of the twentieth century when Kolkata Urban agglomeration was the only one with million population in India, Delhi Urban Agglomerate had a population component of a meager 0.2 million and trailed far behind of Chennai (0.5 million) and Mumbai (0.8 million). It was in the post independence period that Delhi doubled its population from 0.7 million to finally emerge in the million category in 1951 with a population of 1.4 million (Table 1). Since then there was no looking back and Delhi kept on adding population from 8.5 million in 1991 to 12.9 in 2001 and 16.3 million in 2011 trailing behind Mumbai by only a 2.1 million population.

Therefore, a capital city which remained at the foci of all policies and programme implementation can't be let go with such inherent squalor in urban space. Even after the completion of the JnNURM, the condition of Delhi in respect to the presence of such urban canker has not been eradicated and therefore needs to be addressed.

The Study

The present cross-sectional study has been taken up in 13 slums located in the National Capital Territory. The study was conducted between 2009 and 2010. The slums which were included in the present study are Bakkarwala, Indira Camp,

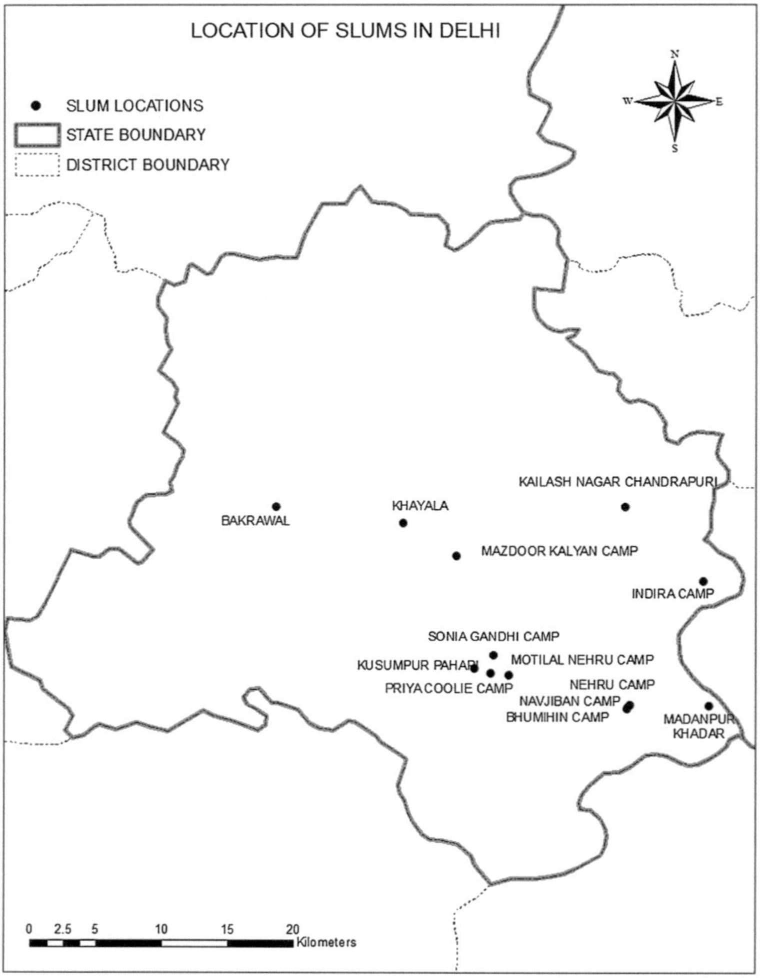

Fig. 1 Location of slums in Delhi

Madanpur Khadar, Khayala, Nabajiban Camp, Priya Coolie camp, Nehru Camp, Mazdur Kalyan Camp, Bhumiheen Camp, Sonia Camp, Kusumpur Pahari, Motilal Nehru Camp, Kailash Nagar Chanderpura. The locations of the slums are depicted in Fig. 1.

The Bakkarwala slum is located in the west of the state of Delhi situated south east of the Mundka Industrial area, Khayala is located in the west of Delhi posited between Kesho Pur DTC bus depot in the west and Tagore garden extension in the east, Kailash Nagar colony aligns the railway line near the Old Yamuna bridge,

Mazdoor Kalyan Camp lies in close proximity to the Inderpuri region, Indira camp lies near Kalyan Puri. Sonia Gandhi Camp, Kusumpur Pahari, Priya Coolie camp and Motilal Nehru camp are all located in the south of Delhi, whereas Nehru Camp, Navjiban Camp and Bhumiheen camp are located in close proximity to the Kalkaji-Govindpuri area and the Madanpur Khadar lies in close proximity to the Okhla Industrial Area.

Objectives

The slums have always come as a blanket category when policy decisions are taken. Whether such a straight jacketing of slums as homogeneous entity is justifiable or they reflect heterogeneity in terms of nature and pattern of the conditions of housing and the other amenities has been considered in the present study. Further, not only inter-slum variations, housing and housing conditions have revealed great degree of variations amongst the slum households. What kind of socio-economic and demographic differences lead to the variations in the availability of amenities has also be addressed. Poverty is one of the significant determinants of the quality of living of the households in the slums and therefore, an attempt has been made to assess the inter-slum and intra-slum variation of poverty at the household level. Quality of living has been attempted to be computed using selected variables and the slums in the present study has been ranked on the basis of the composite score. Attempts have also been made to trace the interrelationship between the socio-economic characteristics of the slum households and their level of available amenities and finally summing up the situation, an attempt has been made to prescribe policy recipes to take care of the situation of those living in blight in a globalized metro like Delhi.

Building from the Past Literatures

The extension of slums in developing countries is a product of twentieth and twenty-first century urban growth and represents the very essence of the Third World city. If the continuous dynamic urban change processes like increase in the urban blight in the form of slums goes unchecked, the process is expected to accelerate in the next several decades bringing in more inconvenience in the holistic growth of the cities in question. In India since independence, the Five-Year plans of the country with their explicit objective to remove poverty have also considered policy measures to improve the living conditions among the urban poor. In the fifth Five-Year Plan, the first formal attempt was made to eradicate poverty by inducting "Slum Clearance and Slum Development Scheme" under the "Minimum Needs Program" which encompasses basic needs in a broader perspective. In the successive plans a greater weightage was given to the provision of reasonable level of living and basic amenities of the poor (Bhusan 2010). The main thrust of the programme was mainly to improve the basic amenities of shelter, drinking water, sanitation, health care and education. Yet, some of the others in addition to the basic amenities took up the employment generation aspect. Generally most of the urban poor reside in the informal settlements, because they cannot afford the high land and housing prices. A lot of indicators point out that the spatial and demographic urban growth in developing countries is characterized by the deterioration of physical, economic and social living conditions for a large part of growing urban population and the non-slum population develop at the expense of the slum population. Evidently the cities are the locations where diverse socio-economic resources are concentrated which can bring substantial benefits in the form of positive social and economic externalities (Montgomery et al. 2004) on one hand, but the lack of access to the infrastructural facilities may lead to a dichotomous existence of the slum and non-slum population in the same urban space which is not a desirable situation. The service-oriented cities that we see today have been marked by squalor, filth and usually speak a lot about deprivation (Gugler 1988). However, the basic services that a city is expected to provide to its residents include a wide range of physical infrastructure starting from supply of water, power, proper drainage and sewerage, street lights and garbage disposal to a range of social infrastructure including education, health, open community spaces and other community services to name a few. It would be really interesting to see how such amenities are made available to the population living in blight in a globalized metro like Delhi.

Discussion

Addressing the problem of the slums require an exploration of the demographic characteristics of the resident population. The socio-economic background of the occupants of the slums is reflected in the type of dwelling units they choose, their living style and conditions of housing. Therefore, attempt may be made to sum up the characteristics of the slum population on the basis of some selected variables before plunging deeper into the conditions of housing and other related issues and problems.

Slums mainly grow in urban areas to accommodate the inflow of migrants who come mainly looking for jobs. Therefore quite likely, the situation may be reflected in the age composition (Table 2 and Fig. 2). It is clear from Table 2, that close to 64.00 % of the slum population belong to the age group of 15–59 years. In all the age groups, male population in the slums has outnumbered the female population. The feature is reflected in the age-sex pyramid illustrated in Fig. 2.

Another significant feature that emerges out of the age–sex distribution is that the sex ratio is skewed in favour of the male in all age groups which is justified by the fact that male population mainly migrate to the cities in search of jobs and are

Table 2 Demographic characteristics of the population in slums of Delhi, 2009–2010

Age group (years)	Male	Female	Percentage in different age groups to total population	Sex ratio
1–4	260	254	8.04	977
5–9	371	335	11.05	903
10–14	434	378	12.71	871
15–19	431	362	12.41	840
20–24	379	327	11.05	863
25–29	316	270	9.17	854
30–34	262	220	7.54	840
35–39	229	222	7.06	969
40–44	225	182	6.37	809
45–49	166	132	4.66	795
50–54	132	75	3.24	568
55–59	76	65	2.21	855
60–64	82	64	2.28	780
65–69	43	33	1.19	767
70+	35	31	13.86	886
0–14	**1065**	**967**	**31.79**	**908**
15–59	**2216**	**1855**	**63.70**	**837**
60+	**160**	**128**	**4.51**	**800**

Source Primary Survey, 2009–2010

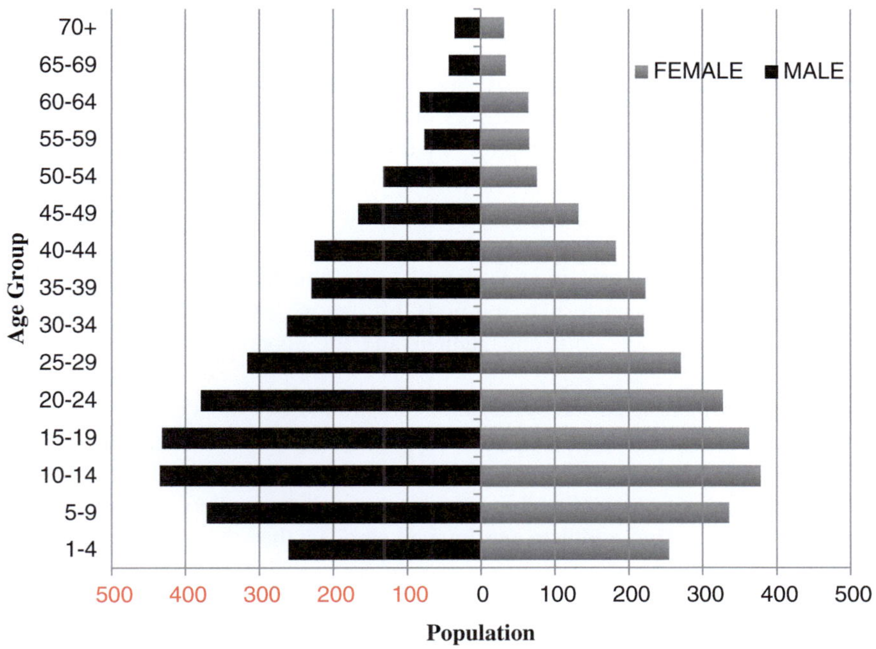

Fig. 2 Age-sex pyramid for slums in Delhi, 2009-10. *Source* Primary survey, 2009–2010

Table 3 Average family size in the slums of Delhi, 2009–2010

Slums	Total households surveyed	Average family size	Percentage of households in different family sizes			
			Less than 3	3–6	7 or more	Total
Mazdoor Kalyan Camp	47	5.94	7.50	55.00	37.50	100.00
Kailash Nagar Chandrapuri	48	5.75	3.76	72.18	24.06	100.00
Madanpur Khadar	222	5.75	1.75	78.95	19.30	100.00
Navajiban Camp	115	5.62	4.58	71.90	23.53	100.00
Kusumpur Pahari	73	5.59	2.08	66.67	31.25	100.00
Nehru Camp	67	5.57	5.48	69.86	24.66	100.00
Bhumihin Camp	40	5.5	4.26	63.83	31.91	100.00
Priya Coolie Camp	40	5.48	8.41	76.64	14.95	100.00
Sonia Gandhi Camp	52	5.48	4.05	65.32	30.63	100.00
Khayala	153	5.45	4.48	68.66	26.87	100.00
Bakrawal	133	5.44	2.61	70.43	26.96	100.00
Indira Kalyan Camp	57	5.39	7.50	60.00	32.50	100.00
Motilal Nehru Camp	107	5.07	9.62	67.31	23.08	100.00
Total	1154	5.54	4.77	69.24	26.00	100.00

Source Primary Survey, 2009–2010

absorbed in low quality of work which deters them from affording decent conditions of living. Thus, such population mainly resides in the squatter settlements.

The dominance of population in the conjugal age is reflected in the average family size of the slum dwellers. A closer look across the slums reveals that in almost all the slums have 5.54 members on an average. The largest family size is reported in Mazdoor Kalyan Camp (5.94 persons per family), followed by Kailash Nagar Chandrapuri and Madanpur Khadar (5.75 persons per family). The lowest family size of 5.07 persons per family is reported to be there in Motilal Nehru Camp as documented in Table 3.

The access to basic amenities is directly or indirectly determined by various socio-economic parameters like religious affiliation, caste category and most importantly the type of work engagement and the economic return from it, to name a few.

In the religious distribution of the slums, it is found that most of the slum population either follow Hinduism or Islam. On an average, 82.42 % of the slum dwellers in Delhi have been reported to be following Hinduism whereas 13.43 % follow Islam. Although not present in all the slums, many slum dwellers have been found to follow Christianity, Buddhism and Jainism amongst the other religious practices as documented in Table 4.

Hinduism emerges out to be the dominant religious practice of the slum dwellers in Delhi, but a great variation is found amongst the different slums. For

Table 4 Percentage distribution of slum households by religious affiliation, Delhi, 2009–2010

Slums	Percentage distribution of households by religious affiliation			
	Hindu	Muslim	Others	Total
Bhumihin Camp	87.50	12.50	0.00	100.00
Bakrawal	91.73	6.02	2.26	100.00
Indira Kalyan Camp	89.47	10.53	0.00	100.00
Khayala	75.16	8.50	16.34	100.00
Kailash Nagar Chandrapuri	39.58	60.42	0.00	100.00
Kusumpur Pahari	93.15	2.74	4.11	100.00
Mazdoor Kalyan Camp	95.74	4.26	0.00	100.00
Motilal Nehru Camp	95.33	1.87	2.80	100.00
Madanpur Khadar	87.39	9.46	3.15	100.00
Nehru Camp	85.07	10.45	4.48	100.00
Navajiban Camp	75.65	23.48	0.87	100.00
Priya Coolie Camp	87.50	7.50	5.00	100.00
Sonia Gandhi Camp	40.38	57.69	1.92	100.00
Total	82.41	13.43	4.16	100.00

Source Primary Survey, 2009–2010

example slums like Mazdoor Kalyan camp, Motilal Nehru Camp, Kusumpur Pahari, Bakrawal, Indira Kalyan Camp, Bhumihin Camp, Priya Coolie Camp, Madanpur Khadar and Nehru Camp are dominated by the Hindus as more than 85.00 % of the residents are found to follow Hinduism. On the other hand, Sonia Gandhi Camp and Kailash Nagar Chandrapuri have reported to have more than half of the population practicing Islam. Therefore, it would be interesting to note whether, such religious practices have any bearing on the access to basic requirements of living.

Affiliation to different caste categories may also be considered if access to basic amenities is being addressed to. In many instances, lower castes are often restricted in the premises where chances of intermingling with the higher castes are there. Therefore, it is necessary to examine the caste composition of the slum dwellers to ultimately note whether there is any specific implication when it comes to the access to the specific amenities (Table 5).

As revealed in the Table 5, the slum population in the present study in Delhi belongs to scheduled caste categories, followed by general category and other backward castes. However, a closer look at the table reveals that there is inter-slum variation in the caste composition to a certain degree. Of the 13 slums that have been studied, 9 slums namely Kusumpur Pahari, Bakrawal, Nehru Camp, Madanpur Khadar, Motilal Nehru Camp, Mazdoor Kalyan camp, Priya Coolie Camp, Navajiban Camp and Bhumihin Camp have reported to have more than half of the population belonging to scheduled caste. However, 50.00 % of slum population belongs to category of general caste in Kailash Nagar Chandrapuri, followed by 43.14 % in Khayala and 42.31 % in Sonia Gandhi Camp.

Table 5 Percentage distribution of households in different caste groups, Delhi, 2009–2010

Slums	Percentage distribution of households by caste groups				
	General	SC	ST	OBC	Total
Bhumihin Camp	27.50	50.00	7.50	15.00	100.00
Bakrawal	13.53	63.16	2.26	21.05	100.00
Indira Kalyan Camp	26.32	43.86	1.75	28.07	100.00
Khayala	43.14	36.60	0.00	20.26	100.00
Kailash Nagar Chandrapuri	50.00	22.92	0.00	27.08	100.00
Kusumpur Pahari	13.70	72.60	5.48	8.22	100.00
Mazdoor Kalyan Camp	29.79	53.19	0.00	17.02	100.00
Motilal Nehru Camp	16.82	53.27	1.87	28.04	100.00
Madanpur Khadar	20.27	55.41	4.95	19.37	100.00
Nehru Camp	28.36	58.21	1.49	11.94	100.00
Navajiban Camp	32.17	50.43	0.87	16.52	100.00
Priya Coolie Camp	27.50	52.50	2.50	17.50	100.00
Sonia Gandhi Camp	42.31	9.62	1.92	46.15	100.00
Total	26.86	50.00	2.43	20.71	100.00

Source Primary Survey, 2009–2010

However, as seen earlier, the average family in the slums of Delhi contains 5 members. It would be necessary to note the kind of family such members constitute. In a way such an analysis would help in identifying the blood relationship that the members share. One of the common features of the slum dwellers is that social networking in the form of kinship ties play a great role in the migration decision of the persons coming to the cities to make a living. Therefore, they often tend to adjust themselves in small dingy tenements as their incomes do not support a comfortable living.

As illustrated in the Table 6, close to 70.00 % of the population residing in the slums belong to nuclear families. However, it is interesting to note that in slums like Bhumihin Camp, Priya Coolie Camp, Khayala, Kusumpur Pahari, Sonia Gandhi Camp, Mazdoor Kalyan camp and Indira Kalyan Camp more than 30.00 % of the families are found to be either joint or extended. Whether staying in such bigger families has any special implication on the access to the basic amenities may be taken up for further exploration.

The study reveals that close to 95.00 % of the slum population are migrants. It may be stated at this juncture that of the remaining 5.00 % who have reported to not have migrated may not have been the first generation migrants, but their ancestors must have done so at some point of time. Though there if not much variation in the migration condition across the slums, Khayala one of the oldest resettlement colonies of the studied slums have reported to have a comparatively lower number of migrant. This may be because of the fact that the present generation of respondents might not be the one who physically migrated, but it might have been their previous generation who did so. An investigation into the reasons behind reveals that most of the slum dwellers had migrated in search of work and the situation is demonstrated in Table 7.

Table 6 Percentage distribution of households by family types, Delhi, 2009–2010

Slums	Percentage distribution of households in different family types				
	Nuclear	Joint	Extended	Single	Total
Bhumihin Camp	60.00	37.50	2.50	0.00	100.00
Bakrawal	75.19	21.05	3.01	0.75	100.00
Indira Kalyan Camp	68.42	24.56	7.02	0.00	100.00
Khayala	64.71	33.99	0.65	0.65	100.00
Kailash Nagar Chandrapuri	83.33	10.42	4.17	2.08	100.00
Kusumpur Pahari	60.27	34.25	0.00	5.48	100.00
Mazdoor Kalyan Camp	63.83	25.53	6.38	4.26	100.00
Motilal Nehru Camp	71.03	24.30	2.80	1.87	100.00
Madanpur Khadar	74.32	22.07	2.25	1.35	100.00
Nehru Camp	74.63	20.90	2.99	1.49	100.00
Navajiban Camp	71.30	24.35	3.48	0.87	100.00
Priya Coolie Camp	62.50	30.00	7.50	0.00	100.00
Sonia Gandhi Camp	65.38	30.77	1.92	1.92	100.00
Total	70.02	25.65	2.86	1.47	100.00

Source Primary Survey, 2009–2010

Table 7 Percentage distribution of migrants by reasons of migration, Delhi, 2009–2010

Slums	Percentage distribution of migrants by reasons of migration				
	Job	Family movt.	Education	Marriage	Others
Bhumihin Camp	92.50	0.00	0.00	2.50	5.00
Bakrawal	90.23	0.75	0.75	0.75	7.52
Indira Kalyan Camp	92.98	1.75	3.51	0.00	1.75
Khayala	92.81	0.00	0.00	0.00	7.19
Kailash Nagar Chandrapuri	95.83	0.00	0.00	2.08	2.08
Kusumpur Pahari	86.30	0.00	4.11	0.00	9.59
Mazdoor Kalyan Camp	85.11	0.00	2.13	0.00	12.77
Motilal Nehru Camp	99.07	0.00	0.00	0.00	0.93
Madanpur Khadar	94.59	1.35	0.00	0.00	4.05
Nehru Camp	89.55	0.00	0.00	0.00	10.45
Navajiban Camp	91.30	0.87	1.74	0.00	6.09
Priya Coolie Camp	90.00	2.50	0.00	0.00	7.50
Sonia Gandhi Camp	96.15	0.00	1.92	0.00	1.92
Total	92.55	0.61	0.87	0.26	5.72

Source Primary Survey, 2009–2010

As evident from the Table 7, more than 92.00 % of the migrant slum population has done so in search of suitable job. However, the situation is a bit different in the slums of Mazdoor Kalyan Camp and Nehru Camp where 12.77 and 10.45 % population respectively have been found to have migrated in response to reasons like kinship ties. What is of more importance is to note whether the ones who have migrated have achieved a desired living and have been assimilated with the mainstream society or still they are striving to subsume themselves with the new urban environment.

Education of the head of the household has a lot of bearing on the access to household amenities. This is because higher the educational attainment of the head of the household, he or she would be better aware of the rights as citizens, their entitlements and are expected to make rational choices from the resources available to them depending on their capacity and further aspire to have a better living. Therefore, it would be justified to take a note of the level of education of the heads of the households in the slums (Table 8).

It is noteworthy, that against the general perception that slum have poor quality of human resources, the educational attainments of the head of the households unfurl a different story. On an average, most of the head of the households

Table 8 Distribution of the heads of slum households by their level of completed education in Delhi, 2009-2010

Slums	Level of education of the head of the household					Total
	No education	Primary	Secondary	Higher secondary	Graduate and above	
Bhumihin Camp	0.00	5.00	42.50	5.00	47.50	100.00
Bakrawal	0.00	9.77	49.62	3.01	37.59	100.00
Indira Kalyan Camp	0.00	5.26	54.39	5.26	35.09	100.00
Khayala	0.00	2.61	53.59	10.46	33.33	100.00
Kailash Nagar Chandrapuri	0.00	0.00	16.67	2.08	81.25	100.00
Kusumpur Pahari	0.00	2.74	39.73	6.85	50.68	100.00
Mazdoor Kalyan Camp	0.00	8.51	51.06	6.38	34.04	100.00
Motilal Nehru Camp	0.00	2.80	42.06	5.61	49.53	100.00
Madanpur Khadar	0.00	4.05	45.95	5.41	44.59	100.00
Nehru Camp	0.00	8.96	34.33	10.45	46.27	100.00
Navajiban Camp	0.00	5.22	48.70	5.22	40.87	100.00
Priya Coolie Camp	0.00	2.50	42.50	0.00	55.00	100.00
Sonia Gandhi Camp	5.77	9.62	38.46	3.85	42.31	100.00
Total	0.26	5.03	45.06	5.81	43.85	100.00

Source Primary Survey, 2009–2010

(45.06 %) in the slums of Delhi have completed up to secondary education and 43.85 % have completed higher education. However, it is good to note that more than 80 % of the heads in the Kailash Nagar Chandrepuri have reported to have completed higher education. Looking at the general distribution of the heads of the slum households by the level of education attained, it is quite clear that they may be expected to be quite aware of their entitlements.

Having noted all these, it would be essential to note the inter-slum variation in some of the selected parameters depicting the housing and the housing conditions. One of the chief indicators of the housing condition is the type of dwelling unit occupied by the residents. If Short has to be believed, "all cities act as gateways for the transmission of economic, political and cultural globalization". In this context, of the megacities in India, Delhi and Mumbai appear to be the chief contenders in the race of *Global cities* and they serve as urban nodes contributing to the alteration of the global economy through the top-down approach of globalization. From this perspective, it would be rather a matter of great despair that these cities still have *kuchcha and semi pucca* dwelling units posited within their urban landscape (Table 9).

A quick glance through the table brings forth one of the dreadful aspects of housing in few of the slums of Delhi like Kailash Nagar Chandrapuri, Mazdoor Kalyan Camp, Priya Coolie Camp and Sonia Gandhi Camp have more than one fourth of the families staying in Kachcha houses. The situation becomes more alarming if the proportion of slum households living in kachcha and mixed houses are combined. It has been found that on an average close to 36.00 % of the slum households reside in kachcha or mixed dwelling units. The situation is worst in the

Table 9 Percentage distribution of slum households by structure of house, Delhi, 2009–2010

Slums	Percentage population in different house types			
	Pucca	Mixed	Kachcha	Total
Bhumihin Camp	87.50	7.50	5.00	100.00
Bakrawal	70.68	21.80	7.52	100.00
Indira Kalyan Camp	54.39	40.35	5.26	100.00
Khayala	97.39	2.61	0.00	100.00
Kailash Nagar Chandrapuri	12.50	29.17	58.33	100.00
Kusumpur Pahari	60.27	34.25	5.48	100.00
Mazdoor Kalyan Camp	17.02	46.81	36.17	100.00
Motilal Nehru Camp	56.07	33.64	10.28	100.00
Madanpur Khadar	82.88	13.96	3.15	100.00
Nehru Camp	46.27	50.75	2.99	100.00
Navajiban Camp	62.61	34.78	2.61	100.00
Priya Coolie Camp	20.00	50.00	30.00	100.00
Sonia Gandhi Camp	36.54	38.46	25.00	100.00
Total	64.21	26.08	9.71	100.00

Source Primary Survey, 2009–2010

slums of Kailash Nagar Chandrapuri (87.50 %), Mazdoor Kalyan Camp (82.90 %), Priya Coolie Camp (80.00 %), Sonia Gandhi Camp (63.46 %) and Nehru Camp (53.74 %) have reported to have more than half of the population living in either kachcha or in mixed tenements.

Though based on their subtle perception, 86.57 % of the slum households have reported to be living in houses owned by them (Table 9). But there are instances which reveal that many of the slum households have been given on rent. What demands attention, is the fact that since the occupancy of the slum dwellings change over time, the beneficiaries to the slum development programme are not fixed as well. In many cases it had been found that many households that originally occupied slum dwellings may often move out by letting off the house ownership though some documentation of transfer. Therefore, the families presently occupying the squatter settlements may not necessarily be the original stakeholders and this becomes a challenge when policy formulations are thought of. The distribution of households by ownership status may be summed up in the following Table 10.

Though on an average, 86.57 % of the slum dwellers stay in self-owned houses, yet a great degree of variation is noticed in the slums of Kailash Nagar Chandrapuri, Motilal Nehru Camp, Bhumihin Camp and Priya Coolie Camp have reported to have 31.35, 29.91, 20.00 and 17.50 % households respectively, living in rented accommodations.

Table 10 Percentage distribution of slum households by ownership status of house, Delhi, 2009–2010

Slums	Percentage population by ownership of house		
	Own	Rented	Total
Bhumihin Camp	80.00	20.00	100.00
Bakrawal	96.24	3.76	100.00
Indira Kalyan Camp	89.47	10.53	100.00
Khayala	86.93	13.07	100.00
Kailash Nagar Chandrapuri	68.75	31.25	100.00
Kusumpur Pahari	94.52	5.48	100.00
Mazdoor Kalyan Camp	89.36	10.64	100.00
Motilal Nehru Camp	70.09	29.91	100.00
Madanpur Khadar	86.04	13.96	100.00
Nehru Camp	88.06	11.94	100.00
Navajiban Camp	92.17	7.83	100.00
Priya Coolie Camp	82.50	17.50	100.00
Sonia Gandhi Camp	90.38	9.62	100.00
Total	86.57	13.43	100.00
Delhi slum total[a]	71.01	19.89	100.00
Delhi non-slum total[a]	67.49	32.51	100.00

Source Primary Survey, 2009–2010. [a]Census of India, H Series: Housing and Housing Amenities (2011), Slum Housing and Housing Amenities (2011)

However, at all occasions when the slums are discussed, they reflect living in dingy tenements in the heart of city with many people co-residing in single rooms which make living a more arduous task for the slum dwellers. Therefore, it would be quite just to have a glance through the number of rooms that the slum households usually occupy and the situation is represented in Table 11.

Clearly evident from the Table 11 is the fact that close to 80.00 % of the slum households lives in two room accommodation. However, the situation is worse in the slums of Kailash Nagar Chandrapuri (93.75 % households), Mazdoor Kalyan camp (91.49 % households), Sonia Gandhi Camp (88.46 % households), Kusumpur Pahari (87.68 % households), Nehru Camp (85.08 % households), Priya Coolie Camp (85.00 % households), Bakrawal (84.96 % households), Navajiban Camp (84.35 % households), Madanpur Khadar (83.33 % households) and Indira Kalyan Camp (80.70 % households) where more than 80.0 % of the households reside in single or double room accommodations.

The situation needs attention when the per room density of the slum dwellers are taken into account (Table 12). Though these population live life of great despair, yet it is quite unhumanitarian to compromise with the dignity and self-esteem and more importantly with the privacy of family life just because of the fact that they live in the slums. To bring out the matter, an indepth analysis of the number of couples per room may be taken into account (Table 13).

Table 11 Percentage distribution of slum households by number of rooms in the house, Delhi, 2009-2010

Slums	Percentage of households by number of living rooms				
	One room	Two rooms	Three rooms	Four rooms and above	Total
Bhumihin Camp	45.00	27.50	15.00	12.50	100.00
Bakrawal	45.11	39.85	8.27	6.77	100.00
Indira Kalyan Camp	40.35	40.35	10.53	8.77	100.00
Khayala	15.69	30.07	22.88	31.37	100.00
Kailash Nagar Chandrapuri	66.67	27.08	6.25	0.00	100.00
Kusumpur Pahari	41.10	46.58	6.85	5.48	100.00
Mazdoor Kalyan Camp	63.83	27.66	8.51	0.00	100.00
Motilal Nehru Camp	44.86	27.10	13.08	14.95	100.00
Madanpur Khadar	44.14	39.19	9.01	7.66	100.00
Nehru Camp	46.27	38.81	8.96	5.97	100.00
Navajiban Camp	35.65	48.70	8.70	6.96	100.00
Priya Coolie Camp	65.00	20.00	10.00	5.00	100.00
Sonia Gandhi Camp	69.23	19.23	0.00	11.54	100.00
Total	42.98	35.44	10.75	10.75	100.00
Delhi slum total[a]	58.55	25.17	8.19	8.08	100.00
Delhi non-slum total[a]	28.75	30.26	21.52	19.47	100.00

Source Primary Survey, 2009-2010, [a]Census of India, H Series: Housing and Housing Amenities (2011), Slum Housing and Housing Amenities (2011)

Table 12 Percentage distribution of slum households by density per room in the house, Delhi, 2009–2010

Slums	Percentage of households in by number of members per room				
	2 members	3–6 members	7–9 members	10 and above	Total
Bhumihin Camp	25.00	70.00	5.00	0.00	100.00
Bakrawal	27.07	63.16	6.77	3.01	100.00
Indira Kalyan Camp	33.33	64.91	1.75	0.00	100.00
Khayala	63.40	32.03	2.61	1.96	100.00
Kailash Nagar Chandrapuri	16.67	64.58	12.50	6.25	100.00
Kusumpur Pahari	20.55	69.86	9.59	0.00	100.00
Mazdoor Kalyan Camp	8.51	82.98	6.38	2.13	100.00
Motilal Nehru Camp	42.06	56.07	0.93	0.93	100.00
Madanpur Khadar	23.42	66.67	7.66	2.25	100.00
Nehru Camp	22.39	65.67	7.46	4.48	100.00
Navajiban Camp	26.96	67.83	2.61	2.61	100.00
Priya Coolie Camp	17.50	70.00	7.50	5.00	100.00
Sonia Gandhi Camp	21.15	67.31	3.85	7.69	100.00
Total	30.33	61.61	5.46	2.51	100.00

Source Primary Survey, 2009–2010

Table 13 Percentage distribution of slum households by number of married couples per room, Delhi, 2009–2010

Slums	Percentage distribution of households by number of married couples per room				
	One	Two	Three	Four and above	Total
Bhumihin Camp	40.00	60.00	0.00	0.00	100.00
Bakrawal	45.11	45.11	5.26	4.51	100.00
Indira Kalyan Camp	40.35	54.39	3.51	1.75	100.00
Khayala	65.79	27.63	3.29	3.29	100.00
Kailash Nagar Chandrapuri	35.42	56.25	6.25	2.08	100.00
Kusumpur Pahari	43.84	43.84	8.22	4.11	100.00
Mazdoor Kalyan Camp	19.15	68.09	8.51	4.26	100.00
Motilal Nehru Camp	45.79	46.73	4.67	2.80	100.00
Madanpur Khadar	37.39	48.20	7.21	7.21	100.00
Nehru Camp	47.76	38.81	1.49	11.94	100.00
Navajiban Camp	49.57	42.61	4.35	3.48	100.00
Priya Coolie Camp	20.00	60.00	10.00	10.00	100.00
Sonia Gandhi Camp	30.77	61.54	3.85	3.85	100.00
Total	43.54	46.49	5.20	4.77	100.00

Source Primary Survey, 2009–2010

One of the disturbing facts that emerge out of the Table 13 is that more than 56.00 % of the households have more than two married couples residing in single room. Looking at the fact that most of the slum population belong to the working age group and further, close to 45.85 %, of the families residing in the slums, belong to the conjugal age categories of 20–49 years, the situation demands special mention when it comes to the number of married couples sharing one living room. The amount of compromise that the slum dwellers have to make with their private life can be imagined from the gruesome story that emerges out of the present discussion. Slums like Mazdoor Kalyan camp, Priya Coolie Camp, Sonia Gandhi Camp, Kailash Nagar Chandrapuri, Madanpur Khadar, Bhumihin Camp and Indira Kalyan Camp have more than 60.00 % of the households having more than two married couples residing in a single room.

Another basic requirement indispensable for a decent living is the availability of drinking water. Since the area of study is Delhi, there is a great variation when it comes to the source of water which to some extent also speaks of the quality of water that the households drink.

It is quite a serious situation (Table 14) that more than 90.00 % of the households in Kusumpur Pahari (100.00 % of the households), Nehru Camp (98.51 % of the households), Kailash Nagar Chandrapuri (97.92 % of the households), Priya Coolie Camp (97.50 % of the households), Mazdoor Kalyan camp (95.74 % of the households) and Navajiban Camp (90.43 % of the households) do not have a

Table 14 Percentage distribution of slum households by presence of water within or outside the house, Delhi, 2009–2010

Slums	Percentage of households by presence of water source		
	Within the house	Outside the house	Total
Bhumihin Camp	12.50	87.50	100.00
Bakrawal	85.71	14.29	100.00
Indira Kalyan Camp	21.05	78.95	100.00
Khayala	96.73	3.27	100.00
Kailash Nagar Chandrapuri	2.08	97.92	100.00
Kusumpur Pahari	0.00	100.00	100.00
Mazdoor Kalyan Camp	4.26	95.74	100.00
Motilal Nehru Camp	22.43	77.57	100.00
Madanpur Khadar	49.10	50.90	100.00
Nehru Camp	1.49	98.51	100.00
Navajiban Camp	9.57	90.43	100.00
Priya Coolie Camp	2.50	97.50	100.00
Sonia Gandhi Camp	17.31	82.69	100.00
Total	37.87	62.13	100.00
Delhi slum total[a]	57.06	42.94	100.00
Delhi non-slum total[a]	89.10	10.90	100.00

Source Primary Survey, 2009–2010, [a]Census of India, H Series: Housing and Housing Amenities (2011), Slum Housing and Housing Amenities (2011)

source of water within the house. It is quite a noted fact that when it comes to collecting water, it is usually the women and children who accomplish the task.

It is quite a known fact that the slum dwellers are a marginalized group in the urban environment. The insufficiency they suffer from the poor economic backgrounds pushes them to a condition where many of the basic necessities remain unaffordable to them. However, it is really painstaking that when it comes to even the most indispensable commodity like drinking water, many of the slum dwellers have reported to have to go for purchasing them from private sources as the water which comes out from the public distribution is beyond the limit of compromise. It would be therefore frenzy to note the different sources of water supply used by the slum households for drinking purpose (Table 15).

Mention may be made of the slums of Kusumpur Pahari and Sonia Gandhi Camp where more than 75.00 % of the households depend on the tankers for the daily supply of water for drinking. It is noteworthy at this instance that the collection of water from such source is not at all an easy task. It may also be brought to notice that 9.01 % of the households in Madanpur Khadar depend on bottled water for drinking. What is indeed painful is the fact that slum dwellers are already in excruciating situation when it comes to living conditions and on the top of that if the most rudimentary requirement like drinking water needs to be purchased, then the pain they take up in making both ends meet can precisely be estimated.

Table 15 Percentage distribution of slum households by source of drinking water within or outside the house, Delhi, 2009–2010

Slums	Percentage of households by major source of drinking water						
	Tap	Hand pump	Bottled water	Tank	Tube well	Others	Total
Bhumihin Camp	77.50	0.00	0.00	20.00	0.00	2.50	100.00
Bakrawal	84.21	8.27	0.00	7.52	0.00	0.00	100.00
Indira Kalyan Camp	64.91	0.00	0.00	35.09	0.00	0.00	100.00
Khayala	92.81	0.65	0.00	6.54	0.00	0.00	100.00
Kailash Nagar Chandrapuri	47.92	20.83	0.00	31.25	0.00	0.00	100.00
Kusumpur Pahari	1.37	5.48	0.00	93.15	0.00	0.00	100.00
Mazdoor Kalyan Camp	63.83	4.26	0.00	12.77	0.00	19.15	100.00
Motilal Nehru Camp	45.79	14.02	0.00	16.82	0.93	22.43	100.00
Madanpur Khadar	9.46	71.17	9.01	10.36	0.00	0.00	100.00
Nehru Camp	68.66	4.48	0.00	26.87	0.00	0.00	100.00
Navajiban Camp	32.17	2.61	1.74	59.13	3.48	0.87	100.00
Priya Coolie Camp	80.00	7.50	0.00	12.50	0.00	0.00	100.00
Sonia Gandhi Camp	13.46	11.54	0.00	75.00	0.00	0.00	100.00
Total	49.22	18.72	1.91	26.69	0.43	3.03	100.00
Delhi slum total[a]	84.26	5.36	–	1.41	6.14	2.61	
Delhi non-slum total[a]	81.54	5.08	–	1.16	8.52	3.60	

Source Primary Survey, 2009–2010, [a]Census of India, H Series: Housing and Housing Amenities (2011), Slum Housing and Housing Amenities (2011)

Table 16 Percentage distribution of slum households by sharing of drinking water, Delhi, 2009–2010

Slums	Distribution of households by sharing of water		
	Individual use	Common use	Total
Bhumihin Camp	10.00	90.00	100.00
Bakrawal	84.96	15.04	100.00
Indira Kalyan Camp	15.79	84.21	100.00
Khayala	93.46	6.54	100.00
Kailash Nagar Chandrapuri	0.00	100.00	100.00
Kusumpur Pahari	0.00	100.00	100.00
Mazdoor Kalyan Camp	4.26	95.74	100.00
Motilal Nehru Camp	5.61	94.39	100.00
Madanpur Khadar	46.40	53.60	100.00
Nehru Camp	0.00	100.00	100.00
Navajiban Camp	2.61	97.39	100.00
Priya Coolie Camp	0.00	100.00	100.00
Sonia Gandhi Camp	13.46	86.54	100.00
Total	33.80	66.20	100.00

Source Primary Survey, 2009–2010

The same kind of pain can be felt from the illustration (Table 16), where more than 66.00 % of the households have to depend on water from a shared source.

Slums like Kailash Nagar Chandrapuri, Kusumpur Pahari and Nehru Camp may be highlighted looking at the fact that all of the houses depend on water from a shared source. Mention may also be made of the slums of Navajiban Camp (97.39 % households), Mazdoor Kalyan camp (95.74 % households), Motilal Nehru Camp (94.39 % households) and Bhumihin Camp (90.00 % households) depend on drinking water from a common source. Keeping an eye on the fact that collection of water is mainly done by the women and children of the family, measures to combat such a dire situation maybe deeply researched.

Having talked of the problem of the availability of rooms, the next situation which demands a look through is the arrangements that the slum households make to manage another priority of living, i.e. food. Therefore, it would be a daunting task to look for the place of cooking used by these slum households (Table 17).

Table 17 brings forth a really gruesome reality, that close to 65.00 % of the slum households have their cooking done in the living room and only 24.78 % have a separate kitchen. Mention may be made of the slums of Kailash Nagar Chandrapuri (91.67 % of the households), Indira Kalyan Camp (91.23 % of the households), Nehru Camp (86.57 % of the households), Mazdoor Kalyan camp (82.98 % of the households), Priya Coolie Camp (77.5 % of the households), Navajiban Camp (77.39 % of the households), Bakrawal (75.94 % of the households) and Bhumihin Camp (75 % of the households) do their cooking in the living rooms. These are the slums which had reported to have a higher proportion of households living in single rooms.

Table 17 Percentage distribution of slum households by place of cooking, Delhi, 2009–2010

Slums	Percentage population by place of cooking					
	Separate room	Varanda	Open place	Living room	Others	Total
Bhumihin Camp	12.50	7.50	5.00	75.00	0.00	100.00
Bakrawal	15.79	2.26	6.02	75.94	0.00	100.00
Indira Kalyan Camp	7.02	0.00	1.75	91.23	0.00	100.00
Khayala	73.20	5.23	1.96	19.61	0.00	100.00
Kailash Nagar Chandrapuri	4.17	0.00	4.17	91.67	0.00	100.00
Kusumpur Pahari	32.88	13.70	5.48	47.95	0.00	100.00
Mazdoor Kalyan Camp	4.26	2.13	10.64	82.98	0.00	100.00
Motilal Nehru Camp	31.78	0.00	1.87	66.36	0.00	100.00
Madanpur Khadar	24.77	4.50	1.35	68.92	0.45	100.00
Nehru Camp	10.45	2.99	0.00	86.57	0.00	100.00
Navajiban Camp	8.70	2.61	11.30	77.39	0.00	100.00
Priya Coolie Camp	0.00	5.00	17.50	77.50	0.00	100.00
Sonia Gandhi Camp	19.23	51.92	3.85	25.00	0.00	100.00
Total	24.78	5.98	4.51	64.64	0.09	100.00
Delhi slum total[a]	46.71	–	–	–	–	–
Delhi non-slum total[a]	84.72	–	–	–	–	–

Source Primary Survey, 2009–2010, [a]Census of India, H Series: Housing and Housing Amenities (2011), Slum Housing and Housing Amenities (2011)

The matter adds to the worries when such a situation is clubbed with the type of cooking fuel used is also taken into consideration (Table 18).

Of all the sources of cooking fuel, Liquefied Petroleum Gas (LPG) seems to be the cleanest. Further, considering the situation where most of the cooking is done in the living room, the situation is really alarming whatever fuel is use. Therefore, the use of kerosene, coal, wood and other fuels may be summed up as unclean ones and close to 30.00 % of the slum households use these for cooking. The situation is worst in the slums of Kailash Nagar Chandrapuri (70.83 % households), Sonia Gandhi Camp (67.31 % households), Bakrawal (46.62 % households), Indira Kalyan Camp (40.35 % households), Priya Coolie Camp (40.00 % households) where close to 40.00 % of the households use coal, kerosene or wood for cooking. What deserves a mention is that the use of unclean fuel affects the women and children the most as they are mostly exposed to such situation. Many of the health hazards like bronchial congestions, allergy of different types are result of such long exposure to the smoke coming out of the usage of such polluting cooking fuel.

Access to toilets and bathrooms also need special mention when the housing and housing conditions are talked of. The presence and access to these amenities have special bearing and implication if the daily lives of the women are taken into consideration. It is really a matter of great shame, that in a capital city like Delhi, that more than half of the population living in the slums do not have toilets and

Table 18 Percentage distribution of slum households by fuel used for cooking, Delhi, 2009–2010

Slums	Percentage of households by different fuel usage						
	LPG	Kerosene	Coal	Electricity	Wood	Others	Total
Bhumihin Camp	75.00	25.00	0.00	0.00	0.00	0.00	100.00
Bakrawal	53.38	24.81	0.75	0.00	20.30	0.75	100.00
Indira Kalyan Camp	59.65	36.84	0.00	0.00	3.51	0.00	100.00
Khayala	98.69	0.65	0.00	0.00	0.65	0.00	100.00
Kailash Nagar Chandrapuri	29.17	27.08	0.00	0.00	41.67	2.08	100.00
Kusumpur Pahari	69.86	15.07	0.00	0.00	13.70	1.37	100.00
Mazdoor Kalyan Camp	61.70	23.40	0.00	0.00	14.89	0.00	100.00
Motilal Nehru Camp	83.18	10.28	0.00	0.00	6.54	0.00	100.00
Madanpur Khadar	81.53	9.01	0.00	0.00	9.01	0.45	100.00
Nehru Camp	71.64	26.87	0.00	0.00	1.49	0.00	100.00
Navajiban Camp	65.22	26.96	0.00	0.00	7.83	0.00	100.00
Priya Coolie Camp	60.00	27.50	0.00	0.00	12.50	0.00	100.00
Sonia Gandhi Camp	32.69	34.62	0.00	1.92	30.77	0.00	100.00
Total	70.54	18.11	0.09	0.09	10.83	0.35	100.00
Delhi slum total[a]	65.10	24.08	0.52	0.12	8.00	1.61	100.00
Delhi non-slum total[a]	93.64	2.67	0.08	0.03	2.53	0.80	100.00

Source Primary Survey, 2009–2010, [a]Census of India, H Series: Housing and Housing Amenities (2011), Slum Housing and Housing Amenities (2011)

bathrooms within the premises of their house (Table 19) and the situation really becomes a matter of concern when the life of women are taken into consideration from the perspective of privacy.

As well depicted in Table 19, close to 70.00 % of the slum households do not have toilets within the house and 55.00 % do not have bathrooms within the premises. Though a bath can be managed in open compromising the privacy aspect to a far lesser degree, the case is not the same when it comes to the non-availability of toilet. It may be further added, that the growing instances of urban crimes and lacking security of the women in the urban space surely calls for larger attention being given to the issue of making toilets and bathrooms available for the women of the households for all ages.

The situation turns more complex when the proportion of households sharing the toilet facility is noted. It is found that more than 70.00 % of the households living in the slums of Delhi have to share the toilet facility. It is not only a matter of privacy, but also a matter of hygiene and cleanliness when this sharing of toilet is taken into account. The situation is worst in the slums of Priya Coolie Camp, Indira Kalyan Camp, Mazdoor Kalyan camp, Navajiban Camp and Bhumihin Camp where more than 90.00 % of the households have to share the toilet facility (Table 20).

The grimness of the situation gets sultrier if the places of defecation are taken into account for the households which do not have toilet facility within the

Table 19 Percentage distribution of slum households by presence of toilets and bathrooms, Delhi, 2009–2010

Slums	Percentage of households by presence of toilets and bathrooms			
	Toilet		Bathroom	
	Yes	No	Yes	No
Bhumihin Camp	10.00	90.00	32.50	67.50
Bakrawal	11.28	88.72	27.07	72.93
Indira Kalyan Camp	3.51	96.49	31.58	68.42
Khayala	98.04	1.96	94.12	5.88
Kailash Nagar Chandrapuri	12.50	87.50	22.92	77.08
Kusumpur Pahari	19.18	80.82	50.68	49.32
Mazdoor Kalyan Camp	4.26	95.74	14.89	85.11
Motilal Nehru Camp	40.19	59.81	60.75	39.25
Madanpur Khadar	36.04	63.96	50.00	50.00
Nehru Camp	14.93	85.07	31.34	68.66
Navajiban Camp	11.30	88.70	35.65	64.35
Priya Coolie Camp	7.50	92.50	25.00	75.00
Sonia Gandhi Camp	42.31	57.69	19.23	80.77
Total	31.54	68.46	45.41	54.59

Source Primary Survey, 2009–2010

Table 20 Percentage distribution of slum households by sharing of toilets, Delhi, 2009–2010

Slums	Percentage distribution of slum households by sharing of toilet		
	Individual	Common	Total
Bhumihin Camp	7.50	92.50	100.00
Bakrawal	11.28	88.72	100.00
Indira Kalyan Camp	3.51	96.49	100.00
Khayala	95.42	4.58	100.00
Kailash Nagar Chandrapuri	12.50	87.50	100.00
Kusumpur Pahari	19.18	80.82	100.00
Mazdoor Kalyan Camp	4.26	95.74	100.00
Motilal Nehru Camp	37.38	62.62	100.00
Madanpur Khadar	33.78	66.22	100.00
Nehru Camp	14.93	85.07	100.00
Navajiban Camp	6.96	93.04	100.00
Priya Coolie Camp	2.50	97.50	100.00
Sonia Gandhi Camp	42.31	57.69	100.00
Total	29.81	70.19	100.00

Source Primary Survey, 2009–2010

premises. The distribution of the slum households by common place of defecation has been summed up in Table 21.

Having discussed about the indicators of housing and housing conditions, discussions on the economic conditions of the slum households may be taken up.

Table 21 Percentage distribution of slum households without toilets by common place of defecation, Delhi, 2009–2010

Slums	Percentage distribution of households without toilets by common place of defecation						
	Community toilet	MCD	Sulabh	Neighbours	Open	Others	Total
Bhumihin Camp	0.00	35.00	52.50	0.00	12.50	0.00	100.00
Bakrawal	4.51	24.06	60.15	0.00	11.28	0.00	100.00
Indira Kalyan Camp	5.26	12.28	77.19	0.00	5.26	0.00	100.00
Khayala	0.00	0.00	1.31	0.00	98.69	0.00	100.00
Kailash Nagar Chandrapuri	0.00	4.17	35.42	0.00	60.42	0.00	100.00
Kusumpur Pahari	0.00	2.74	2.74	2.74	91.78	0.00	100.00
Mazdoor Kalyan Camp	4.26	25.53	53.19	0.00	10.64	6.38	100.00
Motilal Nehru Camp	0.00	18.69	41.12	0.00	40.19	0.00	100.00
Madanpur Khadar	0.00	12.61	41.44	0.45	45.05	0.45	100.00
Nehru Camp	0.00	19.40	65.67	0.00	14.93	0.00	100.00
Navajiban Camp	1.74	26.96	61.74	0.00	9.57	0.00	100.00
Priya Coolie Camp	0.00	10.00	65.00	0.00	25.00	0.00	100.00
Sonia Gandhi Camp	0.00	0.00	9.62	0.00	90.38	0.00	100.00
Total	1.13	14.30	40.99	0.26	42.98	0.35	100.00

Source Primary Survey, 2009–2010

As referred many a times before, slums are not a blanket homogenous category and lot of intra-slum variation may be noticed when it comes to the economic conditions of the households and the housing and housing conditions. The Planning Commission of India has come up with figures for estimating poverty on the basis of the per capita income of the households for rural and urban areas separately. However, the figures for rural and urban Delhi have been fixed at Rs. 1145 and Rs. 1134 at 2011–2012 prices. Taking a note of the fact that the slums are truly an urban phenomenon, an attempt has been made to categorize the proportion of households below and above poverty across the studied slums. The results have been discussed in Table 22.

It is quite interesting to note that the slums vary to a great degree in their level of poverty. But it is disturbing to note that on an average half of the slum households thrive below poverty line and 8 out of 13 studied slums face the brunt of such a critical situation. The situation in the slums of Bakrawal (67.67 % households), Indira Kalyan Camp (64.91 % households), Mazdoor Kalyan Camp (63.83 % households), Navajiban Camp (62.61 % households), Kailash Nagar Chandrapuri (60.42 % of households), Sonia Gandhi Camp (59.62 % households)

Table 22 Percentage distribution of slum households below and above poverty line, Delhi, 2009–2010

Slums	Ranges of per capita income (Rs.)					
	Below poverty line			Above poverty line		
	Less than 500	501–1134	Total	1135–2000	More than 2000	Total
Bhumihin Camp	10.00	37.50	47.50	35.00	17.50	52.50
Bakrawal	12.03	55.64	67.67	23.31	9.02	32.33
Indira Kalyan Camp	12.28	52.63	64.91	28.07	7.02	35.09
Khayala	0.00	21.57	21.57	30.07	48.37	78.43
Kailash Nagar Chandrapuri	16.67	43.75	60.42	25.00	14.58	39.58
Kusumpur Pahari	6.85	31.51	38.36	43.84	17.81	61.64
Mazdoor Kalyan Camp	21.28	42.55	63.83	21.28	14.89	36.17
Motilal Nehru Camp	1.87	32.71	34.58	42.06	23.36	65.42
Madanpur Khadar	10.36	43.69	54.05	35.59	10.36	45.95
Nehru Camp	8.96	49.25	58.21	34.33	7.46	41.79
Navajiban Camp	11.30	51.30	62.61	27.83	9.57	37.39
Priya Coolie Camp	2.50	37.50	40.00	35.00	25.00	60.00
Sonia Gandhi Camp	19.23	40.38	59.62	19.23	21.15	40.38
Total	9.10	41.25	50.35	31.54	18.11	49.65

Source Primary Survey, 2009–2010

and Nehru Camp (58.21 % households) have more than 58.00 % of the households below poverty line in accordance to the bench mark set up by the Planning Commission of India. Mention may also be made of Khayala where a meager 21.57 % of the households are below poverty line in the income range of Rs. 501 to Rs. 1134 per capita per month. Slums like Priya Coolie Camp and Motilala Nehru Camp along with Khayala have more than one-third of the households with more than Rs. 2000 per capita income per month.

Housing and housing conditions is a direct manifestation of several socio-economic backgrounds of the households. However, an attempt may be made to generate a composite index on the basis of some selected indicators of housing and housing conditions enlisted as below.

1. Type of house—pucca and other than pucca,
2. Ownership of house—own house and rented,
3. Presence or absence of toilet facility within house,
4. Toilet facility by individual usage and common sharing,
5. Presence or absence of bathroom within house,
6. Source of drinking water from tap and other than tap,
7. Source of water inside or outside the house,
8. Number of married couples per room taken as one married couples per room and more than one,
9. Presence or absence of separate place of cooking,
10. Usage of clean and unclean cooking fuel,

Table 23 Ranking of slums on the basis of the composite score of housing and housing amenities, Delhi, 2009–2010

Rank	Slum	Composite score
1	Khayala	0.86
2	Bakrawal	0.50
3	Madanpur Khadar	0.47
4	Motilal Nehru Camp	0.44
5	Bhumihin Camp	0.41
6	Kusumpur Pahari	0.38
7	Indira Kalyan Camp	0.36
8	Nehru Camp	0.35
9	Navajiban Camp	0.35
10	Sonia Gandhi Camp	0.30
11	Mazdoor Kalyan Camp	0.26
12	Priya Coolie Camp	0.26
13	Kailash Nagar Chandrapuri	0.22

Source Primary Survey, 2009–2010

11. Presence or absence of Balcony and
12. Number of Living rooms in categories of one or more than one.

The values given to all the amenities available have been made unidirectional in terms of their positive and negative implication on the living conditions of the households. The results may be summed up as follows (Table 23).

The summary of the conditions of housing as illustrated in the Table 23 clearly reveals that there is a sharp divide in terms of the composite score in the different slums that have been taken up for the present study. The values of the score ranges between 0 and 1 and higher value imply better conditions of housing and the condition of living. The old resettlement colonies of Khayala, Bakrawal and Madanpur Khadar have emerged to be in the best state when the housing and housing conditions are taken into perspective. Moderate conditions of living may be experienced in the slums of Motilal Nehru Camp, Kusumpur Pahari, Indira Kalyan camp, Nehru Camp and Navajiban Camp ranking from 4 to 9 and the composite score of housing and housing conditions range between 0.35 and 0.41. However, the most impoverished situation is found to prevail in the slums of Kailash Nagar Chandrapuri with the lowest composite score of 0.22, Priya Coolie Camp and Mazdoor Kalyan Camp with a composite score of 0.26 each and Sonia Gandhi Camp with a composite score of 0.30.

Determinants of the Conditions of Living

As the discussion follows, the condition of living in the slums is not similar in all of the units of study. Therefore, an attempt may be made in delineating the possible causal effect of the determining factors of the differences in the living conditions. A complete set of the selected dependent and the independent variables may be presented in Box 1.

Box 1 List of Dependent and Independent Variables

Dependent variables	Independent variables
1. Whether water facility is available within house (Yes = 1, No = 0)	1. Religion (Hindu = 1, Other than Hindu (Ref.) = 2)
2. Whether toilet facility is available within house (Yes = 1, No = 0)	2. Caste (General = 1, Others (Ref.) = 2)
3. Whether bathroom facility is available within house (Yes = 1, No = 0)	3. Family type (Nuclear = 1, Others (Ref.) = 2)
4. Whether water is for individual use (individual = 1, common = 0)	4. Status of migration (Migrant = 1, Others (Ref.) = 2)
5. Whether toilet is for individual use (individual = 1, common = 0)	5. Sex of head = (Male = 1, Female (Ref.) = 2)
6. Status of ownership of the house (own = 0, rented = 1)	6. Per capita income (< Rs. 500 = 1, Rs. 501 to Rs. 1134 = 2, Rs. 1135–2000 = 3, > Rs. 2000 (Ref.) = 4)
7. Households possessing separate kitchen (yes = 1, No = 0)	7. Level of education of the head
8. Type of cooking fuel used by the household (LPG = 1, Others = 0)	8. Number of working members
9. Nature of house used by the households for living (Kachcha = 1, Mixed = 2, Pucca (Ref.) = 3)	9. Family size
10. Source of water for the slum households (Tap = 1, handpumps and wells = 2, Others (Ref.) = 3)	*Variables 7–9 are taken as continuous variables.*

The living conditions in the present study have been cumulatively represented by the following variables:

1. The **types of houses** summed up as Pucca, Kachcha and Mixed have been considered to reflect the overall living conditions. The Pucca are built with concrete materials, Kachcha made up of non-durable materials in totality whereas the intermediate mixed variety consists of the houses built by the admixture of the two. In order of their degree of reflection of the best possible living conditions, the house types have been ordered as Kachcha, mixed and Pucca.
2. Of the several **sources of drinking water**, tap water has been considered to be the best followed by hand pumps and tube wells followed by the 'other' category cumulatively summed up by sources like bottled water, tank and other miscellaneous sources.

3. **Presence of water facility within the household** has been considered to be the best option reflecting a better living for the households rather than going outside to fetch water.
4. The situation would be much more favourable if the water **facility is available for individual household use** rather than for the community purpose.
5. **Having toilet facility within the premises of the house** is considered to be a desirable situation for the households than having to go outside for the same purpose.
6. Similarly, **the toilet being exclusive for the individual use** is considered to be more preferable than the ones for community use purpose.
7. **Owning of the house** have been considered to be a better situation than the households who stay on rent.
8. Households using **LPG as a cooking fuel** are considered to be in a better situation than the others who are using other kinds like kerosene, coal, electricity, wood, etc.
9. Households having **separate kitchen** are considered to be in a better position in terms of aversion of health hazards than the ones which are compelled to cook in the living room because of lack of space.

To explain the variation in the availability of the above dependent variables logistic regression analysis (binary and multinomial) has been attempted upon by an array of explanatory variables including caste groups, religious affiliation, types of family, status of migration, size of the household, sex of the head of the household, education of the head of the household, number of working members in the household, total household income and expenditure and per capita income and expenditure. The results are presented below.

If the availability of amenities like water, toilet and bathroom are taken into consideration (Table 24), per capita income has a great influence on their availability within the house. It is clear the households having lower per capita income are less likely to have these facilities within their house. If the availability of water source within the house is taken into account, migrant families are less likely to have the facility within house than the non-migrant families, whereas households with large number of working members are less likely to have water facility within the house. On the other hand, households headed by educated heads are more likely to have the water and toilet facility within the house. Households affiliated to category of general castes are more likely to have toilet within the house in comparison to households affiliated to Scheduled castes, Scheduled Tribes and other backward castes.

If the availability of the amenities is considered in terms of the number of users, it is found that migrant households and the ones with lower per capita income are less likely to enjoy the water and toilet facility for individual use in comparison to the non-migrant households. Similarly families headed by educated heads and those with higher number of members are more likely to have amenities for their individual use and the ones with larger number of working members are less likely to have the availability of toilets and water for their sole individual use.

Table 24 Results of binary logistic regression explaining the availability of amenities in the slums of Delhi, 2009-2010

Explanatory variables		No. of households (n)	Amenities present within the house						Water for individual use		Toilet for individual use	
			Water		Toilet		Bathroom					
			Yes = 1, no = 0		Yes = 1, no = 0		Yes = 1, no = 0		Individual = 1, common = 0		Individual = 1, common = 0	
			Sig.	Exp (b)	Sig.	Exp (b)	Sig.	Exp (b)	Sig.	Exp (b)	Sig.	Exp (b)
Religion	Hindu	951	0.092	1.339	0.421	0.865	0.493	1.119	0.291	1.206	0.200	0.793
	Other than hindu (RC)	203										
Caste	General	310	0.679	0.942	***0.006***	***1.519***	0.229	1.182	0.667	0.938	***0.008***	***1.506***
	Other than general (RC)	844										
Family type	Nuclear	808	0.510	0.907	0.787	0.958	0.541	1.091	0.490	0.901	0.414	0.877
	Other than nuclear (RC)	346										
Migration status	Migrant	1087	***0.004***	***0.465***	0.004	0.444	0.093	0.646	***0.000***	***0.380***	***0.003***	***0.437***
	Non-migrant (RC)	67										
Sex of head	Male	1019	0.426	0.853	0.614	0.895	0.506	0.880	0.452	0.856	0.489	0.858
	Female (RC)	135										
Per capita income	More than 2000 (RC)	209	0.001		0.000		0.011		0.000		0.000	
	Less than 500	105	***0.002***	***0.426***	***0.000***	***0.094***	***0.002***	***0.451***	***0.000***	***0.341***	***0.000***	***0.108***
	501–1134	476	***0.000***	***0.522***	***0.000***	***0.205***	***0.007***	***0.622***	***0.000***	***0.517***	***0.000***	***0.218***
	1135–2000	364	***0.004***	***0.588***	***0.000***	***0.391***	0.064	0.718	***0.003***	***0.577***	***0.000***	***0.413***

(continued)

Table 24 (continued)

Explanatory variables		No. of households (*n*)	Amenities present within the house						Water for individual use		Toilet for individual use	
			Water		Toilet		Bathroom					
			Yes = 1, no = 0		Yes = 1, no = 0		Yes = 1, no = 0		Individual = 1, common = 0		Individual = 1, common = 0	
			Sig.	Exp (b)	Sig.	Exp (b)	Sig.	Exp (b)	Sig.	Exp (b)	Sig.	Exp (b)
Education of head	Continuous variables	1154	***0.001***	***1.048***	***0.000***	***1.054***	0.264	1.040	***0.000***	***1.053***	***0.001***	***1.052***
No. of working member		1154	***0.040***	***0.883***	***0.009***	***0.840***	0.220	1.016	0.084	0.898	***0.011***	***0.841***
Family size		1154	0.098	1.062	***0.000***	***1.174***	0.133	0.917	***0.041***	***1.080***	***0.000***	***1.176***

N.B Figures in bold italics depict significant relationship

Table 25 Results of binary logistic regression explaining the ownership of house, availability of kitchen and cooking fuel used in the slums of Delhi, 2009-2010

Explanatory variables		No. of households (*n*)	House ownership		Separate kitchen		Cooking fuel	
			Own = 0, rented = 1		Yes = 1, no = 0		LPG = 1, others = 0	
			Sig.	Exp (b)	Sig.	Exp (b)	Sig.	Exp (b)
Religion	Hindu	951	0.994	0.998	0.675	1.087	***0***	***2.57***
	Other than hindu (RC)	203						
Caste	General	310	***0.038***	***0.664***	0.881	0.975	0.278	1.194
	Other than general (RC)	844						
Family type	Nuclear	808	0.073	0.658	0.842	0.966	0.205	1.23
	Other than nuclear (RC)	346						
Migration status	Migrant	1087	0.919	1.04	0.455	0.801	***0.026***	***0.461***
	Non-migrant (RC)	67						
Sex of head	Male	1019	0.274	1.336	0.529	0.862	***0.015***	***0.571***
	Female (RC)	135						
Per capita income	More than 2000 (RC)	209	0.668		0		0	
	Less than 500	105	0.881	0.937	***0***	***0.141***	***0***	***0.093***
	501–1134	476	0.251	0.743	***0***	***0.164***	***0***	***0.287***
	1135–2000	364	0.586	0.868	***0***	***0.494***	***0.026***	***0.589***
Education of head	Continuous variables	1154	0.173	1.028	***0.001***	***1.054***	***0.001***	***1.052***
No. of working member		1154	0.853	1.017	***0.022***	***0.849***	***0.07***	***0.89***
Family size		1154	***0***	***1.356***	***0***	***1.232***	***0.002***	***1.142***

N.B Figures in bold italics depict significant relationship

Regression results shown in Table 25 establish the fact that the demographic and socio-economic conditions continue to determine the characteristics of the available amenities to the slum households. Hindu households are more likely to use LPG as a cooking fuel in comparison to households following other religions and the households belonging to category of general castes are less likely to stay in rented accommodations. Migrants and Male headed households are less likely to use LPG as a cooking fuel and higher education of the head of the household ensures better amenities like availability of separate kitchen and the use of LPG for cooking.

It is interesting to note that the socio-economic characteristics have significant control on the type of dwelling units.

Table 26 Results of multinomial regression explaining the nature of house used for living in the slums of Delhi, 2009-2010

House type RC = Pucca houses		No. of households (*n*)	Kachcha houses		Mixed houses	
			Sig.	Exp (b)	Sig.	Exp (b)
Education of head	Continuous variables	1154	***0.003***	***0.932***	***0.058***	***0.971***
No. of worker		1154	0.139	1.151	***0.059***	***1.130***
Family size		1154	***0.004***	***0.835***	***0.005***	***0.887***
Per capita income		1154	***0.025***	***1.000***	***0.000***	***1.000***
Religion	Hindu	951	***0.001***	***0.447***	0.073	0.711
	Other than hindu-(RC)	203				
Caste	General	310	0.085	1.477	0.943	0.988
	Other than general-(RC)	844				
Family type	Nuclear	808	0.573	0.871	0.779	1.049
	Other than nuclear-(RC)	346				
Migration status	Migrant	1087	0.259	1.737	***0.022***	***2.354***
	Other than migrant-(RC)	67				
Sex of head	Male	1019	0.240	1.490	0.093	1.485
	Female-(RC)	135				

N.B Figures in bold italics depict significant relationship

As clearly evident from the Table 26, education of the head of the household and family size has great bearing on determining the type of residential units as the households with higher educated head and with larger members is less likely to be in kachcha and mixed houses than in pucca houses. The per capita income though has significant relationship with the type of house used for residence does not explain much. Further, households who have migrated are more likely to stay in mixed houses than in pucca houses in comparison to the non-migrant households.

Similar socio-economic conditions influence the availability of the source of water used by the households in the slums of Delhi. For instance, the households with educated head are more likely to use tap water for their general purpose in comparison to the other sources of water. Households following Hinduism are more likely to use water from hand pumps and tube wells than the other sources of water, whereas the category of general castes population is less likely to use water from hand pumps and tube wells than the other castes in comparison to the other sources of water. The entire results are shown in Table 27 with the help of mutinomial logistic regression.

What clearly emerges from the above discussion is that the socio-economic conditions continue to control the availability of amenities in the slum households. But it is interesting to note that the common notion that increase in income

Table 27 Results of multinomial regression explaining the source of water in slums of Delhi, 2009-2010

Sources of drinking water RC = other sources of water (tankers, bottled and others)		*N*	Tap water		Hand pumps and tube wells	
			Sig.	Exp (b)	Sig.	Exp (b)
Education of head	Continuous variables	1154	***0.043***	***1.032***	0.660	1.008
No. of worker		1154	0.416	0.949	0.378	0.933
Family size		1154	0.671	1.017	0.812	1.012
Per capita income		1154	***0.013***	***1.000***	0.325	1.000
Religion	Hindu	951	0.349	1.186	***0.036***	***1.668***
	Other than hindu-(RC)	203				
Caste	General	310	0.536	1.104	***0.019***	***0.610***
	Other than general-(RC)	844				
Family type	Nuclear	808	0.088	1.324	***0.026***	***1.577***
	Other than nuclear-(RC)	346				
Migration status	Migrant	1087	0.191	0.670	0.569	1.277
	Other than migrant-(RC)	67				
Sex of head	Male	1019	0.482	0.853	0.869	0.956
	Female-(RC)	135				

N.B Figures in bold italics depict significant relationship

positively impact the availability of the amenities have been nullified to some extent in explaining the prevalent conditions in the slums. This may be explained with the logic that change in income may modify the availability of certain amenities and households may switch to better options available but when it comes to amenities like house types and the source of drinking water, mere change in income cannot do much good in changing the choice unless the households shift out of the slum ambience in totality.

Conclusion

Poverty and the access to the available amenities or resources have a great degree of interlinkage especially for the informal workforce in the urban areas (Potter and Evans 1998). This pool of population, for whom their physical labour is the greatest asset, toil hard, put in their labour to make the cities live up with its vibrancy, relentlessly work towards maintaining the beauty of the urban entities and in turn suffer from the inadequacies of the most essential entitlements of their life. Recently, scholars have brought in the concept of *vulnerability,* emphasizing on the ability of the households to cope up with the changes taking into consideration more non-financial attributes like the socio-economic and demographic characteristics of the population (Potter and Evans 1998; Satterwaite 1995; Moser 1995, 1996).

Clearly evident from the above discussion is the fact that there is a great inter-slum variation in terms of the housing and the housing conditions in Delhi. It is reflected that most of the slum dwellers live in abject poverty which in many cases have deterred their access to the basic amenities of a smooth living. Furthermore, post JnNURM and several other urban development programmes in which Delhi had remained in prime focus being the capital of India, does not quite explain the derogatory conditions of the slum dwellers many of whom do not have access to the simple infrastructural facilities. For example, if access to toilet is considered, considering Delhi from the perspective of a *smart city* it is a matter of great humiliation that slum dwellers still have to go to the open to defecate. Moreover, the privacy issues of the women and children in slums are found to be at stake considering the condition that most of the families do not have an in-house toilet and have to share it with many other households. Considering the access to drinking water, which is another indispensable amenity to living, many of the slums households have even reported to be compelled to purchase the drinking water. Living in the margins, the slum dwellers is already pushed to the edge and if such investments have to be made for purchasing the basic necessities, the available disposable income for making the both ends meet is highly questionable. Though several policies have been taken up from time to time, the conditions of the slum dwellers in most of the cases, in terms of access to basic amenities have not changed much. What needs to be taken care of is the fact alongside with providing exposure to earning, vigilant eyes should monitor the access to the basic amenities as well.

Therefore what is required is that, in cases where the individual effort does not suffice to uplift the conditions of the available resources, governmental interventions are recommended. For instance, to improve the conditions of the water supply and free the impoverished population from getting water from sources of poor quality and even go for purchase, government may step into improve the supply of water at least to meet the basic needs of daily life which in some cases had been fixed to be 70 l per capita per day (Bhattacharya 1991) for Indian urban areas. However, for cities like Delhi the per capita per day usage of water has been increasing consistently over the past few years (Mishra and Dung 1990). Most of the working population in the slums are part of the informal labour market and they are in surplus to the real demand for informal workers. Undoubtedly, governmental efforts are there on paper regarding the provision of minimum wages, but many a time's experiences reveal that individuals compromise with the meager amount of money in return of the labour they put into continue earning something to run their family to avoid stiff competition in the market. Governmental interference is also sought in this area to ensure the security at work place and to have a strict vigilance that all get paid equally for similar kinds of jobs negating the impact of the competitive attitudes. Policy measures can also be taken to ensure that the children from these economically weaker sections get assured education and provisions of adult education should also be there. What may be highlighted in this respect is that unlike other slums, the general condition of educational attainment of the heads of the slum households seem to be quite high in Delhi. This surely implies that the quality of human resources is quite high and therefore if policies are undertaken for the general improvement, there is no need to start from the general improvement of the literacy conditions. The apathy of the elderly members in the slum households towards educating their children as wastage of time and resource should be endeavoured to be corrected and this can be mainly taken up by the NGOs and the other organizations working towards the greater good for the greater number of people. Governmental efforts should be there to assist and financially support these organizations wholeheartedly. Special protective policies for the new migrants, members of lower castes and minority religious groups in the slums may also be formulated so that their children get access to education, basic housing and the amenities required for a dignified life.

Having said all these, it is really a matter of dismay that the masses that put their effort in the city building process, ensuring its flamboyance turning urban spaces to *smart-globalized cities* get a step- motherly treatment in their day-to-day life. Projecting the city's splendour in the global space by putting these masses living in blight under cover is not morally correct and is beyond their fundamental rights as citizens guaranteed by the Constitution of India. Therefore to boast the vibrancy and glamour of city which is the *face of India,* Delhi, special care must be taken to the ones living in blight in the nooks and corners to ensure that they are at least endowed with the basic necessities of housing and housing amenities.

References

Bhattacharya, S. K. (1991). Calcutta's urban future: Agonies from the past and prospects for the future. In B. Dasgupta & M. Bhattacharya et al. (Eds.), State Book Board. Calcutta: Government of West Bengal.

Bhusan, S. (2010). Patterns of distribution of basic amenities in different size classes of towns in West Bengal, 1991–2001. (Unpublished Dissertation submitted to Jawaharlal Nehru University for the partial fulfillment of the degree of Master of Philosophy, 2010).

Census of India, Primary Census Abstract (PCA). (2011). Office of the Registrar General of India, Ministry of Home Affairs, New Delhi, 2011.

Census of India, Slum Census. (2011). Office of the Registrar General of India, Ministry of Home Affairs, New Delhi, 2011.

Census of India, Housing and Housing Amenities series. (2011). Office of the Registrar General of India, Ministry of Home Affairs, New Delhi, 2011.

Gugler, Joseph. (1988). *The urbanisation in the third world.* New York: Oxford University Press.

Knox, Paul (Ed.). (1995). *World cities in a world system.* Cambridge: Cambridge University Press.

Knox, P. (1996). Globalisation and the world city hypothesis. *Scottish Geographical Journal.*

Mishra, R. P., & Dung, N. T. (1990). Large cities of the world: changing patterns, functions and structures. In R. P. Mishra & K. Mishra (1998) Million cities in making: growth dynamics, internal structure, quality of life and planning perspectives (Vol. I). New Delhi: Sustainable Development Foundation, Vasant Kunj.

Montgomery, M. R. et al. (2004). Cities. Transformed: demographic change and its implication in the developing world, (for Panel on Urban Population Dynamics, National Resource Council, Earthscan 2004).

Moser, C. O. N. (1995). Urban social policy and poverty reduction. *Environment and Urbanisation, 7*, 159–171.

Moser, C. O. N. (1996). *Confronting crisis: A comparative study of household's response to poverty and vulnerability in four poor urban communities (Environmentally sustainable development studies and monograph series)* (Vol. 8). Washington DC: World Bank.

Potter, R. B., & Evans, S. L. (1998). *The city in the developing world.* United Kingdom: Addison Wesley Longman Limited.

Satterwaite, D. (1995). Viewpoint—the underestimation of urban poverty and its health consequences. *The Third World Planning Review, 17*, iii–xii.

Vinod Kumar, T. P., & Associates. (2014). Geographic information system for smart cities. New Delhi: Copal Publishing Group.

MIX
Papier aus verantwortungsvollen Quellen
Paper from responsible sources
FSC® C105338

If you have any concerns about our products,
you can contact us on
ProductSafety@springernature.com

In case Publisher is established outside the EU,
the EU authorized representative is:
Springer Nature Customer Service Center GmbH
Europaplatz 3, 69115 Heidelberg, Germany

Printed by Libri Plureos GmbH
in Hamburg, Germany